1 MONTH OF
FREE
READING

at

www.ForgottenBooks.com

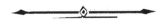

By purchasing this book you are eligible for one month membership to ForgottenBooks.com, giving you unlimited access to our entire collection of over 1,000,000 titles via our web site and mobile apps.

To claim your free month visit: www.forgottenbooks.com/free790656

ISBN 978-0-428-93719-5
PIBN 10790656

INTERNATIONAL DENTAL JOURNAL

A MONTHLY PERIODICAL

DEVOTED TO

DENTAL AND ORAL SCIENCE

EDITED BY

JAMES TRUMAN, D.D.S.

VOL. XXVI

PHILADELPHIA
INTERNATIONAL DENTAL PUBLICATION COMPANY
1905

LIST OF CONTRIBUTORS TO VOLUME XXVI.

ALLAN, CHARLES F., M.D.
ANGLE, EDWARD H., M.D., D.D.S.
BAKER, LAWRENCE W., D.M.D.
BOENNING, HENRY C., M.D.
BOGUE, E. A., M.D., D.D.S.
BRIGHAM, DR. WALTER I.
BROWN, GEO. V.I., A.B., D.D.S., M.D., C.M
BRUSH, DR. F. C.
BYRAM, DR. J. Q.
CARLTON, HARRY P., D.D.S.
CHITTENDEN, CHARLES C., D.D.S.
CROTHERS, T. D., M.D.
CRYER, M. H., M.D., D.D.S.
DAVENPORT, DR. S. E.
DOWSKI, SAMUEL, D.D.S.
FILLEBROWN, THOMAS, M.D. D.M.D.
FOSSUME, DR. F. L.
GELSTON, WILLIAM H., D.D.S.
GOSLEE, HART J., D.D.S.
HAMILTON, DR. HARRY F.
HOWE, HORACE L., D.M.D.
HOFHEINZ, R. H., D.D.S.
HOPKINS, SAMUEL A., M.D., D.D.S.
HURD, LEE MAIDMONT, M.D.
JENKINS, DR. N. S.

LAWSHE, ALLISON, R., D.D.S.
LEDERER, WM. J., D.D.S.
LEONARD, T. M. RUSSELL, L.R.C.P., L.R.C. S. (Ed.).
LEWIS, O. G. L., D.D.S.
MACPHERSON, DR. A. H.
MCLAREN, F. J.
MILLER, WILLOUGHBY D., A.M., M.D., D.D.S., Sc.D.
MCMANUS, DR. CHARLES.
O'BRIAN, DR. L. A.
PALMER, JAMES G.
RHEIN, M. L., M.D., D.D.S.
RICHARDS, GEORGE L., M.D.
ROLLINS, WILLIAM.
SCHAMBERG, M. I., D.D.S., M.D.
SMITH, H. CARLETON, Ph.D.
SPAULDING, JOHN H., D.D.S.
STERN, HEINRICH, M.D.
STRANG, DR. C. W.
TRUEMAN, WILLIAM H., D.D.S.
TALBOT, EUGENE S., M.S., D.D.S., M.D., LL.D.
TRUMAN, JAMES, D.D.S., LL.D.
WEDELSTAEDT, E. K., D.D.S.
WHEELER, HERBERT LOCKE, D.D.S.
WHITLOCK, DR. W. M.
WRIGHT, C. M., A.M., D.D.S.

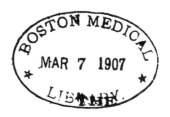
International Dental Journal.

Vol. XXVI.   January, 1905.   No. 1.

Original Communications.[1]

RETARDED ERUPTION OF THE TEETH: THEIR LIBERATION OR EXTRACTION.[2]

BY M. H. CRYER, M.D., D.D.S., PHILADELPHIA.

In order to fully understand this subject one should first be thoroughly familiar with the typical positions of the teeth when entirely erupted and in normal occlusion with those of the opposing jaw. It is also necessary to have a complete knowledge of the internal anatomy of the alveolar process. Therefore, a few illustrations showing the typically erupted teeth, with their occlusion, and the internal anatomy of the alveolar processes will be shown.

Fig. 1 is a side view made from an almost perfect skull of a white woman. The teeth are fully erupted and are almost typical in their position and occlusion. It is evident there has been but little interference with the nutrition of either the jaws or the teeth of this subject. It will be noticed that the mental foramen is on a line drawn vertically downward from between the premolar teeth. This is quite typical and will be again referred to. It is

---

[1] The editor and publishers are not responsible for the views of authors of papers published in this department, nor for any claim to novelty, or otherwise, that may be made by them. No papers will be received for this department that have appeared in any other journal published in the country.

[2] Read at the fifty-fifth annual session of the American Medical Association, in the Section on Stomatology, at Atlantic City, June 7 to 10, 1904.

the external opening of a small tube communicating with the inferior dental canal. For this small tube, which I have described in previous papers, the name " mental tube" is suggested. Its internal opening into the inferior dental canal is situated in the

Fig. 1.

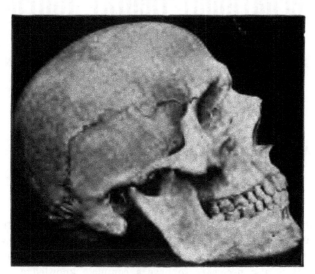

Side view of a typical skull with typical occlusion of the teeth.

movable cancellated tissue near the apex of the root of the canine. If the skull of an infant be examined at birth it will be found that the mental tube, or short canal, passes directly outward nearly opposite the lower portion of the germ of the canine tooth. Then, again, if the skulls of children of various ages, up to adult life, be examined, it will be found that the inlet of this mental tube has been carried forward along with the cancellated tissue of the teeth, while the outlet has, apparently, moved backward, the distance varying according to the age of the child until adult life is reached.

The position of the first molar during its early development was immediately below the upper or inner angle of the jaw. As it increases in size and the other molars are developed, the entire mass of cancellated tissue containing the teeth move forward, the upper portion a little farther than the lower, as is indicated by the curvature of the trabecular and small cribriform tubes passing from the main tube or canal to the roots of the various teeth. To accommodate this growth the mandible proper—the cortical portion—enlarges interstitially as this process is carried on. Interference with this forward movement of the teeth in the cancellated tissue would have a tendency to arrest the enlargement of the jaw, no matter whether the interference be caused by artificial means or by pathologic conditions.

The development of the alveolar process of the upper jaw is somewhat different. While the teeth are developing and erupting the process extends outward and forward without the extension of the maxillæ which is observed in the mandible. When the teeth are finally lost in extreme old age and the alveolar process of both

Fig. 2.

A   B

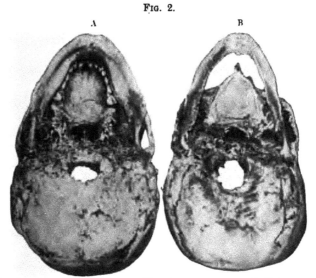

Under view of two skulls. A, from a subject about twenty years old ; B, from one well advanced in years.

jaws is resorbed, the extended rim of the mandible remains, while the upper jaw recedes until the roof of the mouth becomes very small, as is well illustrated in Figs. 2 and 3.

Fig. 4 is made from the skull of a child about six years old.

The external plates of the alveolar process of the upper and lower jaws have been removed exposing the roots of the deciduous teeth

Fɪɢ. 3.

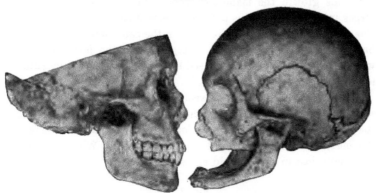

Side view of the two skulls shown in Fig. 2.

Fɪɢ. 4.

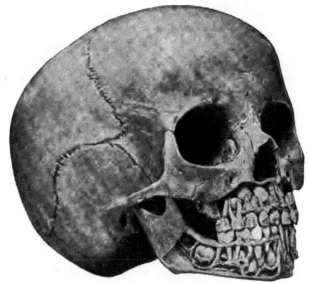

Skull of a child about six years of age, showing all the deciduous teeth with their roots and crowns of nearly all the permanent teeth.

and the crowns of the developing permanent teeth, except those of the lower third molar and the upper first, second, and third molars.

In the majority of children's mouths, at about the age of six, barring accident or decay, the upper and lower teeth (deciduous) are typical in their arrangement in the alveolar process; they are also typical in their occlusion. While pathologic and other disturbances seem to interfere but little in the arrangement of the deciduous teeth, they greatly influence the placing of the permanent teeth.

The positions of the non-erupted teeth shown in Fig. 4 vary in regard to their depth in the bone. Some are deeply set, for example, in this instance the upper canine, while others are quite superficially placed, as illustrated by the lower canine. Others still are found located between the roots of the deciduous teeth, as the crowns of the premolars in the figure. If we take the positions of the developing permanent teeth into consideration, it is comparatively easy to understand why they should often be retarded in their eruption or deflected out of their typical course. If the deciduous teeth are interfered with in such a manner that their physiologic functions are impaired, they, in turn, will interfere with the physiologic functions of the tissue surrounding the permanent teeth.

Local or general pathologic conditions often cause the alveolar arch to become narrowed or shortened, which, in turn, will have more or less influence on the eruption of the permanent teeth. Malocclusion of the teeth is often accompanied by impaction, as will be shown in some of the illustrations. Occasionally supernumerary teeth, odontoma or odontoceles may cause impaction of the teeth.

ORDER OF IMPACTION.

My experience has been that the frequency of impacted teeth is as follows: First, the lower third molar; second, the upper canine; third, the upper third molar; fourth, the upper central incisor; fifth, the lower second premolar; sixth, the upper second premolar; seventh, the lower canine. The first and second groups of this classification will, without doubt, be accepted by all familiar with the subject under discussion. In the museum of the Dental Department of the University of Pennsylvania the following specimens will be found: Twelve impacted lower third molars, nine impacted upper canines, two of which are in one jaw; two impacted upper third molars, both in the same jaw; two impacted lower second premolars.

Examination of Fig. 4 makes apparent reasons for this order

of impaction. It will be seen that the germ of the lower second molar is well back and partly within the ramus of the jaw. The germ of the lower third molar is still farther upward and backward. As these teeth are developed and the jaw grows, the teeth and the cancellated tissue pass forward between the U-shaped cortical bone. If this sliding forward and downward of the tooth be interfered with by reason of inflammatory phenomena within the substance of the jaw, causing the cancellated and cortical portions to become adherent, the already erupted teeth will be prevented from yielding slightly to the eruptive force of the moving molar, and there will be no room for this tooth to slide into its proper position. The lower portion of the capsule is more liable to become retarded or fixed than the upper; consequently, in such a case the upper portion or crown of the tooth is carried forward and downward, causing it in many cases to take a horizontal position. In some instances it is turned directly upside down (see Fig. 5).

If the position of the germ of the upper canine be examined, it will be found on a higher level and deeper in the bone than the other teeth. The first premolar is erupted about three years before the canine and often closes in towards the lateral, erupted five years previously, especially if the deciduous canine has been lost early. Under ordinary circumstances the canine will be forced into a fairly typical position, but if any inflammatory condition of the jaw has been manifested the bone may become firm and the canine more or less impacted. Similar conditions can be predicated of nearly all impacted teeth.

Impacted permanent teeth should, as a rule, be either liberated or extracted. When the impacted tooth can be brought into a useful position through extraction of supernumerary teeth, or by the removal of other causes impeding its eruption, the necessary steps for its liberation should be taken. If left in their impacted state these teeth are liable to prevent the proper nourishment of other teeth and also to interfere with the healthy nutrition of the surrounding tissue. They may press on the branches of the trifacial nerve, producing neuralgia, not only locally, but in remote parts, and through reflex action they may cause various disturbances in and about the head and face. They are liable to bring about inflammatory conditions of this region, produce cellulitis in the tissues of the mouth, neck, throat, and temporo-mandibular articulation, interfere with deglutition, etc. They may cause other teeth to become impacted, or even cause malocclusion of other teeth. Then, again, parts of the roots may penetrate into the maxillary sinus or the nasal chambers, under which conditions, if they become devitalized, they are liable to cause the infection of these cavities.

These four illustrations (Figs. 5, 6, 7, 8) are made from dried specimens. They will give some idea of the most common form of impacted upper canines and lower third molars.

Fig. 5 is from a dried specimen belonging to Dr. T. M. Whitney, of Honolulu. It shows an inverted impacted lower third molar,

Fig. 5.

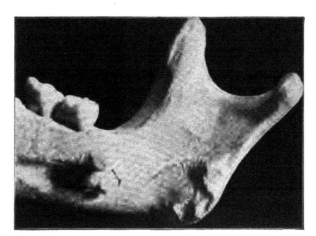

An inverted impacted lower third molar.

the crown of which is partly erupted in the submaxillary fossa. This tooth would be rather difficult to extract in the living subject. From the appearance of the illustration I would judge that it would have to be extracted through the submaxillary triangle.

Fig. 6 shows the anterior surface of an impacted canine tooth resting near the anterior surface of the bone. This tooth could have been diagnosed by the use of an excavator, as the crown was quite superficially covered.

Whenever canine teeth are missing from the arch there is good ground to suspect that they are impacted somewhere within the jaw, unless there is satisfactory evidence that they have been extracted. This is not to be assumed in the case of a missing upper lateral incisor or third molar of either jaw, and occasionally the premolars, all or any of which are often missing through non-development. As an example, I recall the case of a patient about thirty-five years of age, from whose arch the two upper second premolars are missing, and who claims that they have not been ex-

FIG. 6.

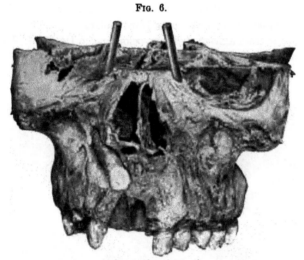

An impacted canine tooth.

tracted. As he suffered from neuralgia in the anterior portion of the maxillæ, I thought that these teeth might be impacted somewhere within the jaw, but a careful exploration with instruments and radiographs, taken at different angles and by several experts, failed to show any evidence of the missing teeth. The failure of these methods of exploration leads me to believe that the teeth in question have never developed.

The extraction of a tooth, such as Fig. 6, would not be difficult. A longitudinal incision could be made over the crown of the tooth, and then by passing a very small spiral osteotome around the crown one would be enabled to pass a universal elevator between tooth and bone. The tooth could then be forced outward; if room could be made so that a small pair of forceps could be used it might be better to use them instead of the elevator.

Occasionally I have found that the bone surrounding such teeth has become very dense and closely adherent to the tooth. Under these conditions the tooth is liable to break, if great care is **not** exercised, and sometimes it is necessary to use a small spiral osteotome to remove the surrounding bone nearly to the apex of the tooth before it can be extracted.

Fig. 7 shows two impacted canines in the roof of the mouth. They were covered principally by bone which extended down nearly

Fig. 7.

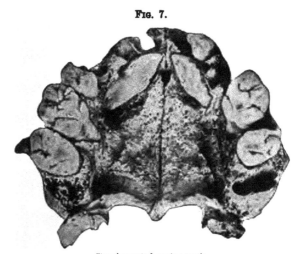

Two impacted canine teeth.

to the point of the crown. These teeth had caused the devitalization of the left first and second premolars and the right first premolar, also of the lateral incisor of the left side. The apex of one of the teeth penetrated the maxillary sinus.

It is more difficult to extract canine teeth when in this position than when situated as shown in Fig. 6, as the danger of causing an opening between the mouth and nose, or mouth and antrum, is greater. It is a good plan to remove the bone from the lingual surface of the tooth, so the tooth can be carried slightly downward and inward without danger of fracture. Usually there is not room to extract it in the line of its axis before it strikes the other teeth or alveolar process.

Fig. 8 shows a common form of impacted lower third molar.

The anterior cusps of the tooth are often interlocked against the concave distal portion of the second molar. In order to extract such teeth it is often necessary to cut these cusps away with either a carborundum disk or an osteotome. When this has been done the instrument can be passed under the tooth, between it and the bone, or both, until the elevator can be passed into the opening. By this

FIG. 8.

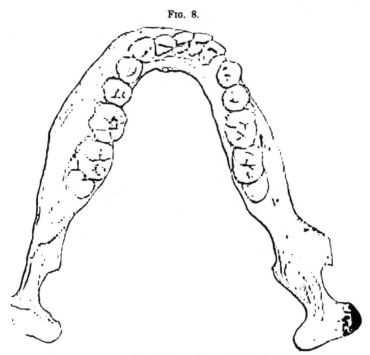

A common form of impacted lower third molar.

means the tooth can usually be removed in a comparatively short time.

The following are from practical cases:

CASE I.—A patient was suffering from neuralgia on the right side of the face. The molar teeth apparently had been extracted from that side of the mandible, but on a closer examination a slight elevation was found about in the position of the right second molar, and by passing an excavator into the enlargement a tooth could be felt. An X-ray picture confirmed this diagnosis. The tooth was removed and the neuralgia ceased. In the X-ray picture the condyloid process is seen plainly resting against the under surface of the eminentia articularis.

In all the radiographs I have seen of this region, when the mouth was wide open, the condyloid process has been found in this position, indicating that the external pterygoid muscles acting together when the angle is comparatively fixed by other muscles, among which are the masseter and internal pterygoid, serve to assist in separating the jaws, by drawing the upper part of the ramus forward, which compels the anterior portion of the mandible to drop, opening the mouth.

CASE II.—Is a patient of Dr. Dray, of Philadelphia. This patient was suffering from neuralgia of the right side of the face. An X-ray picture showed an impacted lower third molar with the crown resting well forward against the distal root of the second molar. In such cases the resorption of this root often takes place, producing neuralgia and devitalization of the tooth. There was a great probability that the second molar was diseased and causing the neuralgia. It was, therefore, thought advisable to extract it, which proved the diagnosis to be correct.

CASE III.—Fig. 9 is made from a plaster cast taken from the mouth of a young woman about twenty-five years old in the practice of Dr. S. Merrill

FIG. 9.

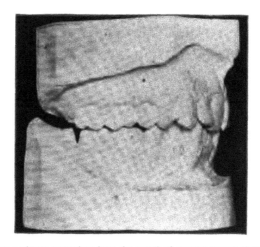

Made from a plaster cast taken from the mouth of a young woman about twenty-five years old in the practice of Dr. S. Merrill Weeks, of Philadelphia, showing an impacted lower third molar.

Weeks, of Philadelphia. The central incisors are erupted with their cutting edges pointing slightly inward instead of outward, probably due to some pathologic condition of the deciduous incisors. The alveolar process around the incisors is harder than normal, which condition prevented these teeth from being carried outward during the eruption of the others. They were thus locked against the incisors of the lower jaw, causing these and other lower teeth to be held back to a greater or less degree, which in turn would cause the impaction of the lower third molars. The right central is directed more inward than the left and in proportion the right lower third molar was more deeply impacted than the left lower third molar. The left impacted tooth was extracted about a year before the casts were made. The right one was interlocked against the second molar. The occluding surface of this tooth was cut away by the use of a carborundum disk, which allowed the crown to rise slightly, as is shown in the illustration, thus making the tooth more prominent and easier to extract.

Fig. 10 is a radiograph taken from a cleaned specimen of the right side of the lower jaw, showing the teeth in position in the cancellated tissue.

FIG. 10.

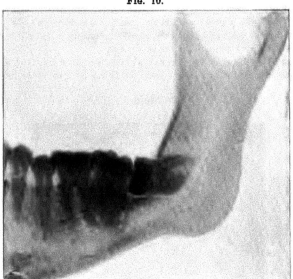

An impacted second premolar and a third left molar.

One might well imagine that a modern orthodontist had moved the first molar "half its width backward" or held it in such a manner that it could not advance. Whether done by mechanical appliance or by pathologic changes, the tooth was held and impaction resulted. If the cancellated tissue be examined, as seen in the X-ray picture, it will be noticed that it is more dense around the first and second molars than anteriorly to these teeth. As the result of an inflammatory condition the cancellated tissue has become united with the cortical bone, thus making another factor in preventing its sliding forward. It will be noticed that the roots of the molar teeth are also thickened by the overaction of the cementoblasts caused by this inflammatory condition.

The inferior dental canal or cribriform tube is slightly deflected from its true course below the roots of the impacted third molar, and is also slightly deflected downward below the roots of the second molar.

It will be noticed that the second premolar stands below the occluding line of the other teeth. It has evidently been retarded in its eruption, perhaps through premature loss or devitalization of the second deciduous pre-

Fig. 11.

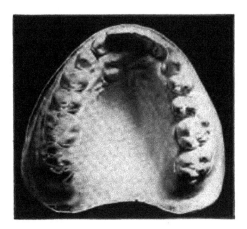

molar. In such cases these roots are resorbed very slowly and often cause inflammatory conditions. It is possible that this was one of the primary causes of the non-eruption of the third molar.

Fig. 12.

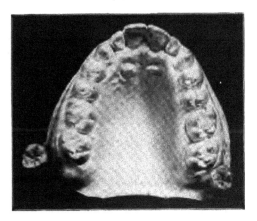

Case IV.—Fig. 11 is from a photograph of a plaster cast of the jaw of a young man about twenty-two years old. Two impacted upper third molars were diagnosed by the use of an excavator. The teeth were afterwards extracted by first removing the overlying tissue and then using small forceps.

Fig. 12 is from a photograph taken of the same cast (Fig. 11), with the extracted impacted teeth placed near the tuberosity of the jaw.

CASE V.—A patient had some neuralgic trouble within the ear, and after having excluded several possible causes, the teeth were suspected, as the upper first and second molars appeared to be sensitive, and a radiograph was taken which indicated an impacted upper left third molar. At this time the patient was referred to me by Dr. George Darby. When one becomes accustomed to examining X-ray pictures it is not difficult to detect a shadow of the crown of a tooth in the region where the upper third molar might be impacted, but this picture gave but a slight indication as to the depth of its occluding surface. No idea was possible as to whether it was near the buccal surface of the alveolar ridge or on the lingual surface. The roots of the tooth, their number, shape, and position, were not shown in the radiograph. All of this practical surgical diagnosis had to be learned by other means. In this case a careful exploration was made with an excavator, and the position of the crown of the tooth was practically located. After the tissue covering the crown of the tooth had been cut away the tooth was grasped with small forceps. The firmness of the tooth indicated that the roots were crooked and held by bone harder than normal. By carrying the handle of the forceps in the line of least resistance, which was outward, backward, and upward, the roots were unlocked from under the over-calcified bone.

Fig. 13 is made from four photographs of the tooth after extraction. A shows the occluding or grinding surface with the points of the roots ex-

FIG. 13.

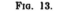

A   B   C   D

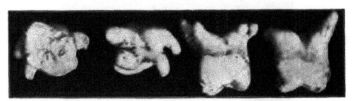

tending outward. B shows the upper surface, or the root end, with the four roots spread outward, approaching a horizontal line. C shows the distal surface, with the hook-like form of the buccal roots, and D shows the anterior surface. It may be interesting to know that the ear has improved since the extraction, and that the other molars appear to have lost their sensitiveness, indicating that the tooth was interfering with the nerve supplying these teeth and through reflex action with the ear.

Fig. 14 was made from a plaster cast of a patient of Dr. G. Marshall Smith, of Baltimore, who has kindly permitted me to use it in this paper. The patient is a girl thirteen years old. Fig. 14 is a side view of a plaster cast of the teeth and alveolar processes. The teeth are undersized, the incisors and canines are too nearly vertical or do not flare enough, especially in the lower jaw. The upper teeth are all erupted, for this age, except the second molars, which are ready to erupt. In the lower jaw they are all

FIG. 14.

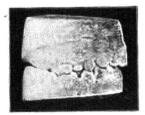

The second deciduous premolar is not in position.

through except the second premolar, which is impacted. The space for this tooth is very narrow, in fact, not sufficient to allow it to take its proper place in the jaw. The description of the teeth on one side of the jaw may also be applied to those of the other side.

If the cancellated tissue in the region of the premolar has become solidified and attached to the cortical bone, this impacted premolar will, to a certain extent, prevent the first and second molars from advancing; these in turn will have a strong tendency to cause the impaction and malocclusion of the third molar.

The primary cause of this pathologic condition of the lower jaw is that the upper anterior teeth have not moved forward in the usual manner, as they bite over the lower anterior teeth, consequently the teeth and alveolar process of the lower jaw are held back, as shown in the illustration, and in order to liberate the second premolar and prevent the third molar from becoming impacted, the upper anterior teeth should be forced forward, which will allow correction to be made in the lower jaw.

CASE VI.—A young man about twenty-one years old, who has suffered from neuralgia of the left side of the mandible. On examination with an excavator, impacted lower right and left one being somewhat broken. The history of the case is that part of the crown of the left third molar has been broken away in an endeavor to extract the tooth, leaving the pulp exposed. A radiograph showed that the crown was deformed, also that the anterior buccal cusp was apparently interlocked under the second molar. By careful examination with an excavator it was found that both of the anterior cusps were so far down in the tissue that a disk could not be used to remove them. The patient being etherized, a mouth-gag was placed in position and a portion of the soft tissue was removed with a small knife. The revolving spiral osteotome was placed within the broken crown, or into the pulp-chamber, cutting almost throu. n the remainder of the crown, and between it and the bone a space was made, partially in the bone, which allowed the point of a universal elevator to pass between the tooth and the jaw.

I seldom use the forceps to remove a tooth after loosening it with the elevator. In using the elevator on the left side, as in this case, it is operated with the right hand, the surgeon standing on the left side of the patient. The left forefinger is placed in the mouth by the lingual side of the tooth, and the thumb is placed on the buccal side of the second molar. This gives steadiness to the jaw and reduces the risk of slipping. As the tooth is raised from its socket the forefinger is placed so as to bring the tooth out of the mouth. If the tooth to be removed is on the right side, the elevator should be used with the left hand, if possible (the surgeon standing on the right side). If the operator must use the elevator with his right hand, he should, however, manage to guard and steady the parts with his left hand.

FIG. 15.

A   B   C

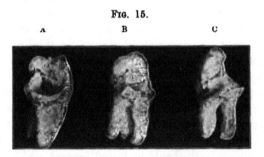

Fig. 15 is made from three photographs of the tooth after extraction. A shows the outer or buccal side of its roots, in about the same position as when in the jaw. The distal cusps were broken away in a former endeavor to extract it. The greater portion of the crown was cut away with the surgical engine. On the side of the tooth there is a groove extending backward, downward and inward, cut by the osteotome. It was along this groove that the elevator was forced under the tooth, causing the slight portion of the crown that remained to fracture. In B the tooth is turned slightly outward, in order to show three roots and the line of fracture which liberated the tooth. In C the tooth is turned on its buccal surface, showing the two anterior cusps which were locked under the distal surface of the second molar.

DISCUSSION.

Dr. Edward A. Bogue, New York City.—What does Dr. Cryer mean by "premolar"?

Dr. Cryer.—A tooth that is in front of the molar tooth.

Dr. Bogue.—Dr. Cryer in his paper used the term "premolar" for a deciduous tooth. I am sorry to hear such misuse of terms. He also stated that Dr. Angle says that if the sixth-year molars are correct in their occlusion all the rest will be right. If he will make further reference to Angle's book he will find that he states that the largest part of irregularities are to be found when the principal molar is in correct, or nearly correct, occlusion. I want to acknowledge my indebtedness to Dr. Cryer; I never hear him without benefit; at the same time, if any defect in his teaching occurs I want to call attention to it, that it may be corrected. As I understand his remarks in regard to impacted third molars he favors extraction. I have a case on hand now in which by tying a small grass line between the impacted third molar and the second molar below I am bringing that third molar to a proper occlusion. I have done this a number of times.

Dr. Cryer.—I said "liberated or extracted."

Dr. Bogue.—I am glad to see that Dr. Cryer's remarks tend in two directions. He advocated the forward development of both jaws. I agree with Dr. Cryer, whose experience is so much greater than mine, that one should be wary of the pressure backward.

Dr. M. L. Rhein, New York City.—Dr. Cryer's idea about the correction of the irregularity early in life and the sacrifice of the third molar later in life is one with which I thoroughly agree. It is expected in these cases of degeneration which cause a lack of space in the mandible itself that there will not be sufficient room for the sixteen teeth to come properly into position. His conclusions, so far as they can be put into practice, I think are the proper ones; that under these circumstances it will most likely be necessary to sacrifice this third molar, and it is the one that can best be sacrificed. I sympathize with all the work that has been done for the preservation of thirty-two teeth in the arch, and especially against the loss of any of the teeth forward of the third molar. There is such a thing as going to extremes on both sides of this question, and if there are any four of these thirty-two teeth to be lost the ones that can be spared with least detriment to the patient are the third molars without the occlusion suffering. In the case of the young Baltimore girl, there seemed to be little question as to what to do. It comes in the category named of gaining sufficient space between the first molar and the first bi-cuspid. If separation is made there Nature will cause that bicuspid to erupt without any difficulty. The undue prominence of the chin and the lack of bone development above it shows to me that it will not make the chin any more prominent. There is plenty of room above the chin for the osseous development, if this forward move-ment is brought about. I have had a number of cases in which after space was provided Nature brought the teeth into position.

Dr. Mihran K. Kassabian, Philadelphia.—The dental and medi-cal professions have derived equal benefits from the introduction and application of the X-rays. The diagnostic value of the rays in cases of unerupted teeth is shown by Dr. Cryer's cases. The ordinary methods of probing with an explorer did not locate the absent teeth, which in some cases were bicuspids and third molars. These had insinuated themselves deeply between other teeth, and the alveolar process was so dense that nothing but the X-ray could locate them. I employ two methods for skiagraphing dental con-ditions, the intraoral method and the extraoral or buccal method. In the intraoral method a small piece of film (which is light and moisture-proof) is placed over the gum tissue at a point where trouble is suspected, placing the tube in such a position that per-pendicular rays will be cast on the teeth and film. This method covers a smaller area, but produces a picture with very sharp details, and is especially recommended for anterior teeth. The extraoral or buccal method requires that a plate 5 x 7 be brought in contact with the jaw at the region of the suspected trouble. The patient inclines the neck and head to an angle of about forty-five degrees. The tube is placed over the shoulder to the opposite side at a distance of twenty inches from the face to avoid superim-position of the jaws. This process produces a picture of greater area and is intended for bicuspids and molars. Two skiagraphs are taken from two angles or directions to determine whether we have a buccal, lingual, distal, or mesial presentment, and I might mention here that Dr. Cryer suggested that I make stereoscopic skiagrams which permit viewing by a reflecting stereoscope, and as a result, instead of observing flat pictures, we obtain a relief or stereoscopic perspective effect, which shows the exact position of the teeth. I have received very good results with my stereoscopic skiagrams at the Philadelphia Hospital, where I used a special table which I had built for the purpose. There is no danger of X-ray burns in skiagraphing these conditions; the time of exposure is short, being from one second to two minutes.

Dr. T. C. Stellwagen, Philadelphia.—The important illustrations made by Dr. Cryer explain how great damage has been done by meddlesome dentists. "Orthodontia" is an incorrect term; the correct one would be "taxidontia." By attempts to correct dental irregularities without a proper knowledge of the development of the jaws an amount of mischief has been done which the profession does not take into account. Early in my practice there occurred a number of instances of patients saying that they had had irregularities corrected, and that since then they had suffered more or less pain and soreness about the teeth; conditions resembling those following fracture or sprain when the weather seems to bring about a neuralgic state. Very often the violence used for such correction has been sufficient to cause permanent inconvenience. Many of the cases, credited to the efficiency of the appliances used, would have been better if left to Nature. Dr. Cryer shows us that the development and growth of the jaws are not confined to any particular locality, but are general throughout, and that under peculiar circumstances we find certain centres of growth arrested, just as we see in hip-joint disease, and then permanent deformity results. The interesting question in connection with the case of the Baltimore child is, can we awaken that trophic influence? Some years ago the permanent cuspid teeth of a patient had failed to erupt, still the deciduous cuspid teeth were *in situ* to work on. Irritation of the teeth until they evinced considerable pain and soreness failed. Ligatures tied around them, hoping thereby to revive or reawaken this trophic force, failed. Extraction of one deciduous canine failed. So far there is but little, if any, hope of ever stimulating these trophic centres. The case mentioned is of interest, as the lad had spasms, caused seemingly by the canine pressure on filaments of nerve in the jaw. The spasms came only occasionally, it is true, but so growth has remissions of energy. I believed that we could do nothing better than to look forward to the time when the growth and alterations of the permanent canine teeth would cease, somewhere about his twelfth year. For about forty years, although still living, the patient has been free from spasms. That the reawakening of the trophic force could have been brought about in his case I very much doubt.

Dr. Bogue.—In a case of a child twelve years of age, in whom the left central incisor had not developed, instead of tapping on that bicuspid tooth, as did Dr. Stellwagen, I put in wedges and spread the right central and left lateral widely apart, and inserted a large central on a rubber plate. The left central came down, even at that age, into correct position. I have done the same thing in the last six months. In other words, I got the room which Dr. Cryer has been telling us we ought to get. The plaster cast of impaction shown us by Dr. Cryer shows also a retracted condition of the incisors, and I think he is mistaken as to the cause. It seems presumptuous for me to question Dr. Cryer, but he must not draw conclusions from the facts he presents to us, unless he expects to be criticised. The irregularities of the incisors in that case seem to me to have nothing to do with the other irregularities which he showed us.

Dr. Stellwagen.—There was abundant room for the cuspids to come down, the teeth were separated and had enough space.

Dr. Eugene S. Talbot, Chicago.—Dr. Cryer's specimens are fine and show many pathologic conditions. The explanation of an individual case does not, however, give accurate information as to the etiology. To understand the etiology, the evolution of man, including heredity and neurasthenia in the parent as well as in the child, must be considered to show the production of these conditions. If there were time, I should like to go over these slides and from these basic principles show how these deformities are produced. Starting with the evolution of man, the face and jaws, like the vermiform appendix, small rib, little toe, and other structures of the body are degenerating under the law of economy of growth for the benefit of the organism as a whole. At about four and one-half months of fetal life, the first period of stress occurs. At this period, owing to the neurasthenia of the parents and improper nourishment, arrests take place. Owing to the transitory nature of the face and jaws, they are more easily affected than permanent structures of the body. Arrests of development of some parts and excess of development of others (due to an unstable nervous system) account for all malformations. The point brought out by Dr. Stellwagen in regard to pain in the alveolar process is not uncommon. It occurs after teeth have been regulated, and the question naturally arises when and how far we are warranted in the correction of irregularities, owing to the interstitial gingivitis produced. This pain occurs in ordinary forms of interstitial gingivitis, as well as in interstitial gingivitis due to injury. This disease is associated with the alveolar process through life. Pain may be experienced at any period. The cribbing of the horse when returned to the stall after a summer's outing and disuse of the anterior teeth is a marked illustration of this pain. The eruption of the cuspid tooth seems to be a providential process by which the anterior and posterior teeth are, in a measure, moved forward or backward for the purpose of enlarging the dental arch.

Dr. Cryer.—In regard to the use of the term "premolar," I perhaps should not use this word before a dental society, as I believe they have arbitrarily adopted another term, which, however, I can not accept in my writing. A premolar is a tooth anterior—in time or position—to a molar tooth. Dr. Bogue says we have not a deciduous premolar. In one sense, all the deciduous teeth are premolars, but the term is more especially and more properly applied to what are commonly called, by the dental profession, the deciduous molars. If I understand the meaning of deciduous, it means not lasting but destined to be lost or shed in time. The deciduous (premolars) molars are shed and their places taken by the permanent premolars, or as they are known in accepted dental nomenclature, the bicuspids. The lower jaw certainly grows forward. The upper jaw I claim does not grow forward, but its alveolar process does. It extends forward, and its base is the upper jaw. The upper jaw is one thing; the alveolar process and its teeth are distinctly another. When teeth are lost, and the alveolar processes are resorbed, the rim of the lower jaw, which has gone forward, remains there, while the upper jaw, not having gone forward. is found to be almost the same as in early life. I want to put it on record that four years ago the city authorities of the Philadelphia Hospital recognized the dental profession by adding four doctors of dental surgery to the medical staff of that great hospital, giving them the same standing as the medical men.

Last year, at the suggestion of the dental staff, an extensive apparatus for X-ray work was added to the already well-supplied hospital, and the dental department was put in the highest possible condition for usefulness. Dr. Kassabian has spared neither time nor energy in working up the use of the X-ray for the benefit of the dental students who have attended the dental clinics given at the hospital.

A NEW PORCELAIN FOR PROSTHETIC PURPOSES.[1]

BY DR. N. S. JENKINS, DRESDEN, GERMANY.

So soon as porcelain enamel had been proved to completely answer the requirements for restoring decayed or broken teeth to health, beauty, and usefulness, I began to occupy myself with the question of producing a porcelain which should simplify prosthesis and make porcelain crowns, bridges and continuous gum work easy to the general practitioner. It was a task, lightened, indeed, by previous experience, but presenting difficulties of no inconsiderable magnitude. The materials employed in making dental porcelain have hitherto been worked somewhat crudely. It has been rare to find a completed product sufficiently free from foreign matter or possessing the desired homogeneity. For this the manufacturers are not to blame. Their object has been to supply what they believed the profession to demand,—viz., cheap materials with which fairly good results can be obtained. No manufacturer, whose legitimate purpose is commercial, can be expected to carry on year-long experiments, at large expense, in the vague hope of supplying a superior material when he has no reason to suppose that there is, or will be, a demand for it. Our debt to the dental manufacturers is exceeding great, but there is much work which only a dentist in actual practice can do. for only he can know exactly what the practising dentist needs, and therefore it is vain and unreasonable to look to any other than a dentist to accomplish such work.

I have been so fortunately situated as to make experiments in porcelain my natural contribution to the progress of our pro-

---

[1] Read before The New York Institute of Stomatology, October 4, 1904.

fession, and it has been solely owing to these favorable circumstances that I am able to present to you to-night a product which seems to me to completely solve the question of porcelain prosthesis. For more than two years I have been able to produce it in the small quantities of laboratory experiment, but only recently has it been found possible to manufacture it in larger quantities. This delay is, however, no cause for regret. During this time I have not only been occupied with the question of manufacture, but also with the methods of applying this material, and those methods are now well systematized. At the very foundation lies the importance of a proper alloy of platinum-iridium. For plates, for caps and bands, ten per cent. of iridium is essential. For posts, twenty per cent. of iridium is necessary. Pure gold should be used for solder.

Prosthetic porcelain begins to melt at 950° C. The heat may be continued up to 1000° C., at which point the electric current should be suspended, and, usually, the piece can then be cooled rapidly. The melting-point of gold is, approximately, 1075° C. At a temperature of 1000° C. not only is there no danger of remelting the solder or volatilizing the gold, but under this heat the above alloy of platinum-iridium does not bend nor change its shape, and if this temperature is not exceeded, the life of the platinum wire of an electric furnace is greatly prolonged. The heat should be determined by a pyrometer. One cannot too greatly insist upon this point. Here is a simple, scientific method, through which it is possible to obtain exact results, without exception. No man who does this class of work, and every dentist ought to do it, can afford to leave anything to chance or to imagination. To be sure, through experience, one can easily learn to work prosthetic porcelain without a pyrometer, but, with the greatest care, the greatest expert will sometimes fail to recognize sudden changes in the electric current, which the pyrometer infallibly records.

Prosthetic porcelain may be used alone, but most dentists will find it desirable to use it in combination with artificial teeth. It combines perfectly with all porcelain teeth, in any proportion. from a delicate jacket crown to a massive molar. It can be used to supplement, to support, to extend, and to broaden teeth, or even to restore the lost glaze of an artificial tooth, with perfect confidence. It is far stronger than the strongest artificial teeth, and in a close bite can be safely used in a thickness of three millimeters. Crowns and bridges, which were formerly made of gold, can be made of platino-iridium, and so built out with prosthetic porcelain that no suggestion of artificiality can be discovered, and the work will be stronger and more cleanly. In fact, it enables any capable dentist to completely conceal his art in prosthesis and to restore the mouth of his patient to its original beauty and usefulness, for he can obtain, with certainty, any desired color, any necessary form, a density which makes grinding and subsequent polishing possible, enduring strength and hardness, and a brilliant and indestructible glaze. There is no limit to its usefulness or to the gratitude of the patients who have experienced its advantages, and it supplies one more step toward the proper remuneration of an overworked and underpaid profession.

SHOULD THE DENTAL PRACTITIONER CONCERN HIMSELF WITH THE CHEMICAL EXAMINATION OF SALIVA OR URINE?[1]

BY H. CARLETON SMITH, PH.D., NATICK, MASS.[2]

UNLESS I am mistaken, and I hope I am, an unqualified affirmative answer to the question presented for our consideration to-night would meet with considerable objection.

The reasons given might be, first, that such examination is not practicable, or, second, the information so gained may be better obtained in some other way; third, such information has slight bearing upon the problems and conditions constantly presenting themselves to a busy dentist.

In regard to these objections, the first one of non-practicability is valid only to a limited extent, and the difficulty here is not so much in making the analysis as it is in getting the samples to analyze. Under the existing social and professional usages we can imagine circumstances when it would be a little hard for a

---

[1] Read before the American Academy of Dental Science, October 5, 1904.
[2] Instructor in Chemistry, Harvard School.

dentist to secure samples that the physician asks for almost from habit. But this would pass.

The second objection, of better ways to the same end, has but little of truth behind it, and that little is constantly decreasing as we learn better and more complete methods of chemical investigation.

The third objection is a reasonable one, and merits our consideration; we might take it for our topic and restate the question for discussion: " Is a knowledge of the relationship between the chemical constituents of urine and saliva and the diseases of the oral cavity of practical value?"

I am a firm believer in the soundness of deductions from analogies. I believe in the first part of the theory of evolution because the last part is before our eyes, and, because the threefold nature of the material world and the threefold nature of man are so plainly manifest I claim a foundation for, and a right to believe in, the threefold nature of some other things concerning which we have less positive material evidence, and so, from among the lesser things of this class, I would call attention to the threefold nature of dental disease, or, better, of the three causes of dental disease which are not nearly so independent as it may at first seem.

Disease may be due, first, to an influence wholly external to the tissues involved, and which we may regard as a mechanical or, in a restricted sense, a chemical cause, as mechanical abrasions or chemical erosion. This is perhaps the least important, and appears as a primary factor in the smallest number of cases; second, to the growth of specific foreign organisms, bacteria, fungi, etc., which is also chemical and may be both external and internal as regards the tissue involved; and third, to malnutrition of the part which is a factor, perhaps in some instances secondary, but nevertheless a factor in *every* disease the nature of which is in any degree chronic.

Again, let us neglect the first two and for a little consider the third part of the proposition before us.

Malnutrition is not necessarily *lack* of nutrition, but often the wrong kind of nutrition; that is, the blood may be abundantly supplied with all the essentials to a vigorous maintenance of its physiological integrity, but the proportion of acid-forming elements may be in excess of the normal, the chemical equilibrium is disturbed and conditions are produced favorable to the development of dental disease,—pyorrhœa, for instance.

Again, there may be a very evident lack of some particular tissue constituent, such as the phosphates, and for some reason the phosphates taken into the system with a view to the correction of such lack pass into the fæces, with but very slight absorption. A case of precisely this kind came to my knowledge during last winter.

Now, is a knowledge of conditions such as these of value to the dentist? It seems to me so, especially if he realizes that his profession is not a trade, but a specialized department of medicine, as is surgery, or bacteriology, and in no way inferior to them or to medicine itself in its opportunities for profound scientific investigation or in its demand for an ability to draw *correct* conclusions from observed phenomena.

If there are diseases of the oral cavity which a dentist is expected to treat, and which may have their etiology in some systemic derangement not easily apparent, then in such cases it becomes the business of the practitioner to inform himself as thoroughly as possible as to the exact conditions existing in the patient's system, and, more than this, as to the tendencies or "diatheses" which will probably produce conditions favorable or detrimental to the future development of such diseases. In other words, if diseases of systemic nature or origin are to receive the attention of the dentist, he should obtain all possible light on his case, and the analysis of the urine throws considerable on diseases of this class. The examination of the urine, however, may be of little or no value if made with a view to the diagnosis of renal disease, and it is usually from this view-point, and in too many instances from this alone, that the physician makes his analysis. If, on the other hand, the examination of urine is made to obtain the greatest possible amount of information regarding vital processes and the body metabolism, it should be of considerable value, at least in any case where there is a possibility of constitutional disturbance.

Urine analysis may be made in different ways to tell different kinds of stories. Not different stories with contrary indication, but different kinds of stories, supplementary to each other. The dentist is not benefited in his work by a knowledge of just the variety of acute nephritis from which his patient may happen to be suffering; in fact, the patient with acute nephritis or acute anything else, unless it be a toothache, usually postpones his visit to the dentist, and acute disease (not dental) is of little importance, except for its history; but the case is different when we come to the consideration of chronic maladies. The chronic disease means impaired function and diminished vitality somewhere or somehow, and its effect on the proper nutrition of teeth and gums is worthy of consideration.

Dr. Metcalf, of New Haven, puts it well when he says that " We do know that normal function is dependent upon normal structure, and it follows that, disease being the perversion of function, and normal function depending entirely upon healthy or normal blood supply, an intimate knowledge of the chemistry of blood and nerve supply would seem indispensable."

The diseases of nutrition and faulty metabolism are receiving a constantly increasing amount of attention; but positive conclusions of a practical nature are difficult to obtain, because experimenting for long periods of time upon human subjects is impracticable and in many particulars impossible, and because the parallelism between laboratory or animal experimentation and corresponding conditions in the human organism may be very far from perfect.

We have referred to pyorrhœa, and there is no disease better suited or upon which more work has been done or may be done to demonstrate the affirmative side of the question of the evening.

I quote the following from a review in the *Dental Cosmos* of an article in the *New York Medical Journal* by Geo. F. Souwers, of Philadelphia: " The cases of pyorrhœa alveolaris which have come under the author's observation have led him to attach considerable importance to the constitutional factor, rheumatism, gout, etc., as bearing upon the etiology of this malady. Pyorrhœa alveolaris of the constitutional type should be treated systemically. If rheumatism or some other vitiated state is found to be a factor in the causation of the disease, a treatment should be instituted having in view the eradication of the constitutional taint." Analyses of urine and saliva will determine the existence of " vitiated states." While I have used this quotation because it supports my own theories on the subject, I fail to understand how the author can refer to rheumatism as a factor in the causation of pyorrhœa, or how a Boston dentist, in a paper recently read before the Northeastern Dental Association, can seriously ask the question, Why, if pyorrhœa is of constitutional origin, do not the gums show signs of some increased irritation in cases of acute rheumatism or gout?

As I understand pyorrhœa, it is a disease of itself, that is, a product of faulty conditions of some sort, and not secondary to gout or, of necessity, to any disease. If this is true, it is as proper to speak of Riggs's disease as the cause of gout as is the converse, or there is as much reason to question that gout is a uric acid disease because people suffering from acute rheumatic affection do not show indications of gout. Because the excess of uric acid in the blood is going in a given direction is, of itself, a reason why it should not at the same time go in another direction. Rheumatism and gout are seldom simultaneous manifestations of the uric acid diathesis. This may be too much of a digression. I do not care to provoke a discussion of the etiology of pyorrhœa, but I *do* want to cite a few cases, as of one of the diseases where an analysis of the urine will be of assistance to the dentist. This will be particularly true if, as I believe, there may be cases of pyorrhœa which are *not* caused by uric acid poisoning.

During the past year I have examined the urine from a number of patients suffering from pyorrhœa, and in the great majority of cases the results would justify placing uric acid among the probable causative factors of the disease. A patient of Dr. V. C. Pond showed increased uric acid in nine out of ten analyses made since June, 1902.

I have had a number of specimens from Drs. C. P. and E. C. Briggs, and of these all have shown excessive amounts of uric acid, with one exception; this happened to be among the first received, and was unmarked. Of the other samples received from the Drs. Briggs, I note particularly three marked Mrs. C. S. D., M. C. G., and Mrs. C. S., in all of which the uric acid was very high and the hyperacidity very marked.

Dr. L. M. Miner sent a sample marked J. M. M., also showing high uric acid, and excessive acidity; incidentally it may be stated that the acidity is *not* due, more than to slight extent, to the presence of uric acid. The uric acid is either combined with the alkaline bases as neutral or acid urates, or if in a free state it is very insoluble in acid urine and appears in crystalline form in the sediment.

Dr. D. W. Dickinson also sent one sample with high uric acid and high acidity; this case also contained sodium oxalate; it was marked J. B. I have noted the presence of oxalates in other samples which have shown high uric acid, but cannot say from my observations thus far how general the occurrence may be.

Samples have also been received from Dr. H. W. Hardy, marked G. I. O., and from Dr. H. E. Kahn, marked D., in which the uric acid was very high, but increase of acidity was not so strongly marked. I have mentioned the initials with which these samples were marked, hoping that some of the doctors from whom they were received would be present to-night and perhaps add a word of subsequent history of the cases. These are all supposed to be cases of pyorrhœa, and an anti-uric acid treatment has been recommended. As previously intimated, laboratory experiments along these lines are not practicable, and preponderance of evidence furnished by cases in actual practice will give the most satisfactory and I believe the most conclusive information on the subject; and along this line Dr. J. Warren Achorn contributes the following: Record of three cases where Riggs's disease was materially benefited by an anti-uric acid diet, which was given for other purposes, the benefit to teeth and gums being purely incidental.

First, a woman of forty-five, weight ninety-eight pounds, sent by Dr. Robert Upham. History of canker of the tongue, had Riggs's disease of three years' standing; had been in the habit of eating in the morning red meat and coffee with considerable sugar. For lunch meat again, beef broth, and coffee; at night, roast beef or lamb, a lot of tomatoes, and strawberries whenever available.

For this was substituted a breakfast of cereal carrying a large amount of gluten, fish boiled or broiled (not fried), eggs twice a week, cestus bread and cestus phosphated crackers, cooked fruit, and cereal coffee. Lunch: White meats, chicken, turkey or game birds; fish, crackers and milk, berries (except strawberries), white grapes, and nuts. Dinner: A more extended course of the same general sort and including soups, raw oysters, plain lobster, little-neck clams, vegetables, and to a very limited extent the red meats, tomatoes, asparagus, etc. The result of this treatment for four months was marked improvement according to her dentist, not according to the physician, for he did not follow the case, but the dentist complained that this system of diet had lost him a patient.

A second case was Mr. C. H. R., of North Adams, cured of chronic recurrent lumbago in one year's time by diet similar to above but adapted, of course, to the peculiarities of the individual, as every diet list must be. At the beginning of the treatment the patient had pyorrhœa; at its finish the gums were hard and firm.

The third case was Mr. C. A. V., of Boston. Weight two hundred and thirty-three pounds; a large eater of sweets and meat. Had Riggs's disease and a tendency to apoplexy. He was treated for obesity, and out of regard to the apoplectic propensity special care was taken to reduce the blood-pressure as far as possible, and to this end all highly nitrogenous foods were eliminated from the diet, with the result that Mr. V.'s weight was reduced to one hundred and ninety pounds and his Riggs's disease was cured.

Dr. Alexander Haig, of London, a great English authority on dietetics, says, in the *Medical Record* for October 31, 1903, that " the chief advantage of a bread and fruit diet is seen in the collæmic, or *high blood-pressure group* of *uric acid food poisonings.* Such used to be called diseases, and were reckoned under the names of headache, epilepsy, obesity," etc. From such cases as those above cited, which I have every reason to believe have been accurately stated, from the testimony of physicians and dentists, from books and articles on the subject which I have had time to read, and from my own results in examinations of urine and saliva of afflicted individuals, I have come to believe in the following summary of doctrine:

First: The great majority of cases of Riggs's disease are accompanied by conditions of hyperacidity of the stomach and by high arterial tension.

Second: That this disease (which I have used to illustrate my point simply because data concerning it was most easily available), if not due to, is usually accompanied by, and aggravated by the presence of excessive amounts of uric acid in the blood, and properly comes under the above classification made by Dr. Haig, although not specifically mentioned by him.

Third: That such conditions may be shown by analyses of the urine and saliva, and may be greatly benefited by a carefully restricted diet based upon a study of the general metabolism of the patient.

Fourth: That the more complete the knowledge of the case in all its details and complications, and the more closely the patient follows exactly the doctor's directions, when based on such intimate knowledge, the better the results.

This fourth statement may seem self-evident and unnecessary, nevertheless it is a very important and a much disregarded fact.

I believe most emphatically that the up-to-date dentist of the future will make dietetics and body metabolism an important part of his study in every case dependent upon constitutional conditions. Further, physicians are more and more turning over to the dentists their patients with any sort of mouth-disease, and where complications of a systemic nature occur, the dentist must make his investigation as thoroughly as the physician in order to treat the case as intelligently.

Now I want to spend a few moments in considering *how* this information may be obtained by the dentist.

Dr. Joseph P. Michaels, of Paris, Dr. E. C. Kirk, of Philadelphia, and many others are putting considerable time and study on the relation of salivary analysis to dental diseases, and among the methods they employ a few simple tests may be selected which are easily made and will mean more as our general knowledge of the subject broadens.

Dr. Michaels first notes the physical properties of a sample of saliva,—its color, its taste (which we omit), its appearance, consistence, and odor; also the appearance under the microscope and the micro-polariscope.

Then the chemical examination, consisting of a five-drop test for five different chemical principles. The first drop is tested for acidity or alkalinity with litmus. The second for ammonium salts with Messler's reagent. The third for sulphocyanates with ferric chloride. The fourth for chlorides with silver nitrate and potassium chromate. The fifth drop for glycogen with Gram's reagent (aqueous iodine solution with potassium iodide).

To these five I would add a sixth, made with equal ease and sometimes giving indications of importance,—that is a test for acetone. The test is made by dissolving in the drop of saliva a small crystal or fragment of potassium carbonate; then a small drop of iodine solution (Gram's) will develop the odor of iodoform if acetone is present. The iodoform separates in small yellow starlike crystals. which may be easily observed under the microscope.

The picture shown by the micro-polariscope is one of great beauty, besides being intensely interesting. A great variety of crystalline forms present themselves, but with the exception of a comparatively small number their significance has not been clearly demonstrated.

The oxalates (sodium), lactophosphate, and urates (sodium) I can show you.

Dr. Michaels says, " The presence of biliary pigments in the saliva is beyond any doubt. These substances can be seen in histological preparations of the saliva of diathetic individuals; also in pathological products of diseased blood and pus of alveolo-dental pyorrhœa. The pigments are perfectly characteristic and it depends only on the technique to discover them." Now, this is one of the things I am particularly anxious to have you teach me about. I have never seen them to know what they are. I do not reflect on the accuracy of the quotation, but I have probably not yet stumbled upon the " technique."

It is along this line of investigation I would ask your assistance. I shall be glad to examine any sample of saliva which you care to send to the Laboratory of the Harvard Dental School, and which in your opinion will show marked departure of some sort from the normal. If the saliva can be accompanied by a twenty-four sample of urine, additional light can undoubtedly be thrown upon the case. These examinations I am glad to make free of all expense throughout this month of October at least.

ELECTROLYSIS FOR THE TREATMENT OF PERIDENTAL INFLAMMATIONS.[1]

BY DR. A. H. MACPHERSON, PHILADELPHIA.

ELECTROLYSIS comes to our profession as a new treatment for inflammations arising in the peridental membrane. It simply does its own work, with no tendency to crowd out other curative agents. Immediate relief may be given in all stages of inflammation; if little or no pus has formed, electrolysis will hasten the formation and draw it to the surface. Where there is much swelling and accumulation of pus, electrolysis will cause the pus to discharge where the electrode is placed; the swelling will disappear, the muscles relax, the flow of blood will be increased, and pain will

---

[1] Read before the Academy of Stomatology, Philadelphia.

cease. Where there is intense suffering from pyorrhœa the treatment will give immediate relief and remove any accumulation of pus.

Electrolysis is the dissolution of a chemic compound by an electric current. The current passing from the positive pole to the negative pole passes through resistant tissue, stimulating the flow of blood, or foreign matter, that may exist in its path. The blood-vessels keep the blood from coming to the surface while pus, which is found in a free state, will flow where the electric current may direct. The direction of the current is toward the negative pole and nothing can prevent its progress. Pus that may exist in the body will be found and brought to the surface where the negative electrode is placed.

Electrolysis is master of the situation, and its work is thorough and complete, marvellous as it may seem. This wonderful power we are permitted to control, and by it relieve days of suffering. The operation is from fifteen to twenty minutes duration and almost painless. Electrolysis used in dental practice stimulates the flow of blood, and the patient realizes the good effects through the entire system.

Electrolysis may only be used from a series of batteries giving a moderate amount of voltage without a series current controller. The amount of current is obtained by a cell selector, or the electric light current may be passed through a genuine shunt controller. The positive pole is applied with a sponge at the nerve-centres at the back of the head, or preferably held in the hand, any rings worn being first removed; the negative electrode is applied where it is desired to remove pus.

One hundred volts will destroy tissue, while it only requires from five to twenty volts for this work. Electrolysis has been used by the medical profession for the past twenty-five years for the removal of tumors, superfluous growths, and birth-marks. This method was discovered by Mr. F. Geiger, an electrician of Philadelphia, who has had many years of experience in medical electricity. For fifteen years Mr. Geiger has applied electrolysis to relieve abscessed conditions of his teeth, and always found relief from untold suffering.

The polarity should always be tested where the electric light current is used. Turn on all the current and place the poles in a glass of water; the negative pole will produce bubbles. Should the positive pole be placed over the abscess, the pus will be scattered and drain into the system.

What proof have we that it is pus? may be asked. By the relief given, by the quick healing of an abscess, and by chemical analysis made by Dr. I. N. Broomell, who witnessed an application of electrolysis at the Pennsylvania State meeting, last summer, at which time I gave a demonstration. The patient then treated had been suffering severe pain in an inferior cuspid which was badly decayed. The doctor—my patient—said, " If the pain does not stop in the next two hours I shall have the tooth extracted." The tooth had been aching for twenty-four hours, with no sleep for the sufferer. The question presented itself, Has pus formed? A member of the society standing near suggested that no doubt there was some formation of pus. There was no swelling and little or no soreness about the tooth. I applied electrolysis, and in less than five minutes there was pus discharging at the negative electrode. The application was continued for about twenty minutes, twenty-four volts being used. More than a spoonful of pus was removed and the pain relieved. Mr. Geiger claims great results yet to be attained by electrolysis. It is an easy and simple operation for him to cure a boil on the neck, and he has done it scores of times. What is more wonderful, he believes it possible to cure blood-poisoning and lockjaw, and would gladly put his belief to a test.

Gentlemen, there is a thought to which I must give voice, and that is, what a blessing to humanity it would be if it were possible for Mr. Geiger to give all of his time and attention to this work! As it is he has very little time to devote to this branch. I believe his heart is in this work, and that he would gladly give himself to study and research along these lines. I have found electrolysis to be a friend in need many times. Its influence is for good, as it stimulates the dentist to more exacting and thorough work and greater faith and confidence in his efforts to become a master of his profession.

Reviews of Dental Literature.

THE CHOICE AND USE OF MEDICAL LITERATURE.[1] By Hugh
T. Patrick, M.D., Chicago.

The choice and the use of medical literature depend first on
what the physician tries to be; not on what he would like to be,
not on what his ideal may be, but on what he thoughtfully, consistently strives to be.

KINDS OF PHYSICIANS.

Our day-dreams of attainment are much the same, but the daily
walk of physicians varies greatly. Most of us have met a physician
who may be called the family factotum. He hobnobs with fussy
mothers and puttering fathers. He is greatly interested in grand-
ma's cough, knows just how to wash the baby, has his special
poultice, and can take off warts. Dropping in to ask about Aunt
Em's backache, he stays an hour visiting with the folks. He is a
gentle and kindly soul, but his mind is occupied with the trivialities
of medicine and domestic chit-chat.

Then, there is our old friend who in winter airs his surgical
deeds and medical acumen about the drug-store stove and in summer holds a like symposium on the shady side of the street. He
knows a good cigar, is a pleasant gentleman, and harmless in all
things save only the practice of his profession.

We have heard of the affable society physician who dresses well,
talks well, knows the best families, attends receptions, and makes
social calls. We know and respect the God-fearing church physician who teaches the Bible-class, sings in the choir, gets together
the pastor's salary, and finances the church debt. The lodge physician, the sporting physician, and the physician deep in politics
are familiar figures. We know them all. They are of us, members of our honorable guild. With loyalty and affection we take

---

[1] President's address, delivered before the thirtieth annual meeting of
the Mississippi Valley Medical Association, at Cincinnati, October 11, 1904.
[This address is equally applicable to dentists, and its forcible statements
should be read and appreciated.—ED.]

them by the hand. They are good friends and good citizens; but really fine physicians—not one of them. And not one of them has any real use for good medical literature.

But there is another man—the man we would like to be; the capable man who knows his work and does it; the man up with the van, who can talk face to face with the great in our noble profession. He has enthusiastically striven or doggedly persisted until he is the wise, skilful physician who practises with no uncertain hand, but knows when he is right and knows where he is ignorant. To be what he is and do what he does means familiarity with what others have done and are doing. To this there is no exception. He reads. He selects his literature well and uses it wisely.

WISE SELECTION OF BOOKS.

The selection of our books is a task as delicate, a duty as significant as is the choice of remedies for our patients. Every book is a prescription for our mental self. And yet, who can deny that the clever book-agent puts thousands of volumes on our shelves? In this day and generation it is the physician's obligation not only to be able to recognize the good in medical literature, but to know the great and the safe among medical writers. A conscientious physician calls in consultation no unknown man, but, strange to relate, he will blindly follow an author of whom he knows nothing except that he has produced a book.

THE ROLE OF THE TEXT-BOOK.

Another somewhat frequent professional indiscretion, to call it by no harsher name, is the good old student plan of sticking to a text-book. Progress means expansion. The more a man progresses the less prominent is the rôle of the text-book. It is necessary for babes, but not meat for strong men. No text-book physician is an A No. 1 man. The latter needs the treatise, the " system," the cyclopædia, and particularly the monograph.

THE MONOGRAPH.

Of all medical books, the monograph is the best—and the worst. As a rule, it is the product of special interest and the wise employment of opportunity. In it we often find the rich harvest of many years of loving labor by a great mind. In all probability, the author has not only consulted the writings of others, but has acquired a sure judgment in weighing their merits. Unfortunately, sometimes he is an enthusiast without balance, a faddist, a man with a theory, a prejudiced observer, a dealer in sophistry. Then, if in addition he be a positive and clever writer he may do untold harm. I have now in mind an interesting, attractive book which in the last twelve years has led astray thousands of physicians, and I am sure that the next quarter of a century will not see rooted out the fallacies planted by its brilliant author. Why is this? Because thousands of well-meaning physicians bought the book without knowledge, read it without care, absorbed its tenets without proving, and promulgated its dicta without prudence.

DISCRIMINATION IN READING.

If he is to really profit by the precious time spent in reading, the physician must be able to read with discrimination. In medicine there is no such thing as an authority. The critical sense must be keen and ever alert. The reader must learn to be a judge, for the plea of every paragraph is to be adjudicated. And if he feels himself at fault, assistance is on every side. I think there is no case in which those who know are more happy to lend a hand than in the selection and interpretation of medical writings.

MEDICAL JOURNALS.

And next, what of the journals? This is a big question and a hard one; one I approach with considerable feeling, but with no confidence. Nevertheless, I shall not attempt to dodge it; and since to advise is more human than to confess, to find fault more spontaneous than to praise, to say " don't" easier than to say " do," I venture first to advance a few of the " don'ts" in my mind. Be it understood, however, that these are suggestions purely tentative, as the expression of only one of a vast company, and that no remark is meant as criticism of editor, censure of publisher, or condemnation of publication *per se.* All is addressed to the reader. I am not talking of foods, but of diet.

Don't admit to your presence a journal that is not perfectly straight and clean. As the first requisites of the good physician are conscientiousness and strictest integrity, so no journal is safe if it be not honest on every page. Humiliating as is the admission, we must confess that there are mercenary medical men writing subsidized articles for the benefit of tradesmen. We may not be able to stop the practice, but for the love of decency, let us drop the articles into the waste basket as soon as received and bar the journals from our table.

Just to illustrate how vigilant we must be, I may state that one medical screed has appeared in different journals as a straight advertisement, an editorial, an "original," a therapeutic hint, a news item, and a clinical note. Again, of seven so-called original papers in one journal, four were obviously for ulterior purposes.

A thinly veiled deception is that of putting amidst scientific matter blatant advertising quoted from *Der Deutsche Medizinische Schurkenstreich* or *La Nation Médicale Trompeuse*. It is simply knavery with German or French sugar coating.

Another sort of debasing journal is the one that pretends, perhaps honestly, to help the physician to success by means other than pure professional excellence. A type of this kind of thing I recently found in an address to the graduating class of a medical school. I have no doubt the orator thought he was advising tact and inculcating practical methods for the management of patrons, the confusion of competitors, and the increase of income. As a matter of fact, he was teaching those young men deception, subterfuge, and meretricious connivance, to take the place of scientific knowledge and manly worth. Concerning the editor who spreads such pestilence, I have nothing to say. The physician who admits it to his library and his mind not only injures himself, but is recreant to his trust.

Don't indulge in yellow journals—for such there are—of deeper or fainter dye. The more harmless kinds merely present a sort of pseudoscientific vaudeville of striking oddities, rare curiosities, marvellous happenings, and other side-show monstrosities of the medical world. All of this serves only to excite a passing interest, and makes no reader one whit better as scholar or practitioner. The worse kinds, under the cloak of medicine, pander to our appetite for the startling, the scandalous, even the salacious, and appeal to passion and prejudice. They lean strongly to sexual perversion and suggestive gossip. Behind the mask of independent thought they delight in strictures on those high in the profession and even indulge in dirty innuendo. They start hot discussions on ethics and foment controversies over personal rights, privileges, and immunities. And this, God save the mark, is circulated as medical literature, because it is read by medical men.

Don't take a journal which is run as an advertising medium, and do not look at it if it is sent to you. Such publications are of two sorts. One kind is issued by some commercial gentleman to assist in selling his wares. In the guise of a scientific periodical, it is to all intents and purposes a sort of medical almanac, about as wholesome and edifying as the pamphlet for Bonesetter's bitters or the bulletin of Mother Udder's uterine uplifter. The other kind is conducted by a medical man with the dollar mark stamped on his aspirations. The good of the reader is no concern of his. He is after the money of advertisers, all of them. Original communications, editorials, excerpts, correspondence, everything, is arranged purely as a bait to induce the gullible to swallow the ads.

Don't read a journal that accepts abortive papers by undertone doctors. There are journals which systematically encourage that sort of thing. Unquestionably, to report cases and write down his opinions is good for any physician. But how about the reader? When the cases are incompletely studied, the writer ignorant or narrow, his conclusions lacking foundation, and his judgment immature, the contribution is not only valueless—it is injurious. Smooth is the descent that leads to Avernus, and easy the downward road of this damning third-rate literature. It is light and easy reading, but begets self-satisfaction, blunts the critical sense, lulls ambition, dulls observation, stunts mental growth, and before he knows it the reader is found on a low plane of thought and practice—no higher than the twaddle he reads.

Don't waste time on journals abounding in short cuts. They are an abomination unto the mind, a snare for the unwary, and their name is legion. A hint or two will indicate the sort I mean.

Purporting to be practical and immediately helpful, some journals make a specialty of what may be called recipes for disease. And they are very alluring. Instead of learning all about pneumonia, its nature, course, variations, and complications, what methods of treatment have been tried and abandoned and what has been the experience of those seeing hundreds of cases, it is so much easier to take some fellow's or some journal's statement that a peculiar poultice or ambitious alkaloid cures the disease. Stamped deep on my feelings is a paper on dyspepsia in a journal of great vogue. With no statement as to what dyspepsia may be, with no word as to diagnosis, with no allusion to pathology, no mention of gastroptosis, dilatation, hyperacidity, or motor power, and no hint of test meal or examination of stomach contents, the author proceeded to advise the administration of seven different drugs. In spite of the multifarious remedies, such advice simplifies practice to a degree. It is no task simply to remember to give this tonic for appetite, that capsule for digestion, this granule for pain, those drops for nausea, one pill for constipation, the other for diarrhœa, and the powder for flatulence. It is a short cut, but it leads to disaster.

In this same category belong the medical magazines that make a leader of questions and answers; a department modelled on the *Ladies' Fireside Guide,* where anxious inquiries go off at half-cock and the answers pop back as prompt and empty as echoes. A very little reflection will show not only the utter futility of this kind of reading, but how it prevents development by curtailing wholesome mental effort.

Then there is the petty journal corresponding to the family factotum above mentioned. Its short cut is simply the avoidance of the great and profound in medicine. Ignoring such fundamental things as anatomy, physiology, and pathology, oblivious alike to basic principles and the best of accumulated experience, it propagates a sort of family confab on the various superficialities of practice. How to bring out the eruption of measles; what is good for hiccough; the best liniment for sprains; these are cheerfully aired in numerous columns. What do you say to the parturient woman when she grows impatient? What is your favorite catarrh snuff? In the treatment of "threatened" appendicitis should aconite be given the first day and veratrum the second, or *vice versa?* On questions such as these, the editor and his writing readers expend great energy, priceless time, and endless ink. With great zest the contributors, as Charles Lamb says, encourage each other in mediocrity. I carefully went through one hundred and fifteen pages of such a penny-wise, pound-foolish publication, and found just six pages of good stuff. And yet·that journal has an enormous circulation—to the great renown of the publishers and the great discredit of the medical profession.

Don't pay much attention to columns of formulæ, notes on treatment, therapeutic hints, brief paragraphs on recent discoveries, and items on new drugs. Pass over abstracts in which the process of condensation has squeezed the life out of the matter, and skip society reports so meagre as to amount to mere personal mention.

Most of such matter is garbled at the best, has no educational value, and, even when a bit of it has virtue, is pretty sure to just slip through the otic tunnel—in one ear and out the other.

From the foregoing negatives a few positives may readily be inferred. As we are to buy only the best books, so let us take only high-class medical periodicals. And then let us read them well. If there are many poor journals, there is much poor reading done; reading that is casual, unsystematic, careless, superficial, cursory, profitless. We have three sources of information and inspiration, —personal experience, personal contact with colleagues, and reading. The first may be limited, the second unsatisfactory, but the last offers to all the highest inspiration, and knowledge without end. Then let us read up and not down.

There is a certain comfortable ease in reading what we already understand. We may gratify our natural craving for approval by revelling in nice little papers which repeat what we have been saying for years. To tickle our vanity by reading papers so poor that they show the author to be more ignorant than ourselves is a pleasing process. Sometimes we feel luxuriously virtuous when reading a medical journal purely for entertainment and mental relaxation. None of these things should be. One and all they create a slovenly habit of mind. They are destructive of good method, and in the end incapacitate us for good work.

Here I must notice an objection or complaint that we have all heard and most of us have made: "I have no time to read." It is not true. The apportionment of time is not a matter of necessity, but of choice. What do I consider of the greater importance? What do I like and dislike? What do I choose to do? These are the determining questions. And in the modern physician's life there is precious little paramount to study. It pays to read. Besides the pleasure of knowledge and the power that knowledge gives, besides the gratifying sense of achievement and the satisfaction of progress toward a goal, it pays in dollars. In conversation with the busiest, the greatest, and the most successful of our colleagues, I have often been astonished at the amount of reading they do and how they rely on it. Very, very often good reading makes the difference between five dollars and twenty-five dollars for an examination, between fifty dollars and five hundred dollars for an operation.

And now, if I may be allowed four little hints as to the manner of reading, I shall have finished.

One excellent way to use medical literature is systematically to get up one subject well; to investigate it thoroughly; to trace its history and follow its development; to scrutinize diverse observations, review conflicting opinions and weigh different conclusions. Having once mastered the thing, it will be surprisingly easy to follow it through the succeeding years, for the annual increment to any given subject in medicine is astonishingly small. After one topic is exhausted another may be attacked, and so onward.

This method easily falls in with a second good one, namely, to read up fully on cases in hand. Note that I say " fully." Hastily to look up an ointment for eczema or to consult a text-book or two on the diagnosis of iritis may be one of the exigencies of practice; it is not reading. Likewise hunting up a remedy for an obscure case may possibly be a necessary makeshift, but generally it does the patient little good and the physician less. We should read for a perfect understanding of the case, which means a complete comprehension of the subject. No case can properly be considered alone. It is always in relation to variant cases under diverse circumstances. For no patient can there be a paragraph explanation and no recipe treatment.

Now, these two plans of reading naturally lead up to a third— reading to write. Of course, this plan is good only when the writer compels himself to produce really good stuff. This proviso fulfilled, I know of nothing more wholesome than the writing of papers and the reading of them where others may pass judgment. If the first two plans have been well carried out, it is reasonably certain that this one will not miscarry. The man who has excellently well worked up any subject or any case of any abnormal condition, is not only well prepared for the next one of the kind, but he is in a position to tell others something they do not know.

Pursuance of these three plans of reading will almost inevitably produce a most desirable habit,—viz., the keeping of case records. The virtues of this practice are many. Two of them are that it stimulates reading and enhances its value. Accurate comparison of our experience with that of others not only serves to impress the facts, but ripens knowledge into wisdom.

The fourth and last suggestion for medical reading is really but a summary of the other three. It is that we acquire the mental attitude, or aptitude, or habit of reading for reproduction. To be a student is not enough. We must be effective students; student soldiers, if you please, preparing for action. There is a vast difference between the acquisition of knowledge as a mere accomplishment and as a means of accomplishment. It is well for us to regard our store of knowledge not as simply an interesting museum of Nature's wonders marvellous to contemplate, but rather as an armamentarium; an orderly array of goodly weapons ready for instant use.—*The Jour. Amer. Med. Assoc.*

PATHOGENY OF OSTEOMALACIA OR SENILE ATROPHY.[1] By Eugene S. Talbot, M.S., D.D.S., M.D., LL.D., Chicago.

The fact that pathology at most implies a disturbance of balance which causes a conflict of physiologic processes is nowhere more evident than in osteomalacia. The current error which assumes that any process aiding disease must be innately nosologic interferes with diagnosis and treatment alike. The clinical and pathologic work done on osteomalacia has been vitiated by the view-point just mentioned. Osteomalacia occurs from so many nosologic states as to indicate that it arises from a process physiologic in character, but perverted ·to nosologic ends by anything which disturbs the balance struggle for existence between the structures.

Bones do not grow in the ordinary sense, since the bone-cells can not multiply. Apparent growth of bone is caused by destruction of bone already formed and by production of new bone. The production of new bone is one, as Minot (Embryology) points out, first to degeneration of the ossifying cartilage. Cartilage begins to be differentiated earlier than any of the mesenchymal tissues except the blood-vessels, and perhaps the smooth muscle-cells. Cartilage undergoes a degenerative change preparatory to ossifying. This is one of the many instances in the embryo where degeneration of a particular structure is necessary for advance of the body as a whole. There are, as Minot points out, two stages in the life-history of cartilage. The first (in which the cells are large) is the earlier stage, and represents the maximum of development, while the second (in which the cells are shrunken and fatty) represents a

---

[1] In " Interstitial Gingivitis, or So-called Pyorrhœa Alveolaris," I called attention to a form of bone absorption,—osteomalacia or senile absorption. Very little was said at the time, for the reason I wished to do more research work before bringing the subject before the profession. That paper was read before the Chicago Academy of Medicine, December 12, 1899.

later stage with more or less degeneration. In what is called ossification of cartilage (an erroneous term) the cartilage undergoes complete degeneration and disappears. Bone is derived always by direct metamorphosis of embryonic connective tissue or of embryonic cartilage and of periosteum. Bony tissue, as already remarked, does not grow except by additions to its surface. To a certain extent it depends on a balance between the metamorphosis of embryonic connective tissue, the formation of cartilage, and the function of the osteoblasts, which build up, and the osteoclasts, which break down.

These four conditions occur in fracture. The tissue around and between the bone ends is provisional callus. The periosteum forms the external callus and medullary tissue the internal callus. Ossification of internal callus is performed by the osteoblasts, which develop, and osteoid tissue, that later by calcic deposits undergoes a change into true bone. This bone formation is often preceded by tissue of the embryonic connective type. The osteoclasts absorb bony substances in excess. Imperfect work by the osteoblast or excessive formation would reproduce in a fracture the condition of tissue which occurs in osteomalacia. Osteomalacia hence depends on the removal of inhibitions on the physiologic balance between formative and destructive functions.

Inhibitions are exercised through the nervous system. It is not surprising, therefore, to find fully developed osteomalacia connected by many links with trophoneuroses, in which similar local bone changes occur. Prominent among these are paretic dementia and locomotor ataxia. Various changes of the bones and joints, as J. G. Kiernan [1] has pointed out, occur in paretic dementia, either in the direction of osteomalacia, of premature and excessive ossification, or hydroarticuli (thickening of the articular extremities of the long bones). Similar conditions were found previously by Charcot, Ball, and J. K. Mitchell in locomotor ataxia.

In other conditions, where like though lesser disturbances of the physiologic balance of the struggle for assimilable nutriment occur, osteomalacia and its converse likewise develop. In pregnancy such conditions are present. So far as the woman is concerned, pregnancy, as Harriet Alexander [2] has shown, is a patho-

---

[1] Journal of Nervous and Mental Diseases, 1878, p. 253.
[2] Pediatrics, January, 1901.

logic disturbance of balance hitherto existing in the organism. In consequence, nutrition and assimilation are increased, while elimination is decreased. In pregnancy, therefore, occurs an autointoxication which may express itself in major phenomena like eclampsia, or minor phenomena like the destruction of the teeth. From the influence of this last type exercised on bone growth occur not only trophic disturbances, like osteomalacia, but also, as Rokitansky[1] long ago demonstrated, osteophytes (of the cranial bones in particular). This condition, as Ducrest has shown, appears and disappears under pregnancy. While Hohl and Virchow have claimed that this condition bears merely a coincidental relation to pregnancy, corroboration of its frequency by French, German, and Italian pathologists demolishes this criticism.

Osteomalacia (the halisteresis ossium of Kilian) consists anatomically of an osteitis and periosteitis, in which the perfectly hard bones are decalcified and replaced at first by lamellar connective tissue; finally this passes centrally into the round granular medullary cell. The medullary spaces and Haversian canals increase in size; the bone corpuscles partly disappear, but in part become shorter and their processes smaller. The more complete the substitution of connective tissue the more flexible the bones become. In osteomalacia corea they are, as Winckel[2] remarks, almost as yielding as wax and not soft enough to be cut. In fully developed osteomalacia, therefore, the cartilage formation has been replaced by connective tissue.

Winckel has shown that the conditions under which puerperal osteomalacia develops are essentially those causing degeneration. By improvement of hygienic surroundings of Bavarian peasant women, his father was able to lessen the amount of osteomalacia. It does not, therefore, form a single nosologic species. It is clearly connected with the trophic factors regulating bone growth, bone repair, and bone existence. In its essence it is, like cancer, a reversion to embryonic conditions. While to some extent lower, the conditions found in osteomalacia are essentially those of the immature sea-squirt in its prevertebrate period. It is a general law of biology that structures in certain parts of an organism retain for the benefit of that organism lower characteristics. This being the case, there

[1] Thèse de Paris, No. 1, 1844.
[2] Text-Book of Obstetrics (American edition), p. 472.

should be one structure in the body which would give a clew to the etiology and early pathology of osteomalacia. Such a structure is the alveolar process. This is situated on the superior border of the inferior maxilla and on the inferior border of the superior maxilla. While usually considered a part of the maxillary bones, the alveolar process should be considered separately. Its structure, embryology and functions differ completely from the structure and functions of the maxillary bone. The alveolar process is composed of soft, spongy bone of a relatively cancellous structure. As early as the eleventh week of intrauterine life calcification of the deciduous teeth commences, and by the twelfth week calcic material is quite abundantly deposited. The alveolar process, being soft and spongy, moulds itself about the sacs containing the crowns of the teeth and along their roots after their eruption, regardless of position in the jaw. While the alveolar process has grown rapidly, it has developed up to this time just enough to cover and protect the follicles while calcification of the jaw proceeds. When the crowns have become calcified and the roots have begun to take in calcic material, absorption of the border of the process takes place in the order of eruption of the teeth. When the teeth have erupted, the alveolar process develops downward and upward with the teeth until it attains the depth of the roots which, in most instances, extend into the superior maxillary bones in the anterior part of the mouth, and the upper and lower teeth rest at a point in harmony with the rami. The depth to which they penetrate depends on the length of the roots and the alveolar process, and this in turn depends on the length of the rami. The incisive fossa, the cuspid eminence and fossa give evidence of this externally. The sockets are lined with extensions of the process, thus making its upper border irregular.

When the temporary teeth are shed, the alveolar process is absorbed to make room for the eruption of the permanent set. The crowns of these, being larger than those of the temporary teeth, require more space and the process must enlarge to accommodate them. It then is rebuilt about the roots of the teeth on a much larger scale. When the temporary teeth are lost the alveolar process is reabsorbed. It is hence developed twice and absorbed thrice, provided the second set of teeth is lost. The process is a very thin, unstable structure, naturally well nourished with blood-vessels. As the skull and brain are gaining in the struggle for existence between the face, jaws, skull, and brain, the jaws with the alveolar process must decrease in size with advance. This fact and the changes just described render the process a doubly transitory structure. For this reason it is very susceptible to metabolic changes, to mineral and vegetable drugs and poisons, as well as to changes in temperature and climate. This is, in part, due to the readiness with which checked elimination elsewhere finds exit through the mouth and nose. The great supply of blood-vessels in the alveolar process plays a part in determining elimination.

Should man live long enough, and should the physiologic process of involution set in, his second set of teeth would disappear as a consequence of osteomalacia of the senile atrophy type. The lower vertebrates are called *Polyphyodontia,* because there is a continuous succession of teeth, not a separation into two sets. In some mammals this condition persists. The pachyderms and rodents (which are connected embryologically) present phenomena analogous to that of the *Polyphyodontia.* In the rodents, especially the nut-eating rodents, continuous growth occurs in the incisors as they are worn down. Should one of the incisors disappear, the opposing one so grows as to interfere with the gnawing powers. Many a squirrel has thereby lost its life. In the elephant not more than three teeth are in use at a time. Those worn down are shed, while new teeth are added.[1] Thus the whole number of teeth are not in place at one time. In other pachyderms, like the hyrax, similar conditions are found. Among the edentates, tooth conditions form a natural transition to the *Sauropsidæ* and *Icthyopsidæ.* A curious link also occurs in the *Monotremata,* where the duck-bill has deciduous teeth during youth, which are afterwards absorbed to make way for horny plates. Judging from the conditions found in the toothed birds, the same result occurred at a phase in evolution of toothed birds from reptiles. In man, however, this degenerative process (involving absorption of the alveolar process and loss of the teeth) is continuously present in a latent way. The alveolar process is, therefore, more subject to change from altered metabolism, due to trophic disorders of nutrition than other structures. Osteomalacia or senile absorption occurs with greater rapidity, and produces more decided change in the alveolar process than in other bones. Causes which would not affect bone structure elsewhere markedly derange it.

---

[1] Tomes's Dental Anatomy, p. 405.

While osteomalacia may affect the alveolar process at any period of life after the eruption of the first set of teeth, it does not usually occur until the period between twenty-five and thirty-five. Before this the osseous system is in its constructive state and lime salts are being deposited rapidly. Later in life the constructive stage is complete, and material sufficient only to repair waste is deposited. At the periods of stress metabolic changes are most active,—during puberty and adolescence (fourteen to twenty-five), during the climacteric (forty to sixty), when uterine involution occurs in women and prostatic involution in men, and, finally, during senility (from sixty upward), when the disease is always present to a greater or less degree. While in allied conditions men are most influenced in this disorder, the sexes seem to be affected about equally. Here the influence of pregnancy comes into play. Pregnancy disturbs the physiologic balance hitherto existing, especially along the line of assimilation and elimination. The well-known dental efforts of pregnancy (whose underlying cause affects the alveolar process) are due to this factor. This is purely a constitutional affection.

Among the causes are non-elimination of toxic substances, whether due to autointoxication, to bacterial action, or to metallic and vegetable drugs. Disorder or disease of any excretory organ (kidneys, bowels, skin, or lungs) will produce the most marked effect, first, on the constitution of the blood, and secondly, on the alveolar process, with resultant osteomalacia.

The urine, as Bouchard has shown, contains each day in a normal individual sufficient toxins to cause death if not excreted. This condition is markedly increased after prolonged nervous explosions, like those of epilepsy or hysteria. This was pointed out thirty years ago by Meynert, who demonstrated that the status epilepticus (condition of rapidly recurring convulsions) was due to the accumulations of a proteid body in the system. The status epilepticus is preceded by a decrease in toxins in the urine and succeeded by an increase. This is likewise true as to the influence of non-elimination by the other excretory organs (bowels, lungs, and oral cavity), as well as to the non-exercise of its poison-destroying power by the liver. Non-elimination, moreover, interferes with ordinary digestive functions, and hence increases its own extent. Another factor in autointoxication is production of toxic products in such quantity as to prevent destruction by organs like the liver and consequent elimination, since a product to be properly eliminated must be changed to a particular chemical type. Among the factors which affect both these elements of elimination is the power over growth and repair exercised by the nervous system. In part, this influence is exerted through control of blood-supply by the vasomotor nervous system and in part by that direct control of the nervous system over tissue change, which is known as its trophic function.

Both influences are affected by nervous strain. Sudden emotion may, as Bichat demonstrated decades ago, produce marked defects on bile secretion and may occasion jaundice. Cases are far from infrequent in which emotions like jealousy produce a mimicry of gall-stone colic in neuropaths. Murchison, Christison, and Thompson have traced attacks of biliary colic to jealousy. Other liver changes from sudden nervous disturbance, whether of mental type or not, are not rare. As mental impressions are communicated to the central nervous system purely through mechanical changes in the nerves, such influence must be purely material in operation. As the brain exercises a checking influence on the operations of the liver, these mental influences produce two effects. The mental shock increases the checking action of the central nervous system on the local ganglia of the liver and destroys the checking action of the liver ganglia, and in consequence these go too fast, resulting in their exhaustion. Either of these conditions interferes with the poison-destroying action of the liver, and accumulation of waste products is the result.

What is true of the liver is true of the other organs. This is especially noticeable, as Tuke points out, in regard to the kidneys. The action of mental anxiety or suspense in causing a copious discharge of the pale fluid is familiar enough to all, especially to the medical student about to present himself for examination, the amount being in a pretty direct ratio to his fear of being plucked. The frequency of micturition may, however, arise from nervous irritability of the bladder without increase or even with diminished secretion. Still, the action of the skin is usually checked, the extremities are cold, and the kidneys have to pump off the extra amount of fluid retained in the circulation. Elimination of the substance usually separated from the blood is diminished, as compared with the aqueous character of the whole secretion. The odor may be affected by the emotions in man as in animals. Prout is of the opinion that mental anxiety will produce not only non-elimination, but also change in the chemical character, as indicated by odor and otherwise. Disturbances in the medulla produce, as Claude Bernard long ago showed, a markedly pale, excessive urine. These disturbances often arise from intellectual strain or emotional shock. The influence of emotional states on secreting processes and thereby indirectly on autointoxication states, is illustrated in the fact long ago pointed out by Tuke that pleasurable emotions increase the amount of gastric juices secreted, the opposite effect being produced by depressing passions. Beaumont found in a case of gastric fistula that anger or other severe emotions caused the gastric inner or mucous coat to become morbidly red, dry, and irritable, occasioning at the same time a temporary fit of indigestion.

The influence of fear and anxiety on the bowels is as well marked as that on the bladder and kidneys. Apart from muscular action, defecation may become urgent or occur involuntarily from various causes. The increased secretion from the intestinal canal may occur from fear, and in some cases from the altered character of the secretion itself. While in this respect the influence of fear may be inconvenient in man, it naturally assists escape in some animals, as the skunk.

Emotions powerfully excite, modify, or altogether suspend, as Tuke has shown, the organic functions. This influence is transmitted not only through the vasomotor nerves, but through nerves in close relation to nutrition and secretion. When the excitement is of peripheral origin in sensory or afferent nerves, it excites their function by reflex action, so that as emotion arises it may excite the central nuclei of such afferent nerves, and this stimulus be reflected on the efferent nerves, or it may act directly through the latter. Pleasurable emotions tend to excite the processes of nutrition, hence the excitement of certain feelings may, if definitely directed, restore healthy action to an affected part. Violent emotions modify nutrition. Various forms of disease originating in perverted or defective nutrition may be caused primarily by emotional disturbance. Emotions by causing a larger amount of blood to be transmitted to a gland increase sensibility and warmth, and stimulate its function or directly excite the process by their influence on nerves supplying the glands. Painful emotions may modify the quality (*i.e.*, the relative proportion of the constituents) of the secretions.

Imperfect elimination of effete matter from the lungs is a fruitful source of autointoxication. The more marked forms are those of tuberculosis, in which there is great debility and in which there is greater waste than repair. Self-poisoning is continually going on, and will continue until death. The chest capacity for the inhalation of pure air is almost *nil*, hence the blood is improperly oxygenated and soon ceases to convey nutriment to the tissues. Eighty per cent. of criminals who die of tuberculosis in prisons have undeveloped chest walls. Degeneracy, therefore, cuts quite a figure in the rôle of autointoxication. Degenerates with contracted chest walls are, however, more frequently found. Many undeveloped individuals in every walk of life for this reason have tuberculosis. People with undeveloped chest walls and chest capacity may not have tuberculosis and yet may suffer from autointoxication. Those who have had pneumonia with adhesion, and who are thus unable to oxygenate the blood, are subject to this disease. Asthmatics and hay-fever patients suffer from autointoxication and alveolar absorption. When the skin is overstrained as to excretion through the kidney and bowel overstrain, the lungs are forced to take on increased work with imperfect oxygenation as a result. This is noticed in the odor of the breath in Bright's disease and in the air-hunger of diabetes, etc. In nerve-strain states and in the condition described by Albu, not only do excretory organs suffer, but the secretions of those glands, like salivary and buccal glands, are so altered as to become irritants. These excretory conditions not only result on autointoxication states, but are modified by trophic nerve function alterations. By trophic changes are meant such tissue alterations as occur in morbid conditions from disordered function of the centres of nutrition. Peripheral as well as central may be involved. The well-known law of Wallerian degeneration of nerve-fibres is an illustration, the posterior spinal ganglion acting as a trophic centre for the fibres of the posterior root in the cord itself. Trophic action may, therefore, be peripheral, though in extensive changes, as a rule, central (cerebral or spinal) origin should be looked for.

The constitutional result of acute and chronic infections and contagions is apt to be an autointoxication plus the action of the germ toxin. All the exanthemata have at times been followed by wasting or necrosis of the alveolus. Here the condition is notably symmetric, and accompanied by disorders of the osseous system elsewhere. The same is true of la grippe and tuberculosis. The well-marked disorder known as Riggs's disease has been charged by Peirce, Kirk, Rhein, Robin, and Magitot to the direct influence of an arthritic state (gouty and rheumatic), and regarded as a special type of arthritic manifestation. The alveolus is clearly vulnerable to the toxins of many infections. It is likewise quickly affected by some autotoxic influences from disordered metabolism. Its vital resistance to these agencies is less than of other tissues. It is the earliest sacrifice when these or any toxins disturb the harmony of the organism.

A cause other than the action of toxins exists for implication of these parts. Whenever tissue waste, whether local or general, exceeds repair there is trophic change. This latter depends directly on disordered local or general nervous functions. Trophic alterations from the first cause appear in growth disorders of the nails and loss of hair (alopecia) after fevers, the most familiarly obvious examples of this pathologic process. Of the other type are localized atrophies, where the direct intervention of toxins can be excluded. The alveolus is liable to the first form of trophic deterioration. The influence of acute diseases on the alveolus is probably thus exerted in many cases rather than by direct infection. Where no cause has been ascertained, examination directed to this factor would probably reveal it. The general failure of the trophic centres after the prime of life (in senile states), which is attended with loss of teeth and wasting of the alveoli, is the most obvious instance of trophic failure affecting the part. Even simple anæmia may thus give rise to alveolar wasting.

The more marked forms of constitutional disorders (typhoid fever, pneumonia, tuberculosis, syphilis, indigestion, pregnancy, etc.) produce intense results.

The second form of trophic failure in the alveolus is less prominent, since it generally coexists with overshadowing disturbance elsewhere, which it creates to a certain extent. Cruveiller noticed its occurrence associated with simple paraplegia, regarding it as of nervous causation. In facial hemiatrophy, local wasting of the alveolus has appeared before the disorder has involved the jaws generally. This is sometimes due to a local cause, but its occurrence and association with other neurotrophic symptoms are suggestive.

The causes which act locally to produce direct autointoxication are the toxic effects of mercury, lead, brass, uric and other acids, potassium iodide, and allied agencies, acting in a similar manner to scurvy. While it is not the intention to discuss at length the toxic action of these substances, a case may be cited in illustration of their similarity of action and results on the tissue. Garnier and

Simon have observed the case of a boy suffering from an obstinate enteritis. Milk was found to disagree, so a purée of vegetables and chopped meat was given. The boy improved for a while, but hæmatogenous jaundice occurred. On investigation the jaundice was found to be due to the action of lead on the liver, the lead having been introduced into the food through a meat-chopper. In this case, the usual symptoms of lead poisoning were absent, but through its action on the liver jaundice had appeared. Scurvy produces the same train of symptoms as the metals, through its disturbance of the metabolism.

The jaws of the hereditarily defective, whether defect be in the direction of advance or degeneracy, are fruitful soil for the development of osteomalacia. In the mouths of the congenital, deaf, dumb, blind, feeble-minded, and delinquent children, osteomalacia attacks the alveolar process before the osseous system has reached its growth. Here, as a consequence of trophic change, metabolic action and premature senility, osteomalacia may occur with the first set of teeth at two years, or at any period thereafter. This may be called juvenile osteomalacia. Regulating teeth and senile absorption are predisposing causes to osteomalacia.

Osteomalacia of the alveolar process is almost as common among domestic and wild animals in captivity as it is in man. Wild animals in zoologic gardens without proper exercise, in close confinement, with impure air, and fed on too easily digested food, naturally acquire autointoxication resulting in osteomalacia. This is particularly noticeable in monkeys, whose changes of environment render them very susceptible to disease, especially tuberculosis. Trophic changes and impaired metabolism are thereby so impressed on monkeys that not infrequently the first teeth become prematurely loose and drop out. The horse and cow are prone to this disease. Cattle returned to the stable after a summer's sojourn in the field, and then being fed on a changed diet without the usual exercise of cutting grass with their teeth, undergo a reaction in their jaws, and osteomalacia results. " Cribbing" of the horse is a marked illustration of the uneasy feeling resultant on this reaction. Cattle fed on brewers' grain and slop suffer most. Dogs afford the best opportunity, however, for studying inflammation and osteomalacia among animals. Nearly every dog in the dog hospital suffers with this disease; twenty-five per cent. of roving curs at four years of age have the disease; eighty per cent. of eight-year-old, at least ninety-five per cent. of twelve-year-old, and all fourteen-year-old dogs have the disease. House dogs suffer to a marked extent with osteoma-

FIG. 1.

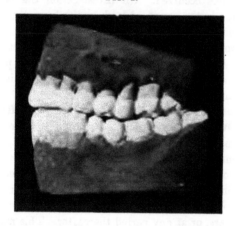

lacia of the alveolar process, no doubt from being trained to house cleanliness, which interferes with natural excretion, causing auto-intoxication and odor.

FIG. 2.

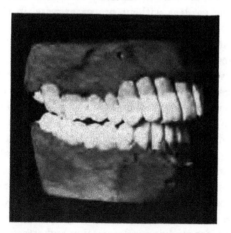

The following models show the action of osteomalacia on the jaws and teeth: Fig. 1 is that of a physician thirty-six years of age. Fig. 2 is that of a physician thirty-eight years of age. Both of these gentlemen are apparently in the best of health. One has slight indigestion, which is the cause of absorption; the other took calomel for malaria fifteen years previous, this being a predisposing cause. In each case all the teeth are involved both inside and out. Some of the teeth are becoming loose. There is no pus in either case. The gums are apparently healthy.

Fig. 3.

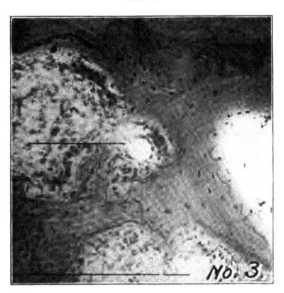

In consulting the literature on the subject, I find that absorption of the alveolar process and recession of the gums have always been attributed to the severe use of the tooth-brush. There are certain conditions in which the tooth-brush will assist absorption of the alveolar process. These are easily observed. I refer to the position of the cuspid teeth, where they stand prominently and are the most conspicuous part of the alveolar process. The bone over the roots is as thin as tissue-paper, and the slightest friction causes a low form of inflammation, which in turn produces absorption of the bone, exposing the root. The brush never, however, produces senile atrophy in other parts of the mouth.

The absorption of the alveolar process in osteomalacia is not always uniform, as sometimes only one or two teeth are involved.

Local conditions modify the extent of the disease. In most cases, however, there is a gradual absorption of bone about all the teeth.

The pathology of this disease about the teeth is not unlike that of osteomalacia of the pelvis, spine, and other bones of the body, as demonstrated by Hektoen, halisteresis being the principal form of absorption. Perforating canal absorption, as described by Volkmann, is very common, passing through fragments of bone. Lacunar absorption is also present, and osteoclasts are frequently found. Howship's lacunæ, containing osteoclasts, are found in the margin of irregular islands of bone. This form of absorption,

FIG. 4.

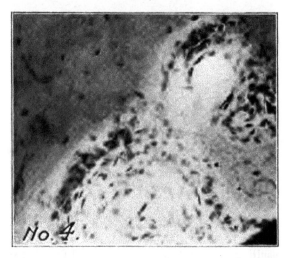

while not always present, does not cut so much figure as halisteresis, it being much slower in its action. New osteoid tissue is rarely ever seen, since this absorption is a natural destruction of bone and is never reproduced.

Here, then, is the basic explanation of interstitial gingivitis or so-called pyorrhœa alveolaris—osteomalacia or senile absorption is the underlying basis of this disease.

The preceding illustrations represent the alveolar process of a man forty-eight years of age, killed in an accident. The teeth and bone decalcified in the usual way were prepared for the microscope. Fig. 3 shows four areas of bone absorption called halisteresis (melting away of bone substance). The waste products become irritants in the blood-stream, and set up a low form of inflammation in the Haversian canals. The inflammation thus set up produces rapid absorption. Each of these local areas enlarges until they join. In this way large areas are produced. In the centre of this illustration is seen an Haversian canal with active inflammation around it. The bone is absorbed. The inflammatory process is in the trabeculæ or fibrous part of the bone. Adjoining is a large area with bone absorption, but the fibrous part of bone remains unbroken. The inflammatory process is seen throughout. At the lower border of the picture are two large areas of bone absorption. The trabeculæ

FIG. 5.

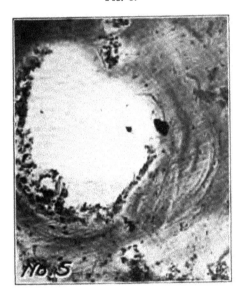

are seen, with round-celled infiltration, while the centre is destroyed. At the right absorption and destruction of the trabeculæ are seen to the margin of the bone.

Fig. 4 shows halisteresis at two Haversian canals. One area is much larger than the other. Both have met, and the area of inflammation will be much enlarged. The trabeculæ are present and filled with round-celled infiltration.

Fig. 5 illustrates a large area of absorption with destruction of the fibrous tissue to a larger extent. Around the border is seen a small amount of inflamed fibrous tissue. An artery, once an

Fig. 6.

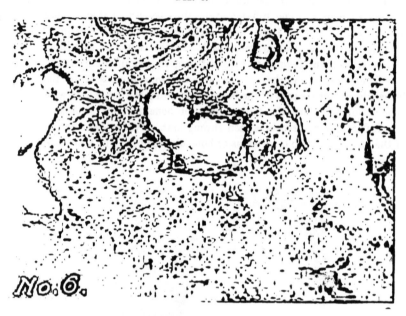

Fig. 7.

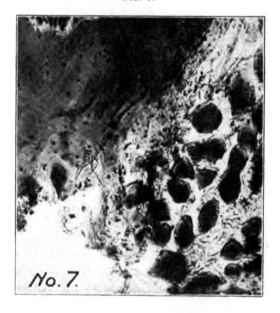

Haversian canal, is also seen. About the large area are also seen three Haversian canals with the inflammatory process just beginning.

Fig. 6 shows four centres of absorption at Haversian canals. Through the picture may be seen dark lines running in all directions. These are vessels of Von Ebner, through which Volkmann's canal absorption takes place. A beautiful illustration of this is the canal running from one large area of absorption to the other.

Fig. 7 shows the third form of bone absorption,—lacunæ or osteoclast absorption. Here a large area of bone is destroyed by these large cells.

Fig. 8 is a low power, showing the distribution of the alveolar

FIG. 8.

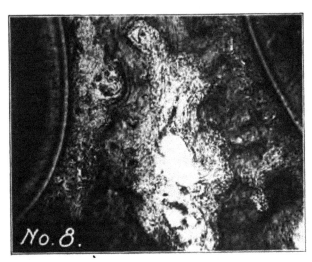

process between the roots of two teeth. Very little of the bone remains. When the trabeculæ or fibrous tissue is destroyed in large areas, and especially in transitory structures, it is rarely restored.

Does it not seem reasonable, therefore, that the etiology of osteomalacia of the pelvis and other bones of the body is the same as that of the alveolar process, since the pathology is the same, namely, faulty metabolism and elimination, autointoxication, and drug poisoning?

A relationship exists between Dercum's disease (adiposis dolorosa) and osteomalacia, according to Pennato,[1] who finds several cases on record in which changes in joints occurred. Bone nutrition is regulated by the trophic centres markedly affected in Dercum's disease. A case of a thirty-five-year-old woman, observed by Pennato, was that whose first adiposis appeared at twenty-three. She slowly developed adiposis dolorosa and lost her teeth, except the inferior cuspids and one molar, although caries did not occur. Symptoms referable to the bones appeared almost at the outset, consisting of distortion of the right knee, curvature of the leg, some years later fracture of a clavicle, and still later of the left humerus. When Pennato saw the case the legs and thighs were semiflexed. Complete extension was impossible on the right side, on account of rigidity in the knee, with partial dislocation of the tibia inward. Such cases bear out the position that autointoxication is the initial cause of osteomalacia, since in obesity or lipomatosis the products of autointoxication are always present in the alveolar process, and since Dercum's disease is an exaggeration of the nutritive degeneracy which tends to appear at the second dentition.[2]

RÉSUMÉ.

1. Osteomalacia may and does exist for years in pelvic and other bones before the symptoms can possibly be recognized by the physician or surgeon.

2. The object of this paper is to show that osteomalacia can be studied earliest in the alveolar process.

3. The alveolar process is the most transitory structure in the body. It develops twice, and is absorbed thrice if the second set of teeth are shed. The evolution of the face, whereby the jaws are decreasing in size, with the many complications thereon resultant, renders the jaws and alveolar process increasingly transitory.

4. In the evolution from the lowest vertebrates up there has been a continuous succession of teeth (polyphyodont), as found in some selachians; a partial continuous succession, as in some mammals; and a comparatively permanent set of teeth, as in man. This shedding of teeth, due to a process called senile absorption, atavistic in type, takes place in every one to a greater or less extent

---

[1] Medical Bulletin, April, 1904.
[2] Kiernan, Alienist and Neurologist, 1900.

after forty-five years of age. Should man live in a comparatively healthy state long enough he would lose all teeth from this process.

5. Degenerate children from precocity, due to arrested development at the senile or simian period of intrauterine life, may show symptoms of this disease in connection with the first set of teeth at from six to ten years of age. A monkey which died of tuberculosis at one year had osteomalacia, which exposed the roots of all the temporary teeth, while three had dropped out.

6. Constitutional causes like autointoxication and drug poisoning are the etiologic factors. Even the mildest types of autointoxication, due to indigestion, change in climate from hot to cold, and *vice versa,* with corresponding change in food, giving more work to some eliminating organs and less to others, as well as to mild forms of drug poisoning, may be potent in this particular.

7. The effect of autointoxication and drug poisoning is first irritation through blood-streams, often causing endarteritis obliterans. Since the arteries are terminal, irritation readily causes inflammation and halisteresis.

8. Osteomalacia is as common among wild animals in captivity as in domestic animals.

9. The influence of bacteria as a cause has not been demonstrated by Koch's law.

10. If due to autointoxication, the effete matter should be removed from the system.

11. Osteomalacia or senile atrophy is the basic explanation of interstitial gingivitis, or so-called pyorrhœa alveolaris. Will not the same line of reasoning hold true of osteomalacia of the bones of other parts of the body?

Reports of Society Meetings.

THE NEW YORK INSTITUTE OF STOMATOLOGY.

A MEETING of the Institute was held at the "Chelsea," No. 222 West Twenty-third Street, New York, on Tuesday evening October 4, 1904, the President, Dr. Brockway, in the chair.

The minutes of the last meeting were read and approved.

The President then introduced the essayist of the evening, Dr.
N. S. Jenkins, of Dresden, Germany, who read a paper on " A
New Porcelain for Prosthetic Purposes."

(For Dr. Jenkins's paper, see page 22.)

DISCUSSION.

Dr. F. T. Van Woert.—It would be hard to express gratitude
at being present this evening and at the demonstration this afternoon. I personally feel under a deep obligation to Dr. Jenkins for
his work in this line.

In the early days I was very sceptical as to the practical value
of porcelain as a filling-material, and to the present just as sceptical regarding porcelain for bridge-work. But after seeing the
demonstration this afternoon I am convinced that I shall have to
take the matter up, as there seems a bright prospect for its success.

In the past I have considered porcelain bridges impracticable,
on account of the ease with which they are broken. Dr. Jenkins
assures me that with his new porcelain there is no such danger.
This being so, it eliminates one of the most serious objections. I
have thought of late that they might be practicable if set with the
Evans cement, which I have found most admirable, in gold bridge
cases.

In cases of a break-down, with this cement the bridge can be
easily removed, and this, in consideration with Dr. Jenkins's new
product, may make porcelain bridges practical.

I cannot see wherein there is very much to say except in commendation of Dr. Jenkins's work. I do not see any chance for a
discussion, and I cannot find any fault.

The inlay material introduced by Dr. Jenkins is a very excellent
one for adapting crowns to the roots. It will stand grinding and
polishing and leave as smooth a surface as when first fused.

Dr. C. F. Allan.—Dr. Jenkins, with his years of laboratory
experiments. pursued with the most patient care and at great personal sacrifice, is an apt illustration of the idea expressed so well
in his paper, that " dentists themselves are the best judges of dentists' needs." The first sugestion of inlay material came to the
essayist doubtless from his desire to do away with the unsightly
display of gold in the mouth, his needs at first being only in the
line of æsthetics and the imitation of nature; but he has builded
so well that besides accomplishing this great purpose he has given

us a material of the very first quality from the point of view of tooth preservation, and especially is it useful for those cases of large proximal and occluso fillings in the back teeth where much contouring is necessary and which could only be done in an inferior manner with gold at an enormous expenditure of time and labor on the part of the dentist and great suffering and nervous strain to the patient. Now, Dr. Jenkins has supplemented this great boon by adding this new material, of which he speaks to-day. He tells us that it is much stronger than the porcelain teeth we use, and will bear a heavier strain than the porcelain bodies.

The flowing of the material as demonstrated this afternoon is all that could be desired; it flows easily, stays put as you want it, and is tough and homogeneous.

It has been the opprobrium of our profession, especially in this country, that we have not imitated nature. All praise now to Dr. Jenkins, who has given us the means for holding the mirror up to nature; and the opprobrium in the future will be the greater if we do not take advantage of such means.

Dr. H. L. Wheeler.—It has given me much pleasure to listen to Dr. Jenkins this evening, and I think he deserves credit for so persistently advocating the æsthetic in dentistry. His constant endeavors can hardly fail to have a beneficial effect in persuading members of our profession to try to imitate nature more closely, and so minister to the beautiful; and as a man I admire him.

Upon reading this paper over several times, in the hope of finding some scientific statement that would admit of discussion, I have been unable to do so. In the first place this is an unsupported statement of an interested party and owner of a secret formula advocating this article as superior to everything else just as every man has done since commerce began. Under the circumstances it is difficult to discuss this paper as scientific papers usually are discussed. But there are some statements in this plea for the use of prosthetic porcelain to which I wish to call attention. For instance, in the statement that "materials employed in making dental porcelain have hitherto been worked somewhat crudely," I suppose he means porcelain used for dental purposes. There might be some difference of opinion concerning this if some of the other manufacturers were heard from. It is doubtful in my mind if prosthetic porcelain, so called, is a porcelain at all. I submitted a sample of porcelain enamel, which fuses at about 200° F. below prosthetic enamel, to one of our most distinguished and possibly the greatest authority on porcelain in this country, and he pronounced it glass. I have tried strenuously to get samples of this material of Dr. Jenkins's to experiment with, but find it is not obtainable. Its fusing-point, 1075° C., which, converted into Fahrenheit according to the essayist's statement, is from 1678° to 1768°, which is nearly or quite 200° below the lowest of the highest fusing bodies, would indicate that the fusing-point of the silicates had been considerably lowered by the addition of artificial means, or the doctor is using a silicate, that is, a feldspar containing an excessive amount of potash or soda, or some other alkaline material to lower the fusing-point, or he could, by breaking up and finely pulverizing and rebaking a number of times, secure similar results. In either case the results would not vary greatly. It is not impossible that his statement of its great strength is erroneous, for I am informed by men of ability, whose work is what might be called mineralogical chemistry, that either of the above-mentioned processes decreases the strength of the material. The statement that it can be used safely at a thickness of three millimetres, which, transposed, is about one-eighth of an inch, does not indicate that it has great strength. The inner cusps of bicuspid or artificial teeth are ground much thinner than this and last for years.

As to the question of the gold volatilizing, it is a matter of indifference if it does. I have put pieces of platinum together, using pure gold as a solder and run the heat up to 2600° F. The gold has apparently disappeared, but the pieces of platinum were held together as though they were one piece. The statement that the fusing-point of gold is 1075° C. (1903° F.) is, according to such authorities as I have been able to find, 113° out of the way. They give the fusing-point of pure gold as about 2016° F. Now, our essayist may make mistakes, as this shows, and it would not be the first time a good man had been in error, and it seems to me that it might be well to be cautious in the use of this material, at least until it shall have time to prove its merits, if it have any.

That the material may prove to be useful does not in my estimation warrant its unlimited use until its lasting qualities are better known. Although proprietary compounds may be very useful and of great benefit, the burden of proof is upon those who advocate their use. In regard to iridio-platinum for full upper plates, I have known of this being used in artificial dentures, and although there is great difficulty in swaging it, it can be used successfully where a vulcanite attachment is used. But as for heating it, in order to solder artificial teeth to it, the evidence thus far seems to be that it will spring badly and ruin the fit; hence I doubt its practicability.

Dr. Houghten.—I would like to ask Dr. Jenkins what the percentage of shrinkage of his porcelain is?

Dr. Jenkins.—Every porcelain has a certain amount of shrinkage if it is really fused. You can take some so-called porcelains and subject them to a very high degree of heat without fusing them; indeed, there are so-called porcelains that no amount of heat will thoroughly fuse. It is always a question of the way in which the materials have been treated. In order to have a porcelain adapted for practical use, it must fuse to a very great extent, and such a porcelain will shrink. The percentage of shrinkage of this porcelain is very similar to that of the inlay porcelain or of any porcelain that is thoroughly fused. However, this is a thing that is of no great consequence in the practical working of the porcelain. Shrinkage is so uniform in any one grade of work in ceramics that no very great attention is paid to it after the first experiments with any particular body are made. It makes some difference as to how moist the piece is. In this material I am presenting to you the degree of shrinkage has never been measured. It is not really a practical question.

Dr. George S. Allan.—I should like to hear a little more definitely from Dr. Jenkins in regard to this iridio-platinum that was negatived by Dr. Wheeler. Dr. Jenkins says that iridio-platinum with ten per cent. iridium, is essential in work with this prosthetic porcelain. As I understand it, he has had two years' actual practice with this metal. The more or less constant use of a material is pretty conclusive as to its merits. When Dr. Jenkins first made the statement to me that he used platinum with such a high percentage of iridium in alloy, the question naturally came to my mind as to how this could be swaged. Dr. Jenkins tells me that it is not so difficult a matter. He uses Melotte's metal dyes. He did not allude to this springing quality mentioned by Dr. Wheeler. All of those present at the demonstration at my office were highly delighted with the simple and easy way in which this porcelain could be manipulated. I know very little about ceramics, and so do not pretend to criticise, but I look upon Dr. Jenkins's

3

two years' use of this material in combination with the platino-iridium base as practically settling the question of its usefulness.

Dr. Gaylord.—I simply wish to add my personal experience with this prosthetic porcelain to what has already been said in favor of it. It is one thing to listen to remarks upon a subject, and another to experiment with your own hands. If any of you will procure some of this material and try it in your own laboratory, you will realize to your own satisfaction its great strength and its perfect adaptation to whatever it comes in contact with. The matter of shrinkage seems to me to be of very little concern. Its great strength and the character of work it will enable us to do is highly gratifying. I believe Dr. Jenkins is too well known to bring forward anything that we cannot endorse. If he indorses it, it is sufficient for me.

Dr. George S. Allan.—Just one more point. All bodies that are used for artificial teeth and continuous gum work are hard and brittle. This body, as I understand Dr. Jenkins, is hard and tough and not as easily broken as former bodies.

Dr. Stockton.—I have always been a kind of hero-worshipper. I like a man who leads. I think that is why I have always been such an admirer of Napoleon. That is why I admire Dr. Jenkins.

I had the pleasure of being at the dental clinics at St. Louis, and the centre of attraction of these clinics was the inlay work. The appearance of this work alone is enough to attract us to it. The only question that comes up with this and all porcelain work is, " Is it strong enough to last?" Whatever Dr. Jenkins tells us we can rely upon, and he tells us that it is strong enough to stand the strain for which it is intended. The interest is so great in inlay work that our humble society in New Jersey, the Central Dental Association, is to have the first clinic it has ever devoted entirely to this work.

Dr. Palmer.—I cannot let the occasion go by without speaking of this work. Fourteen-odd years ago I was forced to take up a different line of bridge-work because of difficulties with the International Tooth Crown Company. Since that time I have used various bodies for bridge-work, but none which were satisfactory. Some few months ago my attention was called to this porcelain of Dr. Jenkins's, and I succeeded in getting some of it. I have used it in a good many small pieces, and have found it excellent, even using plain rubber teeth without having any trouble whatever. With it

I have had so much better results than with anything else that I am delighted. With all due respect to Dr. Wheeler, it does not make any difference to me whether it contains any glass or not; it looks better than anything I have ever used, and I believe it is going to wear better.

Dr. C. F. Allan.—Dr. Jenkins recommends using pure gold for solder. There is nothing better. I have had some experience with platinum gold solder, and it has been very unsatisfactory. It does not flow in the beautiful manner that gold does, and does not begin to be as strong, and as the strength of the framework is essential in the use of porcelain for bridge purposes, I would give this word of warning.

Dr. Jenkins.—I wish to thank Dr. Wheeler for his kind criticism. If he has interested himself in ceramics he must know that the materials of which all the finer porcelains are made are always essentially the same,—silica, feldspar, and kaolin. It is only a question as to how they are prepared, in what proportions they are compounded, and how they are fluxed. The production of a high-fusing porcelain is an exceedingly simple matter. As ordinarily produced, the high-fusing porcelains are but the threshold of a perfect material. There goes into this porcelain that I have prepared for prosthetic work at least twenty times as much work as is necessary to produce the ordinary high-fusing body. It is so complicated a process that if I were to take Dr. Wheeler into my laboratory and give him the materials and set him to work, I venture to say that it would take him two years before he could learn just when and how to unite the different ingredients. These things can be brought out only by painstaking and complicated experiments. In producing your results in this work you must simply pay no attention to time or expense. It is not only a question of the proportion of the .ingredients, but of the different degrees of fineness as well.

Referring to the melting-point of gold, I beg leave to say that no one in all the world has yet been able to say what the absolute melting-point is. I believe that the Germans are conceded to be authorities on this subject, and in Germany it is stated to be 1075° C. There have been within the last few years a series of experiments made in England, and it has been announced there that the melting-point of gold must be conceded to be between 1064° and

1065° C. But the balance of authority I may say is with the German chemists who state it at 1075° C.

What I have endeavored to produce is a material that the ordinary man can use. When I spoke of high-fusing porcelain I did not mean to imply that it is crude, and of course it is a porcelain indispensable in certain forms of work, as, for instance, in the manufacture of porcelain teeth where an indestructible form is necessary. The requirements for a prosthetic porcelain are essentially different. It must be a porcelain which, when fused, will flow into the minutest crevice, which shall perfectly attach itself to the porcelain tooth around which it is placed so that it cannot be separated with violence. You can break away the tooth, but cannot break away the prosthetic porcelain. It is also of great importance that it possess great tenacity. There is an enormous difference too between the kind of glaze a porcelain takes, whether it is produced as a natural result of the fusing of the material or whether it is an enamel put on after the piece is practically finished. The prosthetic porcelain is of one consistency throughout, which makes it exceedingly enduring. You have all seen pieces of continuous gum baked after the old method, where the piece was first biscuited and then covered with a layer of enamel, and where after a time the enamel had worn off leaving the more porous porcelain exposed, and which in time became offensive. This cannot occur with the prosthetic porcelain, because it is the same throughout.

There were so many things mentioned, and there are so many things about it that I could tell you did time permit, that I shall have to ask you to take it upon faith. I can only tell you that I believe you will find it an indispensable adjunct to your practice, and that by means of it you will be able to eliminate any appearance of artificiality from the mouth. Even a clasp can be so completely covered up by this material that it becomes invisible. Of course, it must be a rigid clasp.

One word regarding platino-iridium. There is no question at all but that a properly alloyed platino-iridium can be swaged up. If one wished to strike up a cap, a band or half band, or a plate, either full or partial, ten per cent. platino-iridium can certainly be worked, perhaps not quite so readily, but when accomplished it is stiff and does not change with soldering or repeated meltings without any investment. In these cases there is no union between the alloy and the porcelain. Only perfect adaptation. Perhaps an attachment might be made by roughening the surface of the platinum, but it is seldom necessary.

I am very much obliged, gentlemen, for the patience with which you have listened to me.

Upon motion of Dr. F. Milton Smith, the Institute expressed to Dr. Jenkins its gratitude for his valuable discussion and demonstrations.

Adjourned.

FRED. L. BOGUE, M.D., D.D.S.,
Editor The New York Institute of Stomatology.

Editorial.

THE FIFTH YEAR OF THE CENTURY.

THE average person, very naturally, grows somewhat sentimental at the opening of a new year in the calendar, but this seems unreasonable in view of the fact that every hour and every day should be held responsible for the development of human life.

The fifth year of the twentieth century! How many who now walk the world's pathways will be here when its last hour is rung out by the clanging of bells announcing its passage into oblivion and the birth of the twenty-first century of the Christian era? The human mind is incapable of realizing the full significance of that hour, the story which it will tell of the progress, the development of the human race.

It is possible to draw a picture of the future from the record of the past. The nineteenth century and its work will enable the philosophic mind to solve this in part, the destiny of this the twentieth century, which should be as much in advance as the former in all that makes for the progress of the world.

Professionally it is the part of wisdom not to indulge in, possibly, vain predictions. Indeed, the mind does not exist sufficiently clairvoyant to anticipate the progress hoped for and confidently expected in all branches of the healing art.

When the nineteenth century was young medical men were

floundering in a wilderness of guesses as to the etiology of disease. The pathology of the period might be resolved in a series of negatives. " I don't know" was practically over every physician's doorway. That classical writer and profound medical teacher, Thomas Watson, in his celebrated " Lectures on the Principles and Practice of Physics in 1836," says, " During life it is often no easy thing to determine whether the parts of which the functions are disturbed preserve their integrity of structure or not, and even when the peccant organ is placed before our eyes after death, and the most careful scrutiny fails to discover in it any faultiness of texture, there may still be ground for suspecting that some material change, too subtile for detection by our senses, may have been wrought in its finer and more delicate organization."

Read the same author on the " Cause of Disease" and how poor it all seems in comparison to the knowledge obtained in the subsequent half-century upon the same subject. He says, in part, " The atmosphere may be a source of disease in consequence of its being loaded with impurities. Malaria, contagions of various kinds, and noxious gases in general may be considered as so many poisons." The word *may* indicates the sum total of the knowledge of the time in this direction. It can be said, with some degree of positiveness, that the genuine pathology of the human organism has all been worked up during the last half of the nineteenth century, and that all preceding this was but the shadow of the substance, that came rapidly in succeeding years.

That which is true of medicine is equally true of dentistry; indeed, it is true of all the specialties of the art of healing. While each and all of these are indebted to the past more than words can recount, yet the true renaissance did not appear until the professional mind became dissatisfied with the old pathology based upon mere guess-work.

This could not be said of practical dentistry. It grew upon a substantial foundation of fact, but these facts were limited. Its trade secrets led to no broad generalizations, and apparently were simply a means to gain the daily bread and butter and were without value in a professional sense. That came with the rise of medicine, and with it the stomatologist of the period is capable of developing the cause of disease in his domain of work on far more certain lines than was possible prior to 1850.

Men are living to-day, and actively engaged in professional

work who are very familiar, from personal observation, with all the modern changes in medical knowledge and practice. These have come so rapidly that the student of the period regards them as having always been part of medical knowledge. They forget that the time from Leeuwenhoek to Cohn means an interval of innumerable investigations into the character and life-cycle of low forms of life. To the latter belongs the credit of increasing the interest in these problems, but from Koch (1881) the bacteriologist must date the beginning of bacteriology as a science.

Roswell Park, in his " History of Medicine," writing in 1899, says, " In civil hospitals, as well as in general and private practice, the mortality from these diseases (zymotic) was, until twenty-five years ago, simply frightful; while frequently, and over wide areas of territory, endemics and epidemics of puerperal fever would result in the death of almost every lying-in woman. In consequence of this terrible death-rate, surgeons were afraid to operate, and cer-.tain classes of. operations, especially those on the abdomen and joints, were never performed except under the most exacting circumstances."

Thus prior to 1874 the germ theory of disease was practically an unknown factor in pathology, and from that period became an important subject in the curricula of the medical schools, as also did that of its sister science, histology.

Dentistry rapidly appropriated this valuable knowledge and dental pathology assumed an importance unknown in its past history, and the work of a large body of devoted laborers in this field of investigation have built a system through scientific development that has made dentistry a profession worthy the respect of this and future generations.

Combining these facts as a basis for prophetic knowledge, we can confidently look forward to the coming years as being full to overflowing of accurate information concerning the human organism in health and disease. In all directions this is being studied with an enthusiasm and self-devotion that insures an open way and a clearer understanding of the pathological problems that are, as yet, but a stumbling-block to the practitioner.

Hence we open this new year with hope. The year 1904 has been one of discouragement.

The golden era in dental education is not to be achieved by looking backward, but that has been the attitude of dental educators. They have gone back to the days of 1850, and have gloried in the results. The writer is not, however, disposed to pessimism. There are subtle forces at work in the world that no antagonisms can stifle. The laws of progress are eternal, and these will be obeyed and the efforts of the demagogue, the man of narrow ideas, the one who holds that "the ideas of the fathers are good enough for me," will be of no avail to force back the eternal roll of the ages to the new day and the higher conditions belonging to the more exalted ideas of a broader civilization.

It requires no prophet to foretell the destiny of the world, for past history demonstrates it. The refining processes that have been silently progressing for untold ages, from the coarser fibre of the flora and fauna of the carboniferous period and long antedating this, prove with mathematical exactness the progressive stages toward a higher standard of mentality in man and in everything in the physical world below him. Man's puny efforts to roll back this great ocean of progressive refinement will avail nothing, for all his efforts in this direction will but hasten the day of more perfect regeneration. Hence each recurring year is not a sad reminder of passing activities, but is a new source of satisfaction that we are one year nearer the goal, the final destiny of the human race; and not only this, but the entire world and all it contains; and as this law of progress applies to one world, so must it equally be part of the expansion of the universe.

BRITISH DENTAL ASSOCIATION.

WE are in receipt of a letter from the Secretary of the British Dental Association, W. H. Dolamore, of which the following is the substance:

"I have the honor to inform you that at a meeting of the Representative Board of this Association, held on October 29, it was resolved: That an invitation be extended to the National Dental Association of the United States, the Dental Association of the Dominion of Canada and other British Colonies, to attend the annual meeting of the British Dental Association, to be held at Southport, on Saturday, May 20, Monday, 22, and Tuesday, 23, 1905."

Whether it will be possible for the Executive Committee of the National Dental Association to accept this invitation remains to be seen.. It is to be hoped it will devise some plan to secure the sense of that body, for it seems to the writer very important that this should be accepted at this time. Every effort should be made to draw the English-speaking race closer together, and this is one of the means to accomplish this professionally.

Bibliography.

ORTHODONTIA AND ORTHOPÆDIA OF THE FACE. By Victor Hugo Jackson, M.D., D.D.S., Member of the National Dental Association; Professor of Orthodontia in the Dental Department of the University of Buffalo; Fellow of the New York Academy of Medicine; Member of the American Medical Association, etc. With seven hundred and sixty original illustrations. J. B. Lippincott Company, Philadelphia and London, 1904.

The dental profession has for several years been very familiar with the author's work in orthodontia, through his articles in the dental periodicals, and have come to regard him as an authority in this particular line of dental operations. It is, therefore, with unusual satisfaction that he has concentrated his long experience in book form to be readily accessible to all workers in this direction, and this includes, in degree, the entire dental profession.

There is no branch of dental work that has attracted more attention than that of the regulation of malposed teeth. The books devoted to this subject, both in America and Europe, attest the importance of this branch of dental procedures. This should have been expected, for the disfigurement of the human face through irregular dentures has demanded the highest attainment in skill in its treatment. The earlier efforts in this direction lacked system, and the development of methods was of very slow growth; and, further, the philosophic discussion of the subject was not, to any extent, embraced in the earlier teachings. The works of Farrar, Talbot, Angle, Guilford, and others in this country have broadened the subject until it has become very attractive for the thoughtful and inventive mind, for each new case presents difficulties to surmount and interest.

Dr. Jackson's work is eminently practical. He does not enter into wide discussion of the probable etiological factors that lead to irregular development, but is mainly satisfied with a comparatively brief allusion to these, covering some fifty-four pages. The fact that the teeth must be returned to normal positions and the lines of beauty restored, seems to be the paramount idea in the author's mind.

Dr. Jackson is known as having developed a system. It cannot be said he originated the idea of springs, for wires and springs have been used more or less satisfactorily since the period when it was first attempted to regulate teeth. While this is true, these efforts were but a crude application of force, as a rule, and were very often more productive of injury than of benefit to the patient. Dr. Jackson's system has, however, moulded these earlier efforts into procedures that give to all the appliances originality, and exhibit the active and earnest study of an inventive mind.

The author says of his system, " For many years I have applied in my own practice the principles explained in this book, and the results warrant me in giving a detailed description of my system. In the mean time I have been urging upon the profession, in writings and public demonstrations, the use of the spring as a force in regulating, and it is especially gratifying to note its more general adoption in place of screw-pressure.

"Evolution is the law of our science as of other studies. To realize this, one has but to compare the methods of a few years ago with those of to-day. As it stands, my system of correcting irregularities includes important modifications of the appliances originally presented by me. The changes are in the line of simplicity and practicability."

The care taken by the author in the study of cases is evidenced by the following quotation as to his method of procedure in each case. He says, " The first thing that strikes us favorably in a face is exactness of proportion, then harmony of the features. When a case is presented for the regulation of the teeth, it is important that the contour of the features be studied before the mouth is examined or models are made. Careful note should be taken of the apparent changes required; these should accord with the type and temperament, whether well nourished or developed; the profile, including the size of the nose and the orifices, the width between the alæ nasi, the prominence of the cheek-bones, and the fulness or recession in the region of the upper lip. The relative position of the chin to the forehead should be noted to determine where the deformity is situated, and whether the upper or lower arch should be made more or less prominent. The features should be studied both in repose and when animated, especially when laughing."

These are valuable suggestions to the beginner in this work, the neglect of which has oftentimes produced deformity in attempted regulation. In the reviewer's opinion, upon this will mainly depend whether the operator should spread the jaw, or attempt other means to overcome a contracted arch. Whether extraction should ever be resorted to in regulating must largely depend upon the conclusion arrived at after the study, advised by the author, has been completed.

The difficulty in removing plaster impressions is overcome by the author through forcing water under the lip with the force of a syringe. He regards this "as an invaluable procedure."

Under the head of "Anchorages and Appliances" the author sums up the advantage of his system:

"First. The simplicity and ease of construction of the apparatus.

"Second. It is equally applicable for the regulation of the teeth of the child or the adult.

"Third. It is suitable for all forms of irregularity, doing away with the use of a plate in a large majority of cases.

"Fourth. It is well retained in apposition with the teeth, and when the appliance is properly made it causes no inconvenience. It does not interfere materially with speech or with the occlusion of the teeth, even when an apparatus is used in both the upper and the lower arch at the same time.

"Fifth. While the anchorage is sufficiently firm for all practicable purposes, the appliance can usually be removed by the patient, thus favoring cleanliness.

"Sixth. It can be so arranged that some of the teeth to be moved later in the process of regulating can be employed to assist the anchorage, thereby lessening the disturbance of the anchorage-teeth when extreme force is applied."

He further contends that the force is well under control, and "the appliance can be made of almost any of the precious metals that are springy or base metals." The "attachment base wire and spring wire" are simple and quickly prepared. Almost any of the appliances can be continued in use as retainers.

On page 134 the author shows a decided antagonism to the jack-screw, for he says, " I have not found the jack-screw of especial value in any case, and owing to its interference with the tongue in pronunciation and mastication, suggest that its use, both for pushing and pulling the teeth, be discontinued in favor of methods more agreeable to the patient." While he thus objects to its use, and recognizing "that some operators employ it," he gives illustrations of its employment in several special cases. He states with emphasis his objections to the screw or intermittent pressure for regulating purposes as advocated by Dr. Farrar in what he terms his "positive system." The author says, "The law of nature is, that alternating pressure and relief cause hypertrophy, increased growth, and hardening, while constant pressure causes atrophy or absorption." While this may be true of alternate periods of irritation and rest, it does not seem to the reviewer to apply to the Farrar system. Theoretically the intermittent pressure should produce a hardening of the tissue, but in no sense is this pressure delayed to a period injurious, for the benefit of short periods of partial rest seems of special value to the overstrained nervous system of the patient, while the constant pressure may produce serious lesions in careless hands. This has so repeatedly been observed by the reviewer, that while he is not devoted to any one method of moving teeth, yet he must object to the inculcation of the idea that "the tissues involved in regulating are tolerant of any kind of direct moderate force, whether constant or intermittent." The author seems to contradict this positive assertion in another part of the book, for he there states: "The too rapid movement of the teeth is always objectionable. The alveolar process is gradually absorbed as the roots of the teeth are moved toward one another, and if the apices of the roots are moved too rapidly through the process there is always danger of strangulation of the pulps." This latter is the ever-present danger in inexperienced hands.

The face-masks, illustrated by the author, beginning on page 242, with insets, are of special interest, representing, as they do, the original deformity with the appearance after correction. These give a better idea of the defect, with the improvement, than a photograph of the face could possibly present.

On page 253 (Fig. 281) is a very interesting illustration of an original design by the author to break up the habit of thumb-sucking. It consists of a thumb-cot with a small serrated leather strip attached to the cot, and this again attached to a bracelet at the wrist, held fast by a small padlock, the key of which was kept by the mother. It broke up the habit in a few days.

" General Orthopædia of the Face," including " Nasal Deformities," might, as a chapter in a book on regulating, be profitably omitted. It belongs more properly to the work of the surgeon, and will not, in all probability, come within the province of the orthodontist.

The book as a whole must impress the practical man as one well adapted to his needs. It covers, in its cases, all that the operator will ever have fall into his hands for regulating. The author has spent but little time in theorizing as to the cause of these abnormal conditions, but recognizes the importance of this in his chapter on " Etiology." His desire has been apparently to show in the most direct and simple manner how the irregularities may be remedied by his system, and the reader must acknowledge that his application of force reduces the regulation of teeth to very simple and inexpensive appliances.

It is thought that this book will have a wide circulation; indeed, its original character will compel every practitioner to make it part of his library for frequent reference. It is impossible to have too many of these practical works. They will eventually fuse, as it were, into each other, and in time we will have, not a series of systems, as is the case at present, but one system that can be taught successfully to the coming generations of orthodontists.

The students at our colleges will need this book to broaden their knowledge in a practical direction. There is too much dependence upon certain methods at the present time. Teaching, to be of value, must have elasticity and be prepared to meet all difficulties as they arise without an entire dependence on any one system or any one theory.

The book is prepared by the J. B. Lippincott Company, in type, paper, etc., in their usual excellent style of work. Some of the illustrations are not altogether satisfactory from either a dental or artistic view, but these are probably old cuts used by the author to illustrate his papers. The more recent illustrations are well prepared.

THE PHYSICIAN'S VISITING LIST for 1905. Fifty-fourth year of its publication. P. Blakiston's Son & Co., Philadelphia.

This more than a half-century old publication is offered again for the use of physicians for 1905.

It is doubtful whether any other of similar character can show as long a period of usefulness. For the medical practitioner, for whom it is specially arranged, there would seem that there could be no better arrangement for daily memoranda.

Obituary.

SAMUEL JOHN HUTCHINSON, M.R.C.S., L.D.S. (ENG.).

MR. HUTCHINSON was born at Helmsley, in Yorkshire, in 1848. He obtained his early education at a local school, and afterwards became a pupil of the late Mr. Jonathan Hooten, of Manchester, where he earned the reputation of being both clever and industrious. This character was maintained upon his arrival in London, where he pursued his studies at University and King's College Hospitals and the Dental Hospital of London. In 1872 he obtained the L.D.S. (Eng.), and two years later the M.R.C.S.

He was one of the early students of the Dental Hospital of London, then in Soho Square, and subsequently became assistant surgeon and surgeon to that institution. He resigned his appointment on becoming lecturer on Dental Surgery and Pathology, which post he again resigned on being elected one of the examiners in Dental Surgery to the Royal College of Surgeons of England. At the date of his death he was consulting dental surgeon to the National Dental Hospital and the University College Hospital.

Mr. Hutchinson may be said to have filled every post of trust and honor that the profession had to offer. In the Odontological Society of Great Britain he was successively member of council, honorary secretary, curator, president, and treasurer. To the

British Dental Association he also gave freely of his time and talents, and had filled the post of chairman of the representative board. He was president of the association at its last annual general meeting in London in 1901. He was also a trustee of the benevolent fund.

His commanding position in the profession was obtained by tireless energy and dogged perseverance. Notwithstanding the cares of a large private practice, he constantly took an active part in his profession's public affairs, and faithfully discharged all the duties of the many offices he held.

His health was at no time robust, and it is possible that he was at times overtaxed. Some years ago he suffered from a severe attack of tachycardia, from which he appeared to have made a complete recovery; recently, however, signs of valvular incompetence became apparent, and rapidly increased, and to this he finally succumbed.

He died at his residence, " Ford," Branksome Park, Bournemouth, September 15, aged fifty-six, and was buried on September 20, 1904, at Hampstead Cemetery.

He left an estate valued at over one hundred and fifty thousand dollars. His will provides that should his children die without leaving issue, the Dental Hospital of London, Leicester Square, and the North London or University College Hospital, will each receive five thousand dollars; the Dental Benevolent Fund of the British Dental Association, the Epsom College Benevolent Fund, and the Society for the Relief of Widows of Medical Men, in the same contingency are to receive five hundred dollars each. (The *Dental Record,* and the *British Journal of Dental Science.*)

LADY TOMES.

Another link with the past is severed by the decease of Jane, widow of the late Sir John Tomes, F.R.S. Lady Tomes passed away on October 16, 1904, at the ripe age of eighty-one, at her beautiful home, Upwood Gorse, Caterham Valley, England. (*Dental Record.*)

W. H. T.

Miscellany.

AN INTERESTING FACT IN HAYDEN'S LIFE.—We find an enter-
taining story about a once widely known book in the *Cincinnati
Enquirer.* Two great-granddaughters of Dr. Horace H. Hayden,
it seems, discovered in the Mercantile Library of St. Louis a copy
of their great-grandfather's "Geological Essays," for which they
offered to pay $500. The offer was declined, as the books in the
library are not for sale. We fancy that by judiciously using the
weekly Book Exchange column of the *New York Times Book Review* Dr. Hayden's granddaughters might be able to secure a copy
for a much smaller price. "Geological Essays: An Inquiry into
Geological Phenomena to be Found in Various Parts of America,"
was published in Baltimore in 1829. There may be many copies
extant. Horace Hayden was born in Windsor, Conn., in 1769, and
died in Baltimore in 1844. He was a school-teacher and an architect before he took up the study of dentistry after his twenty-first
year. He became a successful and famous dentist. He studied
medicine, too, and served as an army surgeon in the War of 1812.
His favorite avocation throughout his life was the study of geology.
Though he wrote books on dentistry and other subjects, his fame
as an author is chiefly associated with his "Geological Essays,"
which Benjamin Silliman said "should be used as a text-book in
all our schools."—*Exchange.*

Current News.

PENNSYLVANIA ASSOCIATION OF DENTAL SUR-
GEONS.

THE fifty-eighth annual meeting of the Pennsylvania Association of Dental Surgeons was held at the Continental Hotel, Philadelphia, October 11, 1904. The following officers were elected for
the ensuing year: President, Dr. M. I. Schamberg; Vice-President, Dr. Albert N. Gaylord; Secretary, Dr. J. Clarence Salvas;
Treasurer and Librarian, Dr. Wm. H. Trueman.

J. CLARENCE SALVAS,
Secretary.

THE

International Dental Journal.

VOL. XXVI.   FEBRUARY, 1905.   No. 2.

Original Communications.[1]

THE RELATION OF THE DENTIST TO THE NOSE, THROAT, AND EAR SPECIALIST.[2]

BY GEORGE L. RICHARDS, M.D., FALL RIV 1, MASS.[3]

GENTLEMEN,—I have long been of the opinion that the separation of dentistry as a branch of medicine from general medicine and general surgery is a mistake. I believe that dentistry should be considered only as one of the departments of general medicine and surgery in the same manner that the practice of the diseases of the ear, nose, and throat is so considered. I believe that the time will come when the dentist will first be graduated in the general medical course, or at least carried farther in it than he is at present. The Harvard Dental School requires much more than the average, in that the first year in the dental school and the first

---

[1] The editor and publishers are not responsible for the views of authors of papers published in this department, nor for any claim to novelty, or otherwise, that may be made by them. No papers will be received for this department that have appeared in any other journal published in the country.

[2] An address delivered before the Harvard Odontological Society, December 15, 1904.

[3] Otologist and Laryngologist to the Fall River Union Hospital; Fellow American Otological Society, American Laryngological, Rhinological, and Otological Society, etc.

year in the medical school are one and the same as to course. I think the time will come when the institution will go still farther and that the rudiments at least of general medicine and surgery will be taught to the students of the dental school.

I have long believed that it would be better for our patients if we who are workers in the upper air-tract, the so-called nose, throat, and ear specialists, had a better knowledge of the teeth and their influence relative to these affections, and I think it is equally true that the dentist ought to know more of the affections of the nose, throat, and ear than he does at present.

I therefore welcome this opportunity to speak to you in regard to some of the affections in the treatment of which it seems to me we meet or ought to meet on a common ground.

AURAL NEURALGIA OF DENTAL ORIGIN.

It is well known that the fifth or trifacial nerve has very intimate relationships with all the rest of the face through its various ganglia, its own complex mechanism, the extent of its distribution, and its relations with the sympathetic. Many cases of facial neuralgia have their entire origin in the teeth, even though the patient makes no complaint whatever of the teeth.

I have also found that quite a number of ear-pains have their point of origin in the teeth, although I have been able to find but little touching this subject in the various treatises on diseases of the ear. In my own clinical experience it has seemed to me that those cases in which the teeth are in direct relationship with the ear have more commonly affected the lower jaw than the upper; in fact, the three cases which I recall at this moment have all been connected with the lower jaw. The anatomical reason for this is probably that the otic ganglion, which is situated immediately below the foramen ovale, and in close relation to the structures of the middle ear, the tensor tympani muscle, and the auriculo-temporal nerve, is directly connected with the internal pterygoid branch of the inferior maxillary nerve. Exactly why pain in connection with the teeth should be referred back to the ear rather than any of the other of the points with which the inferior maxillary nerve is in relation, I cannot say. The following three cases will give evidence of this relationship.

CASE I.—A Jewish woman around thirty-five years of age,

came complaining of severe neuralgic pain in the right ear. Examination of the ear showed no inflammatory action whatever, and after seeing her for a couple of times I was very sure in my mind that the cause of the pain was not in the ear. I referred her to a dentist, who removed a lower molar very much out of shape and pressing directly upon the inferior dental nerve. With the removal of this tooth all symptoms referable to the ear immediately disappeared.

CASE II.—A woman about the same age came complaining of severe, somewhat intermittent neuralgic pain in the ear. Examination of the ear showed no inflammatory action visible in connection with the drum, and I referred her to a dentist who removed the tooth and found the whole difficulty to be in connection with it. When I find severe neuralgic pain referred to the ear, where there are no objective symptoms suggestive of middle ear or drum inflammation, I always refer the patient to the dentist.

The third case was one somewhat different. A boy of about twelve, as a result of a cold, had an acute inflammation of the middle ear, accompanied with very severe pain. Incision of the drum was done, but there followed no relief whatever from the severe pain, which continued a number of days and required morphia hypodermically for its relief. As the boy had had a little trouble with his teeth, his dentist was called in, who found that a filling had come out of one tooth and that there was a delayed eruption of one of the bicuspids. He was very doubtful whether either one or the two together was sufficient to explain the intense pain, but after free incision of the gum and the putting in of a temporary filling in the tooth, the pain entirely disappeared, although the ear symptoms as such continued and the case later showed inflammation of the mastoid, for which a mastoid operation was done. The point here is that the severe middle ear pain which in my experience I have found to be invariably relieved by a free incision of the drum, was in no sense relieved by this, and there was no relief from the pain whatever except by the administration of morphia, until the visit of the dentist, after which the severe pain entirely disappeared. Hence it seems to me that the ear and the teeth have sufficient connection one with the other so that the aurist ought to have a certain amount of knowledge of the teeth and ability to locate in the teeth those pains for which he cannot or does not find sufficient cause in the ear; also that the dentist should recognize that certain cases of tooth trouble may produce severe ear symptoms, and be able to work intelligently with the aurist in his endeavor to locate the source of the pain.

RELATION OF MOUTH-BREATHING TO TOOTH-DEVELOPMENT.

November 21, 1895, I had the pleasure of reading before this Society a paper on the causes of mouth-breathing and the treatment to be directed for the correction of that. In the nine years which have elapsed since then, the influence of faulty nasal development and adenoid growths, not only as a cause of mouth-breathing, but as a very important factor in improper development of the upper jaw and the palatal arch, have been universally recognized, and when the dentist now looks in the mouth and finds a high, narrow arch, irregularly developed teeth, and imperfect normal occlusion, he begins to suspect that the conditions of breathing are faulty; and that there is trouble either in the nose or nasopharynx, and is quite apt to suggest that the child consult his physician or the nose and throat specialist with reference to the correction of the condition. That the adenoid growth or the imperfect nasal development is the only cause of a high arched palate or faulty normal occlusion, I would not wish to state, but that the habit of mouth-breathing dependent upon these conditions, continued during the early years of life, is an important factor in the production of this condition, is not, of course, denied by any one. When the breathing is constantly done through the mouth, the nasal passages do not develop; the floor of the nose is unduly high, and the normal nasopharynx becomes unduly small. The earlier in life the correction of this condition can be made, the better the development not only of the palate but also of the teeth.

I have in a few instances been called on to do an adenoid operation on adults of fifteen years and upward in which all the objective appearances suggested adenoids, and yet have found on examination of the nasopharynx that it was perfectly clean, contained no excess of adenoid tissue, and that the facial appearance was wholly due to faulty occlusion of the teeth, high-arched palate, and the inability to close the jaws properly, whereby the lips had a tendency to remain open. Careful teaching of these patients has usually brought about nasal respiration as there has been in each case suffi-

cient room, and in a few instances I have found, on referring the
patient to the dentist for the correction of the faulty tooth occlusion, that very much could be done for the comfort and good appearance of the patient. These cases, however, only prove the necessity
of attending to such conditions at the earliest possible moment, with
the presumption also that all of these patients, had they been seen
in the early ages, say from four to ten, would have shown the
presence of adenoid growths, as it is a well-known fact that in
many cases, perhaps the majority, there is a tendency to the disappearance of these lymphoid masses around the age of puberty,
though this by no means always occurs, as I have removed as large
masses of adenoid tissue from full-grown, fully developed adults
as I ever have from children.

The dentist therefore has it in his power, by going a little
farther in his examination of the mouth than the mere attention
to the teeth, to direct the individual or his parents to see to the
correction of all those conditions tending to interfere with normal
facial and nasal development, and the prevention of conditions
which are so difficult to correct around the age of puberty and
thereafter. In other words, I think it is the dentist's duty, when
he has a child who is manifestly a mouth-breather, to suggest to
the parents that that condition ought to be corrected, not only in
the interests of the child's whole development, but in the interests
of the teeth as well.

The influence of the general mouth secretions has a marked influence upon the condition of the teeth. I regard the enlarged,
chronically inflamed tonsil as a menace to the well-being of the
teeth and the comfort of the individual. While it is no doubt true
that individuals live along very comfortably with enlarged tonsils,
constantly secreting foul cheesy masses, yet the holding of these
masses in the crypts tends to a foul condition of the mouth, which is
often brought to the observation of the dentist when the patient
himself would not seek advice therefor, and does not really recognize the condition, having become used to the discomfort. When
the patient's attention is brought to this condition by the dentist,
advice from him with reference to its correction will usually be
welcomed. It is not always necessary that the gland itself be
removed, although those of us who have been in the habit of removing tonsils for many years always find the condition of the

patient better after their removal. A good deal can be done in the way of local treatment, in the cleaning of the crypts, and in the shrinkage of the tonsil by proper local measures.

It seems to me, therefore, that it lies within the province of the dentist to notice these things when he works in the mouth, and to suggest to his patient that such conditions are deleterious to the teeth and that his family physician or some specialist had better be consulted in relation thereto.

EMPYEMATA OF THE ANTRUM.

The question of the origin of antral empyemata is one that has occasioned considerable discussion. Originally the dental profession had the entire field, but of late the nose and throat specialist is probably seeing relatively more cases as an individual than is the individual dentist, and whereas originally we thought most of them to be of dental origin, at the present time I think the consensus of opinion would rather be that the majority of them would prove of nasal rather than of dental origin, although when one comes to search the literature in regard to it, one meets with the most various opinions, varying somewhat with what has been the author's individual experience. Without wearying you with citations from a large number of authors which would have no especial value, I nevertheless wish to make a few quotations from the recent literature on the subject from three authors, and then wish to give you my own personal observations in regard to the subject.

In the *Monatsschrift für Ohrenheilkunde* of June, 1904, Dr. Alexander Strubell, of Dresden, has a very exhaustive article on the relationship of the vessels of the antrum to those of the teeth. Finding that there was the greatest variation in the opinions expressed by so-called authorities; finding also that there are apparently cases of dental origin of antral empyemata in which there is no communication with the antrum to be seen, and yet in which the clinical history would seem to admit of no doubt that such cases of empyemata had originated from the teeth, he set out to see if he could not anatomically find some relationship between the vessels of the teeth and those of the antrum, or at least some condition that is not as yet fully understood, by which the pathogenic focus could be carried to the antrum mucous membrane. There being no especial lymph-tract, only the blood-current was left, and

the question then was whether there were any existing anasto-
moses between the blood-vessels of the alveolus and the mucous
membrane of the antrum sufficiently related together to render the
theory of infection from one channel to the other plausible.

In most anatomical writings there is nothing concerning this,
although Zuckerkandl, in his article in Scheff's "Handbook of
Diseases of the Teeth," states that the vessels that supply the
alveolus communicate with those of the external periosteum; that
in the upper jaw there is in addition to the external periosteum an
inner one, namely, the deeper layer of the mucous membrane of
the sinus, to which at the same time the arteries of the bone lead,
and the veins from which lead to the bone. In a previous publication Zuckerkandl had briefly referred to something of the same sort,
but as Strubell could find nothing further in anatomical and clinical
literature touching this point, he made personal studies on this
matter in Professor Zuckerkandl's own laboratory. Tandler's
method of injection with sodium iodine, gelatin, and Berlin blue
was used, and the posterior alveolar arteries were injected. The
specimen was then fixed in formol, the lime salts removed in caustic
potash and treated with alum, after the method of Schaffer. The
sections were made from celloidin. As a result of the examination
of the specimens, he found that there were three vessel systems,—a
long narrow one extending to the deeper layer of the mucous membrane of the antrum, that is, its periosteal layer; a coarse-meshed
vessel system of the spongy bone of the upper jaw, and a fine-
meshed one corresponding to the alveolus and the covering of the
tooth-root; that individually these were very characteristic, but that
with one another they had such a close connection that it was very
difficult to absolutely differentiate them one from the other. The
junction of the vessels of the mucous membrane periosteum with
that of the bone is brought about through numerous short, thick
vessels coursing at short intervals in canals at right angles to the
direction of the bone, while the obliquely coursing arteries of
moderate size that bring about the communication between the
blood system of the spongy bone with that of the alveolus are
re-enforced by a large number of the finest blood-vessels. Here
it is seen that the fine capillary system of the spongy bone, whose
vessels lie in the marrow of the bone, are connected with those
of the alveolus, and prove substantially the theory that the three

systems are in foundation one and the same. Hence it seems proper to say that the nourishment of the antrum and its periosteum, the spongy portion of the upper jaw, and the teeth in the alveolus all come from one set of vessels which anastomose with one another in the most extensive way. Hence it is easy to see that inflammation may travel from the antrum to the teeth or from the teeth to the antrum without there being a direct continuity of surface or a direct infection from one diseased area to the other.

Strubell then goes on to discuss the question of the relative preponderance of origin between dental and nasal causes, giving the statistics which follow, all of which from European authorities I take from his article with the exception of those of Tilley and Lermoyez, the source of which is stated.

Bayer, of Brussels, thought the most frequent cause of empyema to be disease of the teeth.

Grünwald considered twenty-one out of thirty cases to be dental in origin.

Schiffers, Goodwillie, Moreau, Schmidt, Baginsky, Lublinski, M. Schmidt, Krieg, Schütz, Christopher Heath, Scheff, Heryng, and Schmiegelow, as the result of their clinical observations, consider the teeth to be an etiological factor.

In an article read before the Odontological Society of London, November 23, 1903 (*Laryngoscope,* February, 1904), by Herbert Tilley, a prominent London laryngologist and surgeon to the Golden Square Hospital for the nose, throat, and ear, the one founded by the late Sir Morell Mackenzie, Dr. Tilley reports briefly on sixty-four cases of antral suppuration seen in private practice, and eighteen hospital cases seen since January 1, 1902. Of the sixty-four cases seen in private practice, upon which his paper is based, he found diseased bicuspid or molar teeth to be present, or by their absence implying previous removal for disease, in every case, with one exception, upon the side corresponding to the antral suppuration. He says, further, that during the past ten years, during which he must have seen at least three hundred cases of antral abscess, he has only met with one patient, a girl aged twelve, in whom the teeth were quite healthy.

B. Fränkel, as a result of his clinical experience states that in by far the larger number of cases disease of the teeth and alveolæ were the causative factor. For his position he states that he had never seen a case of empyema of the antrum in which the corresponding tooth had not been previously extracted or was at least diseased. This would agree with the observation of Herbert Tilley just quoted. And his final conclusion is that empyema of the antrum usually has its origin through the alveolus of the teeth.

Hartmann, in one article, stated that in sixteen empyemata only one case originated from a carious tooth. He reported one case of empyema of the antrum where, as the result of a filling, or following the filling of a second upper molar, pus developed. The tooth was extracted. It was then easy with a few turns of the borer to go directly from the alveolus into the antrum, after which quite a quantity of foul pus was removed. Under daily washing, healing followed a few weeks after. In another article Hartmann stated that in most cases carious teeth formed the etiological moment for the antral empyema, but that it was not always possible to determine whether the inflammation of the tooth was the real cause of the inflammation of the antrum. In only two cases after extraction of the tooth did he find an opening directly into the antrum. The fact that, in spite of a previous inflammation of the roots of the tooth, healing of an empyema of the antrum has been brought about through washing out of the nasal cavity, allows us in many cases to say that there is probably no direct union of the antral cavity with the carious process. In one-third of Hartmann's cases there were polyps in the nose, and in these he thought there was a nasal origin of the affection. In twenty-three out of thirty-two cases healing was brought about through regular washing out through the middle fossa of the nose.

Lermoyez (*Journ. Laryngology*, 1902, p. 576) states that dental origin is more frequent than nasal origin. This is due to the sudden rupture of the radiculo-dental periapexial abscess into the cavity of the sinus. It is only subsequently that the empyema is transformed into a chronic sinusitis.

Those authors who think that the inflammation comes from the teeth base their propositions on the fact that many tooth-roots, especially those of the first and second molar, reach almost to the periosteum of the antrum and are separated from it by a very thin plate of bone, while in others even this thin plate is not present and the roots lie in direct contact with the soft parts of the antrum. Caries of these teeth, therefore, leads easily to the periosteum, and not seldom to the formation of pus. Inflammation, therefore, can go directly to the mucous membrane of the antrum. Inasmuch, however, as almost all people have carious teeth, and as empyema of the antrum is comparatively seldom, this argument rather loses its force. It is perfectly possible that a carious condition can be present before the toothache appears. Even if after the extraction of a tooth an empyema appears evident that previously has given no particular signs of its presence, nevertheless it is perfectly possible that that empyema could have lasted several years. The communication between the teeth and the antrum can have grown up, and this be reopened by the extraction of the tooth. I think that in many cases of chronic empyema this is probably just what happens.

Coming next to the other theory,—namely, that the inflammation can pass from the nose directly to the antrum,—I think that the majority of present-day authors would rather hold to the preponderance of the nasal origin of antrum trouble.

The anatomist Zuckerkandl considered that antral empyemata of dental origin occurred very seldom. In his anatomy of the nose he speaks of the importance of the dehiscence of the infraorbital canal in the antrum, and states that in such cases the entire tract of the tooth nerves is in direct relationship with the antrum covering, and in case of disease of the sinus the mucous membrane can be pressed upon or infected. When this occurs, there would, of course, be pain, first referred to the tooth and supposed to be a toothache, especially if there should happen to be on that side a bad tooth. As a proof of his belief that the inflammation could pass directly (especially purulent inflammation) from the nose to the antrum, the following facts are cited.

First, the presence of cases of empyema that followed sound teeth.

Second, purulent inflammations of the sphenoid and frontal sinus.

Third, the presence of primary and inflammatory inflammation of the nasal mucous membrane.

Dmochowski examined three hundred and four maxillary sinuses without seeing a single case of empyema of dental origin, although he always chiselled away the maxillary process.

In thirty-nine upper jaws examined by Weichselbaum he found

the first bicuspid carious in six cases, absent in eight cases, sound in twenty-five cases; second bicuspid, carious in ten cases, absent in seven cases, sound in twenty-two cases; first molar, carious in fourteen cases, absent in eleven cases, sound in fourteen cases; second molar, carious in nine cases, absent in nine cases, sound in twenty-one cases.

Krause considered that carious teeth did not bring about empyema.

Jeanty, in twenty-one cases where there were carious teeth, in connection with twenty-two cases of empyema, considered that in no case were the teeth the causative factor.

Moreau, in twenty-one cases of empyema, found only eight connected with caries of the teeth.

Killian reports forty cases of inflammation of the antrum,— fifteen men, twenty-one women; with forty-four antral empyema, —eighteen right, twenty-six left. Concerning the dental origin, the history of many was in doubt. Several thought the disease to have been due to ulceration of the teeth or brought about by tooth extraction. In several there was not the slightest complaint of the teeth. In four acute cases three had toothache; one with entirely sound teeth. Killian thinks the only way to get solution of the problem is not through the varying clinical observations, but through direct pathological and anatomical examinations to find a direct way in which an inflammation can travel from the teeth to the mucous membrane of the antrum, by examination of properly prepared specimens as well as through bacteriological work.

In four of Killian's patients, after extraction of the teeth there was direct communication with the antrum. In two there was only a very thin mucous membrane and a very thin bony layer between the tooth and the antrum. In this case it was the second bicuspid. In four it was the first molar, and in another the second molar.

As the observations seem to render probable the infection of the antrum from diseased teeth, one has also to think, in the case of inflammation from the teeth (especially in cases where the bottom layer or even the mucous membrane of the antrum touched the tooth), whether, as a matter of fact, an empyema must be produced. Killian doubts this, for an abscess at the root of the tooth can last a long time without breaking through into the antrum. In such a case the mucous membrane itself can be pushed far forward, and it is also possible to imagine that the tooth can be extracted and the abscess wall opened without breaking through into the antrum. In the case of granulations or fungosity of the roots, as in the case seen by Killian, where the second bicuspid was carious with a hazel-nut granulation on the root, this opened directly into the antrum, and after its extraction there was a correspondingly large communication between the alveolus and the antrum; nevertheless the washing out of the antrum gave no sign of any pus.

Finally, one must also consider the possibility that an inflammation of the nasal mucous membrane itself can be brought about as a result of the antrum empyema, the same way as by influenza. If the nose is absolutely sound; if influenza and the like can be ruled out, and where there is nothing to be considered except the diseased tooth, then it is more than probable from the clinical stand-point that the tooth was the cause.

Hajek, one of the principal workers at the present time in rhinology, thinks the presence of an alveolar sinus with a very thin lamella of bone over the tooth to be the principal cause of the origin of dental empyema. The infection of the antrum can be brought about by abscess of the tooth, inflammation of the pulp as the result of caries or from filling, purulent inflammation of the periosteum of the alveolar process, and cysts of the root with purulent contents. Oftentimes the empyema manifests itself through the extraction of a tooth because at the same time the antrum is opened and allows the pus to come out. In only thirteen cases out of approximately two hundred antrum cases that Hajek has seen in the last eight years, does he regard the origin of the same to have been due to dental causes.

Zuckerkandl and Dmochowski also advance the proposition that it is perfectly possible that many cases of empyema may be not the result of the tooth affection, but, on the contrary, that the tooth affection may be the result of carious and pathological processes in the antrum itself, since the nerves and vessels of the antrum which supply a portion of the teeth have direct relations with the soft parts of the maxillary sinus, the deeper parts of the bone.

I have quoted thus somewhat freely from Strubell's article, interspersing it with comments of my own, because the subject is one of considerable importance, and I think these quotations show that any definite statement in the mass as to whether empyemata are of dental or nasal origin is positively worthless. Each individual case must be worked out for itself, and it is in the working out of the individual case that I think the co-operation of the rhinologist and the dental surgeon is required. The dentist must not lose sight of the fact that many cases of empyema are of extra-dental origin; the rhinologist must not lose sight of the fact that not all cases of empyema are of nasal origin.

Coming from foreign to American authors, I think it will be found, on careful scanning of the latest literature, that the prevailing opinion among rhinologists is coming to be that the majority of cases are of nasal origin. In Cryer's book on the " Anatomy of the Face," he states, page 73: " This close proximity between the apical portions of the roots of the teeth and the sinus gives the impression that the maxillary sinus is oftener infected from diseased teeth than from any other source, some authorities claiming that three-fifths of the diseases of the antrum are brought about in that way. The writer thinks this is a mistake. Though recognizing that diseases of the antrum do arise from the teeth, he believes that, aside from constitutional diseases and malformations, it is more often through the common communication between the nasal chamber, the frontal sinuses, the ethmoidal cells, and the maxillary sinus that infection is conveyed to the antrum from diseased cells and sinuses above it. It is the writer's observation that there are more cases in which teeth are lost through diseases of the antrum than cases in which the teeth are primarily diseased, causing infection of the antrum and associated cells.

" Pus or infected matter will, of course, pass in the direction of the least resistance. When the investing tissues of a tooth become so infected, the osteogenetic layer of the muco-periosteum stimulates renewed activity, with the result that a new layer of bone is produced by it which covers these parts and protects this cavity so that abscesses, with but few exceptions, point and break into the mouth.

" Careless operation by the dentist sometimes causes infection of the sinus, as drilling through the tooth and the floor of the sinus, or forcing the root of a tooth into the sinus, through fracture of the wall in an unskilful effort to extract, or carelessness in driving artificial crowns or bridges upon the teeth or roots."

I have tabulated thirty cases of empyema of the antrum seen

by me in private practice in the last eight years, with the following results: Sixteen of them were chronic cases of undoubted nasal origin in connection with general ethmoiditis, with inflammation of the frontal sinus, or with atrophic rhinitis. One of these had syphilis, but the syphilis seemed to be a coincident condition rather than in any way the cause of the general ethmoiditis. Three were the result of influenza of nasal origin. One was traumatic, the result of a railroad injury. One was luetic, the syphilis causing a breaking down of the naso-antral wall on one side and a great thinning of it on the other. Six were of undoubted dental origin, while three were possibly of dental origin. Or, reduced to percentages, 63.3 per cent. were undoubtedly of nasal origin; thirty per cent. of possible dental origin; 3.3 per cent. traumatic; 3.3 per cent. luetic.

It is extremely difficult in many cases where the empyema is a chronic condition and diseased teeth and general ethmoiditis are both present to determine which was the primary cause and which was a coincident or subsequent condition. Since carious teeth are very common in persons who do not have and never have had any nasal trouble, it is quite possible that the two processes could work along independently of one another. I think this probably occurred in one of the cases which I have stated to be of dental origin, and that really the nasal condition was the primary cause. In one of the cases which I have stated as distinctly of dental origin, this might reasonably be doubted, as no distinct trouble could be found with the tooth on its removal, and the dentist who removed it hardly considered that there was anything the matter with it. At the same time there was no general ethmoiditis, and the removal of the tooth relieved the condition of pain which was present in the antrum. On the whole, I think that in my analysis I have allowed quite as many of my cases to be of dental origin as the facts would warrant. In a recent article (" Pus in the Nose," *Medical News,* December 24, 1904) I stated that I thought my experience had shown that approximately fifty per cent. of my cases were of dental origin, but a careful scrutiny of them shows this percentage to have been altogether too high. From twenty-five to thirty per cent. is probably much nearer the correct figure.

There are many cases of acute inflammation of the antrum of influenzal origin which are seen by every rhinologist, but of which no account is made here. In the three acute cases which I have tabulated pus was actually washed out of the antrum. The acute cases in which there were antral pain and all the symptoms of acute non-purulent inflammation of the antrum I have disregarded.

So much, then, as to the origin of these affections. We come next to an equally important section of the subject: What shall be the treatment of the empyema of the antrum when the diagnosis is made? If we look up the history of cases reported even as late as five or six years ago, we will find that, preceding the days of more radical nasal surgery, the majority of these cases were all treated through openings through the alveolar process made by the extraction of the tooth, with an enlargement of the opening and its maintenance by means of a tube. In process of time a good many of them got well. Others, however, were condemned to wear the tube almost indefinitely. Tilley reports only five cases out of twenty-two that could give up the tube after having used it a long time. Of twenty-seven alveolar cases, fifteen had worn the tube with careful irrigation for at least six months. One patient had worn it ten years; another three and one-half years, and another two years.

I think we have now come to the point where this method of treatment in cases which have lasted any length of time must be considered as distinctly obsolete. Any one who has done a number of radical operations on the antrum, and has seen the character of the degenerated mucous membrane which is found there, often the entire antrum being filled with numerous polyps and various low formations of granulation tissue, will thoroughly appreciate the uselessness of expecting to get any cure through a small tube opening into the mouth, even though that tube may satisfactorily drain the pus. Again, why should a patient be compelled to syringe out his antrum, day in, day out, when a radical operation, the healing of which will be complete in a few weeks, can be performed and the case be disposed of once for all?

Without discussing further this subject of treatment as to its pros and cons, I will tell you the method which I am in the habit of pursuing and which I believe, in the light of our present knowledge, is the proper one. Given a case of supposed antral empyema, first, as to diagnosis. The presence or absence of pus can be determined pretty quickly and very easily by puncturing underneath the inferior turbinate as high up as possible and at the junction of its anterior and middle thirds, although there will be a few cases in which the antrum may be so filled with polypoid growth, with comparatively small secretion, that the diagnosis here may for a short time be somewhat in doubt. In most instances, however, the diagnosis is definite enough.

In the second place, have the case examined carefully by a dentist to see if there is any trouble with the teeth. If the tooth is at fault, extract it. See whether it opens into the antrum. Assuming that it does, and that the tooth is the causative factor, is the antrum acutely or chronically affected? If acutely affected, it will get well in a short time with daily washings out with the usual antiseptic fluids. If it lasts more than a reasonable time, two or three weeks, or even less, without manifest cessation, I regard the case as chronic, and further treatment by way of the teeth as useless. At the same time that the dentist was treating the teeth, if the patient was under my own observaion, I should have enlarged the original exploratory opening made in the nasal wall of the antrum, by means of curettes and alligator cutting forceps, so as to get a free opening from the antrum into the nose, thus securing free drainage, which drainage is very much superior to that through the mouth. The short curettes, bent slightly on the shank, which are used for the radical mastoid operation and are of various sizes, and the smallest and second size Myles's aligator cutting forceps answer very well for this purpose. If the case lasted any considerable length of time, I should next do a radical operation, taking off, under ether, sufficient of the front wall of the canine fossa, so that free inspection of the antrum cavity could be had; its entire contents, including the mucous membrane, removed if necessary, and a large counter-opening then made directly into the nose underneath the anterior end of the inferior turbinate; the natural opening also enlarged, and the whole antrum cavity packed with gauze. The canine fossa opening is allowed to close in a few days, thus sealing off the cavity of the mouth, and the nasal opening is retained as the permanent one. The details of this operation I have described in my book on the nose and throat[1] and in the article in the *Medical News* already referred to.

This operation, of course, lies in the province of the rhinologist rather than of the dentist, but the entire working out of the pathol-

---

[1] "Nose and Throat Work for the General Practitioner," New York, 1903.

ogy and treatment in the borderland cases should be made by the dentist and the rhinologists together.

There is another class of antrum cases which might have been considered in our discussion of the etiology,—namely, those in which the antrum is infected from the frontal sinus by reason of the drainage of the pus from frontal sinus empyemata, down through the infundibulum, and then into the natural opening of the antrum, or directly into the antrum, a condition which occurs, and so frequently that I now believe that all cases of radical operation of the frontal sinus should have at the time of operation, or previously, exploratory puncture of the antrum to determine whether or not the antrum is at the same time affected.

The after-treatment of the cases in which a radical operation is done is comparatively simple, does not last a great while, and has in my hands been invariably successful.

SURGERY OF THE ALVEOLAR PROCESS.

The rhinologist comes in contact with the dentist in another division of his work,—namely, in alveolar abscesses, the extraction of teeth, and affections of the jaw. In quite a number of instances in the last few years patients have come to me complaining of pus underneath the mucous membrane of the upper jaw, in which the history seemed to show a certain degree of infection of the parts at the hands of the dental surgeon. In nearly all of these instances it seemed to be due to the laudable endeavor of the dental surgeon to save teeth which, from the stand-point of the rhinologist, had better have been extracted. I am quite aware, so far as this phase of the subject is concerned, that there may be great difference of opinion, and I will probably be told that the dental surgeon saves a great many teeth which the rhinologist would have pulled, and that in only a few instances is there any after-trouble.

I have recently had as a patient a boy of twelve or fourteen. He had had a tooth extracted some eight months before, a first left upper molar, and later developed a small abscess of the cheek. He was seen by two other dentists, neither of whom seemed to be able to cure the condition. He was referred to me by a general surgeon, into whose hands he fell, as a probable case of antrum trouble. At the time he came he had a granular ulcer the size of a ten cent piece disfiguring his cheek, at the bottom of which ulcer cavity some bare bone could be felt, but which did not penetrate the antrum.

There was nothing in the contour of the upper jaw to suggest that there was any tooth-root present. A competent dental friend of my acquaintance, to whom I took the case and to whom I suggested that there might be a tooth-root there, doubted its presence. I took the boy to the hospital, etherized, curetted, and extracted a carious tooth-root with an abscess at its tip. The further history of the case is uneventful. Suffice it to say that we fortunately got healing with comparatively little scar.

Another instance. A patient came with severe pain in the upper jaw, with all the signs of an alveolar abscess, but with no pus evident and no swelling. I punctured through the alveolus, found pus bathing the tooth-root, extracted the tooth, and found that the dental surgeon, in getting ready to cap this tooth, had drilled through it instead of up to the apex of the root, and had infected the surrounding tissue with the result as stated. He had seen the case two or three times before it came to me, but had neglected to do anything. I would like to make the criticism here that, as I see them, the average dentist is not sufficiently courageous in his surgery of the region around the teeth; that when he opens an abscess he does not make a sufficiently large opening; that when he drills through the alveolar process to a tooth-root in the endeavor to save that tooth, his opening is too small; that his entire surgery, the moment he is away from the tooth, is too timid. The larger the opening, the less the pain, and as in modern days we have to anæsthetize more or less anyway, if we do anything that is likely to produce pain, it means but little more primary pain to the patient to make a good opening, whereas afterwards the comfort is much greater. These last two cases are only examples of quite a number which have come under my observation.

SYPHILIS.

The last topic which I think is of common interest relates to the subject of syphilis. I wonder how many of my dental friends feel competent to diagnose the mouth lesions of syphilis; and if there are any here who do not, I would suggest that they take a course in it at some one of the dispensaries, or study up the subject with some physician of their acquaintance who is versed in the subject.

We have come to pay more and more attention to the care of our instruments, apparatus, etc., and I presume there is no dentist present who would endanger his patients in any way by the using of one set of instruments on another without their thorough sterilization. But beyond that there is the danger of the dentist's infecting himself from the syphilitic mouth and from the syphilitic saliva. In working on the mouth it is very easy to get a slight abrasion in one's own fingers or the fingers of one's assistant, and the syphilitic virus is quite as easily transmitted by way of the mouth tract as by the more commonly supposed one of the sexual act. I think that every dentist owes it to himself and his patients to recognize on the first inspection the commoner syphilitic lesions of the mouth. Within a fortnight a patient has come to me with a sore throat showing most beautifully all the secondary lesions of syphilis, its most contagious stage, with mucous patches on both tonsils, and as I finished with him he said, " Well, I am going to the dentist's now to have a tooth pulled." I inquired what dentist he was going to, but he didn't know. Had it been one of my own friends I think I should have sent a special messenger to him to take extraordinary care. Within a few years I have had another well-marked case of syphilis tell me that she got it through unclean instruments used by the dentist in the extraction of a tooth. More careful inquiry, however, revealed the source had been somewhat otherwise.

That this problem of the syphilitic virus in the mouth probably is of more moment than is generally considered, and that the dentist more often operates on the syphilitic mouth than he thinks, may be proved by the fact that in a single morning in my own private practice I have seen five cases of syphilis of the upper air-tract, and that in an ordinary private practice not exceptionally large I have always under my care from one to three or four such cases. In my own practice my assistant is always informed of the nature of the case, so that she may take extra precautions in reference to instruments, linen, and everything which touches such a case. No linen or towel is ever used on those cases except such as is thrown away, and the table and everything in connection is especially prepared.

The time at my disposal does not allow me to go into the details as to the diagnosis of these conditions. That can be obtained easily in the treatises on syphilis and from the text-books on the nose and throat. I would urge, however, upon every dentist that he make himself perfectly familiar with the commoner lesions of secondary and tertiary syphilis, and this is not difficult.

REPORT OF THIRTY CASES OF EMPYEMA OF THE ANTRUM.

Name.	Age.	Sinus involved.	Operation.	Date first seen.	Date last seen.	Result.	Remarks.	Origin.
Mr. F. W. N.	82	R. frontal. R. antrum.	Right frontal operated on by external incision. Antrum washed out.	Nov. 4, 1898.	Jan. 7, 1901.	Cured so far as known.	Antrum was originally free from pus; became infected from frontal.	Nasal.
Miss M. B.	25	R. antrum.	Exploratory puncture underneath inferior turbinate. Daily washings.	Sept. 25, 1896.	May 11, 1897.	Cured so far as known.	Had atrophic rhinitis also.	Nasal.
Mr. D. H. C.	66	R. antrum.	Exploratory puncture under inferior turbinate. Silver canula. Daily washing.	Oct. 8, 1896.	Mar. 14, 1898.	Cured so far as known.	Is in apparently good health.	Nasal.
Mr. W. H.	82	R. antrum.	November 4, 1902, puncture of antrum showed pus. Daily washing without effect. December 15, 1902, radical operation through canine fossa with extraction of first molar tooth.	April 18,1898. Complained of catarrh.	May 28, 1903.	Cured.	First molar tooth penetrated floor of antrum and had a pus pocket attached. Antrum walls not specially diseased.	Dental.
Mrs. S.	64	L. antrum.	Exploratory puncture; daily washing for two months. Improved, but no cure. Then removed second molar, and made large incision through the alveolar process. Cure in a few days.	Feb. 5, 1897.	May 8, 1897.	Cured.	Complained at no time of tooth which was filled with amalgam.	Dental.

	Age	Location	Operation	Date	Date	Result	Remarks	Cause
Miss J. S.	24	R. antrum.	Puncture underneath the inferior turbinate and washed out cavity.	June 17, 1899.	Dec. 9, 1899.	Slight discharge at time case lost sight of.	No trouble with teeth. Antrum very small.	Nasal.
Mr. G. D. F.	28	R. antrum and R. frontal.	Washed out antrum to no purpose; then did radical antrum and radical frontal.	June 21, 1899.	April 6, 1904.	Cured.	Case traumatic in origin from railroad accident.	Traumatic.
Mrs. M. G.	37	Both frontals. Both antra.	Various operations on frontal sinuses; antra secondarily infected from these.	Oct. 17, 1899.	July 12, 1904.	Cured.	Extensive ethmoiditis several years duration.	Nasal.
Mrs. F.	41	L. antrum.	Radical from antrum through canine fossa, syringing having failed to effect cure.	Dec. 18, 1899. Then occasionally until Apr. 11, 1904, when radical operation was done.	Oct. 28, 1904.	Cured.	Originally thought was case atrophic rhinitis simply. Pain from pressure on infraorbital nerve a prominent after-symptom. Disappeared in three weeks.	Nasal.
Mr. M. S.	24	L. antrum. L. frontal.	March 7, 1900, radical through canine fossa. Antrum filled with soft, pulpy granulation tissue. Second bicuspid absent.	Mar. 2, 1900.	Sept. 1904. Antrum clear.	Cured as to antrum by first operation.	Frontal was afterwards operated on, and again three years later. Permanent cure now effected.	Nasal.
Mrs. N. A.	25	R. antrum.	Radical through canine fossa and also through alveolar process at site first bicuspid previously removed.	June 9, 1900.	Aug. 4, 1900.	Cured.	First and second bicuspids and first molar absent at time of operation.	Nasal or dental (probably dental).

Name.	Age.	Sinus involved.	Operation.	Date first seen.	Date last seen.	Result.	Remarks.	Origin.
Mrs. A. C.	39	L. antrum.	Radical through canine fossa and also through alveolar process at site first bicuspid previously removed.	June 12, 1900.	Nov. 4, 1902.	Cured.	Wore gold tube through alveolar opening for awhile as no opening was made into nose. It would have been better to have made one.	Dental.
Miss M. D.	29	L. antrum.	Exploratory puncture.	April 5, 1902.	Under treatment for atrophic rhinitis, but antrum has no pus.			Nasal.
Miss A. A.	24	L. antrum.	Exploratory puncture.	Oct. 23, 1902.	April 16, 1903.	Cured.		Nasal.
Miss H. D.	26	Both antra. Had general ethmoiditis with polyp formation.	Radical both antra. April, 1904.	Nov. 21, 1902.	Sept. 8, 1904.	Cured.	At time of operation three carious roots were found penetrating left antrum. As both antra were diseased and no trouble with teeth on right side, doubtful if tooth was cause.	Probably nasal, perhaps dental.
Miss O. M.	17	R. antrum. R. frontal.	Radical operation frontal sinus and antrum.	Feb. 11, 1902.	June 9, 1908.	Cured.	Operated on frontal first, then did radical antrum as pus discharge did not stop. Think frontal infected antrum.	Nasal.

Name	Age	Location	Operation			Result	Notes	Type
Mr. W. G.	29	R. antrum. R. frontal.	Radical for each.	Mar. 22, 1908.	Dec. 14, 1904.	Apparently cured.	Impossible to say whether frontal or antrum primary source of trouble. Had general ethmoiditis.	Nasal.
Dr. G. L. R.	40	L. antrum.	Exploratory puncture. Daily washing.	Jan. 1908.	Three weeks duration.	Cured	Absolute cure in three to four weeks.	Nasal (influenza).
Mr. A. J. F.	25	R. antrum	Exploratory puncture.	Mar. 10, 1908.	Mar. 12, 1908.	Cured.	Acute case influenzal origin.	Nasal.
Mr. E. P.	21	Both antra.	Exploratory puncture L. Right side naso-antral wall already perforated.	June 27, 1908.	Nov. 7, 1908.	Improved.	Result tertiary lues.	Luetic.
Mr. L. W. J.	24	Both antra. Both frontals.	Radical operation all four cavities June 17, 1908. All sinuses filled with polypi and degenerated mucous membrane.		Dec. 1904.	Cured apparently.	No tooth complications.	Nasal.
Mr. M. W. M.	25	L. antrum. L. frontal.	Exploratory puncture antrum showed pus. Frontal sinus also involved.	Oct. 24, 1908.	Nov. 24, 1908.	Relieved.	Middle turbinate was removed. This improved drainage. No other treatment allowed.	Nasal.
Mr. H. S. H.	85	R. antrum.	Radical operation R. antrum.	Feb. 10, 1908.	Dec. 22, 1908.	Cured.	Luetic with general ethmoiditis and polypi each nostril. No tooth symptoms.	Nasal. Luetic.
Miss E. A.	49	L. antrum.	Removed portion middle turbinate followed by radical antrum operation.	April 21, 1908.	July 14, 1908.	Cured.	Had first molar tooth pulled but root found to be healthy and not penetrating antrum.	Nasal.

Name.	Age.	Sinus Involved.	Operation.	Date first seen.	Date last seen.	Result.	Remarks.	Origin.
Mrs. W. W.	68	R. antrum.	Exploratory puncture and daily washings; removal middle turbinate.	Nov. 19, 1903.	Dec. 12, 1903.	Improved.	Had many nasal polypi and extensive ethmoiditis. On account of very poor general health no further operation allowed.	Nasal.
Miss M. T.	32	L. antrum.	Exploratory puncture and daily washing out with canula.	Mar. 5. 1904.	Mar. 19, 1904.	Cured.	Acute case from influensa. No return eight months later.	Nasal.
Miss F. H.	36	R. antrum.	Second bicuspid extracted; showed old inflammation at root but did not penetrate the antrum. Then drilled into antrum. This opening closed in two days. The exploratory opening from the nose then enlarged with curettes and cutting forceps.	May 24, 1904.	Sept. 3, 1904.	Cured.	This may have been primarily of dental origin as pus had lasted some time. After establishing free nasal drainage cure was rapid.	Nasal or dental.
Mrs. N. B. B.	50	R. antrum.	Removed first molar; showed root abscess with opening directly into the antrum.	April 18, 1904.	May 20, 1904.	Cured.	After treatment through root cavity only.	Dental.

Mrs. D. V. C.	30	R. antrum.	Exploratory puncture through nose. Second bicuspid, a capped tooth, then removed. No abscess, but penetrated antrum.	April 2, 1904.	April 15, 1904.	Cured.	Influenza closed natural opening. Pus probably of dental origin, but gave no sign. Many patients do not notice slight purulent discharge, considering it a symptom of what they call catarrh. [Dental.]
Mr. W. E. Y.	87	R. antrum.	Exploratory puncture under inferior turbinate. Removed second bicuspid. No apparent connection with antrum but relieved pain. Cut away portion naso-antral wall with cutting forceps.	April 28, 1904.	Sept. 10, 1904.	Cured.	Had complained of catarrh for some time with some discharge. Possible dental. No ethmoidal trouble.

NOTE.—Since tabulating the above a case of double empyema of the antrum in a young woman of twenty-three has come under observation. All of the teeth in the upper jaw were sound. The antral empyema seemed secondary to a general ethmoiditis with polyp formation. A portion of the naso-antral wall was cut away under the inferior turbinate, and treatment carried out through the nose.

CHANGES IN THE SALIVARY SECRETION, AFFECTED BY SYSTEMIC DISEASE.[1]

BY HEINRICH STERN, M.D., AND WILLIAM J. LEDERER, D.D.S., NEW
YORK CITY.

COMPARED to other subjects of interest to the stomatologist, only a few papers of practical value have appeared on this subject as yet. Various experiments, and conclusions drawn therefrom, are scattered throughout medical literature, but these are of no great practical value, as the investigations were carried on at different times, under varying conditions and on different subjects.

The task which the writers have undertaken is to study the saliva in a number of systemic diseases under as analogous conditions as possible, which is rendered more difficult by the fact that the literature existing on the subject is so little congruous and the results so far obtained are at a great variance.

For example, if we study the investigations of the saliva in febrile conditions, what a chaos confronts us. If investigators do not agree on the modifications of the salivary secretion in so ordinary a condition as a febrile disturbance, how much more lacking in unity must be the results of investigations of the oral fluid in chronic affections which present so many different phases and aspects.

The conclusions of this paper are the results of investigations which were carried on under as uniform and congruous conditions as possible concerning the saliva in: *a,* diabetes mellitus; *b,* uricacidæmia; *c,* gastric disease.

It is not our intention to enter into the details of this vast subject, as time is limited, but we simply present the results of certain examinations, which will be fully described and published in various journals at a later period.

Before studying the salivary secretion as it becomes modified by systemic disease, it is, perhaps, not out of place to define normal saliva.

Saliva, in the strictly physiologic sense of the word, implies the

[1] Read at the fifty-fifth annual session of the American Medical Association, in the Section on Stomatology, Atlantic City, June 7 to 10, 1904, copied from the Journal of the American Medical Association.

secretions of the parotid, the submaxillary, and sublingual glands. Ordinarily, however, the term denotes the aggregate secretions of all the glands pouring their contents into the buccal cavity; the sum total of all these secreta shall be spoken of as saliva in this paper, as it is impossible to obtain saliva in that condition in which it is secreted by the salivary glands proper, and before it becomes admixed with the other fluids and factors introduced into the mouth.

In order to collect any amount of saliva for measuring or examination, it becomes necessary either to introduce a sponge into the mouth to collect the fluid, or to instruct the subject, from whom the sample is to be taken, to keep the mouth open for some time, without swallowing, so as to permit the secretion to accumulate. Anything or any method that may be employed to collect the saliva directly, will act as a stimulant to the gland, by contact or reflexly, and when nothing is employed and the mouth is simply kept open, the muscular exertion of keeping the jaws apart, the air striking the oral mucous membrane, as also the psychical influence, will act as stimulants, and the saliva obtained is not true physiologic saliva, but saliva obtained by stimulation; hence the output of the gland is augmented and more fluid is obtained than would be secreted without the stimulant. However, as the fluid medium is but water, and the chemical factors and active principles are held in solution or suspension therein, it will facilitate matters, by only considering these organic and inorganic constituents of the secretion, irrespective of the solvent medium, and to define physiologic normal saliva as:

" The total amount of organic and inorganic material, elaborated and secreted by the salivary glands under normal conditions, *i.e.,* without undue stimulation by either drugs or other factors, irrespective of their fluid medium and without the admixture of excessive amounts of histologic elements."

Under normal conditions, but varying diet, the glandular cells may be taxed to perform varying amounts of work, for the ingestion of large amounts of soluble, assimilable elements which enter the blood-current may be followed by an increased output of salivary solids. As long as the system retains perfect metabolic equilibrium, and as long as no local disease obtains in the salivary glands, it does not matter how large the excretion of solid matter may be. The greater the amount of the solvent medium, up to a certain limit, the more perfect may be the excretion. However, it will always remain an open question whether the salivary solids should be completely excreted, or if a residue in the gland, of the same composition and concentration, is normal or not.

The variations that the saliva may be subject to in health may either be a change in the quantity secreted or an alteration in the composition. In order to ascertain any deviation from the normal, it becomes necessary to establish a standard as normal.

The actual amount of saliva secreted during twenty-four hours has been expressed in varying figures by different authors. However, as the activity of the glands is modified by many conditions, all of which must be considered normal, as diet, amount and nature of ingesta, the manner of eating and masticating, and also the psychic condition of the subject, and as all these factors do exert a positive influence on the organism and actually modify the secretion, and as it is impossible to have all these conditions congruous in any two cases, and as the results under unlike conditions must vary, figures are but relatively correct and cannot be accepted as the absolutely physiologically correct standard of the amount of fluid secreted. As figures will not express the normal amount of saliva secreted, for stated reasons, it will, perhaps, be physiologically correct to define the normal output of saliva as follows:

" The normal amount of saliva secreted is that which is put out without artificial stimulation (by drugs or any factor that will act as an irritant to the gland directly or reflexly) without the subject being aware of its secretion, irrespective of figures."

Having determined what can be called the normal output of saliva, what will be abnormal and what will be pathologic, and which can be classed as either?

Any condition beyond those productive of normal secretion will, of course produce an abnormal or pathologic action of the gland, but how to distinguish between these two, what is abnormal, what is pathologic?

" An abnormal secretion is one produced by artificial stimulation, as by drugs or any other factor producing an altered secretion."

" A pathologic secretion is one produced or altered by local or systemic disease."

Another property of the saliva that is expressed in greatly varying figures is the specific gravity of the fluid. Inasmuch as this property depends on the amount of solids contained in the secretion, it (specific gravity) also is subject to many modifications, and the absolute physiologically correct standard can only be obtained by determining the amount of solids in a given amount of normal saliva.

Experiments in this direction will also appear at a later period.

To study the question of modified saliva from all points of view would necessitate an accurate quantitative and qualitative analysis of the secretion in a normal state and the same examination of the fluid as secreted in disease. To do this at the present is impossible, as the glandular activity and the secretion itself are subject to many and rapid changes, so that no two examinations would show like results. Therefore, we confine ourselves to the study of such eventual alterations of the oral fluid which are not accidental and thus may become of practical value to the medical and dental diagnostician.

ALTERATIONS OF THE SALIVARY SECRETION IN DIABETES MELLITUS.

The saliva of one hundred and fifty-eight cases of diabetes mellitus was examined; altogether three hundred and eighty-four tests were made, from which the folowing data were obtained:

Alterations of the Quantity secreted.—The amount of saliva was found to be decidedly increased in six cases, decidedly diminished in eighty-nine cases, normal in sixty-three cases.

The subnormal secretion was very likely due to the same causes as is the diminution of the secreta of other glands in this disorder, namely, the increase of the urinary water.

In making these quantitative examinations, the samples were always obtained about two hours after breakfast (except where otherwise stated). In order to avoid any secretory changes due to psychical influences, the patient was requested to expectorate into a watch-glass, while being engaged in conversation. This was measured by a standard obtained by taking many hundred samples in the same fashion from healthy individuals. If the patient could bring forth but a few drops of saliva after repeated efforts, the secretion was called decidedly diminished; if, on the other hand, the amount expectorated would fill or flow over the watch-glass, it was termed decidedly increased.

The Reaction.—Acid in forty-seven cases (two hundred and fifteen examinations); alkaline in ninety-two cases (one hundred and sixteen examinations); neutral, eight cases (fourteen examinations; not examined, eleven cases.

The tests for the reaction were litmus paper and phenolphthalein.

ALTERATIONS IN COMPOSITION.

Glucose was found in the saliva in eighty-five cases (one hundred and eighty-one examinations), and no glucose was found in seventy-three cases (two hundred and three examinations).

The examinations for glucose were made with Nylander's solution, and with phenylhydrazin.

The diastatic quality was found unchanged in about ninety per cent. of the cases examined. A quantitative test for the conversion of amylum into maltose, glucose and dextrin was not made on account of the small amount of secretion obtained at a time.

Trommer's test was employed in these examinations; the tests were made at 40° C.

One gram of amylum was boiled with ten cubic centimetres of water and ten parts of the starch solution were mixed with one part of saliva and kept at 40° C. To this Trommer's solution was added. If the diastatic quality of the saliva is normal, a yellow precipitate, which later turns red, is formed in from fifteen to forty-five minutes. If the changes take place in from five to fifteen minutes, the diastatic property is increased, and if it takes longer than forty-five minutes for the reaction to take place, the diastatic property is subnormal.

All the cases in which glucose was demonstrated in the saliva were of undoubted genuine diabetic character, and in those cases where glucose could not be found in the oral secretion, although it was excreted in considerable amount in the urine, the glycosuria of some was apparently of non-diabetic origin. The cases of true diabetic glycosuria, after a rigid antidiabetic diet had been pursued for some time, so that the urine became free from sugar, exhibited the same changes in the salivary secretion, so that no salivary glucose could be demonstrated after the urinary sugar had disappeared. This fact would evidence the common hyperglycæmic origin of the glucose in both fluids. Again, the appearance of salivary glucose is by no means indicative of the severity of the diabetic condition, for the degree of the diabetic condition does not depend on the degree of hyperglycæmia. The milder cases of diabetes, at least those cases of well-established diabetes not influenced by dietary regulations, are often characterized by the excretion of very large amounts of urinary and salivary glucose. The reduction of the carbohydrates often causes a secession of the sugar in both fluids. In some of the graver cases of diabetes no glucose was found whatsoever in the saliva on any occasion. In one instance more than twelve examinations were made, and salivary glucose could not be demonstrated. These are the cases where, very likely, secondary glandular changes, sclerotic in character, had taken place and where no secretion whatsoever was going on.

ALTERATIONS OF THE SALIVARY SECRETION IN URICACIDÆMIA.

Twenty-eight cases were observed; fifty-nine examinations were made. These cases examined partly manifested symptoms of arthritis uritica, partly of chronic affections of the upper air-passages, and partly of contracted kidney and its consequences.

The saliva was found to be increased in not one case; was diminished in only one case.

The reaction was obtained by the same tests employed in diabetics, was found to be alkaline in fifty-two examinations, acid in five examinations, neutral in two examinations.

The diastatic quality in but eighteen examinations made was found normal thirteen times, somewhat subnormal three times, and decidedly subnormal twice.

Biliary pigments were looked for at fourteen examinations, and demonstrated but once by Gmelin's test.

Uric acid was looked for fifty-nine times, and demonstrated in the saliva but twenty-one times, the murexide test having been employed.

ALTERATIONS OF THE SALIVARY SECRETIONS IN SOME GASTRIC DISEASES.

All the examinations of the saliva in gastric disease were undertaken after the diagnosis had been made and before treatment had been begun, as medication would influence the saliva both systemically and locally.

Acute Gastritis.—Twenty cases were examined.

The quantity of saliva secreted was found to be increased in nine cases; in the others, about normal.

The reaction was found to be acid in eight cases, alkaline in twelve cases; acidity was found to be due to lactic acid in two cases.

Uffelmann's test was employed (modified, as it has been used in Dr. Stern's laboratory for some years; that is, salicylic acid is substituted for carbolic acid). Twice the acidity was found to be due to acetic acid (ferric chloride test), and in four cases the character of the acidity was not determnied.

Hyperchlorhydria.—One hundred and eighty-two cases examined gave the following results: An increased secretion was found in twenty-seven cases; the others showed a fairly normal secretion.

The reaction was found acid in seventy-one cases, alkaline in forty-one cases, neutral in five cases; amphoteric in all others, or in sixty-five cases,—that is, the secretion was both alkaline and acid; in other words, red litmus paper turned blue and blue paper turned red.

These facts are of interest to the stomatologist, as it shows that a hyperchlorhydric stomach does not always produce an acid saliva; also is it important to always use both red and blue litmus paper in testing the reaction of a secretion, as one or the other, used alone, is liable to mislead the examiner.

The acidity was found to be due to lactic acid in twelve cases, acetic acid in twelve cases, lactic-acetic acid in nine cases, inorganic acid (HCl) in six cases (Günzburg's test); in the others it was not demonstrated.

Hypochlorhydria.—Twenty-three cases were examined.

The quantity of saliva secreted was found to be decidedly increased in but one case; the other cases showed a fairly normal quantitative secretion.

The reaction was found to be acid in two cases, alkaline in fifteen cases, amphoteric in six cases; acidity was found to be due to lactic acid in one case, formic acid in one case.

Pyloric Stenosis.—Fifteen cases examined.

The secretion was found to be increased in three cases; balance fairly normal.

The reaction was found to be acid in five cases, alkaline in eight cases; in two cases the reaction was not determined. Acidity was found to be due to lactic acid in two cases, acetic acid in two cases, lactic-acetic-formic acid in one case.

REMARKS.

In presenting these data, obtained from over thirteen hundred individual examinations, we do not claim to have brought forth anything new or startling, but have applied old principles in a new direction, and the results obtained may not be of direct value presently, but they open new avenues for investigation which in course of time may become instrumental to shed light into pathways that at present are somewhat dark,—namely, the coherence or non-coherence of systemic and oral disease, what *rôle* the salivary secretion plays in these derangements, how it is affected by either, and the disclosure of this will entail new, better, and perhaps more successful treatment.

DISCUSSION ON PAPERS BY DRS. ALLAN AND STERN AND LEDERER.

Dr. Eugene S. Talbot, Chicago.—So far as malposition is concerned, the extraction of a tooth or teeth has great influence on the alveolar process and the dental arch. The irregularity of the arch (other than the local causes) is due to an unbalanced nervous system. The teeth that decay the most in this country and Europe are in those persons who suffer with nervous difficulties. They are found in the insane hospitals, schools of idiocy, and all institutions for degenerates. In a study of the teeth of nationalities it is found that the English lose their teeth sooner and irregularities are more common among them because evolution has gone on to a greater extent. Decay of the teeth next in frequency is in New England, and in the older parts of the country. Irregularities are also greater there than in the newer parts of this country. In pregnancy teeth decay faster; in neurasthenia the teeth begin to decay rapidly, and the same condition obtains in grief. How far the environment and the saliva have to do with this matter is a question. I believe these factors have something to do with it, but the experiments shown do not indicate the saliva has very much to do with the conditions. If the saliva be at fault, why does the decay not occur except at the approximal surfaces and the crowns? Why does it not occur at certain periods rather than others? These things must be taken into consideration in regard to the general condition of the system. I have been experimenting along certain lines to show from my stand-point why decay occurs in certain mouths more than it does in others. I believe that in disease, pregnancy, and in conditions of neurasthenia there is a want of resistance in the pulp which has as much to do with decay as any other cause. It is not often that acidity of the salivary glands takes place to a marked degree. It is unlike the urine, which

5

carries off the waste products. The saliva is a physiologic secretion for the purpose of digestion, and therefore diseased conditions are not expected to be found in the saliva of mouths where changes have taken place in the system, as in the urine.

Dr. Edward A. Bogue, New York City.—I hope that Dr. Talbot will not regard as unfriendly anything I may say. He has been for years gathering facts. These facts we accept, but not his conclusions. In the past twenty years not a child who has ever come into my hands and stayed there has ever had the toothache or ever lost a tooth. Not only that, but during that twenty years only five adults who have been in my hands have lost a good, firm tooth. Three of these were impacted molars; one was an upper wisdom-tooth and one was a right lateral incisor from a lady having an irregular row of teeth from which a number of teeth had been already lost. Dr. Talbot's remarks are so mingled with splendid truth and possible error in his statement that evolution shows loss of teeth that I cannot accept his conclusions. Whether the removal of the last molar which has been so extensively practised is going to result in nature excluding that tooth is a question. He also says that teeth are not necessary. Perhaps that is true, and perhaps not. For the present time we may look on teeth as necessary for our healthful existence, and the better we can keep them the better it will be for the individual's health. He also said that perfect occlusion was not necessary, and that what it had to do with decay of the teeth he could not see. Dr. Talbot says that the English people lose their teeth most frequently, and next in frequency the New England people; and he had just said that loss of teeth was especially noticeable in degenerates, *ergo,* the English people and the New England people are degenerates. That being the case, and these being the head nations of the earth, with them the whole world is degenerating. Dr. Talbot said that the loss of pulps and the destruction of the resisting power of the pulps tended toward decay. With this I heartily concur. He did not seem to know that that is in opposition to the statement of one of our profession who says that teeth do not need pulps after adult life. I also agree that prophylaxis begins as far back as Dr. Rhein has suggested, and as far back as Dr. Talbot suggests in his book, long before birth. And this brings us to Dr. Allan's paper. If the child is born in good health and has a constitution which is adequate to the eruption of good temporary teeth which perform their function in life and are shed at the proper moment and replaced by the permanent teeth in their proper position, there is no reason why those teeth should not last during the threescore years and ten almost without care. I have before spoken of a man fifty-two years of age who told me he had never had a tooth-brush in his mouth. Yet that man's teeth were clean and in good condition. The dental apparatus was so admirably arranged for the purpose of mastication that it not only did that part of the work thoroughly, but in the very act of mastication the teeth were cleansed by the flow of the saliva and by the friction of the food taken in. When civilization came and gave us soft food instead of hard, cooked food instead of fibrous and raw food, it did us a damage so far as the teeth are concerned. I find that where the occlusion and the arches are perfect there is very little decay; and acting on that principle during these last twenty years my results have been attained.

Dr. M. H. Cryer, Philadelphia.—Dr. Angle and others have used a picture made from a photograph of a negro skull which indicates considerable prognathism to illustrate the typical and normal occlusion of the teeth. In my paper on " Retarded Eruption of the Teeth: Their Liberation and Extraction," will be shown a fairly good illustration of the teeth of a Caucasian, which, in my opinion, gives a better standard than this photograph of the negro. Dr. Allan spoke of the teeth moving forward in the jaws. He said the crowns move forward, while the roots do not, thus causing the tipping of the teeth. In the normal jaw where there has been but little interference with its physiologic functions, the roots will advance in the same proportion as the crowns. The cancellated tissue of the alveolar process, in which the teeth are developed and retained, moves forward in mass, but when the physiologic functions or any portion of this cancellated tissue has been interfered with by either pathologic means or mechanical appliances, then the crowns may tip forward or twist because the cancellated tissue, holding the roots, is more or less withheld.

Dr. N. S. Hoff, Ann Arbor.—I think the value of a perfect occlusion of the teeth is one of the most important facts that Dr. Angle has brought into prominence by his work. It has its bearing not only as a prophylactic measure, but on operative procedures in filling teeth. Much injury has come to the teeth by the use of amalgams, cements, and other plastic filling-materials, because it is impossible to restore the contour of the teeth with them. We all know that amalgam is liable to change form, and that cements are transitory in character. The teeth tip out of their normal positions because an incline plane is made as an occlusal surface where a cusp is the natural condition. There is but one material that can be successfully employed to restore the cusps of the teeth as they ought to be, and that is gold. Many operators prevent recurrence of decay with gold fillings which securely stop the cavity, but the occlusal surface of the tooth is put into such form that it changes its place or position in occlusion. It does not occlude in a proper manner to perform its function. Many a filling, for lack of contour, provides a condition between the teeth which favors destruction of the gum, by irritation, or perhaps ulceration, which may result in so-called pyorrhœa, which is often nothing more than an inflammatory condition caused by the impact of food in the interdental spaces. The attention of the profession has not been properly called to the value of restoring the cusps of the grinding teeth to their original form for the purpose of preserving the surrounding gum tissue and also for preserving these teeth in their proper articular relations. Dr. Allan said it could be done with porcelain. I have no doubt it can in a measure be done with higher fusing porcelain, but the tendency of porcelain is to flatten in fusing and thus lose the valuable cusps. The crown surfaces are too often made without regard to their articular relations; inlays are made to conform to cavity margins only. The restoration of natural cusps is one of the most important features in operative dentistry, and I would emphasize the necessity for it because I think it is being overlooked in the present agitation for cavity extension, and in the increasing use of the plastics and inlays which are made only to accurately fit cavity margins.

Dr. G. V. I. Brown, Milwaukee.—It seems to me that Dr. Lederer is in a way to reach the pith of the question. What we want to know first of all is the relation between urine, an excretory product, and saliva, that which is simply a secretion for a specific physiologic purpose. I believe that the work which Dr. Kirk has done is going to give our branch of this great profession a standing which it has never had, and I believe examination of saliva will ultimately be accepted as one of the standards of physical diagnosis. I speak of it to illustrate the broadness of this subject and to warn against using terms, such as perfect occlusion and various other expressions, that may be construed in a narrow way and misunderstood when they get into cold print. It seems to me that "typical occlusion" and "perfect occlusion" are vastly different. I have an illustration of a condition due to malocclusion pure and simple. Dr. Talbot will tell you the condition is due to degeneracy. Dr. Cryer will tell you that he can prove conclusively the influence of the want of development and the want of symmetry, and both would be right, yet we, in our treatment of the case, depended simply on correction of the occlusion. Another illustration is along similar lines and represents a case of nervous spasm, tic douloureux, cured by grinding down the teeth and removal of the pulp. Another is apparently the same condition associated with disturbance of the salivary secretion, which was markedly different from other saliva. Another condition represented is due, as we believe, to miliary tubercle, from which the patient finally died. Another is due to malopposed teeth. We ought to be particular about cataloguing such things all under one head.

Dr. *M. L. Rhein,* New York City.—I sympathize with Dr. Brown's desire that we should be very particular about our statements. I agree with him about the question of a perfect occlusion. I think that a perfect occlusion is too radical a remark. I have made a chemical analysis of oral secretions in a number of cases of diabetes mellitus and simple glycosuria, but I have never published the result. Dr. Lederer speaks of "salivary secretions." He has no right to make use of that term. It is saliva mixed with oral secretions, and to a large extent is the secretion from the mucous follicles. I may be at fault in my criticism.

Dr. *Brown.*—When we speak of a condition due to pathologic change of some organ or organs of the body, and undertake to show that coincident with such disease there may, by examination of the salivary secretion, be determined certain distinct pathognomonic changes in its character under chemical or microscopic study which can be recognized by reaction or the form of crystals, or in any other way as sufficiently indicative to warrant dependence in basing a diagnostic opinion, then it goes without saying there must first be accurate methods of excluding from the tests all results of mixtures with other fluids and agents in the mouth, since saliva, as we recognize it, is a mixed product, and since it is equally true that dependence in leading to diagnosis of more or less remote disease must be placed on results apparent from the true physiologic secretion of the salivary glands, and until this can be done the results must be largely influenced by oral conditions and necessarily variable.

Dr. Rhein.—In order to speak of saliva, it is necessary for us to draw that saliva from the ducts or the glands as the catheter would draw the urine from the bladder before it passes through the urethra and is not allowed to come into contact with the urethral glands. The catheter-drawn urine and the ordinary urine are different. In the mouth the difference is still more marked. Dr. Lederer speaks of examining the saliva by having the patients spit. It is impossible for that to be saliva. I have devoted a vast amount of attention to the clinical observation of the fluids of the mouth, and have examined over five thousand cases of guinea-pigs infected with tuberculosis, and the clinical observation in every one of them was identical, and it has been of such value to me that I can tell a case of tuberculosis of the lungs at once by inspection of the mouth. This is not necessarily saliva. The saliva, so far as we can judge from our clinical experience with the salivary glands, is one that is less apt to be infected by general pathologic conditions than the mucous follicles of the mouth and the other secretory organs which do not excrete materials, especially for physiologic functions. Until a method can be evolved by which the secretion from the salivary gland can be examined without mixture with the other fluids of the mouth, all the statistics that Dr. Lederer has presented to us are absolutely valueless. They do not at all correspond with facts according to my observations. The very things he tells us in regard to the acidity and alkalinity in the same line of cases illustrate that there is something substantially wrong. The error lies in the fact that a great many of these cases are of acid reaction from the mucous follicles where there is likely nothing of this kind from the saliva itself. The prophylactic care of the mouth—and I prefer that term to prophylaxis, because I do not think the noun is well adapted to the purpose—has been very well presented to us by Dr. Allan. To preserve the occlusion as nearly akin to perfection as possible, it must naturally be started almost, as Dr. Bogue said, before birth. Dr. Talbot misunderstands my views in regard to the value of the pulp. I have never said that the teeth of adults would be better off without the pulp. No one appreciates the value of the pulp in the tooth more than I do. What I have said is that in a large number of diseases, especially of the arthritic and sclerotic types, when we see pulp-disease inviting constant trouble, removal of those pulps is of the utmost value to the patients. I agree with Dr. Hoff relative to the filling up of the cusps so that the occlusion will be perfect. I have replaced the rubber dam many times on an operation to add to the cusps of my molars or bicuspids where I failed to get the occlusion that should be normal under such circumstances. I do, however, disagree with him when he says that only the high-fusing porcelains can be used. I have too many cases of the Jenkins body that had been used in bicuspids and molars where I have absolute restoration of occlusion. There is an objection to the use of porcelain in these cases. The number of favorable cases, as Dr. Allan has outlined, is rare, because of the difficulty of obtaining the filling as near perfection as possible. I claim that when a porcelain inlay is inserted it should be so closely adapted to the margin of the enamel that the line is almost imperceptible. If that is not obtainable, a gold restoration is by far the more serviceable.

Dr. Vida A. Latham, Chicago.—I would like to draw the attention of the Section to work done by Dr. Joseph M. Flint in the *American Journal of Anatomy,* vol. i., No. 3, on the structure of the submaxillary gland. It is one of the most profound histologic researches ever made in this connection. There are new theories, new facts, and new methods of investigation which will certainly make a great difference in our future work. He is now, I believe, at work on the second part of the contribution. I should like to ask, How much do the deposits that occur on the teeth bear on the question of salivary or oral secretions? There are cases where a set of teeth may be typical to that type of person. There has been no disturbance, when suddenly the teeth become sensitive and there is a discharge of secretion from the glands of the gingival surfaces. The condition may be due to the saliva which produces irritation. I have a case now in which a V-shaped piece is dissolved or eroded at the cervical border, and if teeth are extracted the patient is relieved from neuralgia. I simply bring this question up, because there is something in the relation of the deposits of the teeth with prophylaxis.

Dr. Brown.—I have been criticised, and I want to make myself clear. It seems to me that the remarks are unnecessary, because the author very clearly distinguishes between saliva of the mouth and of the glands. Until we can distinguish these differences which are due to mixture and to other conditions of the mouth from the saliva pure and simple, we are not warranted in ascribing the condition of the saliva to constitutional diseases.

Dr. Rhein.—I think it is wrong to speak of the oral secretions and claim that they are saliva.

Dr. Allan.—It is such investigations as those of Dr. Lederer, involving great labor and serious inroads on one's time, that dignify our profession and lead to practical results. In relation to the use of the word "saliva," which has been so much criticised by one of the speakers, I wish to say that there is the best of authority for such use. Gould ascribes saliva as "the mixed secretion of the parotid, submaxillary, and sublingual glands and the small mucous glands of the mouth," and Gould is supported by general usage. Dr. Hoff said that porcelain restoration, such as I have referred to, would have to be made by the use solely of high heat porcelain; but, as Dr. Rhein has so well observed, it can be as well or better done by low heat porcelain and with equally good results.

Dr. Lederer.—In answer to Dr. Rhein, I would say that he came in late, and did not hear the first part of the paper, therefore he cannot accuse me of using a misnomer. No one has as yet made an accurate quantitative or qualitative analysis of any oral secretion, and as we can only work with what can actually be obtained in a normal condition, we must be satisfied with the mixed secretion of all the oral glands. I think Dr. Rhein is doing a great injustice to humanity at large by not telling how he is able to diagnose tuberculosis and diabetes by simple oral inspection; he is withholding a good thing, of inestimable value, from the general medical profession.

PROPHYLAXIS: ITS VARIOUS PHASES IN RELATION TO CONSERVATION OF THE TEETH.[1]

BY CHARLES F. ALLAN, M.D., NEWBURGH, N. Y.

I WANT to make a broad distinction between reparative and restorative operations, and to weigh relatively the importance, from a tooth-saving point of view, of some prophylactic measures.

---

[1] Read at the fifty-fifth annual session of the American Medical Association, in the Section on Stomatology, Atlantic City, June 7 to 10, 1904, copied from the Journal of the American Medical Association.

Broadly speaking, prophylaxis, the prevention of disease, should be the highest aim of the physician. In our specialty of medicine we are nearer, perhaps, concrete facts than the general practitioner; the organs that furnish us our principal work are in sight and lesions are generally visible and within reach, and possibly it is not asking too much of the average patient to expect more of us in the way of prevention than in the warding off of disease by the family physician. Certainly if we do not accomplish quite as much, we are very culpable.

Prophylaxis is prevention—prevention of what? Not simply the loss of teeth by caries, nor added to it the loss of few or many teeth by pyorrhœa, but it means the prevention of the loss of the full comfortable use of thirty-two teeth through the whole or main part of possibly a long life. I do not think this at all a too high ideal to have before us. At present, in a large majority of cases, we certainly will not reach to this standard.

The great controlling factor in relation to immunity or non-immunity from caries has reference to the condition of the secretions of the mouth. We are now in the early stages of our examinations in the histo-chemistry of the saliva, and though we have a limited knowledge of the conditions making for decay, we are as yet unprepared and unable to change those conditions to one of immunity. Often we will not have the complete support of the patient in the matter of hygienic cleanliness, without which we are powerless to accomplish the best results; and it will also generally be impossible for any one person to have the consecutive management of many mouths extending over a series of years dating from childhood, without which the best services canot be rendered.

Still, prophylaxis is steadily gaining; hygienic cleanliness is being more and more insisted on by the dentist and more and more practised by our patients, and this greatly offsets environment. With better modes of treatment and a more careful living up to the high ideals of nature, we have every reason for encouragement.

The high standard of success here outlined in the salvation of the teeth involves of necessity a knowledge of the perfection of the normal conditions of the tissues and organs of the mouth; this in the environment of the teeth, in the teeth themselves and in their arrangement, and in the relation of the teeth of one jaw to the teeth of the opposing jaw.

I have placed at the head of these phases of necessary normal conditions that of environment; and yet if I am asked to describe what I consider a normal environment, mainly, of course, with reference to the juices of the mouth, I can only say I cannot tell. So far the chemical constitution of what may be called normal saliva has, to my knowledge, never been described and I think cannot be; that is, in its exhaustive and ultimate analysis within the varying limits of what still may be termed normal.

We occasionally hear of the rare case of an aged person who has never been to a dentist and who never has lost a tooth, and very, very much more rarely we meet such a person, but in what respect the saliva of this *rara avis* has differed from the mouth secretions of the ordinary individual we do not absolutely know.

We do know that Dr. Michaels (to whose investigations in the histo-chemistry of the saliva I will shortly refer) found that a hypoacid condition of the saliva was generally associated with rapid destruction of tooth tissue, and the hyperacid condition was associated with comparative immunity from decay. The researches of Drs. Kirk, Kyle, and others confirm those of Dr. Michaels. We know also that the immunity from caries in the rare cases I have referred to has not been as the result of extraordinary cleanliness. The deduction seems obvious.

The researches of Black, Williams, and others have proved to us that, in the main, the physical conditions of the teeth of different individuals of adult age are substantially the same, and the facts that are before us every day, showing the wide difference of conditions of tooth preservation, all point to a cause for tooth destruction, outside of the teeth themselves; this means, of course, in their environment, and this is now universally recognized.

In August, 1900, before the Third International Dental Congress, Dr. Michaels, of Paris, read a paper on " Sialo-Semeiology," which was a record, with deductions therefrom, of a long series of examinations and analyses in connection with the histo-chemistry of the oral secretions. The limits of my paper preclude even a *résumé* of this paper, but he clearly proved the intimate relation of immunity from caries with certain conditions found in the saliva, and he found radically different conditions of the saliva where caries in a mouth were rampant.

Though by no means exhaustive, Dr. Michaels's investigations were most carefully made, and his results and deductions have been amply confirmed by other investigators.

To quote a truism of medicine put in simple words, " It is a well-known clinical and laboratory fact that a study of the products of the secreting organs, which in their excreting functions throw off waste material, gives us by deduction a fair idea of what process is going on within the body." This being true, why, as an index of systemic condition, would not the study of the saliva give as good an idea as the study of the urine, especially as the latter is solely a waste product, while in the saliva, swallowed as soon as excreted, we have products of metabolism which return into the system as a part of a physiologic process?

The bearing of all this on tooth destruction is, of course, even more intimate than I have suggested above in connection with general systemic conditions, for the teeth are bathed in the secretions of the mouth and are exposed continuously to the fermentative and bacterial results of their environment.

The present relation of prophylaxis in this connection is as follows: We know the distinctive condition of the saliva, as found by Dr. Michaels and others, when related to rapid decay of the teeth; we know another distinctive condition of saliva seemingly always associated with immunity from decay; but I am afraid to say that as yet we know how to influence nutrition to that point that we can change the one undesirable condition to the one that means tooth preservation.

The study of the histo-chemistry of the saliva is one involving organic chemistry of the most intimate nature, and requiring an immense amount of laboratory detail and the study of formulæ and analyses requiring any amount of time. The advance already made is very great, and the introduction of the micropolariscope, according to Dr. Kirk, is a most valuable aid. To know the actual condition from which we require relief is a great point gained.

Drs. Kyle, Milligan, and others, in connection with hay-fever, ozæna, and diathetic and nervous diseases of various kinds, have gathered diagnostic indications from the saliva that have secured successful treatment and have proved to them of the greatest professional value. We are pointed in the right direction, with a solid substratum of facts to work up from. Laborers in this field are very necessary, and the reward, how to help secure immunity from caries, is the greatest that can be put before the dentist.

We cannot conceive of any period when absolute hygienic cleanliness in the mouth will not be necessary, but up to that time in the future when we shall be able to change by treatment the destructive character of the mouth secretions, this same hygienic cleanliness, as advocated and practised by its well-known exponent in Philadelphia, is, and will be, our best sheet-anchor for the preservation of the teeth. So much has been written by him, and his principles and practice are so well approved by the profession in the main, though not in all details, that it would be supererogatory for me to add any words.

Normal occlusion, that is, occlusion as opposed to malocclusion, as described so well by Dr. Angle in his record work on "Orthodontia," is a very necessary factor in prophylaxis. The knuckling up of the several teeth against one another, thereby securing for each tooth under stress the support of all the teeth of the arch, is most necessary and most helpful, and is provocative of comfort and tooth preservation. Now, when we add to this the perfect normal relation of the teeth of the mandible to the teeth of the upper jaw, that perfect relation of the planes and cusps of the teeth of the two jaws to one another, we have an ideal arrangement, a perfection of mechanical adaptation and artistic lines better than which we cannot conceive of; so, when we have before us a case of malocclusion to correct, it is this perfect ideal we must try to work up to, and we must always remember that the Almighty found thirty-two teeth none too many for the purposes of his perfect work, and it is not at all likely that we can do as well with less.

Now, the practical application of this matter of normal occlusion to prophylaxis lies in the interdependence of one tooth on another, as mentioned above. It lies in the fact that each tooth in a normal arch is necessary to the best welfare of every other tooth, and that you can not remove one tooth without injuring all. The natural tendency of the back teeth, in the absence of mesial support, is to move forward, and unfortunately that tendency is not to move *en masse,* but to follow the line of least resistance and seemingly pivot on the ends of the roots, the crowns tilting, with the effect of not only destroying to a great extent the mutual support of adjoining teeth, but also destroying more or less that perfect relation of the teeth of the two jaws to one another.

All irregularities of the teeth, and especially all losses of teeth, are provocative of further trouble. The proper interdigitation of the cusps of the teeth of one jaw in the sulci of the teeth of the opposing jaw is interfered with, the area of masticating surface is reduced, and what remains is usually not in as good condition for service. Some of the teeth no longer have the stress of use along the line of the axis of the roots, and the tilting continuously increases. The malocclusion affects also certain teeth that otherwise would be in normal health by putting on them unusual strain, and that strain in a direction the teeth are not expected to bear, with the result of loosened teeth in diseased sockets. The tendency of all such maloccluded teeth is to get lame and loose and to be early subjects for pyorrhœa, and in the end the forceps. Teeth irregularly placed in the jaws are difficult to keep clean, and are much more prone to caries, and in more ways than I have time to speak of malocclusion tends to tooth loss. Proper occlusion, especially when attended to early in life, is an eminently important factor in prophylaxis.

Tooth loss is mainly occasioned by departure from the high ideals established for us by Nature. The teeth, generally erupting with normal shapes and with normal structure and physical conditions, are, by reason of perverted environment, subjected to caries. Caries generally means repair, and, in the fullest sense of the word, should mean restoration; and it is this in many cases incomplete repair and hardly at all restoration that is a great cause of tooth destruction. To give a broad generalization in one short clause, we should live up to nature.

All of these many years, in which we have made so many and great advances as a profession, we have been handicapped by the fact that we have had no filling-material that was at all ideal. Amalgam, tin, gutta-percha, cements, have all done us great and good service, and, above all, gold. The latter is a royal metal, and has done our patients a royal amount of good, but restoration has been a restoration of contour only; not a restoration of color and appearance; not a restoration of thermal non-conductivity; not a restoration of the vitreous polished enamel surface which is of such immense importance; and this lack of restoration has generally been at the expense of serious distress to our patients; often of serious physical and nervous strain to the operator. Drs. Varney and Webb, and others as well, practically gave their lives to establishing their high ideals of tooth restoration, and then their ideals failed in the above-mentioned serious respects. All glory to them, however; they were in advance of their fellows, and we are greatly better dentists by having had their ideals to work up to.

Now the relation of all this to prophylaxis lies in the fact that in just these important matters in which tooth restoration fails with gold, it is a success with porcelain. The vitreous polished surface, practically continuous with the enamel surface, the non-conductivity of the material, its comparative ease of insertion at an immense saving of time, pain, and nervous strain, are all important respects in which the prophylactic value of porcelain transcends that of other materials.

Again, I cannot go into details, but it is entirely practical in the great majority of cases to fill the occluso-proximal cavities of the bicuspid and molar teeth with porcelain, at a great saving of strain and pain to the patient, with a perfect restoration of contour made in the furnace and not in the patient's mouth. Some of you, I fear, will dissent from this statement, but I want to go on record as saying that it is practical, and that such restorations, if properly made, will be permanent.

For the sake of brevity, I have instanced only occluso-proximal cavities, because they are, possibly, the most difficult and the necessities of such cases are greater, but the principles involved are the same with all proximal fillings, and the essential saving conditions are just as evident.

The last few years have developed an immense amount of literature on prophylaxis, but it has been of the narrow kind that has seen but one phase of the subject, and for that has claimed the earth. All of you know that prophylaxis is many-sided,—has, indeed, many more sides than I have had time to indicate,—and that though hygienic cleanliness is one phase, and that a very important one, it is still not all there is that stands for the prevention of the loss of the teeth.

The investigations of Michaels, which include an immense amount of painstaking laboratory work, have opened up a field of activity whose promise is very great.

In the language of the very reserved and modest claim made by the eminent editor of the *Dental Cosmos,* " Dr. Michaels has thrown a ray of scientific light on the problem of dental prophylaxis, and has clearly indicated the direction from which greater light on the problem may be expected to come."

Dr. Angle, in his great work on malocclusion, has treated his subject in a scientific manner quite beyond anything hitherto attempted, and in the simplicity of his classification and in the clear idea he has given us of the ideal we are always to work up to, with methods and apparatus most simple of use, has given the profession great aid in treatment, which in so many cases makes for prophylaxis.

To this should be added a word of tribute to the enthusiastic and earnest labors of Dr. Jenkins, stretching over many years and all to the end that tooth-structure might be imitated and that tooth repair might mean tooth restoration in the fullest and best sense of the word.

Other names could be added to this brief list, but these I have mentioned seem to me typical of the best, in that they have obtained their important results only because of great labor, backed up by most earnest enthusiasm.

It is such enthusiasm that in the end will conquer for tooth salvation. It is such enthusiasm that always conquers.

Reports of Society Meetings.

THE NEW YORK INSTITUTE OF STOMATOLOGY.

A MEETING of the Institute was held at the " Chelsea," No. 222 West Twenty-third Street, New York, November, 1904, the President, Dr. A. H. Brockway, in the chair.

The minutes of the last meeting were read and approved.

The regular business of the evening was opened by Dr. J. F. P. Hodson, who presented several useful appliances and methods.

Dr. Hodson.—I shall present this evening a number of little helps that are familiar to me in my practice, but some of which may be new to you.

First.—A combination of flexible steel holding point, with ball and socket jointed mirror, to hold in the left hand while starting gold fillings in deeply placed approximal and posterior cavities, until the fillings shall have become self-anchored.

Second.—A little thin, saucer-like attachment to be slipped over the back and edge of the mouth-mirror for catching pieces of amalgam as it is being carried into a cavity, or bits of gold while cutting out a gold stopping, instead of letting them drop into the mouth or on the dam. It can be slipped on or off from the mirror in an instant. Every operator should accustom himself to operating in the mirror, held in the left hand to reflect the operation; it transforms difficult of access, posterior cavities into easy ones, and even when not so needed, is still of great value in the left hand for throwing a ball of light upon the work.

Third.—An old engine hand-piece that has been locked, making an excellent socket for a hand bur.

Fourth.—For very many years I have had manufactured for me the round cedar sticks for cleansing teeth. I still use them for that purpose, and I have found, when they have worn short, that a convenient way of lengthening them is to put them into an ordinary penholder with the pen part removed.

Fifth.—A pair of amalgam carriers, that I use more than all my other amalgam carriers put together, one for forward and the other for backward work.

Sixth.—In connection with amalgam, some know, and some do not seem to, how to trim the margins of amalgam stoppings under the gum, judging from the ragged masses which we often see hardened under the gum. The best instrument for that purpose is a thin, round, flexible, old-fashioned canal-plugger, which, carried along that edge, will clean the margin perfectly, and, followed with a thin, flat burnisher, will leave as perfect edges under the gum as above it.

Seventh.—A mouth-mirror with the glass broken out makes an excellent scoop for catching up bits of amalgam or gold from the rubber dam.

Eighth.—A rubber apron, that I always adjust the moment the patient gets into the chair. A so-called improvement has been made upon mine by some one, consisting of a pocket to catch the saliva and hold it. I think that is merely filthy. With this apron the patient's clothes are kept neat and clean from drops of water, saliva, etc. The patient is made comfortable with the thought that her clothes will not be spotted. The white towel is of course placed over it. I get this material by the yard at a very small price, and all the work of making them consists in sewing on the neck tape.

Ninth.—To go back to amalgam stoppings, for finishing them off and wiping margins I use a piece of wet spunk instead of cotton, as it gives a much finer grain and is much smoother.

Tenth.—The paper points for drying root-canals that I presented to you a good many years ago are an illustration of a principle that I apply as such very largely in my practice,—the principle of capillary attraction. It is astonishing what can be done by means of it. In drying out root-canals a piece of cotton on a broach will push material ahead of it, possibly carrying the septic material beyond the apex of the root, while these paper points made from bibulous paper will attract the moisture and absorb it instead of driving it ahead. Syringing a root-canal will never cleanse it, but three or four floodings alternated with the paper point absorbings will certainly do so. The points are made from the French bibulous paper. They are also sold by Johnson & Johnson.

Eleventh.—The principle of capillary attraction suggests conditions allied thereto. For instance, I never find it necessary to make retaining points in building amalgam on to an old amalgam stopping for the purpose of repairing it. It is sufficient to first make the surface of the old filling, in that part where the repair is to be made, perfectly bright and clean, and then tinning that surface with a portion of very thinly mixed amalgam. The new amalgam takes perfect hold of this, being a cold soldered joint.

Twelfth.—I also use this principle in filling thin, winding root-canals, and, in fact, all others as well. I fill my root-canals with chloropercha and gutta-percha. By wetting a fine smooth broach with the chloropercha and carrying it to the end of these small canals, and in this position touching it with a drop of chloropercha, capillary attraction will surely carry it to the end of the canal. This, however, is in my hands only the preparation for the root-filling. The chloropercha is merely to cement the gutta-percha point that I stick to the end of a nerve-canal instrument and gently carry to the end of the canal. The root is thus filled surely to the end, no air-bubbles, and the minimum of the chloropercha.

Thirteenth.—Many years ago Dr. Merriam showed us a method of making gutta-percha stoppings stick in wet cavities by taking a piece of gutta-percha on the proper instrument, warming it, and carrying it to the cavity immediately after having dipped it in oil of cajuput. As the surface of such gutta-percha stoppings will not wear well, it is best to use this method only for very temporary stoppings or for the first part of a stopping where it is intended to dry out the remainder of the cavity and fill with a stronger gutta-percha. I have sometimes filled the collar-like cavities around the necks of teeth with a modification of this method, drying out the cavity as well as possible, then touching with the oil of cajuput and applying the stopping. It is astonishing how well the gutta-percha will stick with this method.

Fourteenth.—Another bit of advising born of my own experience as a patient. When I was a boy student a dentist who at that time stood in the very front rank for ability and skill, while condensing a gold filling in my mouth, brought all his power upon the instrument held *off hand,* and the instrument slipped and went through my cheek. Since which time I have never made even the smallest move in the mouth which was not guarded by a fulcrum or rest, formed by the third finger end on the teeth for fingers grasp, and by the thumb for the fist grasp of the instrument, and I can truthfully say that in consequence I have never in my life let an instrument slip to hurt a patient.

Fifteenth.—Speaking of slipping instruments reminds me of a matter somewhat akin to it. It may happen at very rare intervals, even with the most skilful operator, that in the hurried changing of an instrument during an operation he may catch it in the rubber dam and make a rent. The need for a stopper is most instant and urgent. I suggested such a remedy many years ago. It consists of a section sawed from a cork, filed oval on both sides, and a deep groove running all round the edge, thus making it like two thin oval buttons placed back to back. A half-dozen sizes kept at hand will fit all possible rents, and the proper-sized one quickly stretched therein will effectually dam out all moisture,—will hold its place perfectly and all without being in the way, even though it be in the immediate vicinity of the filling.

Dr. G. W. Weld.—I wish first to mention one little point in connection with Jenkins's little tray for fusing inlays. The trays that come with the Jenkins outfit are composed of some composition other than platinum, and repeated heating quickly burns them out. I have remedied this by riveting to the bottom of the little pan a platinum disk. I find this will stand the heat splendidly. It will be necessary to put five rivets in; this makes practically a platinum pan.

What I wish to show specially is home-made impression cups for porcelain inlays. The subject is not entirely new, and these cups have been placed upon the market, but I have found them of little practical value to the dentist. We all know that the foundation of a perfect inlay is a correct impression or a correct matrix, or both. If the matrix can be taken directly from the cavity it will save time, and is often done. I have done it myself, and have had beautiful fits. But there are thousands of cases where this cannot be done. But with a correct model of the cavity set in a piece of plaster it is very easy to tease the matrix away from it, whether it be of·gold or platinum. Therefore, when I can I use an impression. It follows that to take an impression of a cavity you must have a proper cup to do it with. Take, for instance, two approximal cavities between the central incisor teeth, where the front plate of enamel is intact but extremely thin. Porcelain inlays are indicated here for the reason that there is great danger in fracturing the enamel walls in putting in a gold filling. A right and left impression cup is here needed. They are made of platinoid, but can be made from German silver. A little piece of the platinoid is cut out the proper size and shape, and to this is soldered another piece of the same material to serve as a handle. In this way a perfect impression cup can be made, using the smallest quantity of impression material possible; a surplus being as bad as an insufficiency. The impression is then set with the convex surface upward in a little plaster, and after that has hardened the surface is painted with talcum powder. Stiff Harvard or Ames cement is then pressed down on the impression and allowed to remain for some time. When hard, the model thus made is set in a piece of plaster. Then the gold can be easily teased away without injuring its shape.

The most simple cavities are the cavities on the labial surfaces of the front teeth. Here it is easy to take the matrix directly from the cavity. Indeed, there are cases of compound cavities where I have succeeded better with this direct method. Sometimes it is better not to make the little holes in the cup, designed to hold the material better, thus allowing the cup to be removed first, and taking out the impression afterwards.

Dr. W. D. Tracy.—Inasmuch as this society seemed last year to take such an active interest in orthodontia, I thought it would not be amiss to show some little instruments I have devised to assist in the adjustment of the Angle bands. The set consists of three instruments, which I shall pass around together with a band fitted upon a model. The conditions on the model are somewhat exaggerated for illustration. The working face of the instruments are finely serrated, so that they will not slip when used with heavy pressure to carry this band in contact with the tooth.

Dr. Hodson spoke of trimming the cervical margin of amalgam fillings with a canal-plugger.

In my own experience something more rigid than the instrument shown by Dr. Hodson is necessary, because the amalgam, being packed quite dry, hardens quickly. To meet the requirements of trimming all kinds of fillings on the approximal surface I have had made this pair of right and left trimmers, which I submit to your criticism.

Dr. S. H. McNaughton.—I wish to present some two-angled excavators—hatchets and hoes—which have been very useful to me. In the preparation of cavities in the approximal surfaces of teeth in which plastic fillings are to be inserted, and where it is desirable to save as much enamel as possible as a protection to the filling, by means of these instruments all the angles may be reached and all the decay removed without the necessity of much loss of enamel. The width of blade is three-, four-, or five-tenths of a millimetre, the length of blade three times the width; the first angle (the angle nearest the cutting edge) is twenty-five centigrades (ninety degrees), the second angle is twelve and five-tenths centigrades (forty-five degrees)—and should be the length of blade from the first angle; the direction at this angle should be to the left, or to the right, or in same direction as at first angle. These constitute the three shapes and sizes which are indispensable to me.

In filling large occlusal cavities where one or both approximal surfaces are involved, where the walls are frail and badly broken away, especially lower molars, I make use of a combination, filling in the following manner: I use a matrix made from a section of a ping-pong ball. Instead of first placing zinc phosphate over the floor and partly on the buccal and lingual walls, as is ordinarily done, I first pack amalgam against the gingival wall, the matrix to the occlusal edge, and the margins of the buccal and lingual walls. When this has been done I have a cavity with four walls and a floor, which may be filled two-thirds or entirely with zinc phosphate. If but partially filled with the zinc phosphate, it may be completed with amalgam, in which case it has the appearance of an all-amalgam filling. The advantages of a filling of this kind are: The amalgam is keyed in by the cement; it is held while setting in perfectly close contact with the walls, so much so that in removing one of these fillings it seems to adhere to the walls as tightly as does a copper amalgam plug. There will be no washing out at the gingival margin, as is likely to be with zinc phosphate; it holds its shape better than gutta-percha. There are other classes of cavities in which this method or variations of it may be used.

As an investment for soldering I use a mixture of equal parts of modelling clay, coarse powdered pumice, and ground asbestos, which I keep wet in a fruit-jar, by which means it is always ready. It is especially good for small pieces, and it holds very tightly. It does not set. As a support for it a piece of coarse iron wire netting is used. Wax will be burnt off in the heating.

Dr. F. L. Fossume.—Right lower central incisor missing, and patient wearing a small rubber plate with an artificial substitute. This rubber plate impinged on the gums and lingual surfaces of the necks of the teeth which were denuded. The teeth were slightly loose but otherwise in perfect condition.

I inserted a dummy in the following manner: The central and lateral incisors on either side of the space were ground lingually in the centre at the cutting edge, forming a hollow into which pure gold 40-gauge was burnished. Rivet holes were bored near the wall approximating the space. Platino-iridium wire about the thickness of the pin in a rubber tooth was forced through the gold into the holes and bent so as to meet the backing of the dummy to be inserted. The gold lining and pin in position, they were tacked together with hard wax and soldered; then they were placed back on the teeth and an impression taken in plaster. The dummy was now ground, backed, and waxed into place. The whole piece was invested and the backing soldered to the rivet wire and gold, with 22-carat solder. Solder was allowed to flow on the gold only along and over the platino-iridium wire. The cavities prepared in the cutting edges were now undercut at sides distally to the approximating space, where the rivet holes were bored. After polishing the backing, the piece was cemented into place and the thin gold hammered into the undercut and built up with gold-foil the same as in any other cavity. The whole thing was then polished and burnished; the only gold visible was a small half-moonshaped filling on the cutting edge on the central and lateral on either side of the dummy.

Dr. F. Milton Smith.—Previous to entering upon the discussion of these various subjects, I have the privilege of presenting to the Institute some radiographs sent me by Dr. C. Edmund Kells, of New Orleans.

While Dr. Kells did not send these for exhibition, I have taken the liberty of bringing them here, that you may get an inkling of Dr. Kells's work in this line.

Dr. J. Bond Littig.—I can verify Dr. McNaughton's statement with regard to asbestos and clay as an investment. I have used for many years a little ordinary moulding sand with asbestos. I put it upon a piece of wire gauze and put the piece to be soldered right into it, and without waiting for it to thoroughly harden heat it up and let the moisture dry out. In ten minutes I can have my piece soldered. I have, as I say, been doing this for many years, and you can find it published in "Catching's Compendium," 1890.

Dr. Chas. O. Kimball.—I have lately encountered a case where the X-ray was of great assistance. A little girl about nine years old presented with a left lateral in a very markedly crooked condition. When we came to get a radiograph of the condition, it was found that the canine on that side, which was yet up in the tissues, was misplaced and was bearing in an abnormal way upon the root of this lateral, causing the peculiar irregularity. It is easy to imagine what my difficulty would have been had I tried to regulate that tooth without knowing the condition causing the irregularity.

Dr. F. Milton Smith.—I wish to express my extreme gratitude to Dr. Hodson for the comfort and help I have derived from the combination mirror he has shown us to-night. I have used it, more or less, for twenty years.

Dr. F. C. Brush.—Regarding investments for soldering, I have found that a combination of two-thirds plaster and one-third ashes is excellent. It makes a very hard investment that will not change in shape or crack under the heat of the blow-pipe. The ashes should be in the form of the fine powder obtained from ordinary coal ashes.

Upon motion of Dr. F. Milton Smith, a vote of thanks was extended to the gentlemen who so kindly assisted in the helpful entertainment of the evening.

Adjourned.

FRED. L. BOGUE, M.D., D.D.S.,
Editor The New York Institute of Stomatology.

Editorial.

THE FADDIST IN DENTISTRY.

It is a peculiar trait in human nature to run in droves and to become infatuated with one thing until exhausted. This is common to the race, but more pronounced in some sections than in others. This may be due to climatic conditions, and possibly it may furnish the explanation why the people in this part of the world exhibit this trait to a greater extent than more conservative peoples elsewhere. " To run mad" after a new thing is a common expression, but it very nearly describes the mental attitude of the masses under the hypnotic influence of a peculiar stimulus.

This wild enthusiasm in the adoption of a new idea, which so much prevails, is not without its redeeming quality. Were it not for this, much that has made the new life in this country so full of vigor, with a readiness to receive new impressions and to evolve new conceptions, would have been lost to the world. Indeed, it is feared that modern civilization is hardly cognizant of the debt due to this vigorous concentration of mind in the investigation of unsolved problems, so prevailing in American life. The new inventions, the discoveries that have had their origin here, and which have so much influenced the civilization of the nineteenth century, could not have been accomplished but for this spirit that has become intense with life in this people and. is beginning to infuse its power into the conservative elements of older civilizations.

That this has induced an enthusiastic tendency is not singular, for it may be found in all phases of mental activity. It only requires a leader of unusual mental force to point out the way, to be followed by a rush of converts, whether this be to the temples of religion, to the doubtful arena of politics, or the more quiet avenues of science and philosophy.

The history of dentistry is replete with this tendency to grow unduly enthusiastic over a new theory, new method, new process, or new appliance. The earlier history of pulp-capping is very instructive and full of minor instances of this tendency to hastily accept a new idea without due reflection. How many methods were devised for the salvation of pulps, and how the dental operators would go, almost in a body, to examine and adopt this new revelation, to be forced, in the end, to acknowledge that empiricism led where experience and wisdom demanded results.

Perhaps no better evidence of the faddist tendency was ever given in dentistry than was manifested upon the introduction of cohesive gold. Dentists became enthused with this as the greatest blessing ever vouchsafed to an overworked body of men. Everything could be accomplished with this, it was asserted, that had ever been done with non-cohesive gold, and that with less labor and with more certainty as to results, and we all, including the writer, became enthused over gold and nothing but gold. The huge fillings of that day, placed in with so much toil and skill, attest this almost insane devotion to one material. The conservative man who still adhered to old methods, with non-cohesive gold as the best for his patients and himself, was looked upon as non-progressive, and was the subject of the sympathy and pity of his associates.

This enthusiasm worked its way until more reasonable views began to change the minds of dental operators. They were forced to recognize that this supposed perfection in filling-material had its weak points. That it required more skill to insert and a sacrifice of time injurious to the operator and exhausting to patient, physically and financially, and this brought a return wave of mental objections resulting in the era of plastics. The much-abused amalgam, through the "New Departure" fad, became reinstated in favor, and men rushed into this old method of filling teeth, and the older ideas relating to gold for large cavities were regarded by many as an unwise procedure. No one claimed that amalgam was artistic, or even wholly satisfactory, but it relieved the operator and the patient of an onerous burden, and was, equally with gold, a preservative from decay. The amalgam craze has had its day, and is now on the decline; in fact, no one writes papers on its shrinkage, or how it may be avoided through certain alloys, or how the material should be inserted, yet its use will remain as one of the important materials for filling defective teeth.

It does not require a long memory to go back to the wave of enthusiasm and hope that filled the professional mind upon the introduction of the method of overcoming the hypersensitiveness of dentine through cataphoresis. The supply houses could not readily supply the demand for appliances, yet the unfortunate results are too fresh in the experience of many to need extended notice. It was unfortunate, for cataphoresis is, and must always remain, a valuable aid in the treatment of sensitive teeth, but it is not a process for ignorance to handle, and this was too much the case with the majority who attempted its use. The possible dangers of the electrical current in connection with a delicate organ, as the pulp, were not sufficiently understood, hence frequent devitalization followed, and cataphoresis was relegated to the few who appreciated its value and understood the proper methods of use.

Now we are in the storm centre of another method of filling. It has grown more slowly than any other fad in dentistry. It began years ago at a time when dentists would aim to fit a portion of porcelain into cavities on the labial surfaces of incisors, and for years this was the ultimate of the ambitious practitioner. Suddenly a tidal wave, figuratively, came across the Atlantic, and, singularly, not from a foreign mind, but from the progressive intellect of an American, weary with the inartistic productions of gold. The Jenkins low-fusing body started a furor for all sorts of inlays, low fusing, high fusing, new combinations of porcelain, new methods of forming matrices, shaping cavities, etc., and very little is heard now in our conventions but porcelain for all sorts and sizes of cavities. So much has this developed that the average dentist cares but little for anything but this and bridge-work. These are the fads of the hour.

The programme of a prominent dental society lies before the writer, in which the meeting, it is stated, will begin with a paper on " Porcelain Problems," to be followed by fifteen separate clinics on porcelain inlays and crowns, with two of gold inlays. Thus an entire afternoon and evening will be consumed with this subject. No objection could be made to this if it did not sacrifice, for the time, all interest in the scientific side of dentistry, so important in its several relations.

It must be said, however, that this porcelain craze should be encouraged, for, in proportion as it becomes perfected, will be removed from dentistry one of its most laborious operations, as well as the opprobrium heaped upon it for its disfigurement of the mouth through a lack of artistic methods. If it can infuse a better taste in our operative work, it will be worth all the time spent in its development.

The enthusiasm of the faddist is not, therefore, to be cast aside as unworthy a body of intelligent workers. It is the stimulus to progress, and should be encouraged in spite of possible injury produced through the crude efforts of the unskilled. There is a great stimulus in the combined mental effort of many. It forces the masses to active competition, and, while it may result in a relapse, it will leave an impress for good not to be eradicated by time, but will leave a healthier state than was manifest at the close of the nineteenth century.

That which is true of porcelain can be said equally of all the apparently wild impulses of dental workers. The results have justified the energy displayed, faulty though it may have been, and which has led the profession of dentistry upward to a higher standard of thought and practice.

IDENTIFICATION THROUGH THE TEETH.

Upon another page will be found a communication from the chief of police of Colorado Springs, requesting dentists generally to assist him in the identification of the body of a woman found dead in that vicinity. This identification it is hoped may be secured through an examination of the accompanying diagram of the teeth. As this woman seems to have been in charge of a competent dentist, it ought not to be difficult for one who has kept careful records to identify the work.

The fact that when all other means of identification have been exhausted, the examination of the teeth has alone accomplished the solution of the problem is of great importance. The cases on record are many in proof of this, but the celebrated case of Webster-Parkman will be remembered by many, where Dr. Keep was enabled to identify the remnants of the incinerated jaw as that of Dr. Parkman, through the models he had kept, and it was principally on this evidence that Webster was convicted.

The possibility of being called to testify in similar cases should cause great care in keeping records in prosthetic work, as well as in operative procedures. This is certainly more carefully looked after at the present time than in former years, as the active practitioner has found it necessary for his own protection; hence the identification of the dead through the examination of the teeth has become part of dental jurisprudence, as officials recognize the importance of this class of evidence.

ACKNOWLEDGMENT.

OUR readers from time to time have been, it is hoped, interested, and certainly instructed, in a series of papers read before the Section on Stomatology of the American Medical Association, at its last session, at Atlantic City, in June, 1904. We are indebted to the courtesy of the editor of the official journal of that body for the privilege of reproducing these valuable papers. It is thought that there has been very much gained by giving these articles a wider publicity in the pages of a journal more directly interested in the work of the Section originating them.

The series are now about concluded, and it is, therefore, deemed proper to give credit where credit is justly due. The thanks of the INTERNATIONAL DENTAL JOURNAL are extended to the editor of the *Journal of the American Medical Association,* and also to the officers of the Section on Stomatology, for the privilege accorded.

Bibliography.

NOTES ON X-LIGHT. By William Rollins. Boston, Mass., MCMIV.

The readers of the INTERNATIONAL DENTAL JOURNAL have from time to time been made familiar with " Notes" by William Rollins. All of these have been of an eminently practical character, and especially valuable for their originality. All may not be aware that Dr. Rollins has, aside from his professional labors, a wide reputation as a worker in electrical problems, and of recent years he has been more directly connected with the study of the X-light.

In a former number of this journal the interesting and valuable work of Williams on " The Röntgen Rays in Medicine and Surgery" was reviewed, and much of the apparatus used by that author was from the inventive mind and manipulative mechanical skill of Dr. Rollins.

The author has evidently no love for wordy dissertations. His notes are generally very brief, but in the condensation nothing of importance is omitted.

This large book of four hundred pages and one hundred and

fifty-two pages of plates is introduced by the shortest preface
coming within the observation of the reviewer. It covers just six
lines, and may be copied entire:

"In these notes are recorded some impressions derived from
experiments made after the day's work, as a recreation, yet with
the hope of learning to design and construct apparatus for my
friend, Dr. F. H. Williams, who has done most to show the importance of X-light in medical diagnosis."

The notes are throughout very technical in character, and yet
from first to last are of vital interest to the student in X-light
problems. The number of these, while comparatively limited, at
present are constantly increasing and more and more capable of
appreciating an original work of this character.

It seems impossible for those who read the pages of this book
not to feel a degree of admiration for the self-sacrificing devotion
that has led the author to devote his hours of recreation to experimenting and devising apparatus to render the X-light more
efficient and to reduce its manifest dangers. The average individual would recoil from this continuous labor supplementing the
exhaustive professional work of the day.

The Notes are not strictly subject matter for review. They have
had their origin in the laboratory, and are the product of a mind
intensely active and devoted to the subject, hence there is no room
for criticism, while there is much for approval from those who are
prepared to follow Dr. Rollins and make use of his apparatus to
assist them in their work.

These Notes have been originally published in the INTER-
NATIONAL DENTAL JOURNAL, *Electrical Review, American X-Ray
Journal, American Journal of Science,* and *Boston Medical and
Surgical Journal.*

Those who have confined their reading upon this subject to its
application in dental lesions may have but a limited appreciation
of the extended use to which the X-light has been applied. This
will be best illustrated by one quotation as typical of this taken
from one of the Notes, "On seeing and hearing your heart beat."

"By placing a mirror in proper relation to a luminescent screen,
a man can see his own heart beat. By combining the mirror with
the instrument (Plate 19), he can both see and hear the heart.
A nervous patient whose organs are sound, is sometimes much com-
forted by being shown through his own eyes that all is well."

The following interesting facts connected with " Vacuum Tube Burns" are worthy of note in this connection. " The first report of burning from a vacuum tube was probably by Hawkes, in the *Electrical Review* for August 12, 1896. Tesla, in the same journal for December 2, 1896, said they were not due to X-rays, but to ozone, and possibly to nitrous acid.

" In the experiments four strong guinea-pigs were used. Two were exposed to X-light under the conditions mentioned in the Notes of February 14 and 28 and March 28, 1901, for protecting them from the effects of ultra-violet light, electric induction, and convection. The others were subjected to the same treatment and handling, except that no X-light was allowed to shine upon them. . . . When a pig was being exposed, his nearest side was fourteen centimetres from the radiant area of the target. It will be observed before the X-light could shine on a pig it passed through two thicknesses of aluminum, the outer one connected with the earth by a metal wire. It should also be remembered Tesla and others have stated a single thickness of aluminum was a protection against ' X-ray burns.' These experiments showed burns could be produced and animals killed by X-light after it had passed through two aluminum screens."

The author follows these with elaborate tables showing the effect on the pigs each day.

In a note on " The Effect of X-Light on the Crystalline Lens," the author states that " No X-light should strike a patient except the smallest beam that will cover the area to be examined, treated, or photographed. . . . An experimenter who works much with X-light should use a non-radiable face-mask, the eye-holes of which are glazed with thick plates of heavy lead glass."

It is impossible to quote extensively from this unique volume, but the temptation is to give the short, crisp, and valuable ideas a wide publicity. Those interested in the subject will find the study of these Notes not only instructive, but interesting, and another evidence, if any be needed, of the wonderful progress made in the development of the X-light since Röntgen startled the world by the announcement of his discovery.

Not the least interesting part of the volume will be found at its close, covering one hundred and fifty-two pages of illustrations of appliances for the use of the X-light. They very perfectly explain the text and the use to which they are to be applied.

The University Press of Cambridge, Mass., is responsible for the printer's part of the work, and this has been very perfectly met. It is artistic throughout in type, press-work, and paper.

Domestic Correspondence.

LETTER FROM DR. TALBOT.

CHICAGO, December 14, 1904.

To THE EDITOR:

SIR,—In the November INTERNATIONAL DENTAL JOURNAL, under "Bibliography," page 895, in reviewing Dr. Otto E. Inglis's work on "Dental Pathology and Therapeutics," the reviewer says, "The editor separates 'interstitial gingivitis,' as named by Talbot, from pyorrhœa alveolaris, making it a distinct disease. This is not as Talbot intended, for he distinctly renamed pyorrhœa alveolaris by this term, and it is difficult to understand how any pathologic distinctions can be made between these two as described by the editor."

In the same journal, on page 866, "Reports of Society Meetings," Academy of Stomatology of Philadelphia, appears the following:

"*Dr. M. Schamberg.*—There is a case which should be reported by Dr. Fogg. He brought to my office about a week ago a patient who had rather a peculiar condition upon the root of a central incisor tooth. He noticed a swelling upon the gum overlying the root of that tooth, and upon testing it found it to be vital and decided that the condition must be a pericemental abscess. He was very anxious to find some cause for the trouble, and a radiograph was taken which showed a large area of tooth destruction. This destruction indicated resorption. The tooth was kept under observation for quite a while. Yesterday, the doctor told me that, in addition to this tooth, quite a number of the other teeth exhibited this irregular resorption, to such an extent, indeed, that the tooth-crown was lost. It is the only case of the kind I have ever seen, and it is of such an unusual type that I thought it might be interesting for the Academy to hear of the case. I would be very glad to know whether any have met with a similar condition.

"*Dr. E. T. Darby.*—Were they all vital teeth?

"*Dr. Schamberg.*—They were in the main vital. In some of the lower teeth the pulps were dead.

"*Dr. James Truman.*—How old was the patient?

"*Dr. Schamberg.*—The patient was about thirty-two or thirty-five years old.

"*Dr. H. R. D. Swing.*—Was there any pyorrhœa?

"*Dr. Schamberg.*—There was no pyorrhœa, but there was a certain amount of recession. The tooth was vital up to the time of its removal.

"*Dr. I. N. Broomell.*—Had the alveolar bone filled in the space?

"*Dr. Schamberg.*—No; the alveolar process in most cases was resorbed over the site of the root resorption, due more to infection which reached the part in consequence of the food débris entering the spaces. Almost every surface of the molar teeth affected showed resorption."

The two quotations bring into view the entire pathology of the alveolar process. There seems yet mystification as to etiology, progress, and termination of the inflammation of the alveolar process. Dr. Inglis's arrangement is an improvement over other works on pathology. There was no intention on my part to "rename" as "interstitial gingivitis" "pyorrhœa alveolaris," except as this term is loosely and popularly used to indicate a specific disorder. Pyorrhœa alveolaris is the result of disease, and therefore a secondary state. Interstitial gingivitis is a disease, just as interstitial nephritis is a disease, which affects the deeper structures of the kidney. If the disease be due to local causes, such as tartar, a tooth cavity, unfinished fillings, etc., there is, first, gingivitis, then interstitial gingivitis, and last pus infection or pyorrhœa alveolaris. If pus germs occur in the proximity, the part may become infected at either stage of the disease. The patient from pregnancy, or from drug poison, scurvy, or auto-intoxication, may and frequently does have interstitial gingivitis. The gingivitis is secondary to the interstitial stage because the deeper structures are first involved. This is due to the exceedingly transitory nature of the alveolar process and to the alveolar process holding the roots of the teeth (virtually foreign bodies), thus being an end organ. In the second expression of the disease there generally is the infection constituting pyorrhœa alveolaris.

Employment of the term pyorrhœa alveolaris, except where pus flows from the sockets or gums, is not justifiable. The term should be restricted to its proper place and proper time by teachers of pathology. Interstitial gingivitis is an inflammation of the alveolar process which attacks every mouth after the alveolar process has obtained its growth. In a majority of cases there is no gingivitis. Absorption of the alveolar process begins as soon as the building up process ceases. When a tooth erupts, there is interstitial gingivitis. When a tooth is extracted, absorption is produced by interstitial gingivitis. When a patient becomes infected by syphilis or gonorrhœal germs, interstitial gingivitis occurs and the teeth become more or less loose. Underlying the trophic tooth and jaw changes of the great neuroses, tabes dorsalis, paretic dementia, etc., is interstitial gingivitis. ·

Change of climate and food, with slow adjustment of the organs of the body, as observed in the English soldiers and women and children in the concentration camps of South Africa, American soldiers in Cuba and the Philippines, miners in the Klondike, and men working on the Jungfrau Railroad in Switzerland, produce interstitial gingivitis.

The best illustration of interstitial gingivitis is the inflammation of the peridental membrane and alveolar process in the formation of an alveolar abscess. All inflammation of the alveolar process from any cause is an interstitial gingivitis.

Since every one has potential interstitial gingivitis after the alveolar process has obtained its growth, the severity of the disease depends upon the etiologic moment. Only a very small per cent., say five, has the secondary symptoms, pus infection.

The nature of the case of Dr. Schamberg, quoted above, is now clearer. This patient was the victim of extreme interstitial gingivitis, not pyorrhœa, just as Dr. Schamberg stated. This was due to some systemic condition which skiagraphy would not solve. Osteoblasts and osteoclasts build up or tear down tooth or bone structure by a process of inflammation. Here, as in pseudohypertrophic paralysis, two opposite processes arise from the same inflammatory process. Exostosis and root absorption are liable to occur. Since the cause of the interstitial gingivitis is systemic or constitutional, we would expect all the teeth to be absorbed more or less. It is also to be expected that the alveolar process is absorbed about the roots, if not entirely, not from " infection" due to " food débris," but from interstitial gingivitis.

In the same manner absorption of the temporary teeth occurs. The permanent crowns start to erupt. They set up an interstitial gingivitis. The interstitial gingivitis sets the osteoclasts at work, and the roots of the temporary teeth are thus removed. The question naturally arises, Why are not the roots of the temporary teeth whose pulps are destroyed absorbed? Occasionally they are; now only a small portion, then in most cases not at all. The reason is that irritation and infection produced by the decomposition of the dead pulp is so severe that interstitial gingivitis is extensive. Not only has an alveolar abscess formed, but bone absorption area is quite large. The trabeculæ are thus destroyed and the osteoclasts deprived of a resting-place near the root, hence absorption is impossible. The term pericemental is used. Here a proper knowledge of pathology is wanting. Since interstitial gingivitis is, as a rule, general and not circumscribed, the abscess may be located at any point where the infection is the greatest. I have demonstrated these points of infection and abscess on the outer surface of the alveolar process as well as at the centre. The term " peridental," therefore, is more to the point than " pericemental."

EUGENE S. TALBOT.

[Dr. Talbot's assertion in the foregoing, that " There was no intention, on my part, to ' rename' as interstitial gingivitis, pyorrhœa alveolaris," is somewhat at variance with his published work. The reviewer of the Burchard-Inglis " Dental Pathology" accepted Dr. Talbot's statements on the title-page of his book and in the introduction as conclusive. He names his work " Interstitial Gingivitis, or So-called Pyorrhœa Alveolaris," and in the " Introduction" he says, " With a view of clearing up this question at the outset by the use of a proper title, I have adopted as a designation for the condition hitherto known as pyorrhœa alveolaris, the term " Interstitial Gingivitis." It seems impossible to give any other meaning to these quotations except that it was the expressed intention to rename this pathological condition. The frequent use of it by writers in place of the old term seems to accentuate the position taken by the reviewer.—EDITOR.]

6

Miscellany.

New Appliances advertised in the English Dental Journals, 1904.—The Dental Manufacturing Company, of London, Manchester, and Dublin, offer the following:

A pure nickel flask, suggested by Mr. G. Brunton, for vulcanizing repairs, small dentures, and regulating appliances which can be made on the model, and which do not require the rubber to be packed under pressure. This is a method of constructing vulcanite pieces which has not been generally adopted on this side. With some repair cases flasking can be avoided by packing the rubber in place; small dentures and regulating appliances can be made by cementing the rubber onto the model, building it up into the desired form and shape, and after covering it with tin-foil embedding it in powdered talc or French chalk, and immediately placing it in the vulcanizer. This flask is designed for this purpose, and consists of a cup-shaped vessel made of pure nickel and provided with a tight-fitting cover held in place with spring clips. Mr. Brunton claims that this is much cleaner than flasking in plaster in the ordinary way, and that the quality of the finished product is better.

A renewal flask, suggested by Mr. Boucher. This is a gun-metal flask, square in shape, and very deep, and is especially designed for flasking cases nearly vertical to facilitate renewing the pink rubber rim representing the gum. Its shape and roominess make it a desirable addition to laboratory appliances.

The "accurate flask," suggested by Mr. W. Paton Scott. This flask, instead of the usual bolts, has side lugs on the upper half through which screws pass into the sides of the lower half of the flask. As these screws are in place when the flask is filled with plaster, and cannot be replaced after the case is packed unless the upper and lower sections are precisely in the same position as they were when the plaster was placed in, it is claimed that breaking of models by overpressure, or raising of bites from the flask not being completely closed is absolutely prevented. There is no means provided in the flask for closing it during packing; this is presumed to be done with some kind of a press.

The Brunton soldering appliance. This is a stand very much like a chemist's retort stand, supporting a large clay crucible fitted with a Bunsen burner, which is fed with gas through a rubber tube. The work to be soldered, inverted as is usual, is placed on a grid which rests inside the crucible over the flame. When ready for soldering the gas is lighted, the work placed in position, and a crucible cover placed over the crucible. When the case is sufficiently heated, the crucible, which rests in an iron ring attached to the stand, can be slightly raised and tilted to either side, thus enabling the blow-pipe to play on the parts to be soldered. When the soldering is completed the cover is replaced and the case allowed to cool down. It is a handy appliance, and easily made when it cannot be had, but the price at which it is offered is so close to that of the required material, it is economy to purchase.

The Parris lower molar crown, devised by Mr. Stanway Parris. This molar crown resembles a Logan crown without a dowel. The part fitting onto the root is provided with a large recessed cavity coinciding with the pulp-chamber of the tooth. It is held in position by a double-headed stud made by soldering two pieces of metal to a wire, or it may be turned from wire of sufficiently large diameter. The root is prepared by grinding off the remains of the crown level with the gum, and as flat as possible. The crown is then fitted so as to make a close joint. The pulp-chamber is enlarged to accommodate the stud, and recessed. The cavity in the root and that in the crown is filled with cement in which the stud is embedded, and the crown is then forced into place. The idea seems to be excellent for cases where it is inexpedient or inconvenient to adjust dowels to the pulp-canals. Whether the stud is a desirable addition may be questioned; so large a body of cement will in most cases be amply strong, while the stud, by becoming slightly displaced, or by failure to completely embed in the cement, may prove an element of weakness. The idea somewhat resembles one suggested by Dr. Horatio C. Merriam, Salem, Mass. (*Dental Cosmos*, vol. xxviii., August, 1886, page 493.)—W. H. TRUEMAN.

Current News.

JOINT MEETING OF THE SOUTHERN BRANCH OF THE NATIONAL DENTAL ASSOCIATION AND TENNESSEE DENTAL ASSOCIATION.

THE eighth annual meeting of the Southern Branch of the National Dental Association will take place jointly with that of the Tennessee Dental Association at Memphis, Tenn., February 21 to 23, 1905. Special railroad rates, one and a third, certificate plan.

Following is a partial list of the papers and clinics:

Dr. Jules J. Sarrazin, New Orleans, La., Chairman, Report.

Dr. B. D. Brabson, Knoxville, Tenn., "Prophylaxis in Dentistry." Discussion opened by Dr. N. N. Vann, Atalla, Ala., followed by Dr. Robin Adair.

Dr. Robin Adair, Atlanta, Ga., "A Successful Introduction of Oral Prophylaxis Treatment into Practice." Discussion opened by Dr. N. N. Vann, Atalla, Ala., followed by Dr. B. D. Brabson, Knoxville, Tenn.

Dr. R. Boyd Bayle, Chairman, Report.

Dr. August F. Sonntag, Chairman, Report.

Dr. M. F. Fennily, Washington, D. C., Report.

Dr. E. P. Beadles, Danville, Va., "A Few Points in Inlay Work."

Dr. S. D. Ronebo, Marietta, Ga., "Gold and Tin and Amalgam and Gold at Cervical Margin as an Excellent Material for saving Teeth."

Dr. T. T. Moore, Columbia, S. C., "Insulating Deep-Seated Cavities."

Dr. B. Holly Smith, Baltimore, Md., title not given.

Dr. J. E. Chase, Ocala, Fla., Chairman, Report.

Dr. Geo. S. Vann, Gadsden, Ala., Chairman, Report.

Dr. F. M. Milam, Little Rock, Ark., "Orthodontia."

Dr. W. E. Grant, Louisville, Ky., "Orthodontia, Surgical and Mechanical."

Dr. J. Lewis Walker, Norfolk, Va., "Orthodontia: Successes and Failures."

Dr. H. H. Johnson, Macon, Ga., Chairman, Report.

Dr. R. K. Luckie, Holly Springs, Miss., Chairman, Report.

Dr. Geo. W. Dick, Sumter, S. C., Chairman, Report.

Dr. Burton Lee Thorpe, St. Louis, Mo., "The Masters of Early Dentistry," with lantern-slide pictures.

Dr. Arthur Hynes Fleming, Louisburg, N. C., "The Problem of Education."

Dr. W. G. Mason, Tampa, Fla., "Dental Education."

Dr. A. W. Meyer, Chattanooga, Tenn., "Diseases of the Antrum: A Practical Case."

Dr. J. C. Bogue, Harriman, Tenn., "The Education of Present and Prospective Dental Patients."

In addition thirty-nine clinicians will give demonstrations in an unusual variety of operations together with original appliances.

From the interest manifested, this promises to be the largest meeting in the history of the two Associations. The railroads have given a rate of one and one-third fare on the certificate plan. The meeting will be held at the Hotel Gayoso, rooms $1.50 and $2.00 per day, European plan. Accommodations can be had at other hotels on the American plan at $2.00 per day. The exhibits of the various supply houses will be exceptionally attractive, embracing everything of interest to the dental profession.

J. A. GORMAN,
Corresponding Secretary.

ASHEVILLE, N. C.

KENTUCKY STATE DENTAL ASSOCIATION.

THE next annual meeting of the Kentucky State Dental Association will convene at Lexington, Ky., May 15 and 16, 1905. We anticipate a most pleasant as well as profitable meeting, and a cordial invitation is extended to the profession.

W. M. RANDALL,
Secretary.

MASONIC BUILDING, LOUISVILLE, KY.

DESCRIPTION OF NUDE BODY OF MURDERED WOMAN FOUND ON CUTLER MOUNTAIN,
DECEMBER 17, 1904.

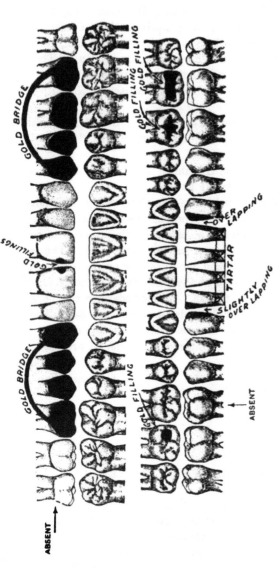

THE body was that of a woman well developed and apparently well kept, but discolored from fire and exposure to the elements. The face, nose, lips, chin, left side of neck, both ears, shoulders, and breasts were burned so as not to be recognizable. She was probably between twenty-five and thirty-five years of age, weight about one hundred and twenty to one hundred and thirty pounds, height five feet two or three inches, light auburn or ash-blond hair, part of which was burned off; skin evidently fair, with no birth-marks or scars showing; small bones, limbs well rounded, hips and thighs large, very small hands, nails clean, long, and well manicured; feet small, toes even and straight, nails manicured; probably wore a No. 2, 2½, or 3 shoe.

Teeth.—The teeth were large, white, and chalky. In the upper jaw on the right side the wisdom-tooth had never developed; the second molar was present with no fillings. A bridge extended from the first molar to the cuspid. This bridge was of solid gold and worn on the linguo-mesial portion of the crown. The first and second bicuspid being absent, their places were supplied with solid dummies. Two gold fillings of medium size in the mesial of the upper centrals or incisors. The upper teeth protrude slightly. In the left upper jaw a gold bridge extended from the first bicuspid to the second molar; a peculiarity of this bridge is in the fact that the second molar is made of a bicuspid dummy. The third molar or wisdom-tooth on this side is present. In the lower jaw on the right side the third molar or wisdom-tooth is present; the second molar has a gold filling in the mesio-occlusal surface. The first molar is absent, evidently for some years, as the space is almost closed. Slight overlapping of cuspid on lateral. Pyorrhœa of lower teeth,—centrals and laterals,—with considerable tartar, showing that they had not been cleaned recently. Left side: considerable overlapping of cuspid on lateral; all teeth present on left side of lower jaw. First molar, large gold filling on occlusal surface; second molar, large gold filling on occlusal surface; extending on to the distal surface; third molar or wisdom-tooth undeveloped, that is, partially covered with tissue.

All clothing, finger- and ear-rings, and all other means of identification had been removed from the body, and no trace of same have been found, and up to the present time we have been unable to identify her.

The above description and diagram is the only evidence we have for identification.

Kindly call the attention of dentists in your city to the above description and diagram. If possible, have your newspapers print it.

Address all information and inquiries to

W. S. REYNOLDS,
Chief of Police.

COLORADO SPRINGS, COL., December 28, 1904.

THE FRATERNAL DENTAL SOCIETY OF ST. LOUIS, MO.

AT the annual election of the Fraternal Dental Society of St. Louis, December 20, 1904, the following officers for the ensuing year were elected:

President, Burton Lee Thorpe; Vice-President, E. P. Dameron; Secretary, S. H. Voyles; Treasurer, W. E. Brown.

Executive Committee.—E. E. Haverstick, W. L. Whipple, T. G. Donnell.

S. H. VOYLES,
Secretary.

A FREE DENTAL SERVICE AT THE HOMES OF THE SICK POOR.

THE Dental School of Harvard University has recently organized its free dental service at the homes of the sick poor so as to be of greater efficiency than heretofore. The Dental School is now prepared to send a dentist, who is a graduate of the School and registered by the State Board of Registration, to the homes of the sick poor or to hospitals for the purpose of relieving pain originating from the teeth. This service does not extend to the filling of teeth or making of plates for artificial teeth. Its object is simply the relief of pain; a more extended treatment of the teeth being postponed until the patient may have recovered, and can visit the Infirmary of the School. The service here described can be obtained by telephoning the Harvard Dental School, North Grove Street, Boston, or by letter.

EUGENE H. SMITH,
BOSTON, November 1, 1904.   *Dean.*

GOLDEN ANNIVERSARY AT NEW ORLEANS.

ON February 21, 1905, a golden anniversary banquet will be tendered by the dentists of New Orleans to Dr. George J. Friedrichs, who graduated in dentistry February 21, 1855.

L. D. ARCHINARD,
For Committee of Arrangements.

THE

International Dental Journal.

VOL. XXVI.   MARCH, 1905.   No. 3.

Original Communications.[1]

DISTAL AND MESIAL OCCLUSION: SOME CAUSES AND SOME RESULTS.

BY HORACE L. HOWE, D.M.D., BOSTON, MASS.

IT is an undisputed fact that of all the different classes of mal-occlusion of the teeth, the two forms which tend to mar the facial expression the most are distal and mesial occlusion.

The open mouth, the protruding upper teeth, the undeveloped nose, and vacant expression of the mouth-breather with distal occlusion is a sight familiar to us all. Hardly less familiar is the bull-dog expression of the prognathous lower jaw with mesial occlusion.

Admitting that the face is the mirror of the soul, hence the outward expression of the mental processes, it becomes of especial interest to us as dentists to recognize and to study the abnormal conditions which tend to distort the normal facial lines, and, if possible, to rectify the malocclusion; thus enabling the person to breathe normally, to masticate food perfectly, and at the same time improving the powers of expression both by voice and by the countenance.

---

[1] The editor and publishers are not responsible for the views of authors of papers published in this department, nor for any claim to novelty, or otherwise, that may be made by them. No papers will be received for this department that have appeared in any other journal published in the country.

To avoid confusion, let us first consider distal occlusion. This condition is nearly always associated with mouth-breathing, which is usually first caused by adenoid growths in the nasopharyngeal vault. These growths are most commonly seen in the North Temperate Zone, and occur from infancy to puberty. Their cause is conceded to be due to an hypertrophy of the tissues brought on by inflammatory changes resulting from colds. In most cases they disappear at puberty, largely due to a diminution of the morbid activity of the tissues.

If these growths do not disappear in childhood either naturally or by surgical operation, the person will continue to breathe through his mouth; first, because of the physiological law, " That the use of a part tends ·to stimulate its growth and development, and disuse to lack of development and atrophy."

The nose, unused, becomes undeveloped and blocked. Second. the relaxed state of the muscles of the lips, and the abnormal pressure of the muscles of the cheeks, together with lack of occlusal support, causes the contraction and protrusion of the upper arch and the recession and distal occlusion of the lower arch. Consequently, the child in this state will breathe through the mouth because it is easier and of his inability to close his lips over the protruding front teeth.

Again, distal occlusion may be caused by some seemingly slight habit of the child when very young, such as sucking the thumb and the rubber tubes and nipples of nursing-bottles.

These are undoubtedly great factors in causing the deformity. Is it not reasonable to suppose that the lower jaw might be pushed backward in its socket by a heavy nursing-bottle hanging from it and left there for hours at a time, especially when we consider how much the flexible bones of babyhood may be changed?

For instance, the abnormal shapes of the skulls of the ancient Peruvians and Flat-Head Indians were caused by simply bandaging the heads of their children when very young.

Lastly, when there is a decided irregularity anterior to the sixth-year molar, the premature extraction of the temporary teeth accounts for this type of distal occlusion. Mouth-breathing does not usually accompany this type of distal occlusion.

To illustrate this form of distal occlusion, let us consider Fig. 1. This slide was made from a specimen obtained from the Warren Museum of the Harvard Medical School. The subject was evidently

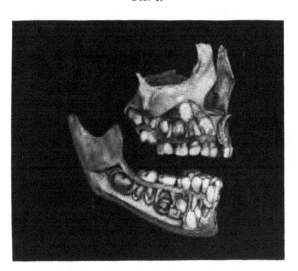

Fig. 2.

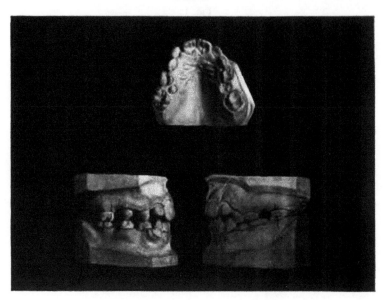

FIG. 3.

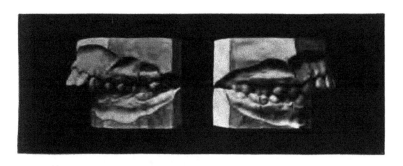

FIG. 4.

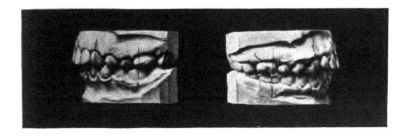

FIG. 5.

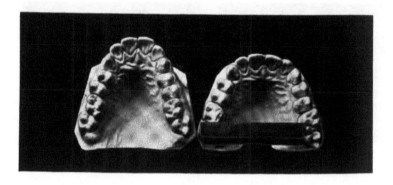

FIG. 6.

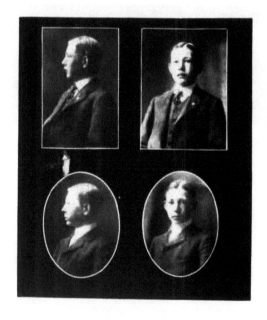

a child about six years old. All of the temporary teeth, excepting the two inferior centrals, are in position; the sixth-year molars of the mandible have erupted, while those of the maxillæ have partly erupted. The permanent teeth are beautifully shown partially formed, and which will succeed the temporary ones in their normal positions, providing nothing is done to disturb their course of eruption. But we can easily understand, if the second temporary molar was extracted prematurely, the sixth-year molar would erupt forward of its normal position, and its distal buccal cusp would engage in the buccal groove of the lower molar instead of its mesial buccal cusp. This necessarily would cause an irregularity anteriorly.

Case I.—Fig. 2 shows a typical case of this kind. The right second superior temporary molar was extracted two years prematurely. The sixth-year molar erupted forward in its place, causing the second bicuspid to erupt out of line, as is shown by the palatal view. Upon the left side the condition is better, but owing to the badly decayed second temporary molar, the sixth-year molar is a trifle mesially dislocated.

Case II.—The models shown in Fig. 3 represent a case with typical distal occlusion. The patient, a boy of fourteen, had the habit of sucking his lower lip almost constantly. Probably adenoids were formerly associated with the case. You will notice that every tooth of the lower arch occludes *distally* instead of *mesially* to its corresponding fellow of the upper arch. The first lower molar, for instance, occludes distally to the upper first molar, and so on.

Fig. 4 presents the case three months from the time the previous models were made. Normal occlusion is established, with the result that the facial lines are improved and the boy can breathe normally through his nose.

Fig. 5 shows the palatal view of the two previous models compared.

Fig. 6 shows the photographs compared.

Case III.—Fig. 7 illustrates another case of typical distal occlusion. Patient twelve years of age. Notice, if you will, the remains of the right, second temporary molar.

Fig. 8 shows normal occlusion established with the exception that the second right upper bicuspid has not fully erupted.

Fig. 9 is a profile view showing difference in facial lines. Observe, if you please, that the shape of the nose is even changed. The drawn expression and hollow cheeks have disappeared, all the change taking place in six months' time.

Fig. 10 shows a front·view of the photographs compared. This case illustrates the advantage of correcting the malocclusion as soon as possible after being recognized, that the face may develop along normal lines as the child grows older, instead of along abnormal lines.

CASE IV.—Fig. 11 is a very interesting case of a child three and a half years of age. This case goes to confirm the theory of Dr. Henry Baker that mesial occlusion is often caused by habit. This child had the habit of protruding the lower jaw forward so that the lower front teeth would lock in front of the upper incisors. The jaw became accommodated to its new position, so that the child was unable to bite normally. Her family physician noticed the deformity and remarked upon it. She came under my observation, and I instructed the parents of the child to tell her to bite back as much as possible. The result was that within two months the child was able to bite normally, as is shown by the model upon the left.

The tendency to mesial occlusion was undoubtedly inherited, as both parents have slight mesial occlusion. This case, with others, convinces me that mesial occlusion is usually caused by the jaw being too far forward in its socket, rather than by any abnormal development of the jawbone itself.

CASE V.—Fig. 12 shows a case of mesial occlusion. The patient is a man twenty-eight years old, who when young had the habit of protruding the lower jaw forward and sucking his fingers with the tips behind the lower incisors. In this case the patient was unable to project his jaw any farther forward than he usually held it.

Fig. 13 shows the improved occlusion, although not perfect. This condition was obtained without grinding the back teeth at all. The condition is improving constantly rather than growing worse, as the case would have been providing nothing was done. The facial lines show a marked improvement, although I have not the privilege of showing photographs.

I am indebted to Dr. W. H. Parker for the privilege of showing the following case. The patient, a girl of fourteen, recently came to him for treatment with the teeth in the condition that we see them in Fig. 14, caused, the mother said, by the child's sucking and pulling upon the rubber tube of a nursing-bottle. Three years ago she was evidently in the hands of an enthusiastic extractor, as

Fɪɢ. 7.

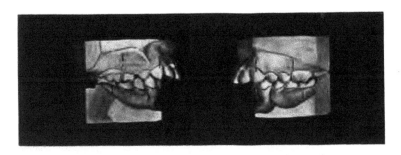

Fɪɢ. 8.

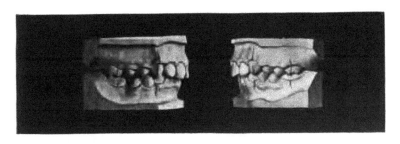

FIG. 9.

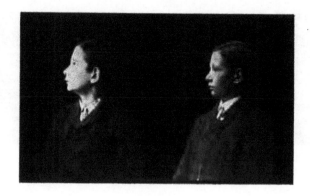

FIG. 10.

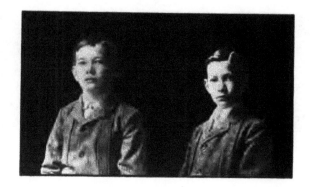

Fig. 11.

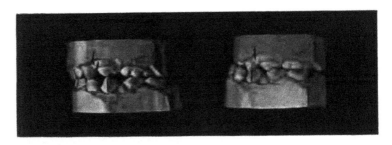

Fig. 12.

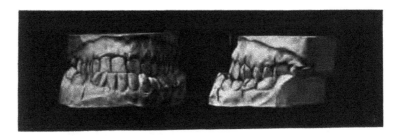

Fig. 13.

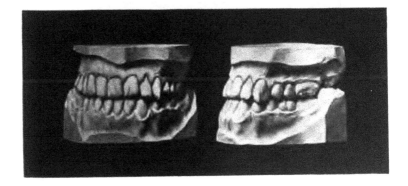

FIG. 14.

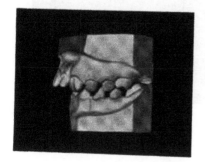

FIG. 15.

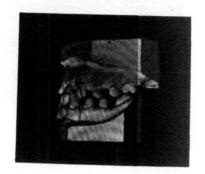

FIG. 16.

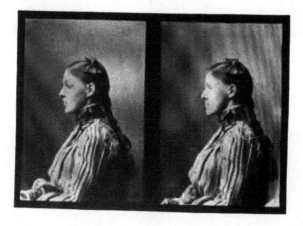

the four perfectly sound sixth-year molars were removed to correct the protruding front teeth. The dismal failure we can all see.

The remarkable feature of the case is that a year ago the child was told that if she would close her lips it would improve her appearance. She bravely made the attempt, and protruded the lower jaw forward so that the teeth occluded, as we see them in Fig. 15, thus enabling her to close her lips. The girl therefore came to have practically two bites,—the old bite, to which she was forced to return for masticating, and the forward bite, which enabled her to close her lips and to breathe normally.

Incidentally, the mother stated that the child could endure having her teeth regulated now better than she could a year ago, as her health was much better.

But in the attempt to conceal one deformity the child developed another, not as marked, perhaps; still the facial expression lacks harmony, as we can all see by Fig. 16. The facial expression of the picture upon our right is that of a typical prognathous lower jaw, it being caused by her extreme forward bite.

From these cases we are able to draw several conclusions. First, *that distal occlusion* may be caused by the lower jaw being forced backward in its socket by the same means that force the upper teeth forward.

Second, *that the improvement in general health* which invariably follows the establishment of normal occlusion is not accidental, but due to normal breathing through the nose, improved nutrition resulting from better mastication of food, and because the stomach is less contaminated by the foul secretions of the unused nose.

Third, *that the muscles, the condyles, and the teeth* of the lower jaw will accommodate themselves to new positions of the jaw. This is especially true if the teeth of the upper arch are made to give occlusal support to the teeth of the lower jaw in its new position.

In a previous part of this paper I stated that it becomes of especial interest to us as dentists to recognize and to study these deformities, and, if possible, to rectify the malocclusion, thus enabling the person to breathe normally, to masticate food perfectly, and at the same time improving the powers of expression both by voice and by countenance.

We have reason to be proud of the fact that a Boston man, Dr. Henry A. Baker, has given to the profession the intermaxillary elastics which afford a practical method for the correction of these cases. Dr. E. H. Angle in a recent article said, " The Baker anchorage has revolutionized the practice of orthodontia." I can say no more in appreciation of their value than to simply indorse this statement.

Finally, the results of distal occlusion with consequent mouth-breathing may be far reaching. Breathing through the mouth from necessity is shallow breathing. The air is drawn into the lungs without being filtered, warmed, or moistened. From lack of deep breathing the lungs become small and contracted, and the person hollow-chested. The blood is not properly aërated. The whole vitality is lowered, and the powers of resisting diseases are impaired, hence there is a greater susceptibility to all diseases, especially diseases of the air-passages.

Altogether the mouth breather is poorly equipped for life's work. To have a perfect working machine, the most minute parts are looked after and kept in order. If one tiny wheel goes wrong, it impairs the total work of the machine. If not set aright, it will be but a short time before the whole machine is useless. Why not as true in the case of the human machine, the most wonderfully constructed of them all?

The influence of health upon the career of the individual is aptly shown by John Tyndall in his address to students, where he says, " Take care of your health. There have been men who by wise attention to this point might have risen to any eminence,—might have made great discoveries, written great poems, commanded armies, or ruled states, but who by unwise neglect of this point have come to nothing. Imagine Hercules as oarsman in a rotten boat; what can he do there but by the very force of his stroke expedite the ruin of his craft? Take care, then, of the timbers of your boat, and avoid all practices likely to introduce either wet or dry rot among them. And this is not to be accomplished by desultory or intermittent efforts of the will, but by the formation of habits. The will, no doubt, has sometimes to put forth its strength in order to strangle or crush the special temptation. But the formation of right habits is essential to your permanent security. They diminish your chance of failing when assailed, and they augment your chance of recovery when overthrown."

It is unnecessary perhaps to say in conclusion that habits which impair the vital functions of nutrition and respiration must influence the health and hence the career of the individual.

THE RADICAL TREATMENT OF THE MAXILLARY ANTRUM.[1]

BY LEE MAIDMENT HURD, M.D.[2]

THE antrum of Highmore, as we all know, is liable to become the seat of a suppurative inflammation either acute or chronic. Of the chronic, which we are about to consider, nearly one-half are secondary to an inflammatory condition about the roots of the teeth, and practically all the others are of nasal origin. The chronic cases may begin with an acute inflammation which subsides into a chronic condition, or it may be insidious from the beginning.

The more prominent symptoms are a purulent discharge from the nose, sometimes so slight as hardly to be noticeable; in fact, the most frequent cause of one-sided purulent nasal discharge is antrum disease. Nasal obstruction on the affected side, sometimes on both sides, is frequent. Pain around the eye is found in a great many cases, but pain in or over the antrum is rare and is only caused by retention of the pus under pressure or a neurasthenic tendency in the patient. Trigeminal neuralgia, pain in the vertex or occiput, are frequently present when the sphenoid is involved, and pain to the inner side of the eye generally means that the anterior ethmoid cells are affected. Tenderness on pressure over the canine fossa is generally present, but not invariably. Gastric disturbances are frequently present from the swallowing of pus at night; also a bad taste in the mouth in the morning. Sometimes frontal headaches are present, but more frequently infraorbital neuralgia or shooting pains in the teeth. This dentalgia does not necessarily mean that the antral trouble originated in the teeth. The pus in the nose sooner or later sets up a chronic rhinitis. Once in a great while eye symptoms develop, affections of the tear ducts, a recurring iritis, or a chorioretinitis.

In regard to diagnosis, pus under the middle turbinate may come from the frontal or anterior ethmoid cells as well as from the

---

[1] Read before The New York Institute of Stomatology, December 6, 1904.

[2] Assistant Surgeon, Manhattan Eye and Ear Hospital.

antrum. As the antral orifice is near the roof, the head held horizontally and to the opposite side will increase the flow of pus, if it is not too viscid. A small silver canula can sometimes be passed through the antral orifice and the cavity either inflated with compressed air or irrigated, which will bring out whatever it contains and give valuable aid in arriving at a diagnosis. It is justfiable to remove part of the middle turbinate to gain an entrance to the antral orifice. If you still fail, an exploratory puncture through the wall of the middle or inferior meatus or through the canine fossa may be made. This is done with a trocar and canula or an especially devised steel exploratory needle. In using the middle meatus route care should be taken not to enter the orbit by mistake.

I prefer the canine fossa or inferior meatus routes, for then one can inflate with compressed air and drive the contents of the antrum out through the normal opening. Aspirating is not very reliable, as the membrane is liable to be quite thick and the needle may not pass through it; and again, the pus may be so viscid that it will not pass through the needle; but by inflating or douching through the needle or canula you will break through whatever membrane may cover it and drive the thick secretion out through the normal orifice, taking for granted that it is open because of the pus in the middle meatus.

Transillumination is of some help, especially where the affected side is quite dark, but is not at all reliable. It may be a rudimentary antrum that causes the darkness, for example.

If there is an opening through a tooth socket from which pus is flowing, then there is not much doubt about the diagnosis.

The hardest part of all is to determine whether the antrum is truly the site of the inflammation or only a reservoir for pus coming down from the frontal or ethmoid cells. This is at times a difficult point to decide, which may require repeated examinations and sometimes treatment of the frontal or ethmoid cells.

In treating the antrum, most of the cases of nasal origin get well spontaneously or with nasal douching. Those of dental origin, as a rule, do not, but treatment of the roots of the affected tooth and the necrotic bone about them, with irrigations through a tooth socket (Cowper's operation) or through the canine fossa, will cure a large per cent. of them. If this method is not successful at the end of three or four months, it never will be. Of the chronic cases, very rarely will a case recover with nasal irrigations alone.

A certain number will be cured by irrigations through a tooth socket. Of those of nasal origin, part will get well by making as large an opening as possible into the antrum through the middle or inferior meatus (Mikulicz's operation), with irrigations and the application of antiseptics. But there are a number of cases in which none of these procedures will effect a cure, and a more radical operation must be performed.

Caldwell, Luc, Boenninghaus, and Jansen at about the same time began to adopt more radical measures. The operation I am about to describe follows the method of Jansen nearer than that of the others. Before giving the technic of the operation I will present the histories of two cases, to illustrate some of the points in diagnosis and the result of operation.

CASE I.—C. I., male, aged twenty-four years. Consulted me October 22, 1903, because he had lost a rubber drainage-tube into the antrum that he had been wearing in an opening through the tooth socket of his second molar. The antral trouble dates back three years, when he had a decayed tooth removed, part of the root remaining until about one year after the removal of the tooth, when he began to have a purulent discharge from the nose. He had the root extracted, a hole bored into the antrum through the socket, and a rubber drainage-tube inserted, which he wore until it slipped into the antrum six weeks ago. During the time he had the tube in place the discharge greatly diminished, but never entirely ceased. When I first saw him he was thin, anæmic, had gastric disturbances, headaches, pains about the eyes, a bad taste in the mouth, purulent discharge from the nose and alveolar opening, and nasal obstruction. On examining the nose, the membrane over the turbinates was swollen, middle more than the inferior, and pus was emerging from the middle meatus. Operated upon October 23. The antral mucous membrane was found in a state of polypoid degeneration from one-quarter to one-half of an inch in thickness, with the rubber tube in the cavity. No necrotic bone was found. The patient was out of bed the next morning, and the only evidence of the operation was some swelling of that side of the face, and he left the hospital the next day. November 13 the discharge had ceased, and he has gained fifteen pounds since the operation.

The preceding case is a clear one of antrum disease of dental origin. The following case shows the difficulty at times of arriving at a diagnosis and source of the trouble.

CASE II.—W. Z. M., male, aged twenty-two years. Consulted me because of an offensive odor and purulent discharge from the nose, with severe headaches and vomiting. Two years previously he had an ulcerated tooth removed. He first noticed purulent discharge from the nose about three months later, but just previous to noticing the discharge he had his nasal septum operated upon and wore a nasal splint afterwards. Under these circumstances it is hard to say which was the cause of the infection, except that if it was caused by the nasal operation it probably would have subsided spontaneously. The patient himself thinks that the tooth caused the trouble. On examination, I find the affected side of the nose very narrow from the septum deviating to that side; the upper part of the nose filled with creamy pus, with an offensive odor of dead bone. The nose was so narrow and the mucous membrane so swollen that it was hard to make out the landmarks. There was a swelling of the mucous membrane in the region of the ethmoidal bulla and middle turbinate, with a perforation near the centre of this swelling leading into the antrum, and, on probing, dead bone was felt, but the pus coming from so high up in the nose led me to believe the trouble might be in the frontal sinus, but as that was the only symptom of frontal disease present I continued my investigation of the antrum, by puncturing the canine fossa and inflating the antrum, which caused the nose to fill with very offensive pus. Transillumination gave no aid, there not being much difference between the two sides. As I was sure of the antrum trouble, I operated upon that first. As a preliminary step to give me room in the nose, I straightened the septum. On entering the antrum I found the lining membrane from one-quarter to three-eighths of an inch in thickness, and necrosis of the upper portion of the nasal wall and of the ethmoid cells. The packing was removed on the fourth day and the nose douched thereafter.

The operation is performed under ether anæsthesia with the jaws held apart by a mouth-gag placed on the opposite side to the trouble, the choana on the side of the lesion tamponed, and a gauze packing placed between the cheek and the jaws well back to prevent blood from running into the pharynx. The cheek is retracted upward and outward with a blunt retractor placed in the angle of the mouth.

This gives a very good view of the field of operation. The incision is made from the last molar to the canine tooth, about one-quarter of an inch below the gingivo-labial fold, down to the bone. Then the periosteum is elevated over the entire anterior wall of the antrum, and as far on the lateral wall as necessary. Now, by placing the retractor into this incision and elevating the soft parts a good view is obtained of the canine fossa. With a chisel an opening is made at the most depressed portion of the fossa, large enough to admit a rongeur, with which the entire anterior and part of the lateral wall of the antrum are removed, care being exercised not to wound the membranous lining of the antrum, thereby avoiding troublesome hemorrhage. Now that the bony walls are removed, incise the lining mucous membrane and examine the interior of the antrum for granulations, character of membrane, foreign bodies, etc.

Remove the entire membranous lining of the antrum, giving especial care to the superior internal and external angles. The bone may now be examined for necrotic spots, which are more frequently found about the roots of the teeth, or on the upper nasal wall. Necrosis is frequent in the cases operated upon. It is almost needless to say that all necrotic bone must be completely removed, down to healthy tissue, and any partitions or ridges in the antrum should be broken down and made smooth with the walls. The next step is to remove the bony nasal wall completely, from the floor to the roof, from the anterior margin to the posterior. This is accomplished by placing the little finger into the nose, to act as a guide, and chipping the bone away with a curette or forceps. After a little practice this can be done quickly without injuring the mucous membrane. The inferior turbinate bone should also be shelled out in the same manner. The next step is to examine the ethmoid cells, and, if affected, they should be removed with a curette or forceps, and if the sphenoid sinus is involved, the anterior wall and lining membrane should be removed. Now, with the mucous membrane remaining on the nasal wall, flaps are made to help line the antrum. If you have all the membrane from the middle meatus to the floor, including that of the inferior turbinate, two large flaps can be made, one to partly cover the roof and external wall, and one for the floor. I divide the membrane from its anterior attachment and then make a horizontal incision just above the membrane of the inferior turbinate back to the attachment to the bone. The upper flap I place partly on the roof and partly on the external wall and suture the end to the periosteum at the external angle of the incision. The lower flap is laid on the floor of the antrum and sutured in a like manner to the periosteum, as far externally as it will reach.

I now pack the cavity firmly with iodoform gauze in such a way that it can be removed through the anterior naris, and then I close the buccal wound with silk sutures. On the fourth or fifth day the packing is removed and not replaced, also the sutures, the cavity simply being douched thereafter several times daily with a normal salt solution.

There is considerable swelling of the upper lip and cheek from the stretching received during the operation. Some cases need an opiate to relieve the pain after operation, as the infraorbital nerve is injured during the operation. There is no sensation in the soft parts for a number of weeks. The cases can generally leave the hospital the day after the packing is removed.

Indications for the Radical Operation.—If a diseased antrum has been treated for several months by one of the more conservative methods without result, the radical procedure becomes necessary to effect a cure. In certain cases, that have received no previous treatment, it seems useless to try the conservative operations,—namely, where there is considerable necrosis, which can generally be diagnosed by the odor and probe; or where the ethmoids and sphenoid sinus are extensively involved.

Advantages of the Operation.—You have a full view of the interior of the antrum, and in removing the nasal bony wall and using the nasal mucous membrane to partially line the antral cavity, the antrum, as such, is eradicated and made part of the nasal cavity proper, making a recurrence of the disease impossible, as there is no antrum, only a recess in the nose which is accessible through the anterior naris. The mucous membrane of the inferior turbinate continues to functionate, as is shown in an attack of acute coryza, when it swells, as does the turbinate of the other side. The opponents of this method contend that there are two disadvantages, —one, that it will cause a dry pharyngitis from increasing the caliber of the nasal chamber; in fact, it is not increased as much as they think, as the posterior third of the inferior turbinate remains, and part or all of the middle turbinate, unless the ethmoids have been involved. The other disadvantage, they contend, is that it does not always cure. I have yet to see a case it has not cured where the disease has been fearlessly and thoroughly removed.

SOME STUDIES IN OCCLUSION.[1]

BY EDWARD H. ANGLE, M.D., D.D.S., ST. LOUIS, MO.

MR. PRESIDENT, MEMBERS OF THE ACADEMY OF STOMATOLOGY, AND FRIENDS,—The subject of my paper this evening, as announced, is "Orthodontia," but I am going to take the liberty of modifying this title to one which I think will awaken a keener interest and give a broader understanding of the term "Orthodontia." I shall call it "Some Studies in Occlusion," for I feel that a greater interest should be awakened among you all to that principle which goes back of orthodontia and underlies its very inception and entirety, and not only orthodontia, but every operation which you as dentists are ever called upon to perform upon the teeth. This principle is occlusion, and I will define occlusion as being the normal relations of the inclined occlusal planes of the teeth when the jaws are closed.

I hope that at some day not far distant I may be able to read in the announcement of our colleges that a new chair has been added, a new professorship established, the mightiest of them all,—the chair of the Science of Occlusion,—where the student from the time he enters the school shall be taught occlusion broadly, deeply, grandly, and not only the one link in the chain of occlusion,—the human teeth,—but comparative occlusion from the lowest to the highest. Then he will be impressed with its mighty importance, and so studied, this knowledge of occlusion will be a mighty incentive in governing the plan and performance of his every operation upon the teeth. For were the teeth not created solely for occlusion? Study their shapes, study their forms and proportions, examine them microscopically, study their positions and periods of eruption, and the very structure and arrangement of that wonderful membrane that holds them in position, and, too, that peculiar structure, the alveolar process, that comes at their bidding and vanishes with their going,—all, *all* point to occlusion and the one grand object of its function. Who can estimate the value of normal occlusion in the development and maintenance of the entire physical

---

[1] Read before the Academy of Stomatology, Philadelphia, March 1, 1904.

economy, even reacting on the developing masticatory apparatus itself; or who can estimate the results on the development of the entire physical economy when handicapped by malocclusion? I know you will lightly pass this thought by, but I assure you it is not one to be lightly cast aside by truly scientific men, inasmuch as malocclusion is rapidly growing to be the rule instead of the exception.

When men shall have become impressed with the importance and value of occlusion, then will many questions in dentistry which now agitate and provoke controversy be naturally and scientifically settled. Then will the practice of placing bridges on leaning piers, which in reality serve chiefly the purpose of spanning space and for the lodgement of débris, be changed, and bridges will be constructed for purposes of occlusion and attached to piers that have been first placed from a leaning position to that best suited for occlusion and support. When men shall understand the real meaning of occlusion then will there be vastly fewer bridges and crowns needed, for the jewels in the crown of occlusion will be prized more nearly in accordance with their true worth, and the earliest and most careful attention will then be given, not only to their preservation, but to their eruption and direction into normal positions. Then will their careless sacrifice surely be regarded as a punishable crime, for I believe that, generally speaking, the loss of a first lower molar is really a far greater damage to the physical economy, as a whole, than would be the loss of a finger.

When men shall understand occlusion they will realize that the loss of a tooth is of such serious consequence in its relation to the rest of the dental apparatus that it should and must be immediately substituted by the best that is artificial.

Then the question of extraction for the correction or prevention of malocclusion will be naturally and thoroughly settled of itself, and we shall read with amazement and view with surprise the pictures and discussion of cases treated by orthodontists of these days when extraction was resorted to and defended with all complacency.

When men shall know occlusion, then will the requirement of the natural form to each filling be self-evident, and such monstrosities of form in fillings and crowns as those we now daily see coming fresh from the hands of reputable operators will be regarded with amazement.

When men shall be taught and shall have mastered occlusion then will orthodontia no longer be made subservient to all else in colleges and practice, but it will take its rightful position as the first, the principal, and the most important effort toward the betterment of the permanent human teeth, for then all will be impressed with the mighty importance of teeth being directed into their normal relations, and that, too, not at the age of sixteen, but at the very time of their eruption, for then will it become self-evident that that time is the golden time for orthodontia and the highest possible betterment of the relations of the teeth, and how strange will such advice sound, now so commonly given by dentists to anxious mothers, as " Your child is too young," or, " Wait until all of the teeth are in position." When men shall have mastered occlusion they will realize that perfect fillings can only be made when teeth are in perfect relations, and that the perfect contouring of a filling is essential, not only to the immediate locality of each tooth, but, likewise, to the bracing and maintaining of all the other inclined planes in both dental arches, and that to sacrifice a cusp or any considerable portion of a tooth in a denture normally occluded is soon to result in the modifying of the beautiful, the harmonious, the efficient relations of many if not all of the remaining inclined planes. Then will such questions as " extension for prevention" have a true light thrown upon them by many not now comprehended.

When our new professorship is established,—I mean a *real* professorship with a *real* professor,—then will anatomy and histology have a different meaning to the students. The study of the development of the jaws and the alveolar process will then have a real meaning, as well as that of the pathology of the nose and throat, for their mighty bearing upon occlusion will then be comprehended and its teaching be listened to by students in a different spirit. Then the relation of the dentist and the true rhinologist will not be that of casual acquaintance, but of hearty friendship and co-operation.

Then will the pale-faced, badly nourished mouth-breather, with perhaps only his second molars occluding, now more commonly seen than children with strabismus were thirty years ago, be as rare as these children now are, for since the eye has been scientifically studied and treated at the proper age this formerly common ailment has been largely overcome.

I am also convinced that the study of occlusion goes beyond the study of dentistry, and is a wonderful impetus to the appreciation and understanding of art, for no one can study those wonderful curves and lines of beauty and harmony of proportion of the teeth in normal occlusion, and what this means to the general balance of the rest of the face, without having a keener appreciation of art, for what is art but harmony of proportion of form and color? and I sometimes think that the reason that dentists seem to have such poor ideas of art is their lack of an ideal to work to. Or, in other words, from the nature of things, as dentistry is now practised, the correct form of a tooth and its importance means but little to the dentist. The picture of the surface to be restored is imperfect in his mind, and the malposition of the tooth renders the perfect form of his filling ofttimes impossible, so he works upon an imperfect surface and aims to stop decay, and leaves a surface without regularity of form.

I know that I shall be accused of being an idealist. I hope so, for there is need of a few more in dentistry. I shall be accused of advocating the practice of that which is too ideal and impossible. You will say that we have to work for people who have passed the age for consideration of the ideal or normal in occlusion, and that which will prolong the usefulness of the organs of mastication is all that can be considered. I grant you that this is probably true with many of your patients, but is it not also true that almost daily those youthful patients come to you in whom the golden hours for establishing the normal in occlusion is passing, and are you treating them according to the demands of occlusion? Or are you treating them without consideration for the matchless form of grace and beauty of the surfaces you are restoring, and of what those surfaces mean in that dental apparatus and to that face as a whole? Are you seeing to it that the inclined occlusal planes lock and harmonize in the manner designed by nature for the best use, preservation, and beauty of an harmonious whole? If not, you are neglecting your highest and most sacred duty as dentists, for the period for the normal locking of the cusps of these teeth is one that only comes once, and if you have neglected your duty in the intelligent supervision of this locking and have permitted the beginning of chaos in occlusion you surely are not true to your trust.

In this paper I shall have little to say regarding regulating appliances, for in comparison with occlusion they seem so lacking in importance that I feel it were probably better not to intrude them upon your time, for only after occlusion is comprehended and thoroughly mastered can the proper form and use of a regulating appliance have any true meaning. When occlusion shall be mastered then will the question of concentration or specialization naturally be settled, for then even the colleges will learn that it were far wiser and better to so educate students that they might in their life's work do some one thing well than many badly, as is now the rule. Then will the different branches of dentistry be truly specialized, and occlusion will be the basis of them all and the bond that will bind them all into one harmonious whole.

In the pictures which I have prepared for this evening many are new. Some have been seen by a few of you before, but all have been made to try to tell in a rambling way the story of occlusion, a story which ought to be very old,—which is old in truth,—but one that is far too new to many of those who are intrusted with the care of the teeth.

Following this Dr. Angle showed one hundred and thirty slides of the occlusion and faces of patients treated for malocclusion of their teeth.

SYPHILIS OF THE MOUTH.[1]

BY HENRY C. BOENNING, M.D., PHILADELPHIA.

SYPHILIS of the mouth is of very common occurrence, and of especial interest to the dentist because of his exposure to infection.

The lesions are of the most protean character; some are highly contagious; hence a discussion of the features of this disease is of the greatest practical advantage to the members of your profession.

The question, " What is Syphilis?" has been asked from time immemorial. Syphilographers contend that much of David's physical distress and Job's diseased body was due to syphilis; and that the classics testify to the existence of this disease in the remotest eras of civilization.

---

[1] Read before the Chester and Delaware County Dental Society, October 26, 1904.

Certain it is that syphilis is to-day the most commonly met and most widely distributed disease. It is no respecter of persons, or of rank in society. The rich and high-born share equally with the poor and plebeian the susceptibility to infection.

The cause of syphilis is a germ. This has been established beyond controversy; but whether that germ is an animal or a vegetable micro-organism has not been shown.

From time to time, up to the present, the germ of syphilis has been " announced," only to find that it fails to meet Koch's law, but eventually it will be isolated, and a new treatment, by probably an antisyphilitic toxin, will be inaugurated, to the enormous benefit and relief of the syphilitic, whose afflictions are often greater than those of the leper.

Lustgarten's bacillus, supposed by many to be the cause of syphilis, failed in the laboratory to prove its claims; but with each exclusion we gain a better understanding of the action and probable identity of the germ responsible for this malady.

Syphilis is a disease of different stages. This conforms with nearly every zymotic disease in which the micro-organism has been satisfactorily demonstrated.

But the stages of syphilis extend over periods of months and years; whereas those of most diseases are limited to days and weeks. Thus, in typhoid we have the period of incubation of the germ, the prodromal period, the stage of invasion, the period of intestinal lesions, and the active disease, terminated at the end of three weeks, when begins the tardy and precarious stage of recovery by lysis. In yellow fever we have the stage of invasion, often fulminant, the period of lull or abatement, often deluding the patient into the conviction that recovery has set in, only to be followed in many cases by the dreaded black vomit and death—all phases of the disease terminated in a week or ten days.

In syphilis the stages and periods are as strongly marked but more greatly extended, and are viewed over a long lapse of time. They are months apart, years apart, and often extend throughout life.

Syphilis of the mouth may be of any stage,—primary, secondary, or tertiary; and not infrequently we meet here also the lesions of hereditary syphilis.

Primary syphilis is chancre and bubo. The initial point of infection is the chancre; and about the mouth it may occur on the lips (usually the lower), the gums, the tongue, and the tonsil. Other parts of the oral cavity, however, may be infected.

The mode of infection is direct and mediate.

Direct infection means infection-contact of the primary lesion, or contagious secondary lesion, or infected blood during either of these stages. Infection is greatly facilitated if the recipient has an abrasion of the part infected; in truth, it is held by many that a surface of unbroken continuity is invulnerable to infection, but this is fallacious. A subject with abundant mucous patches of the oral cavity can convey infection by a kiss. Any number of cases of specific infection are recorded in which the subject has been infected by some vessel or agent used by the syphilitic. This is mediate infection.

One of the most extraordinary cases of chancre about the oral cavity I ever saw was the case of a gentleman of unquestionable moral integrity. The source of infection was a mystery. The chancre involved the gum near the lower right lateral incisor. After a week of the most patient inquiry, he came to my office and told me that he had noticed the day previously that the clerk at the desk of the restaurant which he patronized picked a toothpick from the tray on the desk, and, after using it, tossed it back. He saw him do this several times. I instructed him to notify the manager, and, together they watched the cashier, and saw him use toothpick after toothpick, tossing some to the floor and some back upon the tray. The young man was notified to stop the habit he had acquired, and the toothpicks were removed from his desk, and at the request of my patient he was brought to me for an examination. His mouth was everywhere covered with mucous patches, and a general examination showed a virulent case of syphilis of about three months' standing. A contaminated toothpick was, in this case, undoubtedly the mediate means of infection.

Primary infection, the chancre, is then the point at which the syphilitic poison is introduced. This excepts, of course, congenital syphilis.

As has been said before, the donor of the disease may infect the non-syphilitic by the virus from a chancre, by the virus from a mucous patch, by discharges from secondary lesions (the so-called moist, secondary manifestations), by the blood during the primary and secondary stages, but not by the normal secretions, such as the saliva or those of the skin.

The chancre may appear in one of several different forms. Of these the deep, or conical, or Hunterian chancre, the chancrous erosion, and the dry chancre, or infecting papule, are the commonest. They all have one thing in common, and that is in their development they cause such irritation that marked induration takes places about and beneath the base of the chancre.

The chancrous erosion and the Hunterian chancre are those met with about the oral cavity. Very soon after the appearance of the chancre enlargement takes place in the lymphatic glands directly associated with the base of the sore. This is due to a lymphoid adenitis, and to this is due the bubo, or specific lymphatic tumor associated with chancre as primary syphilis.

An ulcer within the mouth or on the lip, of a duration of some weeks, and associated with a tumor of the lymphatic glands in the vicinity, should give rise to a suspicion of the presence of primary syphilis, especially if the person be a young man or woman, and the patient should be carefully examined and interrogated as to the cause of the ulcer.

The induration in chancre, especially of the lip, is peculiar. If it be the deep, or Hunterian type, and you take the parts between your fingers, it feels as if you held a bullet, in the top of which, extending toward the centre, is the ulcerating chancre.

In the chancrous erosion the induration is often referred to as parchment induration—it imparts the feel of a thickened layer. It is superficial, but of considerable area.

The victim of syphilis, after about six weeks of primary syphilis, begins to show some evidences of constitutional infection. He complains of slight fever and a general indisposition. If seen at this time the chancre has probably cicatrized, the bubo diminished in size, but the lymphatic glands at large have become involved, and a general lymphatic adenitis results. The lymphatics can often be felt as thickened cords. Sometimes when the lymphangitis is more marked they can be seen as red lines over various parts of the body. The lymphatic glands above the internal epicondyle and about the neck—especially behind the sterno-mastoid—and the post auricular glands are almost invariably involved, and form valuable diagnostic signs. They feel like small pebbles beneath the skin.

Some morning the patient observes, after exertion, perhaps, or after a bath, that his skin is mottled, and on closer examination he finds himself spotted like a leopard: but the spots are rose-colored.

and disappear temporarily under pressure. This is the earliest syphiloderm, and is usually regarded as ushering in the secondary stage of the disease.

In rapid sequence we have the papular eruption, presenting a strongly marked eruption across the forehead, and known popularly as the "corona veneris." All these syphilodermata have a peculiar dull copper-color, as a rule.

Then the pustular and tubercular syphilides follow, often in rapid succession, sometimes so rapid that the next syphilide appears before the former disappear, and this gives rise to the remarkable appearance of a variety of eruptions *co-existent*, and known as the polymorphous syphiloderm.

Even before the skin manifestations occur there is present pain in the bones, most severe at night.

During this stage we also have the secondary iritis, alopecia, local and diffuse analgesia, and, most important to you, the throat and mouth complications.

Syphilitic sore throat is often an early secondary symptom, and is generally associated with mucous patches of the tongue, pillars of the pharynx, uvula, and inside of cheeks.

These oral patches are virulently contagious. Many dentists have become infected from them,—have developed chancre of the finger, and have gone through all the stages of this disease.

What is the mucous patch? It is a syphilitic rash in those positions where there is heat and moisture—where the epithelium is macerated. Hence it is found about the natural orifices; also beneath the breasts in women; also within the mouth and vagina.

Remember that the secondary moist manifestations are virulently contagious, and that if you put your finger into the mouth of a patient having mucous patches, and you have an abrasion on your finger, you are almost certainly sure to become infected, unless there be some special or exceptional immunity.

Mucous patches within the mouth are grayish-looking, surfaces slightly raised, and showing an abundance of macerated epithelium. They are seldom symmetrically disposed, their irregularity of distribution being a diagnostic sign. A little later they ulcerate, the ulcers frequently existing as fissures. About the uvula they often run a rapid course, and destruction of portions of the soft palate is frequently the result. Deep ulceration of the pharynx is very common. The roof of the mouth is often involved, generally among the later secondary lesions, and frequently coexisting with gummatous nodules of the hard palate. Unless now the most active treatment is employed, extensive destruction of the hard palate may ensue.

Tertiary syphilis may come on as early as the second year of this disease; sometimes it is many years later before its lesions develop.

The tertiary lesions are not generally contagious, and when they develop about the oral cavity are of the gummatous and tubercular varieties. These often lead to extensive necrosis of the hard palate; less frequently of the lower jaw. The bones of the nose are most vulnerable, and the disease often invades the air sinuses at the base of the skull. The tongue and salivary glands occasionally become affected with tubercular syphilis, a condition simulating hard cancer and sometimes mistaken for it.

Hereditary syphilis is, unfortunately, often seen. It seldom appears until two or three weeks after birth, when the infant shows evidences of a rhinitis, and gradually develops a snuffling and discharge from the nose. The victim suffers from malnutrition, looks aged and wizened, and frequently secondary eruptions appear, especially bullæ and vesicles on the palms and soles of the feet. Often destructive infiltrations occur in the septum nasi and other nasal structures, and in the floor of the nose, and the peculiar flat, distorted, sunken nose, with the projecting natiform frontal bosses, form the deformed but unmistakable "facies syphiliticæ."

Fortunately, seventy-five per cent. of these infants die before the second year; but those who live show remarkable changes in the form of the permanent central incisors. These are pegged, or notched, or irregularly developed, and are familiar to you as Hutchinson's teeth.

The subject of hereditary syphilis, you are to remember, is liable to develop any or all of the contagious secondary lesions, including mucous patches, and later the tertiary lesions.

It is contended by Colles that a child may inherit syphilis from the father, the mother remaining immune, immunized by the leucomaines and toxins produced in the infected child entering the mother's blood.

Profeta has shown that a child may be born free of or immune to syphilis, both parents being syphilitics prior to the tertiary stage.

It is contended that tertiary syphilis is not transmissible to the progeny.

These are very important matters in the practical consideration of the subject to the medical adviser and to the bench and bar.

I think I have shown that the dentist must, for his protection, be able to recognize syphilis when he sees it; also, that he must exercise extraordinary care to prevent infection; also, that his instruments are easily contaminated, and must be made surgically clean, to protect the non-syphilitic patient.

A NOTE ON KERAMIC FILLINGS.

BY WILLIAM ROLLINS, BOSTON, MASS.

During the last few years several manufacturers, among whom may be mentioned Ash, Brewster, International Dental Manufacturing Company, Dr. N. S. Jenkins, and the S. S. White Company, have placed within reach of the profession excellent keramic materials for producing fillings for teeth by my method of fusing in foil matrices, and in consequence I have seen in the mouths of patients passing through Boston a considerable number of these fillings. Most of the work has been admirable, but some of the operations have been injudicious. In cases where the edge of the cavity was near or under the gum the work was not always well done, because the difficulties of getting a perfect foil matrix had been too great. As a result the layer of cement between the fillings and the edges of the cavities near the gum was too thick to be durable, and decay had begun. On this account a method of getting a suitable foil matrix from these cavities is given.

From the beginning, to save time, I endeavored to make keramic filling a laboratory method as far as possible, and soon perfected a means of making sharp impressions, which was described in my early papers and is the one used with the method to be described, only, instead of making an electrotype from the impression, a mould is obtained by using a zinc cement of the type described in my paper of 1879 and now known as oxyphosphate. This gives hard and perfect moulds, from the impressions of which there should be several. When the cement is hard the impression compound is removed. The part of the mould representing the gum is then ground away, giving free access to the cavity, thus facilitating the production of the foil matrix. The mould is then fastened by sealing-wax to the centre of a thin board twenty-five centimetres long, which serves as a rest for the hands while making the foil matrix, which is done from the zinc mould instead of from the tooth. The operation is simpler, and as many foil matrices can be made as are desirable, for, the work being done by an assistant, neither the dentist's nor the patient's time is taken. It is usually an advantage to have three fillings baked, as one is often a better color than the others. This method gives good impressions of the edges of cavities under the gum margins because the impression compound forces the gum away from the edges, leaving them sharply defined.

In keramic work I have employed for many years a binocular magnifying glass attached to the head and leaving both hands free. This was made by Heinrich Westien, of Mechlenburg. It has the advantage of allowing the work to be placed at the normal operating distance of about twenty-two centimetres, therefore all muscular movements seem normal. It is of especial value in manipulating the foil matrices and in baking, as it protects the eyes from the heat and allows the operation to be minutely watched during the whole fusion. For keramic material that fuses in gold matrices I have used, since its introduction some years ago, Mitchell's little furnace, which weighs only a hundred and seventy grammes. If the foil matrix is placed two centimetres from the open mouth of the muffle, fusion is perfect and the work can be constantly observed.

Reviews of Dental Literature.

Six Years' Work in Oral Prophylaxis.[1] By D. D. Smith, D.D.S., M.D., Philadelphia, Pa.

The term oral prophylaxis, so recently injected into the vocabulary of dentistry, is endowed with a meaning which as yet seems not well understood.

Prophylaxis is quite commonly confounded with prophylactic,

---

[1] Read before the New Jersey State Dental Society, Thirty-fourth Annual Session, July 20, 1904.

and is used by speakers and writers interchangeably with it, when, in fact, the two words have quite separate and distinctive significations. These terms are also used, apparently without discrimination, as synonyms for asepsis, oral hygiene, oral massage, and whatever is supposed to ward off disease of the teeth.

One dental writer says, " Prophylaxis has invaded the domain of nearly every disease, and its science and practice is daily increasing and its field of usefulness becoming better known."

Prophylactic measures may be employed to ward off some diseases when preventive remedies, from experience, commend themselves, or when experimentation in this direction seems warranted, but to affirm that " *prophylaxis* has invaded the domain of nearly every disease" seems a confusion of terms.

It is to be hoped that the science of prophylaxis is becoming better known, but it cannot at present be said that prophylactic remedies or the prophylaxis treatment is " well understood" in dentistry, or that either is applied or practised as a science.

In defining the terms prophylactic and prophylaxis we would emphasize the fact that prophylactic is a word used both as an adjective and as a noun, and that it relates to therapeutic *remedies*, which may be administered as preventive of disease. Prophylaxis relates to remedial or preventive *treatment*. The dictionaries generally pointed to the signification as here given when the first paper on this subject was prepared and read in 1898, under the caption " Prophylaxis in Dentistry." Only one has been found to give prophylaxis any other meaning; this is as follows: " Prophylaxis, preservative treatment for disease; conservation;" from which one would naturally infer that prophylaxis preserves and conserves disease, instead of preventing it.

Webster's Dictionary, 1901 edition, defines prophylactic as follows: " Prophylactic, a *medicine* which preserves or defends against disease; a preventive;" and " prophylaxis, the *art* of preserving from, or of preventing, disease. The observance of the rules necessary for the preservation of health; preservative or *preventive treatment.*"

Worcester gives: " Prophylactic, an adjective, preventing disease; preventive; preservative." Prophylaxis not defined.

The Century: " Prophylaxis, *n.*, anything, as a *medicine*, which defends against disease; a preventive of disease;" and " prophylactic, *a.*, preventive; defending from disease, as prophy-

lactic doses of quinine." (That is, treatment by therapy; therapeutic treatment.) "Prophylaxis, the guarding against the attack
of some disease;" example: "The germs do not appear to be very
tenacious of life, so that an efficient prophylaxis can be readily
exercised.—*Science*."

Standard Dictionary: "Prophylactic, any medicine or measure
efficacious in protecting from disease." "Prophylaxis, preservative
or preventive *treatment* for disease; especially a particular form
of disease in an individual."

Briefly then, prophylaxis is an art or a surgical treatment, involving manipulative effort, as distinguished from the administration of a systemic medicament or a therapeutic remedy. Hence,
oral prophylaxis implies surgical instrumentation or treatment of
the mouth and teeth in contradistinction to a germicide, a wash, or
any form of medication for the prevention of disease in the oral
cavity.

Although the title of this paper is "Six Years' Work in Oral
Prophylaxis," the time really covered in developing the treatment,
by the author, embraces a period of ten years. Experiments were
carried forward on members of my own family and among friends
for four years prior to the reading of the paper on "Prophylaxis in
Dentistry" referred to above, that theories might be verified before
giving any publicity to the treatment. The results were so satisfactory that in the beginning of the fifth year it was determined to
force recognition of it in general practice, little dreaming what
astounding revelations were to follow.

In reviewing the subject at this time it will be my endeavor, as
in former papers, to present some of the remarkable phenomena
which appear as unvarying results, from a consistent and intelligent
prophylaxis treatment of the mouth and teeth. While these results
are surprising, almost startling, to one who has never witnessed
them, they are but the logical and inevitable outcome of this system
of caring for the mouth and teeth.

PROPHYLAXIS TREATMENT AS APPLIED TO TEETH IN THE MOUTH.

To understand what the prophylaxis treatment in its application
to the mouth and teeth is, we must understand the long train of
unstudied and disregarded pathologic conditions which have their
origin in the undisturbed infection on and about the teeth in the
human mouth.

Calcific deposits are constantly occurring and recurring, and not less the more immediately hurtful acidulated bacterial accumulations; and more dangerous still the inspissated mucus which cements mouth fluids, mucoid excretions, decomposing food particles, and other septic and odoriferous matter upon the teeth; this débris is all maintained in the high normal heat of the mouth—98.6° F.—and furnishes ideal conditions for the proliferation of germs, the induction of decay, and the fostering of disease in the human system. The pathologic states of the mouth and teeth, in the order of their seriousness and frequency, may be defined as follows: pericemento-alveolar inflammations, dental caries, and impeded alveolar development.

Resulting from the first and most important—pericemento-alveolar inflammations—we find gum inflammations, alveolar absorption, pyorrhœa, stomatitis, and pericemental abscess; the latter a serious condition, resulting in the inevitable loss of the tooth. Caries, with its attendant decalcification of dentine, followed by pulp exposure, alveolar abscess, and final destruction of the *crown of the tooth*, although it has engrossed the thought of dentistry in the past and is the embodiment of its efforts in the present, is far less serious in its results. Impeded alveolar development, a common result of mouth infection of childhood, is a cause of many alveolar deformities and many crowded and irregular conditions of the teeth;—conditions which detract from the charm of facial expression, greatly increase infection, incite decay and multiply loss of the teeth.

Whether conscious of it or not, every human being with natural teeth is a sufferer from mouth infection; some to a greater extent than others—the civilized more than the savage.

The oral prophylaxis treatment, as instituted and recommended by the author, has for its object and aim the freeing of the oral cavity of conditions of tooth decay which has become practically universal, and the eradication of infection from the same, to conserve human health and prolong human life. In all stations and conditions the treatment has demonstrated its sufficiency and its reasonable practicability. The benefits accruing to the mouth and teeth, and thence to the general health, are startling in the scope of their marvellous efficiency.

SUBSTANTIATION OF THEORIES RESPECTING TOOTH DECAY AND TOOTH PRESERVATION. .

In previous writings I have persistently maintained that tooth decay always begins on some surface of the tooth which is exposed to the fluids of the mouth. It never originates in the substance of the tooth unexposed, either crown or root. If the decay is in the crown, it begins in the enamel; if devoid of enamel, it may attack the surface of the dentine at any point. Once in the dentine, the decay proceeds along the lines of the tubules in the direction of the pulp. The process of tooth-solution, which we call decay, is largely chemical, and is hindered or opposed by two conditions only: (*a*) the composition or consolidation of enamel and dentine; (*b*) the expression of vital energy interposed by a living pulp—a force often scarcely appreciable. No matter what the physical state of the crown of the tooth, whether hard or soft, good or bad, alive or dead, the agents and agencies which cause decay are in the environment or surroundings of the teeth. Evidence from practical experience in support of this is abundant and unvarying. A simple and incontestable proof is found in the state of an extracted tooth. Let a pulpless, decaying tooth be removed from a mouth where the environments are such that resolution is rapidly taking place, and let it be placed in water, alcohol, or glycerin, or simply exposed to the air, and all decay in that tooth is immediately arrested; further disintegration will come only with the lapse of years.

To institute simulated or artificial decay in a tooth while it is out of its natural environment, as has been frequently done, is wholly unavailing as a matter of scientific investigation. All such processes are but artificial decomposition, and are so unlike tooth-decay in the mouth that true scientific research is not advanced by them. Teeth are the subject of true decay only when they are in the normal menstruum and temperature of the mouth.

The all-important matter for dentistry to consider and determine is, whether oral prophylaxis, understood and properly instituted, will arrest, prevent, or retard decay of the teeth *in the mouth*. To this end there is needed not *theorizing* but clear clinical observation and close study of mouth conditions.

Ten years' experimentation has abundantly demonstrated that while the treatment will not arrest decay which is already in progress, whether as new cavities or under old or imperfect fillings, it will prevent its appearance on surfaces where the prophylaxis treatment has been regularly instituted. It will also greatly retard the progress of decay in open cavities and under old fillings.

An editorial in a recent number of *American Medicine* reads in part as follows: " There are ten millions of them! Everybody knows about them, the disease they spread, their horrors, their worse than loathsomeness! Every one endures, submits in silence, feels himself powerless to remedy. Boards of health cannot, or think they cannot, attack the evil; or they are too busy with things they think are more important. And so the filthy country and village water-closet persists from generation to generation. The intellectual philanthropist is yet to come who shall undertake one of the greatest reforms of the world!"

The greatest sanitary reform of the world is not the abolition of the village closet, but it lies in the herculean task of revolutionizing the unsanitary and infectious condition of the human mouth. Contagion and disease from the latter are a thousand-fold more subtle and dangerous than from the former, for infection in the human mouth is found not in country and village alone, but in town and city—in all places where humanity dwells.

If this be true,—and who shall dispute it?—oral prophylaxis treatment presents itself as a subject of momentous import both for the profession and the public. It is not a matter to be tossed hastily aside because it does not coincide with our prejudices or preconceived opinions; neither is it a matter to be adjudged wholly from the stand-point of self-interest. Theoretical difficulties have been presented and unjustifiable self-interests have been urged against it, until we have sometimes asked with unutterable groanings, " Is dentistry, with such views, worthy to be called a profession ?"

One writer declares, " The great limitation to the universal success of Dr. Smith's method lies in the non-receptiveness of the mass of people to methods involving as much attention to detail as must be required of those patients following his system."

This unjustifiable deduction in the *Dental Cosmos*, from the pen of a professor in dentistry, exhibits not only the prejudice of inexperience, but shows a lamentable, if not inexcusable, ignorance of the whole subject of oral prophylaxis; it is an example of the futility of theory in dentistry *vs.* practical experience.

In reply to the seeming objection respecting " the non-receptiveness of the mass of the people," it may be said, the statement is assertion only; it has no basis in fact.

To "the mass of the people" dentistry of the present extends no benefits, it presents no hope, it affords no relief, save in the one direction,—that of ridding the mouth of aching teeth through extraction. "The mass of the people" are not instructed respecting the teeth; they are wholly unacquainted with the necessities, requirements, or value of these organs. How, then, should they be expected to follow out any theory or give attention to the details of any "system," for their betterment or preservation?

This, however, is true: whenever requisite presentation respecting the infectious states of the teeth in ordinary conditions of the human mouth is made to people of intelligence, with whom dentistry has largely to do, and the relations of these conditions to decay of the teeth has been correlated and explained, the liveliest interest has always been awakened, and patients have been stirred to willing co-operation in all reasonable efforts for the betterment and immunizing of the teeth by the system of prophylaxis treatment I have advocated for the six years just past.

When instructed, patients have been quick to see and appreciate the imminent danger of systemic infection due to septic states of untreated teeth. A set of septic teeth, ordinarily presenting a surface of twenty to thirty square inches in the oral cavity, a cavity which has been aptly designated the vestibule of life, is a perpetual menace to human health.

No adequate consideration has ever been given to the sources of infection inherent in the human mouth, consequent upon the presence of natural teeth. The adverse *local* consequences—decay, alveolar necrosis, pyorrhœa, gum recession, and final loss of the teeth—are as nothing in comparison with the evils to be revealed in the systemic disturbances and diseases which result from the continuous state of infection found in association with the teeth in the human mouth. These conditions, studied by dentistry and intelligently set forth to "the mass of people" would find "a receptiveness" which would not only astonish the opponents of this "system" of preventive treatment, but would render incalculable benefits to general health, longevity, and the happiness of all civilized humanity.

WHAT THE PROPHYLAXIS TREATMENT IS.

Let us here consider the nature and character of the prophylaxis treatment, and what it does for the mouth and teeth.

In general the treatment consists of enforced, radical and frequent change of environment for all teeth and all mouth conditions, and the maintenance of perfect sanitation for the oral cavity. More in detail it is the careful and complete removal of all concretions, calcic deposits, semisolids, bacterial placques, and inspissated secretions and excretions which gather on the surfaces of the teeth, between them, or at the gum margins; this instrumentation to be followed *in every case* by the thorough polishing of all tooth surfaces by *hand methods,—power polishers should never be used,—* not alone the more exposed labial and buccal surfaces of the teeth, but the lingual, palatal, and proximal surfaces as well, using for this purpose orange-wood points in suitable holders (porte polishers) charged with finely ground pumice-stone as a polishing material. Treated in this manner the teeth are placed in the most favorable condition to prevent and repel septic accumulations and deposits, and what is of equal importance, it aids the patient in all efforts to maintain sanitation and cleanliness.

"Brushing the tongue" for the removal of infectious coatings has been advocated more recently. Tongue *brushing* is impractical and devoid of utility. A coated tongue, especially if accompanied with tonsular inflammation, may very properly and advantageously be disinfected (mopped off) by the use of germicidal applications on bibulous paper. I have produced marked beneficial results, when finding the tongue infectiously coated, through mopping it off once or twice a day with phenol sodique. There are other remedies for this purpose perhaps equally efficient.

SOME SPECIFIC BENEFITS.

Studying more closely some of the specific benefits which result from the oral prophylaxis treatment, we notice first those that accrue to the teeth themselves. Three to six months of this treatment consistently carried forward will effectually change the whole appearance, and to some extent the whole character of a set of teeth. This change is seen in all cases, young and old, but it is specially marked in children and youth and in young adults. The dull, opaque, and lifeless aspect of the teeth exhibited in ordinary conditions of nearly all mouths, quickly gives way, under the prophylaxis treatment, to a clear, pure tooth color; the teeth in a limited time become naturally translucent, and present the appearance and true characteristics of living, healthy organs. Teeth that appear as a disfigurement in the mouth, even to disgust and loathing, when subjected for a time to the prophylaxis treatment, become strikingly ornate and attractive. The osseous structures, after a few months, exhibit unmistakably a marked change for the better, and in most cases they become wholly immune to decay. The vital forces within the tooth—the pulp—and those surrounding it—the pericementum and its connections—are stirred and stimulated to new life and activity. Circulation in dentine and enamel is revived and quickened; old, stagnant colors and deposits are manifestly taken up and removed, and new, fresh material deposited in place of them.

It is most interesting and instructive to witness the awakening and revivifying of the life forces of the teeth under treatment, as exhibited in the discharge of this undue and disagreeable color, in the brightening general aspect, and in the cessation of hypersensitiveness and irritability.

An irritating, life-destroying infection continuously adherent to the surfaces of untreated teeth, becomes a condition of violent exhibition in some cases, and when trained to recognize it, it is distinctly manifest in all. This infection retards circulation, hinders nutrition, and greatly interferes with the general health of the teeth. Manipulative treatment and the medication attending its frequent removal stimulates and fosters the remarkable changes and improvements noticed in the character and substance of all teeth which are the subject of this treatment.

The prophylaxis treatment, as yet but very imperfectly understood even by its friends, has been charged as merely a form of "tooth cleaning." Far more than this, it is a manipulative process that positively relieves the teeth from a virulent infection, and introduces a stimulation most beneficial to their internal and external life. If a tooth-cleaning process, it is one of profound significance.

If time would permit, instances might be specifically cited and multiplied in which *no* new decay has appeared in mouths, even with complete sets of teeth, for four, five, and six years; and many others in which but a modicum of decay has been found in the same length of time, and that chiefly around old fillings.

WHAT IT DOES FOR DECIDUOUS TEETH.

The deciduous teeth in all cases are quickly and markedly influenced by the treatment. Of the limited number of children under seven years of age who are under the prophylaxis treatment, not one presents a new decay or a new defect in a tooth.

AN INTERESTING CASE.

One remarkably interesting and instructive case is that of a boy, of strongly marked nervous temperament, brought to me when but three and a half years of age, in delicate health. At this time there were five large cavities—three approximal—in his teeth, and two places exhibiting such predisposition to decay that I prognosed cavities in them within three months. Through exercise of patience and perseverance the cavities were excavated and filled with amalgam. (Perfect operations were impossible.) Immediately following the filling, for an entire year, his teeth were carefully treated every two weeks, barring one month during the summer vacation. Since that time—nearly five years—I have seen him on an average once a month; meanwhile, his teeth have received rather more than the ordinary care of childhood, at home. The boy is now in his ninth year, with this record: excessive nervousness arrested; general health fully established; teeth, as to decay, in perfect condition (predicted cavities did not appear); one new pin-head cavity in distal sulcus of left superior temporary molar (probably started before first five fillings were made); one re-decay around largest and most difficult of the five original fillings. Twelve of the temporary teeth have loosened and come out, every one in nature's own way, through complete root absorption. First permanent molars, inferior and superior permanent incisors erupted, cuspids presenting. The first molars—erupted at five and a half years—have unusually large crowns with strongly-marked, pointed cusps and correspondingly deep sulci and linear markings. Formation, shape, and time of eruption of these teeth presaged early and rapid decay; nevertheless, they are at this writing all in perfect state of preservation, and evidently improving in character. Neither infection nor chemical agents are permitted to fasten upon any of their surfaces, and the life forces are evidently building into them a more compact and decay-resisting structural consolidation.

The benefits resulting from the prophylaxis treatment as exhibited in this case are equally marked in every case where deciduous teeth have been subjected to the treatment.

Another result, convincing as to the benefits of this treatment beyond all others that can be cited, may be witnessed in connection with many cases in which decay, running riot in both temporary and permanent teeth at ten and eleven years of age, has been practically stopped following the full institution of the prophylaxis treatment. The second or twelfth-year molars, erupting into a healthy environment, have been universally found in perfect condition, and have continued thus far devoid of decay, even in the sulci. Not in one instance merely, but in practically every instance, these conditions exist.

Other and most convincing proofs may be seen in connection with the eruption of wisdom-teeth. Perhaps the most noteworthy instance in my practice in this connection is that of a young man, at the time about nineteen, for whom I had operated from boyhood, long antedating the introduction of the prophylaxis treatment. The teeth in this mouth had decayed early and in all directions. Crown, approximal, and labial fillings are to be seen in all parts of the mouth; even the lower incisors and cuspids had not escaped. The four wisdom-teeth appeared about two years after beginning an irregular and unsatisfactory course of prophylaxis treatment, but even with this, the contrast between these teeth and the twenty-eight which preceded them affords a most instructive lesson regarding the benefits of treatment. Despised, misrepresented and condemned to decay and loss, as wisdom-teeth frequently are, these teeth (and I could mention a number of other similar cases), erupting into a mouth which had been quite irregularly under treatment, were perfect. Decay had appeared in every class of teeth which developed before the prophylaxis treatment commenced, but in these wisdom-teeth there was neither decay nor the appearance of it, and this condition pertained until the case passed from under my care.

THE INFLUENCE OF THE PROPHYLAXIS TREATMENT ON SENSITIVE DENTINE.

As a further observation of the benefits of this treatment, I desire to put on record a development of marked significance,—namely, a decided modification noticed in the sensitiveness of the dentine of teeth, especially in children, following the institution of a regular and consistent treatment. Diminishing of acute sensitiveness seems to follow as a general result, and not to be some special temporary condition. The extreme sensitiveness in the dentine of young teeth has been so modified and lessened, apparently by this treatment, that ordinary operations for filling have been performed without the intense suffering usually attending such cases. Children and young people who are under this treatment submit to ordinary operations without compulsion or special complaint.

Operations that under the old *régime* would cause much suffering, if not deemed unbearable, have been greatly mitigated in intensity.

It is an inadequate presentation to say that the prophylaxis treatment is a marked modifier of sensitive dentine, especially in the young, and that it is a mitigator of suffering under all dental operations. This may seem an extreme statement, but when fully tested by experience it will be received as conservatively true.

Hypersensitiveness of dentine is a result of pericemental irritation far more than of pulp irritation. The external and most important life of the tooth—the pericemental life—is markedly influenced by the irritative infection found always at the necks of untreated teeth. Removal of this infection is the removal of the cause of much of the undue sensitiveness of dental tissue.

THE MARKED BENEFICIAL INFLUENCE OF THE TREATMENT IN CONNECTION WITH GUM AND PERICEMENTAL TISSUE.

The benefits which accrue directly to the teeth are not more manifest nor more pronounced than such as immediately appear in the pericementum and gums. The presence of irritative infectious matter on the surfaces of untreated teeth, sufficient to affect the pericementum and surrounding gum tissue, is found in connection with all untreated teeth. It appears coeval with their eruption, and continues, in ordinary conditions, as long as the teeth are retained. It is bounded only by the extent of the dentate surface exposed in the mouth; as a result, the pericemental tissue and gums in ordinary mouth conditions are perpetually in a state of undue sensitiveness, and not less, a condition of undue, often extreme, vascularity. Under the prophylaxis treatment, through which all irritants are removed, these tissues quickly lose their extreme and unnatural sensitiveness, and recover the normal condition of low-grade sensibility. (Gum tissue in a state of health is always without acute sensation.) The circulatory vessels also lose the unnatural distention and tumefaction consequent upon irritation, recover tonicity, and contract to normal dimensions. Three to six months of treatment will remove all marked sensibility and tendency to bleed, and operations for filling at cervical margins, especially on the upper jaw, can be safely and easily performed without the use of the rubber-dam. It is the irritative, toxic matter at the necks of the teeth that occasions the sensitive states and highly vascular conditions of the gums and pericemental tissue. A mouth with teeth freed from this infection and kept in an aseptic condition will have gums tense and hard, without vascularity and without undue sensibility.

We have, then, to commend the prophylaxis treatment: first, for its prevention of decay; second, for its stimulation to external and internal life and health of the teeth; third, for its influence in decreasing sensation in dentine and gum tissue; fourth, for its correction of the undue vascularity in gum tissue; and fifth, for its positive removal of all infection from the mouth and ultimately from the breath.

SELF-TREATMENT BY PATIENTS.

It may be well to enter somewhat into detail respecting the care and co-operation expected, *even required*, of patients under the prophylaxis treatment. In the beginning, for four to six months they are required to present regularly, on appointment, once a month for treatment, which is carefully applied, using only hand methods as heretofore described. Every patient should be armed with proper appliances, especially brush and dentifrice, for cleansing the teeth and mouth, and fully instructed in the use of the same.

The tooth-brush, which is the main reliance of the patient, is at best an inefficient instrument for cleansing teeth. It is, however, the best our civilization has produced, hence until something better is devised, necessity compels the use of it: of the hundreds of shapes, varieties and kinds on the market, very few are suitable for use. Unfortunately the choice and *selection* of tooth-brushes for the general public is now largely relegated to salesladies in the department stores, and the preparation of dentifrices and so-called mouth-washes is in the hands of druggists; a condition of things as incongruous as is the compounding of medicines by the post-office clerk in a general country store. Would not dentistry itself be greatly embarrassed, if not awkwardly handicapped, if suddenly confronted with a demand, from kingly authority, for a really efficient tooth-brush or dentifrice? Probably not one in a thousand could present a clear, consistent idea of what the character or shape of a brush should be to best do the work of cleansing the teeth.

It may be said, without hesitation or fear of contradiction, there is no part of the human body which is so imperfectly and ignorantly cared for as this most important cavity containing the teeth. Attending to the teeth by the patient is a matter which has neither been studied nor taught either by the professionalist or the laity.

The child is *taught* to wash the hands, to bathe the body,—but the human mouth, the very vestibule of life, is left wholly without intelligent care.

Witness the education of the average child in a matter of such vital importance: After breakfast (occasionally), "John (or Mary), have you brushed your teeth this morning?" "No, ma'am." "Well, go right away to the bath-room and brush your teeth." Has the child ever been taught rational methods? No. Examine the equipment placed in the hands of childhood for this important operation. Even when new, a cheap, ill-adapted brush and unusable dentifrice (good enough for the children) is all they can find. This want of intelligent instruction, and these careless methods in childhood, follow through life.

The results are everywhere seen in repulsive exhibits of decayed, infection-coated teeth, offensive breaths, a display of discolored fillings, and that dental monstrosity, so common,—the gold crown.

Solomon said of the teeth of the daughter of Zion, the perfection of beauty, "Thy teeth are like a flock of sheep, even shorn, which go up from the washing whereof every one bearest twins, and there is not one barren among them." A most beautiful description of a perfect, thoroughly cared-for set of teeth.

The general public, compelled to rely on the tooth-brush, is yet without proper equipment for cleansing the teeth. The whole operation soon becomes distasteful, irksome, and generally the merest farce. Patients present with mouths reeking with infection, teeth loaded with deposits that are antiquated, and affirm "that they are very careful about brushing their teeth."

All this should be changed. It can only be done by a process of education, and that through instruction given by dentistry. Every dentist should first inform himself, and then fully instruct individual patients in the details of the care of the human mouth. The people should be taught that cleaning the teeth is not merely the *possession* of a tooth-brush. The best-shaped brush in the world will not clean the teeth in a human mouth unless it is intelligently used.

A tooth-brush should possess the requisites of shape, substance, and stability. In shape it should be plain and perfectly straight, the bristles neither coarse nor fine, set in rows of different lengths; in substance, all of the best materials. There should be no concavity to fit the arch when the brush is at rest; no fancy curves;

no tufts of bristles at the end. It should be of size, in length and width, to form a mass of bristles to cover the teeth and give stability and substance when in use.

In using the brush it should be passed over labial, buccal, lingual, and palatal—or the whole outer and inner surfaces of the teeth, with a vigorous *horizontal* movement, the hand adapting the brush, as far as possible, to all tooth surfaces. With care and a straight brush all parts of the exposed crowns may thus be reached and cleansed as well as a brush can do this office work. Attempting to cleanse the teeth with the vertical movement, using a concave brush, as some teach, on the convex surface of the dental arches, while of little avail, will do no harm, either to the teeth or gums. Such use of the brush in a measure relieves the interstices of food remains, and thus assists in a work that can be much better done with a tooth-pick. The most widely advertised, and perhaps the most popular tooth-brush of the present, is the so-called " prophylactic." This brush, and all similar in shape, is a conspicuous example of lack of adaptation of means to an end. It demands the vertical movement of the brush on the external surface of the arches and on the inner surfaces it presents a double bow, most effectually preventing contact of any considerable surface of the brush with the most uncleanly portions of the teeth. A plain brush, with horizontal movement, is much better and much more efficacious.

It has been urged that the vertical movement of the brush acts as a kind of massage, tending to brush the gums onto the teeth, while the horizontal movement brushes them away from the teeth. This is the merest *theory*, a statement wholly without justification in actual conditions. The vertical movement of the brush is not more a massage of the gums than is the horizontal movement. There is no process of brushing which approximates a massage treatment of the gums, and it would avail nothing if there could be. My patients are always instructed, in connection with the prophylaxis treatment, to use the brush with a vigorous horizontal movement, even when the gums and alveolar process have necrosed until the festoons have become everted, and to continue the brushing until the teeth are not only brushed but *cleansed*. I have never yet seen a case in which reformation of tissue has not followed the treatment, and in all cases not connected with pyorrhœa, restoration of the festoons has been complete and perfect.

The tooth-brush implies a dentifrice, and a dentifrice is demanded for cleaning the teeth. To attempt a review of the compounds under the head of so-called dentifrices would consume far more time than is allotted this paper. We can only say of the tooth-powders, tablets, washes, and pastes sold as dentifrices, while they are manufactured and sold largely through the greatest empiricism, and while some are far more efficient and pleasant than others, few of them can be classed as positively harmful when used within proper limits.

So-called tooth-powders are compounded from some base, generally prepared chalk (*calc. carb. precipitas*), orris root (*iridis Florentinæ*), acidum salicylicum, or some other material. To the base selected may be added, according to the fancy of the druggist or compounder, white sugar, soap, soap-bark, cinchona, cinnamon, cuttle-fish bone (*ossis sepiæ pulveris*), pumice-stone (*lapidis pumicei pulveris*), flavoring and coloring, or whatever may be supposed to make a pleasant and salable preparation, to be advertised and sold " for beautifying the teeth and imparting sweet odors to the breath." We are not altogether decrying these powder preparations, for something of the powder or soap nature is demanded always with the brush. Patients should be taught to avoid all pastes or liquid dentifrices, for they are not only inefficient, but frequently harmful. A good soap, as a pure Castile, may be used *ad libitum,* and always with benefit to the mouth.

The impression very generally prevails that the *time* for brushing the teeth is after meals. This is a fallacy for dentistry to uproot. To receive the greatest benefit from the use of the tooth-brush, the mouth should be thoroughly cleansed always just *before* meals. Infection gathers upon the teeth in the interim between meals, when the salivary glands are at rest and the teeth not in use; it is during periods of rest that the mucous secretion and mucoid excretions from mucous surfaces are lodged upon the teeth in greatest quantity. Cleansing the mouth and teeth from this viscid débris *before* meals prevents the washing of these toxic tooth accretions into the gastro-intestinal tract with the food. Who is not taught to wash the *hands* before meals? Of how much greater importance is the cleansing of the human mouth! If the accustomed method with the brush is not practicable, it may be always practicable to thoroughly rinse the mouth with water and to wipe the main exposed surfaces of the teeth with the corner of a towel or napkin. This method of cleaning the teeth is not enough in vogue. After meals the teeth may be freed of food remains with some form of tooth-pick, preferably the "quill," which is all that is required. Careful cleansing, devoting not seconds but minutes to the operation, should always precede retiring for the night and immediately succeed rising in the morning.

Cleansing the mouth thus frequently, and at stated periods, will greatly tend to preserve the teeth from decay, and surely lessen the inroads of systemic infection.

ANOTHER VIEW OF MOUTH INFECTION.

The photographer who would make sure of a satisfactory picture, having made one negative, will frequently change the position of his subject for another view; he may move the head into another light, readjust the camera and screens, or perhaps rearrange the shading. That we may fasten upon the mind and carry away with us a more vivid and lasting picture of these adverse, repugnant and hurtful mouth conditions, let us here endeavor to secure a picture from another point of view.

A Mr. McC. quite recently applied for relief from one of the most unpromising conditions of pyorrhœa it has been my good fortune to encounter. I say "good fortune," for I regard it as good fortune that through study and practice of the oral prophylaxis treatment the dental profession is now able to throw off the shackles which have so long held it in bondage to the commonly accepted theory that alveolar pyorrhœa is a *disease* of constitutional origin, and incurable. It is good fortune as well as a great pleasure to bring relief to a long list of afflicted ones, and to proclaim the fact that alveolar pyorrhœa is not a *disease* in the true meaning of that term; that it does not result from the gouty or uric acid diathesis; it is a pleasure to proclaim that it is not a result of some "constitutional vice," nor of any special constitutional condition. The glamour and charm of mystery no longer hang over this affection; the light of rational, indisputable, scientific truth shines through the mists and clouds of speculation and theory which have so long enveloped it.

WHAT ALVEOLAR PYORRHŒA IS.

Alveolar pyorrhœa is not properly classified as a "disease." Its very definition—flow of pus—implies that it should be taken from the category of diseases and placed among the inflammations. Properly defined, alveolar pyorrhœa is an inflammation within the confines of the pericemental membrane and contiguous tissues; an inflammation due wholly to the irritation resulting from stagnant septic matter adherent to the surfaces, necks, and roots of natural teeth. It need no longer be said that these are " constitutional conditions, complex in their manifestations ;" neither that their " medical and hygienic management are almost exclusively in the hands of the physician." How utterly absurd is the proposition that the " duty of the dental practitioner is confined largely to the question of diagnosis." Treatment of pyorrhœa relegated to the medical profession! *Neither* diagnosis nor treatment belongs to medicine; it is a mouth disorder strictly within the realm of the dental practitioner. It is to the discredit of dentistry and not of medicine that such inconsiderate and contradictory teachings prevail respecting it. It is a mouth affection in association with the teeth of which medicine, as a profession, has never assumed to know. Occurring in mouths with large, strong, and apparently healthy teeth, how should medicine suspect that it is largely, if not entirely, the prime cause of renal disturbances, uræmia, diabetes, and albuminuria; and many other constitutional disturbances of which we know so little?

I here exhibit casts of the mouth referred to as it presented from the hands of one of the fashionable dentists of Philadelphia. It is a typical case of pyorrhœa. A married man in middle life— thirty-eight years—with hard, strong teeth, crowns large and irregular, roots not long and probably conical, marked cervical constriction, and pericemental tissue scanty. This gentleman is a smoker, but not given to excesses or vices; had brushed his teeth latterly with so-called " prophylactic" brush after approved methods, vertical movement.

As through this case we look upon the horrible conditions in human mouths everywhere, in high and low born, king and peasant, and realize that they are wholly due to states and conditions of natural teeth, and so largely preventable, shall not we rise as witnesses for, and to advocate better things for, neglected, untaught, suffering humanity?

But to return to this typical case of pyorrhœa: The broad-bladed scaler of the Smith set was passed back to the lingual surface of the second lower molar, where it was loaded with years of accumulations of calcic toxins, recent exudations of globules of pus, and gatherings of every variety of mouth débris. This conglomerate mass of revolting matter was held up to view, and the patient asked if he would like to handle it, to smell it, to taste it, to have it returned to the mouth.   To all of these suggestions there was prompt declination.   Then it was clearly explained that matter of similar nature is found on all untreated teeth; and that teeth are not on the outside of the body, *but inside the mouth;* that such conditions exist, not one hour in the day, but twenty-four hours of every day; not one day in the year, but three hundred and sixty-five days of every year; and further, this infectious matter on the teeth, *in the mouth,* is in a temperature constantly maintained at 98.6° F., than which nothing could possibly be more favorable for germ culture, for imparting odors to the breath, or for filling the lungs with infectious emanations.

From the mouth and teeth, septic matter is being conveyed directly into the gastro-intestinal tract, thence to the circulation, whence it may be deposited in any organ or tissue, and become the nucleus of serious chronic, systemic maladies.   To emphasize the continuous presence of this deleterious matter, the patient was told he could at any hour of the day draw floss silk between the teeth, or pass the finger over their surfaces, and discover most repellent odors; or he could recall the unpleasant taste in the mouth on rising in the morning, the fetid breath, especially at night,—due not to stomach conditions, but to the stagnant, odoriferous matter on the teeth.   Becoming dry, through inactivity of the salivary glands, the teeth send out into the breath of the sleeper poisonous emanations to do continuously a work of infection, unnoticed and unsuspected.

I would that it might be recognized by all, that sequences of the universal infection on the teeth in the oral cavity are, in our present civilization, affecting the health of humanity to a greater extent than any other one physical condition.   I could wish nothing grander or better for our profession than that it should see and embrace the magnificent opportunity unfolded in oral prophylaxis to move forward and occupy this new field of untold benefits.

Dentistry, in these revelations respecting states of infection ordinarily existing in the human mouth, has opened a door for general etiological research of far-reaching importance.

The secrets of tooth decay, in and of themselves, are of minor consequence in comparison with the systemic infections due directly to states and conditions of the teeth in the mouth.   We venture to predict that recognition will ere long be made of the fact that tuberculosis,—that decimator of homes,—and possibly other grave chronic disorders, can find no soil for development in a system kept from the contaminations of mouth-infection through a rigorous prophylaxis treatment from childhood.

We have abundantly proved that diabetes and many gastro-intestinal troubles are directly traceable to the mouth-infection of alveolar pyorrhœa; also that many pharyngeal and tonsular inflammations, and many skin troubles, have their origin in infection in the mouth, due to septic states of neglected teeth. We know, also, that mental depression and hypochondria, and many of the perplexing nervous conditions in women, result from the same cause.

Dentistry alone has the power to relieve humanity from the plague of mouth-infection. When shall it command its own rightful place among the specialties of medicine?

Reports of Society Meetings.

THE NEW YORK INSTITUTE OF STOMATOLOGY.

A MEETING of the Institute was held on Tuesday evening, December 6, 1904, at the "Chelsea," No. 222 West Twenty-third Street, New York, the President, Dr. C. O. Kimball, in the chair.

The minutes of the last meeting were read and approved.

Dr. Lee Maidment Hurd read a paper entitled "The Radical Treatment of the Maxillary Antrum."

(For Dr. Hurd's paper, see page 159.)

DISCUSSION.

Dr. T. Passmore Berens.—Dr. Hurd's paper has been such that it leaves but little to be added. However, the subject is one of considerable interest and of such importance that perhaps you will pardon my emphasizing one or two points in the doctor's remarks.

In discussing the subject before us,—chronic empyema of the maxillary antrum,—it is necessary to understand what is meant by chronic suppuration of this cavity. Chronic empyema may be defined as a suppuration that has persisted more than six months, although, as the writer has stated, it may apparently begin as a chronic disease.

The etiology of these cases frequently is remote, but in the majority of instances the infection may be traced to various intra-nasal infections,—*e.g.*, grippe, scarlet fever, etc.,—or to a direct infection by diseased teeth.

The first class of infections of the antrum, those of nasal origin. usually are associated with a more or less extensive infection of all or part of the pneumatic cellular structure of the rest of the accessory sinuses,—viz., the ethmoid cells and the sphenoid sinus; and in many of these cases the maxillary antrum acts only in a passive way as a reservoir for the pus formed in the superimposed ethmoid cells. This pus, in turn, sets up various pathological changes in the lining of the antrum, and usually results in granulations and myxomatous tissues. These changes in the antrum may, and most frequently do, cause various symptoms in the teeth, the most frequent of these being dentalgia. In many of my cases this dentalgia was the most prominent symptom present, and the particular symptom from which the patients sought relief, a relief often too readily but vainly promised by extraction.

A diseased tooth may be, and not infrequently is, the cause of antrum disease, usually of an acute type; and, unless prevented by the proper treatment, this type may rapidly change into a chronic one. Given a tooth with an ulcerated root protruding into the antrum, and allowed to remain until granulations and necrosis have formed about it before its extraction, obviously the extraction of the tooth *per se* may not remove the necrosis and granulations. The necrosis may be extensive and the granulations form a large mass in the cavity of the antrum, and while the extraction permits of. drainage through the tooth socket, this drainage frequently is insufficient to control the spread of the necrosis or the growth of the granulations, and we thus have the beginning of a stubborn antrum disease; again, the incomplete extraction of diseased roots will result in the same condition.

I have seen several instances of each of these conditions. In cases of this character there may readily be an extension of the disease into the other accessory sinuses. A point I wish to emphasize is that a tooth that has been troublesome for a long time,—several months,—if it has caused antrum disease at all, may have caused empyema long before the empyema is suspected, and thus the condition may really be a chronic empyema from a tooth when first it is diagnosed; and, therefore, that a discharge that does not yield readily to treatment after tooth extraction and proper treatment through a drainage opening should be suspected to belong to this class of chronic cases and treated accordingly. Another point I wish to make is that cases of dentalgia accompanied or not by other neuralgias, or by nasal pus, should be suspected as of antral origin, even when in the presence of decayed teeth; that is, that antrum disease and not the decayed teeth may be causing the dentalgia.

To be clearly understood, briefly stated, I believe that antrum disease is caused many times by diseased teeth; but, on the other hand, that many a sound tooth has been sacrificed when proper treatment of the antrum would have saved it. I believe also that extensive disease in the antrum may under certain circumstances cause ulceration and death of a tooth.

During the last two years I have operated on eighteen cases of chronic empyema of the maxillary antrum. Fifteen of these cases were successfully operated upon by the Jansen operation, similar to the operation described by the author. Three cases were operated upon by milder measures. Of all of these cases, twelve had a history of some sort of trouble with the teeth; in four, diseased roots were found on operation lying buried in granulation tissue, and necrosis in the floor of the antrum. In three other cases all of the teeth of the upper jaws had been wrongly extracted years before for cure of the dentalgia; and in one case the teeth were saved from extraction and the dentalgia cured by operative measures.

As to the operation of preference in these cases, there is no rule that can be laid down for our guidance; we must be guided by our general experience, together with a careful study of each case. In advanced cases, and especially when multiple sinusitis is present, as it practically always is, the operation of Jansen, as described so accurately by the reader of the paper, is beyond question, in my hands, the most satisfactory. In less advanced cases the Moure or Caldwell-Luc is sufficient.

In any operation for chronic suppuration, however, it is a *sine qua non* of success that a large free permanent opening be made at the floor of the antrum and between it and the nose. If this opening is sufficiently large and far forward, with proper appliances a good view of the antrum may be had and the result of its treatment noted.

Dr. Dawbarn wished to congratulate Dr. Hurd upon his excellent operative results in a class of troubles where good results and not persistence of lingering annoyance from discharges, etc., means that thorough work has been done. Dr. Dawbarn proceeded to discuss several points of the paper. Alluding to the fact that frontal sinus suppuration is sometimes a cause of antrum infection, and not always suspected where the infundibulum is large and so pus drains freely and without its retention causing frontal pain, he mentioned that the opening of the frontal sinus and that of the antrum lie side by side, the former anterior, in the middle meatus of the nose; so that in dorsal recumbency the frontal pus necessarily drains directly across the antrum opening, or, more properly, openings; for though there is but one in the skeleton head, there generally are two, quite small and close together, in the mucous membrane here.

Dr. Hurd had taken the position, in his address, of believing that disease of the roots of teeth in the antral floor is a very common cause of disease of this cavity. In this he is widely at variance with numerous careful observers, though admittedly he can find others agreeing with him. But in a paper on this disease,[1] Dr. Dawbarn quoted Dr. Stout, of Philadelphia: " Dmochowski, after making one hundred and fifty autopsies (for this purpose), holds that but few cases have a dental origin." Again: " Fletcher, in five hundred skulls, in two hundred and fifty-two of which there were abscesses of the upper molars, found only twelve molars perforating the floor of the antrum." Also: " Carious teeth would appear to be an effect rather than a cause of antritis (Fränkl)." Stout himself states that he has never seen a case caused by carious teeth. However, Mears, of Philadelphia, agrees with Dr. Hurd in thinking the teeth the chief cause.

Dr. Dawbarn called attention to the very severe operations necessary in the cases shown to-night, and said that doubtless Dr. Hurd had not intended to indicate, by not mentioning the mild plans of treatment used in mild cases of antrum disease, that he treated all cases in this manner. On the contrary, a free opening in the anterior wall just above the gum, permitting admission of the little finger, and thus enabling a careful study of the cavity, so differing in different people, and in simple cases draining this and gently packing with mild, soothing antiseptic gauze—this plan

---

[1] " Disease of the Antrum." read before the Central Dental Association of Northern New Jersey, April 16, 1900, published in Items of Interest.

suffices for many cases, gradually to effect a cure. But in the really severe cases, and also those which had become chronic through years of neglect, we are face to face with a problem practically identical in principle with that met by the surgeon in empyema of the pleural cavity,—namely, a rigid walled cavity lined with a membrane discharging pus into that cavity. And where the lung is bound down by inflammatory exudate, mere drainage of that pleural space by excising an inch or two of a rib, low down, to permit of good drainage through tubes would almost never suffice. Either the outer wall must be made to collapse against the inner by dividing a series of ribs, or (as recently is being done) at the same operation dividing, and even stripping off sometimes, the thick, unyielding membrane tightly holding the collapsed lung, this organ quickly expands to meet the ribs; and then a cure follows by " secondary adhesion," the growing together of the two surfaces which so long have formed pus. Now, in the antrum, similarly, given the worst inflammatory diseases of it, we must, as Dr. Hurd's cases show, carry out the same idea, or else expect a permanent continuance of the trouble. As it is not feasible here to remove the rear wall nor the upper, and not, as a rule, the inner (unless these are themselves diseased), there remains the front bony wall; and this is most freely sacrificed, together with the suppurating lining membrane. Healthy flesh fills in the space thus left, and with much less evidence of the operation left than would be supposed. All cutting through the skin can generally be avoided, in such operations, by those experienced in such work; thereby much adding to the patient's gratitude.

Dr. Fossume.—Dr. Hurd's paper is most instructive, and I would like to relate the circumstances of a case that I had under treatment last spring, as we stomatologists are most interested naturally in cases which are in line with our actual professional work. The patient had been suffering a good many years with a continuous pain in the upper right side in the vicinity of the molars. There was distinct heaviness, together with some orbital and frontal pain. The two molars and the first bicuspid were loose, and directly above and between the buccal roots of the first and second molars there was a discharging fistula. She objected very much to losing the teeth. I opened the three teeth and found the pulp of the second bicuspid congested and semivital, and this I extirpated by pressure anæsthesia, and sterilized the canal and filled it. The roots of the molars were partly filled but badly infected, and there was a very distinct putrescent odor. The canals in all six roots were very small, and it was with great difficulty that I cleansed and filled them. As the patient had not the slightest relief after the canals were filled, and the discharge had not abated in the least, I injected beta-eucaine hypodermically around the buccal roots of the molars, and with a long shank bur bored away the alveolus and amputated the ends of the posterior buccal root of the sixth-year molar and the anterior buccal root of the twelfth-year molar. I found these roots penetrating the antrum, and although I do not really believe the case was one of true abscess of the antrum, I feel positive that the lining membrane was affected.

When I syringed the wound, the solution would pass through the nose. In the dressing and the after-treatment of such a case I have found the greatest help and most satisfactory results from using carbolized oil (a solution of 1 in 40), and a little hydro-naphthol. I have substituted at times boiled glycerin and aristol, but have always had to go back to the carbolized oil on account of its soothing influence on the tissues, stopping pain at once. Furthermore the dressing will never adhere to the wound, but comes away readily.

This case was discharged as cured in three weeks, the teeth became perfectly firm, and the abscess disappeared. I have had occasion to see the case this winter, and the teeth are in perfect condition.

Dr. Leo Green.—I am at a loss to understand why the old operation has been so universally condemned to-night as being useless. It has been my fortune to come in contact with several nose and throat men, and I have seen them perform operations in this manner with success. There need be no danger of food getting into the opening during mastication. To prevent this I take an impression of the opening immediately after the operation, with a piece of orange-wood stick, and from this impression make a hard rubber plug to fit the opening, having a shoulder below. This can be removed whenever necessary, to syringe the antrum. I have followed up a number of these cases, other than those upon which I operated, with uniformly good results. I have in mind one case which seemed to call for a radical operation, but to which I was opposed. It was my opinion that the trouble in this case was due to an injury to the nerve in the anterior buccal root of the molar, caused by the bur in drilling into the antrum. The tooth was finally extracted, and this condition was found to obtain. The indications for a radical operation disappeared after the extraction.

Dr. F. Milton Smith.—I do not understand that Dr. Hurd advises these operations unless in extreme cases of antrum trouble where all other measures of a milder sort have failed. My own experience in this line of work has been very limited. I have seen, in my practice of thirty years, four or five cases which in one way or another involved the antrum. I have read some on the subject, talked with those who know of the matter, and have the impression that in years gone by some of our leading men along these lines have taught us that about the best we could do with these old chronic cases was to keep them in as cleanly a state as possible. Of course, the operation Dr. Hurd has described to us to-night is radical, and ought not to be done unless it is needed, but it has seemed to me that as between wearing one of these drainage-tubes all my life and submitting to such an operation, I should prefer the latter.

Just a word regarding some of these simple cases that do not come within the range of Dr. Hurd's operation, where there is possibly simply a puncture into the antrum from an abscessed root or some other cause. I had under my observation some ten years ago a patient in one of whose upper molar teeth the pulp in one of the canals had become devitalized. It had gone on to suppuration, causing a discharge of pus into the antrum. He had called upon a dentist, who had opened the tooth and then sealed it up again and gone away from town. During the week of his dentist's absence he came into my office suffering terrific pain. I could not account for the acute pain until the tooth was opened, when I found live pulp-tissue in the remaining two roots, the extreme pain coming from the pressure of the pus upon this sensitive tissue. After evacuating the pus I treated the canals once or twice and then filled the roots as I would fill an ordinary root. Then through an external opening I treated the antrum a number of times, until one day he appeared for treatment and I was unable to find any opening. It had healed. I have no doubt that if I had not treated as long as I did it would have healed more quickly. This seemed to be illustrated by another case that I had where there was a discharge into the antrum from a suppurating condition of the roots of a tooth. As it was a tooth that had given considerable trouble, I decided to have it out, and after the extraction thought I would see what would happen without any treatment of the antrum at all. The case got entirely well of its own accord.

Two or three years ago a patient had trouble with his antrum. His dentist told him the trouble was caused by the root of a tooth left in after an extraction. He had advised that the antrum be opened and thoroughly treated. He was not willing to have this done, and eventually fell into my hands. I told him that perhaps a mild antiseptic used with the nasal douche might be all that was necessary. He used this for about a week and came back vastly improved. In three weeks' time there was no further disturbance. I mention these cases merely to show that there are cases that do not need operative treatment, and for such cases I am confident Dr. Hurd does not advise the radical operation.

Dr. Hurd.—I believe I stated in my paper that it did not have reference to simple cases. Nearly all of the acute cases will get well without an operation. Of the chronic cases, some will get well and some will not, and it is in these latter cases that we perform the radical operations.

With regard to the walls of the antrum collapsing, I do not see how the anterior wall of the antrum can collapse much.

In regard to transillumination as a test for disease of the antrum, sometimes it fails entirely. In the same mouth I have seen the normal side appear denser than the affected side.

Dr. J. W. Canaday, of Albany, read a paper entitled "A Study of the Dental Club in its Relation to the Dental Society."

The President.—I feel that the great value in the paper will be found, not so much in relation to us here to-night as among the men to whom our voice goes through the country, encouraging them to form dental clubs in the small cities. It is in this manner that the greater value of the paper will be found.

Dr. F. Milton Smith.—The thought to which our chairman has just given expression has been uppermost in my mind during the reading of the paper. We are fortunate in that the proceedings of our meetings go round the world. Papers of this character, if carefully and thoughtfully read, will greatly help the dental profession. It is meeting in this informal way that is going to make better men and better practitioners. I think I feel strongly upon this point because of the great help I have had from the little gatherings I have been permitted to enjoy in this town, perhaps at somebody's dinner-table or out for a walk with some friend.

The President.—Before we adjourn, I wish, in the name of the society, to tender, especially to our two medical friends and to Dr. Canaday, who has come to us from Albany, the most sincere thanks of the Institute for their kindness in addressing us to-night.

Adjourned.

FRED. L. BOGUE, M.D., D.D.S.,
Editor The New York Institute of Stomatology.

OFFICERS ELECTED.

THE annual meeting of the Institute was held on Tuesday afternoon, December 6, 1904, at the "Chelsea," No. 222 West Twenty-third Street, New York, the President, Dr. A. H. Brockway, in the chair.

The following officers were elected for 1905:

President, C. O. Kimball; Vice-President, S. E. Davenport; Recording Secretary, H. L. Wheeler; Corresponding Secretary, J. Buckley Locherty; Treasurer, J. Morgan Howe; Curator, S. H. McNaughton; Editor, F. L. Bogue.

Executive Committee.—F. Milton Smith, Chairman; C. F. Allan, E. A. Bogue.

ACADEMY OF STOMATOLOGY.

A REGULAR monthly meeting of the Academy of Stomatology of Philadelphia was held at its rooms, 1737 Chestnut Street, on the evening of Tuesday, March 1, 1904, the President, Dr. L. Foster Jack, in the chair.

A paper entitled "Some Studies in Occlusion" [1] was read by Dr. Edward H. Angle, of St. Louis.

(For Dr. Angle's paper, see page 165.)

---

[1] This paper of Dr. Angle's was extensively illustrated by the lantern, but as the author has not furnished the necessary photographs, it is presumed he regards the text as sufficiently clear without them. Most of these have been previously published in Dr. Angle's articles on related subjects. They were all to prove that the full complement of teeth is necessary to the best occlusion and best harmony of facial lines in all cases, and that extraction, according to the essayist, is as disgraceful as it is unnecessary and behind the times.—ED.

Dr. M. H. Cryer.—Dr. Angle speaks of moving a tooth backward as if it were an easy thing to do. I believe my friend, Dr. Head, thinks the same. I do not believe that the lower molar can be pushed backward. It can be moved forward, but not backward. The anatomy of the tissues allows everything to go forward, both in the upper and lower jaws, but I do not believe the backward movement can be as easily accomplished as Dr. Angle believes. He states that Nature makes a certain set of teeth for one face and another for another. That is true, but she makes the greatest mistakes in doing it. We would not be here as dentists if it were not to correct Nature. We live in houses to protect ourselves from the cold winters we have. We cross the stormy deep with perfect safety in spite of Nature. There is only one thing yet which we cannot control,—the volcano, such as that at Martinique; but the time will come when we will even harness that as we are doing Niagara, and utilize it.

I have a specimen here of a small mouth of a white person. See the amount of tooth tissue that is in that specimen. There are not only sixteen, but eighteen teeth in the upper jaw. In the small mouth that is uncommon, but Nature has made it. Therefore these teeth ought to be brought into line. If we correct that, we push the teeth forward and carry the lip outward.

Here is a specimen of a much larger mouth. The teeth are almost like deciduous teeth. They are small, with spaces between. This is a lower jaw, and you see the profile that we have. These teeth pass outward, carrying the lips, making the face, as Dr. Talbot, of Chicago, would say, that of a degenerate. The incisors and laterals are a little out of position. Dr. Angle here would say widen the arch. There are cases with which we must work according to the material. I believe there are cases in which we should extract a tooth or four teeth rather than keep them in. I have a patient who has been in the hands of an enthusiastic man following the method advocated by Dr. Angle, and I fear that these lips are going to protrude and that bone will not be developed to support those teeth either upper or lower. These teeth at the present time ought to be almost perpendicular.

The jaw that Dr. Angle showed was not a typical one. Here you have a typical jaw, and not one of a negro. This is a true and typical occlusion.

If I have a patient whose appearance I can improve by extracting four bicuspids and getting the teeth into line, I am going to do it, no matter what Nature has done. I have slides here that I would delight to show where that has been done with improvement to the face.

The President.—You say that you cannot move a tooth backward; when you extract bicuspids, how do you fill the space?

Dr. Cryer.—I said that molars could not be moved backward. You must make some fixed point to prove that you have moved the molars backward.

Dr. S. M. Weeks.—I feel very much embarrassed in speaking on the subject after the remarks that have been made. I have been very much interested in the paper by Dr. Angle, and it can call from me nothing but commendation, though the paper speaks for itself and needs no commendation of mine.

The case spoken of by Dr. Cryer is a patient whom I have had for treatment. I am sorry that he did not have the slides to show this evening. I have the photographs. The patient is twelve years of age. While there may be, as Dr. Cryer has said, a suggestion of too much prominence in the lips at the present time, I believe with Dr. Angle that, with the general development of the bones and soft parts during the coming years, this will be overcome; but only time can settle that fact.

Dr. Cryer.—For Dr. Angle's method of moving teeth and that of Dr. Weeks I have the highest commendation. I concede to Dr. Angle all the way, excepting in those few cases I speak of, and I think I am right; I do not know positively. I am sorry that I cannot stay and listen to Dr. Angle's reply, and am sorry that he is going away so soon. I most certainly appreciate what he has done in coming here, and he is certainly doing a great deal of good work.

Dr. J. Head.—I can only say from my personal experience that in hearing Dr. Angle's paper to-night I have been moved on one side with admiration and on the other with self-condemnation to think that I have done so much harm in the past by not following the lines he has laid down.

Regarding Dr. Cryer's remarks about the mistakes of Nature and the mind of man fighting Nature, it seems to me that the mind of man has a pretty big contract on its hand if it attempts to remake Nature and pick out individual points wherein she has made mistakes. When I was down in Washington last week I heard it declared that the teeth were not necessary for mastication; in fact, that mastication was not necessary for the human health, that frequently people who lost their teeth were much better without them. I also heard that the temporary teeth frequently were not necessary. I have frequently heard that we may extract teeth for the sake of improving the contour of the face. It is a serious thing for us to decide, when the face is yet undeveloped, whether we are going to improve that contour. How can we tell what that face is going to be at the age of thirty? What Dr. Cryer says may be so. There may be cases in which the four molars will change the plan of articulation to a certain extent. These conditions have to be met separately. I do think that too much praise cannot be given to Dr. Angle for giving us a scientific classification. When we find that within the Angle classification we can go forward with absolute safety as to an ultimate outcome, I think we should act on his lines. A tooth put into absolute occlusion will stay in occlusion, and a tooth that is not in occlusion will go into some other position. So much do I believe in the care and preservation of the permanent teeth that I am now instructing mothers to see that with their children of three or five years the silk floss is used between the teeth each day and the teeth carefully brushed afterwards. When the first permanent molars erupt, I watch the child to see that the cuspids come in with proper and normal occlusion. Sometimes the mother thinks the child does not need any care until it is seven or eight years of age. We frequently then find that harm has already been done; that the first molars have slipped out of occlusion. I think a good plan is to take those temporary molars that are going to be lost and put bands on them, and so arrange the cuspids that the child will be compelled to bite normally. In that way, by the time the temporary molars are lost the occlusion will be correct.

Dr. H. E. Roberts.—I wish to speak of a young man who had been under my care since the time he was six years of age. Six years ago he went from under that care, and at that time I believed his teeth to be in perfect occlusion. I saw him lately at twenty-one years of age. At fifteen his teeth were apparently in perfect occlusion; at twenty-one his lower jaw protrudes the full width of the third molar beyond the uppers. I think this Dr. Angle calls the third class. I never have seen a more pronounced case.

The elongation of the molars to correct the bite of the incisors, spoken of by Dr. Angle to-night, I advocated at a meeting at which Dr. William H. Trueman was present, some twenty years ago, and Dr. Trueman has used that method himself. Bring all the bite on the front teeth or the incisors, and the molars will, as Dr. Angle says, in from three to five months' time elongate; you can bring them up almost as much as you choose.

Dr. W. H. Trueman.—During the time I have been in dentistry I have kept my eyes pretty wide open, and I think I have seen some things. When I began I was quite enthusiastic about orthodontia. I think I was very successful. I know I gained considerable reputation with my work and put thousands of dollars into my pocket. As time went on I have seen the result of some of these operations, and I am not now as enthusiastic as before. The question is now asked me by a patient, " Can these teeth be made regular?" I say, " Yes." The reply is, " I shall be glad to have you undertake it." I say, " No, I refuse, because I think they are better as they are." And so I think with a great many regulating cases,—while I yield to no one in my admiration for what Dr. Angle has done,—a great deal of the work is of no real, clinical, practical value. I have watched many cases of my own and of others, and while time has gone on I have been exceedingly doubtful whether any real good has been accomplished. I would like to know what the result has been in these cases reported and illustrated after an interval of ten or fifteen years. I recall one case that illustrates very nicely what Dr. Cryer has said, in which there was a lateral curve instead of an arch. It is an easy matter to regulate such a case, and if when the tooth is brought into position it overlaps the tooth by one-sixteenth of an inch, we would say that that tooth, once brought into position, would stay there. This case I was doubtful about undertaking. The young man was eighteen years of age, and the configuration of his teeth was such as to indicate that it would be difficult to get the tooth to stay; but I succeeded in bringing it about. I put on a retaining fixture and said it would have to remain some months. After six months I removed it. Then I saw him at short intervals to observe that the tooth remained in place. It was there all right for two or three years. In two or three years more it was back where I found it. Why was that tooth moved backward? The lower teeth were in position to keep it in place. Why did it get back to its old position? We

have but to consider what Dr. Cryer said,—that there is something
we inherit from our remote ancestors. There is a constant pushing
forward of all the teeth. In some cases it is more marked than in
others. We cannot by our art go against Nature. We must remember there is constant change.

To illustrate another point. Some years ago a case was brought
to the city for surgical operation and fell into the hands of some
dentists. One of the central teeth had met with an accident. It
was shorter than the others, and it was suggested that this could
easily be brought down. I was present, and I asked whether that
could be safely done? The answer was, "Oh, yes." It was at
about the time that nerve-stretching came into vogue. It was
stated that stretching of these tissues in young people could not
produce harm. Later on I saw the case while the apparatus was
in place, and still later saw it when it was pronounced a complete
success. It was questioned whether the tooth had sustained any
injury, and the statement was that there was only a little change
in color, but no injury had been sustained. A few years later I
learned that the pulp had died, the tooth abscessed, and that, in
spite of all that could be done, it had to be extracted. It would
have been far better had it been left alone, for in time it would
have assumed a somewhat normal position. Interference with it
cost the loss of a useful tooth.   .

In one case I had, in which the upper and lower dentures were
crowded, I took casts and showed them to my preceptor. He advised me to extract the four first bicuspids and the work would be
done. I did not like that. I took these casts to one of our dental
associations and had them carefully examined. I was told to expand the arch. I told my preceptor, and he said, "Take out the
four bicuspid teeth and the work is done." I undertook to do it.
I took out the two upper bicuspids and left the lower ones in place.
I expanded the arch, and brought them into position. I saw the
case at intervals of thirty years. While it was very successful in
so far as it brought me reputation, to me it was not successful.
I had very little trouble with the upper teeth, but much with the
lower, and in fact, forced them into position. I presume that by
this time that jaw is almost edentulous. I would like to see these
cases in which the delicate tissue is stretched ten or fifteen years
afterwards, and know what the result is then, not the result immediately after the operation is done. Occlusion is a very impor-

tant point; but when we secure that perfect occlusion we must ask, Will Nature permit it to remain so?

A gentleman came to Robert Arthur, first graduate of the Baltimore Dental College, some years ago with perfect upper and lower dentures which articulated and occluded nicely. Later, changes took place, not from breaking down, but from normal wear, and the occlusion had become a protrusion. The changes were so great that photographs taken ten years before would hardly be recognized as those of the individual. Nature will assert herself, and I think she will rebel in some cases of regulating which we sometimes think have been so very successful. I would suggest that Dr. Angle let us know what the result is ten or fifteen years after the work has been accomplished.

Dr. M. I. Schamberg.—There is no doubt but that the progressive men of dentistry will give Dr. Angle credit for the advances made in this direction. I would like to ask him whether, in moving the teeth backward for young people, the third molars, which are already crowded, are not likely to give trouble. We find to-day that the jaw scarcely accommodates them, and it is surprising how very many cases require almost surgical means for their removal. Only a person specializing in work of that kind can realize the tremendous number of wisdom-teeth that are impacted, and I was wondering whether Dr. Angle's method would influence those teeth.

In reference to the premature resorption of temporary teeth, I would like to state that I have several radiographs showing conclusively that resorption frequently takes place in the temporary teeth when the permanent are not within reach.

In regard to the habit Dr. Angle speaks of, of a patient with enlarged tonsils throwing the lower jaw forward, causing its protrusion, I would say that I have had several cases sent to me for removal of adenoids and tonsils prior to regulation, and I believe that the throat is so largely filled with tissue, the post-pharyngeal glands, and the tonsils that the patient tries to create a larger breathing space by throwing the lower jaw forward.

Dr. Angle (closing).—It is already late, but I would like to hear from many more. It is not often I get a chance to have people pitch into me, and I rather enjoy it. I have not much to say now, because I tried to bring out in my paper all the points that have been touched upon in the discussion.

First, in regard to Dr. Cryer's criticism. We are not looking for exceptions to rules. There are exceptions to all rules, and it is also said that they prove the rule. Now the exceptions that Dr. Cryer has mentioned do not prove anything. It is true that we now and then find freaks, but they certainly should not be taken as a basis for rules to govern normal people. I do not know of a man on this earth who is more fond of collecting freaks in the way of specimens (especially if they have two or three extra dormer windows in their antra) to offset general rules than my friend Cryer, but this ransacking the whole country to run down freaks in order to prove that it is right to sacrifice these priceless jewels, the teeth, I do not believe in. I am trying in my humble way to prove to you that the sacrifice of teeth for the prevention or correction of malocclusion is wrong, is unnecessary, and that it is followed by such far-reaching and baneful effects that its practice should be abandoned, especially by the intelligent, conservative men of our profession. The "odontocides" should diminish in numbers, and they will diminish in numbers just in proportion as occlusion in all of its bearings is understood, and I dislike to hear even feeble efforts on the part of good men to defend a practice so pernicious. It is of the "old school" and not of the new, the scientific, the progressive in orthodontia. Now, I have shown you the worst cases that have ever come to my practice through the long busy years; in other words, I have put my theory to the severest tests, and in every single instance in all these cases we have found that both the occlusion and art requirements were best fulfilled by simply carrying out Nature's plan of putting all the teeth in their normal positions—normal occlusion.

There is no man in the dental profession for whom I have more respect and for whose work I have a higher admiration than for that of my friend Cryer, and I am surprised when he says we cannot push the molar teeth distally. I showed you several cases this evening where it had been done, and if you will come to St. Louis I will show you hundreds of cases where it has been done. This distal movement of molars has been in my daily practice ever since we have had the Baker anchorage, as it is, also, with my students and most of the members of the American Society of Orthodontists, and I have yet to see or learn of any symptom or result any more unfavorable than follows any other tooth movement.

Dr. Roberts spoke of a case where the lower jaw migrated

mesially after the fifteenth year. I could not venture an opinion without first seeing the case, and probably even then I could not tell much about it, for there are many things about the third class that are still shrouded in mystery. I have been surprised with the ease with which some cases belonging to this class have been corrected, and equally surprised at the difficulties in treatment or even failures met with in other similar cases.

I am impressed by what Dr. Schamberg says in regard to the possible and probable influence that enlarged tonsils and adenoids have in causing some patients to protrude their lower jaws the better to provide for themselves breathing space in this class of cases.

I agree with Dr. William Trueman that we ought to know more about the cases we treat in after years. I am sure there would be revealed a large percentage of failures, but I also believe these failures could be traced to simple causes, either from following an incorrect line of treatment, or from improper methods of retention, and yet there are many, many cases treated that are lasting successes. I could show you hundreds. I did show you one on the screen to-night, but you know it is natural to be more interested in and enthusiastic over the cases we have just completed or that we are still working on. If Dr. Trueman, or any of you, will come to St. Louis, I will be pleased to show you many of them which I believe to be more of successes than your best fillings because they are more permanent. I am surprised to hear my friend Trueman at this day and age speak in such disparagement of the practice of orthodontia. Such advice as he says he gives his patients in regard to treatment might have been excusable twenty years ago.

Gentlemen, I am extremely grateful to you for the attention and interest you have manifested, as well as for your kind words of commendation, and may the interest awakened here this night be fruitful of great good in the uplifting of this beautiful and useful branch of science.

Editorial.

LEWIS AND CLARK DENTAL CONGRESS, PORTLAND, OREGON.

IT is difficult to realize the rapidity with which countries, cities, and peoples develop from primeval conditions to the civilization that marks the progress of the twentieth century. Persons are now living who can remember before Chicago was incorporated into a city, 1837, and when St. Louis was the last fitting-out city for expeditions over the plains, and Oregon the last place on the map where a civilized man would desire to locate. The imagination of the writer was vividly impressed in his youthful years with the published reports of the Lewis and Clark expedition and the subsequent efforts of Frémont and others to solve the problems connected with the great divide which the Rocky Mountains made between the East and the West. The last remnants of the aborigines were a constant source of interest, and the trapper and his perils in his lonely quest for fur were more vividly impressed on the boyish imagination than the dry details of ancient and modern history.

It is, therefore, difficult to realize that the civilization of the past has been transplanted to the Pacific coast, fully armed with all the essentials to meet the demands of an exacting age, and with more of the vigor than is manifested in the older sections.

We have hardly begun to experience a recovery from the strain of the International Dental Congress, held at St. Louis, when word is received that at Portland, Ore., will be assembled, July 17, 18, 19, and 20, 1905, the Lewis and Clark Dental Congress, and if it be possible to judge from the advanced sheets detailing plans, this will be one of the most interesting of the many congresses held, not excepting those of an international character. The preliminary work thus far accomplished indicates this, and promises to those prepared to attend a treat not often vouchsafed to the weary workers in dental conventions of the cut-and-dried character.

Upon another page is presented the names of the officers and general committees, a sufficient guarantee for the success of the Congress.

While membership in this congress requires a recommendation from a member of the General Committee for those living west of the Rocky Mountains, this is not required of those applying for membership from the East. These applications are to be sent direct to the Secretary, to be acted upon by the Executive Committee. The membership fee for the Congress is fixed at five dollars. The officers are very anxious that the representation should be large from the East, and this desire will, without doubt, be seconded by many who will arrange to be present, and the moderate rates from the Middle West should certainly assure an equal reduction from other points, and a large delegation from the eastern sections of the country.

A letter in relation thereto from the Secretary states that "Railroad rates to Portland, Ore., during the Lewis and Clark Fair will be fifty-six dollars for the *round trip from Chicago,* and if dentists residing east of the Missouri River will, instead of taking their vacation in the mountains or in Europe, embrace this opportunity to join with us in the Lewis and Clark Dental Congress, we can show them, besides an interesting professional and scientific programme, a country of exceeding beauty. The tickets will be on sale at all the railroad ticket-offices. The routes may be selected, both coming and going, by the purchaser, and the tickets will be good for ninety days for the round trip. . . . Returning east they can visit Yellowstone Park, Alaska, Puget Sound, see the Columbia River from Portland, and can visit the Yosemite Valley, San Francisco, and Southern California.

"We expect an attendance in the territory west of the Rocky Mountains of at least one thousand men, and, in order to make the programme interesting, are desirous of securing essayists and clinicians among prominent men of the Atlantic coast."

It will thus be seen that the interest involved, outside of the Congress, should be sufficient to attract the professional man confined day by day, and month by month, in one apartment. Those who can take this trip are to be envied by their less fortunate brothers, for it is one that comprises more of real interest to the traveller, in its topographical features, than probably any other that could be taken in the broad domain of the United States.

It seems, aside from this, that something is due the dentists of the Western coast. They have contributed more than their share in making our Eastern meetings interesting, and now that they have a congress worthy of a great effort, let all who can join hands with them and demonstrate that, though leagues separate, professionally and fraternally we are one in spirit and practice.

Domestic Correspondence.

CORRECTION.

To the Editor:

Sir,—In a recent issue of the International Dental Journal you printed a paper which I read last October before the Academy of Dental Science in Boston, the subject of which was, " Should the Dental Practitioner concern Himself with the Chemical Examination of Saliva or Urine." In this paper I gave some of the results of work with the micro-polariscope which has been done by Dr. Kirk, of your city, and Dr. Michaels, of Paris, but I find by some accident my preliminary references to these gentlemen were not published, making it perhaps appear that I claimed an originality in this line of investigation which did not belong to me. I have tried to be particular in this, and trust that you will correct any possible impression of this sort by an explanation in your journal.

My paper was written for the purpose of interesting dentists in Boston in a work which Dr. Kirk had previously interested me in, and which I am trying to carry on along lines laid down by Professor Michaels and Dr. Kirk, hence I do not want it to appear that such investigation was original with me when I was simply trying to extend an interest in the work of others, and at the same time, to be sure, to facilitate my own research.

H. Carlton Smith.

[The foregoing explanation is published with pleasure in justice to all parties interested, but the writer's assertion, " I find by some accident my preliminary references to these gentlemen" (Drs. Michaels and Kirk) " were not published," seems to carry the imputation that the editor of the International Dental Journal. or some one else, had presumed to eliminate an important part of the manuscripts. The author of the paper may rest assured that it *appeared in this journal without any change,* and the original copy received at this office gave no indication of having been subjected to the editing process elsewhere.—Editor.]

Current News.

OFFICERS OF THE LEWIS AND CLARK DENTAL · CONGRESS.

GENERAL COMMITTEE.

NORRIS R. Cox, D.D.S., Chairman, Abington Building, Portland.

ARTHUR W. CHANCE, D.D.S., M.D., Secretary, 809–810 Dekum Building, Portland.

OREGON.

State Dental Association.—E. G. Clark, Portland; W. A. Cumming, Portland; Norris R. Cox, Portland; Walter F. Lewis, Portland; G. H. Nottage, Portland; Arthur W. Chance, Portland.

Stomatological Club.—S. J. Barber, Portland; J. B. Keefer, Portland; Geo. A. Marshall, Portland.

CALIFORNIA.

State Dental Association.—H. B. Carlton, San Francisco; Jas. G. Sharp, San Francisco; C. E. Post, San Francisco.

Southern California Dental Association.—L. E. Ford, Los Angeles; Ray D. Robinson, Los Angeles; G. A. White, Santa Barbara. Los Angeles Alumni, H. D. Regua, Los Angeles.

San Francisco Dental Association.—A. M. Flood, San Francisco; J. S. Marshall, Presidio; F. C. Pague, San Francisco.

Alameda County Dental Society.—J. Loran Pease, Oakland; H. G. Chappel, Oakland; John S. Engs, Oakland.

BRITISH COLUMBIA.

British Columbia Dental Association.—R. Ford Verrinder, Victoria; K. C. MacDonald, Grand Forks; Richard Nash, Victoria.

WASHINGTON.

State Dental Association.—C. S. Irwin, Vancouver; E. S. Barnes, Seattle; C. A. Custer, Seattle.

Seattle Dental Club.—E. B. Edgers, Seattle; J. W. Ball, Seattle; Gregor McGregor, Seattle.

Tacoma Dental Club.—B. S. Scott, Tacoma; J. M. Myer, Tacoma; R. S. Williams, Tacoma.

Spokane Dental Club.—A. Stark Oliver, Spokane; Chas. C. Mann, Spokane; Jos. W. Downing, Spokane.

IDAHO.

State Dental Association.—J. B. Burns, Payette; J. H. Lewis, Nez Perce; E. H. Maberly, Boise.

MONTANA.

State Dental Association.—J. B. Keenan, Butte; R. M. Leslie, Great Falls; A. C. Sandberg, Butte; T. M. Hampton, Helena; J. D. Sutphen, Helena; Joseph Oettinger, Missoula.

UTAH.

State Dental Association.—W. G. Dalrymple, Ogden; W. Lean Ellerbeck, Salt Lake; E. A. Tripp, Salt Lake.

NEVADA.

J. C. Hennessy, Reno.

Executive Committee.—Norris R. Cox, Portland, Chairman; C. S. Irwin, Vancouver, Wash.; Arthur W. Chance, Portland, Secretary; Jean Cline, Portland; E. G. Clark, Portland.

Committee on Essays.—S. J. Barber, Portland, Chairman; C. L. Goddard, San Francisco; B. F. Eschelman, Tacoma.

Committee on Clinics.—G. H. Nottage, Portland, Chairman; J. M. Meyer, Tacoma, Wash.; C. E. Post, San Francisco; A. Stark Oliver, Spokane, Wash.; Claude W. Gates, Salt Lake, Utah; J. H. Holmes, New Westminster, B. C.; A. W. Cate, Boise, Idaho; W. H. Barth, Great Falls, Mont.; F. I. Shaw, Seattle, Wash.

Committee on Exhibits and Manufacturing Clinics.—W. F. Lewis, Portland, Chairman; Woodard, Clarke & Co., Portland; Archer & Schanz Company, Portland; John Welch Dental Depot, Portland; Oregon Dental Supply Co., Portland.

AMERICAN DENTAL SOCIETY OF EUROPE.

THE next annual meeting of the American Dental Society of Europe will take place at Geneva, Switzerland, April 21 to 24, next. A cordial invitation is extended to members of the profession.

CHARLES J. MONK,
Honorary Secretary.

THE

International Dental Journal.

| Vol. XXVI. | April, 1905. | No. 4. |

Original Communications.[1]

THE ETIOLOGY, PATHOLOGY, AND TREATMENT OF TROUBLESOME TOOTH SOCKETS.[2]

BY M. I. SCHAMBERG, D.D.S., M.D., PHILADELPHIA.

SINCE man has been made aware of the worth of his teeth and the advisability of retaining them as long as possible, even at the expense of time, money, and a moderate amount of physical pain, the number of unwarranted extractions has been materially reduced. Coincident with this laudable conservation of these important organs, there is noted a tendency toward the retention for too long a period of teeth, the removal of which would prove a far better service to the patient. The wobbling molar with its pyorrhœal socket, the uncured abscessed tooth with its fistulæ, the impacted wisdom-tooth with its readily infected pocket, and the exostosed tooth with its disturbing influence upon the enveloping bone are all examples of cases which frequently come to the extractor at such a late date that a troublesome tooth socket is bound to follow. It is, indeed, unfortunate that just and prompt dis-

---

[1] The editor and publishers are not responsible for the views of authors of papers published in this department, nor for any claim to novelty, or otherwise, that may be made by them. No papers will be received for this department that have appeared in any other journal published in the country.

[2] Read before the Academy of Stomatology, Philadelphia, November 22, 1904.

crimination cannot always be made between the tooth that will grow well under treatment and the one whose inevitable loss is but a matter of time. It is, however, possible for each and every one of us to make up his mind to cure every abscess, check the pus discharge in every pyorrhœal case, brace every loose tooth, or cause these offending members to be removed lest they menace the health and longevity of their hosts.

Your essayist takes this emphatic stand for the reason that he has observed many cases where the prolonged retention of diseased teeth has not alone endangered the integrity of the surrounding tissues, but has been the cause of constitutional disorders of serious import. The citation of an illustrative case might here be of interest. Mr. H. presented himself for the treatment of an abscess upon the lower second molar tooth. Examination of the mouth revealed a fistula upon the buccal aspect of the alveolus communicating with the distal root. Upon inquiry it was learned that the patient had noticed for two years or more a " small gumboil" in this region. The usual history was obtained that the abscess filled from time to time and would then burst, discharging its contents into the mouth. During this time the patient had been a sufferer from frequent outbreaks of boils and carbuncles upon the neck and other parts of the body. He was treated both here and abroad for this distressing condition, yet no thought had been given the possible connection between this small alveolar abscess and the constitutional poisoning from which he was suffering. His trip abroad and the cures taken there improved his health, but he still suffered from an occasional boil. An effort made to cure the abscess failed because of an obstruction in the distal canal which interfered with its proper cleansing, whereupon the tooth was removed.

Though a year has elapsed, the patient has not had a recurrence of his boils, and his health is much improved. There is little doubt that this general infection was due to the absorption of pus from the alveolar abscess, and that the patient might have been spared several years of needless suffering, inconvenience, and expense had this tooth been removed a few years earlier. The review of this case could be followed by a number of other cases in which the gastro-intestinal tract and the entire system have suffered from the swallowing of pus formed within the mouth, from faulty mastication rendered so by loose and tender teeth.

and from physical exhaustion due to prolonged suffering. Thus far in this paper particular stress has been laid upon the baneful effects of the retention of diseased teeth upon the general health. This is done to emphasize the necessity for removing such teeth unless they respond to treatment within a reasonable period of time. The removal of aching or sore teeth is almost invariably followed by prompt relief. The purpose of this paper is to consider clinically and pathologically the causes of those cases in which relief does not follow the extraction of a tooth. Attention will also be directed to the prevention and treatment of troublesome tooth sockets. For the purpose of systematically dealing with the subject, troublesome tooth sockets might be classified in the following manner:

Traumatic Sockets.
1. Injury to alveolar process.
2. Laceration of soft tissues.
3. Unremoved ends of roots.

Dry Sockets.
1. Interference with the formation of blood-clot
   - through drugs.
   - through suppuration.
   - through hæmophilic tendency.
2. Dense alveolar walls
   - exostosis.
   - impaction.
   - peridental inflammation.
3. Infection
   - pre-existing: abscess, pyorrhœa.
   - operative.
   - post-operative.

To adequately consider these various deviations from the normal requires a full understanding of the uneventful extraction of a tooth and healing of the socket without pathological interference. When a tooth is removed no greater local disturbance should be produced than the rupture of the peridental membrane and the pulp at the apex of the tooth, together with a moderate amount of spreading of the process made possible through the normal resiliency of that tissue. The bleeding which takes place should entirely fill the socket of the tooth with a well-formed blood-clot. This clot is supposed to remain and form a matrix for the new cells which spring from the socket wall and rapidly spread until they have replaced the clot and caused its absorption. Most sockets heal in the manner just outlined. It must be remembered, however, that there are many conditions which tend to alter or interfere with this normal process of healing. Teeth do not always possess the ideal conformation, and are therefore not always removed with as little trauma as characterizes the uneventful tooth extraction. Neither are all teeth free from affections which alter the surrounding structures sufficiently to prevent the normal repair. Again, the mouth of many patients and the instruments and hands of many operators are not always free from organisms which are ever ready to invade the socket and work their noxious effects. Lastly, a proportion of patients, however small, come to the extractor at such a time when their lowered state of vitality tends to unfavorably influence the proper healing of the socket.

By *traumatic socket* is meant an injury to the socket produced during the extraction of a tooth in excess of the rupture of the peridental membrane and pulp and slight spreading of the process. The traumatic socket, next to the normal socket, is the one most often met with, but fortunately it seldom proves to be as troublesome as the dry socket.

1. *Injury to the alveolar process* constitutes a frequent variety of traumatic socket. It consists of an excessive spreading, crushing, or fracture of the process. It may be due to the shape of the tooth, as noted in teeth with exostosed, curved, or flaring roots, to an abnormal position of the tooth, to brittleness of the process, to its adherence to the tooth, to the necessity for crushing through the alveolus to dislodge a root, or to carelessness, haste, or incompetence of the operator. This form of traumatism may cause the part to remain tender for some time, though it seldom, unless complicated by other conditions, causes excruciating or unbearable pain. Small forceps, elevators, the surgical bur, care, and skill will often prevent excessive injury to the process. When the alveolus has been fractured, loose pieces should be removed and sharp edges made smooth so as to cause as little irritation as possible.

2. *Laceration of the soft tissues* usually accompanies injury to the process, though it may occur independent of that complication. It consists of tearing and crushing the gum tissue, and may be due to the gum being adherent to the tooth, to the removal of a piece of process with gum attached, to grasping the gum with the forceps, to crushing through it to reach a root, and to the same faults of the operator, as were mentioned in referring to process

injury. Here the employment of small forceps, elevators, and
the lance will reduce the possibility of laceration to a minimum.
The soreness from injury to the gums seldom lasts very long, and
the repair takes place with promptitude unless interfered with by
continued irritation from projecting process or through suppuration.

3. *Unremoved ends of roots* are always barriers against the
normal healing of the socket. Roots become fractured during extraction, through efforts at hasty removal of teeth rather than a
slow spreading of the process and a gradual dislodgement of teeth
in the direction of least resistance. Exostosed, curved, and frail
roots are naturally prone to this mishap. Impaction, brittleness,
excessive decay, density of the enveloping bone, and non-yielding
process are also conditions which predispose to this injury. Unremoved roots may or may not give trouble, much depending upon
whether they contain exposed portions of vital pulp, abscesses at
their apices, or other peridental disturbances.

It is always well to be sure of the presence or absence of the
ends of roots. This may be accomplished by carefully examining
every tooth removed, by the skilful use of the explorer, by swabbing
the socket with a styptic so as to check all bleeding, by the use
of a good electric mouth-lamp with a mirror to reflect the light
into the socket, and by the use of the X-rays when other methods
fail. It is always best to remove every portion of every root, lest
it immediately or eventually give trouble. *Every root can be
removed. The judgment of the operator must decide whether the
end justifies the means.* When it is decided to allow a portion of
a root to remain until nature makes its removal an easier task the
patient should be kept under observation, and upon the first indication of trouble occasioned by the retained root the same should
be promptly removed.

By *dry socket* is meant a socket in which the normal blood-clot
is absent. This term is a misnomer, for a socket is not necessarily
dry though it be devoid of its blood-clot. The name is here used
for want of a better means of designating the condition and because of its accepted usage.

1. *Interference with the formation of a blood-clot* is the usual
cause of a dry socket, and may follow the use of drugs in the socket,
may be brought about through suppuration, or may be the result
of bleeders' diathesis. In each instance the clot fails to form and

leaves the socket unprotected and open to the reception of saliva and oral débris. Such sockets are usually painful, and can be best relieved by thorough cleansing with peroxide of hydrogen and packing with sterile boric acid or iodoform gauze, or with a tampon of cotton saturated with campho-phenique. This treatment must be applied until the walls of the socket are covered with a layer of healthy granulations, after which time the part is usually able to take care of itself.

In a communication received some time ago from Dr. Louis Jack, in which he requested that I prepare for the INTERNATIONAL DENTAL JOURNAL an article on the subject of troublesome tooth sockets, he says, "Concerning the condition which has been designated ' dry socket,' my observations have led me to consider that it is most frequently caused by the use of such disinfectants immediately after extraction as have stopped the natural hemorrhage and thus prevented the formation of the protective coagulum. The effusion of lymph is also checked.

"This result has repeatedly occurred in healthy and clean mouths, and most frequently after the removal of third molars, more particularly of lower ones. This has been more the case when phenol sodique has been used. The consequence of this unprotected condition of the alveolus renders the process liable to severe irritation, presumably infective. The condition bears some relation to that of compound fracture. If the mouth has been disinfected with dioxide or permanganate of potash, I can see no necessity for the use of active or irritating disinfectants in the sockets. My preference is for the use of the normal aqueous solution of either acetanilide or hydronaphthol in the form of spray. Neither of these interferes with coagulation. The former has the advantage of arresting pain. A solution of two parts of the tincture of calendula to six parts of water, as a spray, is exceedingly useful in mild cases and is especially soothing where laceration takes place."

The substance of the above quotation is deserving of weighty consideration, coming as it does from such a trustworthy and experienced stomatologist as Dr. Jack. His allusion to the destruction of the protective coagulum by the application of phenol preparations and the consequent production of a dry socket is pertinent, and offers food for thought to those who practise the invariable post-operative swabbing of the socket with a disinfectant.

It was upon Dr. Jack's advice that I have long since discontinued this practice, save in such cases in which the existing disease of the socket necessitates active treatment.

2. Dense alveolar walls, such as are formed about exostosed and impacted teeth and those the seat of chronic peridental inflammations, are occasionally found to be the cause of dry sockets. This constitutes probably the most painful variety of troublesome tooth socket, for in such cases there is a total absence of bleeding in the socket and a complete denudation of the socket wall. The cancellated portion of the bone having been rendered dense there is little opportunity for granulations to spring from the socket wall. Such cases can be treated in a similar manner to those in which there is an absence of blood-clot from other causes, but a much longer time is required for the granulations to spread from the edges of the socket. By burring out the dense wall of the socket the cancellated bone is sometimes reached and more rapid healing made possible.

3. Infection of tooth sockets may be due to a pre-existing alveolar abscess or pyorrhœa, to the introduction of germs at the time of the removal of the tooth, and to the migration of organisms into the socket some time after the extraction. Most cases of alveolar pyorrhœa and abscess are immediately benefited by the extraction of teeth involved. There is, however, a small proportion of cases in which the traumatism occasioned by the removal of the affected teeth aggravates the trouble for the time being. In such cases a thorough curettement of the diseased area, followed by cauterization with pure carbolic acid, is usually followed by relief. The socket should be then loosely packed and allowed to heal by gradually filling with granulations. If a clot be allowed to form over an infected area before complete drainage is effected, an extension of the disease is likely to follow. Serious consequences have resulted from infections of the bone brought about in this way. An osteomyelitis so produced calls for an immediate and thorough burring out of the socket with careful antiseptic treatment. Orthoform applied to the socket will relieve the pain when carbolic acid fails.

Operative infection may be due to non-sterile instruments and to an unhygienic condition of the mouth. *Post-operative infection* is usually due to the latter cause. The gravity of infection thus produced will depend upon the character and number of the germs, their virulence, and the resistance offered by the tissues. Fortunately, the staphylococcic and streptococcic infections far outnumber the tetanic, the erysipelatous, the syphilitic, and the tubercular, but the bare possibility of such germs gaining access to the system through wounds created by tooth extraction warrants the utmost care as to the sterilization of all instruments, the disinfection of the operator's hands, and the antiseptic treatment of the patient's mouth.

Miller, in the September, 1903, issue of the *Dental Cosmos,* says, "I have found that the secretions of wounds produced by the extraction of teeth examined three or four hours after operation contain vast numbers of leucocytes, and that in many cases they are loaded down with bacteria." Farther on in this laudable contribution to dental literature, entitled "Immunity to Diseases of the Mouth and Teeth," he says, "The protective powers present in the mouth are not to be accounted for by any antiseptic action on the part of the saliva, but rather by the phenomenon of phagocytosis, by the struggle for existence, and probably by certain forces residing in the soft tissues which have not yet been investigated."

These observations made by Miller warrant the conclusion that in the battle which is waged between the white blood-corpuscles and the bacteria-laden saliva the defence against infection could be materially strengthened by the use of mouth-washes which will dispose of a proportion of the invading organisms. Permanganate of potassium 1 in 1000 is the mouth-wash which I usually employ to precede extraction. It is not a pleasant-tasting wash, but is an excellent oxidizer, deodorizer, and disinfectant, and if vigorous rinsing is encouraged the mouth can be rendered fairly sterile in a few moments. Staining resulting from its use can be promptly overcome by hydrogen dioxide, which makes a good supplementary wash because of its combined bleaching and antiseptic properties. I do not recommend permanganate of potassium to patients for use at their homes after extraction because of the deep staining that will follow its prolonged usage. Patients are much more likely to adhere to instructions if advised to use some pleasant mouth-wash, such as borine, listerine, glyco-thymoline, or the wash to which they are accustomed.

All instruments and appliances used during the removal of teeth, such as forceps, elevators, cotton-pliers, mouth-props, etc., should be thoroughly sterilized, preferably by boiling or by immersion in a formalin solution. The operator's hands should be thoroughly cleansed immediately prior to handling the patient, the use of warm water and a non-irritating soap being sufficient except where special precautionary measures are necessary, when the hands should be dipped in a 1 in 1000 bichloride solution or in an equally efficient wash. The extraction of a tooth being a surgical procedure, its performance should be accompanied by similar precautions to those that are employed in general surgery. *In the light of our present knowledge of the prevalence of germs within the oral cavity, the failure to precede and supplement every operation within the mouth which entails the shedding of blood by antiseptic washing or douching should be stamped as unpardonable negligence.*

GONORRHŒAL ULCERO-MEMBRANOUS STOMATITIS.

BY EUGENE S. TALBOT, M.S., D.D.S., M.D., LL.D., CHICAGO.

SINCE Neisser discovered the gonococcus, in 1878, much light has been thrown upon obscure infection in different parts of the body. This germ is now known not to be confined to the urethral gonorrhœal lesions and discharges, but that nearly every structure, particularly mucous membrane, may become involved. Successful culture methods have added much to diagnosis.

The literature of gonorrhœal infection of the mouth in adults is meagre. W. L. Baum [1] remarks, " Gonorrhœal ulcero-membranous stomatitis is, according to Menard, always due to profound systemic infection, is always a secondary state. This position was opposed by J. P. Tuttle [2] more than a decade ago, who cited in opposition, among other cases, that of C. W. Cutler,[3] where, in an adult, osculation of a gonorrhœic penis was followed in a few hours by a raw, dry feeling in the mouth and in twenty-four hours by the lip vesicles. The gums by the third day were painfully swollen, and on the fifth the mouth was intensely inflamed. A whitish fluid having a disagreeable odor and taste was secreted. The lips cracked and were covered with herpes; the lip and cheek

[1] The Practical Medicine Series, vol. x., 1904.
[2] Morrow's System, vol. i., 1893.
[3] N. Y. Med. Jour., January 25, 1889.

mucous membrane was thickened, reddened, denuded of epithelium in spots, and in patches covered with a false membrane. Cases later reported by R. Larson [1] were of similar type and origin.

"Gonorrhœa, a common epidemic in institutions for children, usually assumes the form of ophthalmia, vulvo-vaginitis, and pyæmia. In a number of cases of infant pyæmia reported by R. B. Kimball,[2] no local lesion was found to explain the entrance of the gonococcus to the general circulation. In Kimball's opinion, the gonococcus may produce stomatitis, from which a systemic infection could arise. Many conditions of the gums and alveolar process, such as occur prior to pyorrhœa alveolaris, predispose to stomatitis, readily forming a culture medium for the gonococcus. Conditions like this in an infant can easily be mistaken for sprue and treated therefor, thus concealing a possible source of systemic infection resulting in pyæmia.

"Gonorrhœal stomatitis, in a case described by Juergens, developed on the gums and cheeks of a man who had recently had gonorrhœa. The resultant dirty gray deposit contained the gonococcus."

Two cases have come to my notice in the past six months. A thirty-six-year-old travelling salesman, unmarried, was sent to me by his physician for local treatment, May 3, 1904. There was a history of gonorrhœa with continual urethral discharge. The mucous membrane on the entire superior alveolar process was involved. The gingival border of the mucous membrane was destroyed and the alveolar process was exposed. Marked inflammation with excessive swelling occurred. Interstitial gingivitis extended throughout the alveolar process, and the teeth were loose. The pain was so severe that sleep was out of the question. Salivation was excessive. The raw ulceration was covered with a glazed surface of greenish-gray color. Local application of glycerol was used for three days, when he left the city, at which time he said the pain was not so severe. The time was too short to notice any improvement of the mucous membrane.

A forty-five-year-old clerk, married, came for consultation, who had contracted gonorrhœa twenty-four years before. He had suffered with gleet ever since. The anterior superior alveolar process

---

[1] St. Louis Med. and Surg. Jour., 1896.
[2] Med. Record, November 14, 1903.

was exceedingly inflamed and raw. It was badly swollen. He suffered severe pain. Interstitial gingivitis was very profuse through the alveolar process. The incisors were loose, two of which I was obliged to remove. The surface was ulcerated and raw with a glazed surface of greenish-gray color. He has been married eight years; has no children. His wife has had local trouble, for which she has had three operations; he does not know the nature of her trouble. He was advised by a former consultant to have his jaw removed, because of its cancerous appearance. Hektoen's examination of the tissue for cancer proved it to be simply inflammatory. I suspected gonorrhœal infection. Examination of the tissue proved my suspicion correct. Applications were first made of glycerol, then silver nitrate. The inflammation subsided in the anterior part of the mouth, but extended rapidy through the vault of the soft palate, which was reached in three weeks from the time I first saw him. On consultation with Dr. Baum, argyrol (twenty-five per cent.) is now used.

Both these men were in the best of health except slight rheumatism. Both seem to have been infected by the fingers as an intermediary host of the gonococcus.

A horny gonorrhœal exanthem is described by G. Baermann.[1] The exanthem was secondary to a severe gonorrhœal attack, and was hyperkeratotic in nature. It bore some resemblance to certain tertiary luetic results and to psoriasis. A bacillus was found which resembled that of the bacillus of the kerosis group. Baermann is inclined to refer the results to this bacillus, as the gonococcus was not found. It would seem more probable, Baum remarks, from the results of Woodruff,[2] that the gonotoxin, which is exceedingly irritating, was the proximate determining cause. The exanthem involved the upper surface of the foot as well as the sole, and was evidently related to the arthritic conditions which appeared in the case.

That the gonotoxin could be drawn to the alveolar process when the elimination is interfered with elsewhere is undeniable. That processes could be set up similar to the hyperkeratotic states ascribed by Baum to the gonotoxin is equally indisputable, still the evidence in my two cases pointed to direct infection.

---

[1] Arch. f. Derm. u. Syph., B. lxix.
[2] Practical Medicine Series, vol. x., 1902.

THE RATIONALE OF PULP EXTIRPATION.[1]

BY HART J. GOSLEE, D.D.S., CHICAGO.

In assuming to interest the members of this distinguished body, I must confess that, even with all the latitude so kindly granted, the selection of a subject which would be even partially commensurate with the honor conferred has occasioned me no little concern.

A discussion of pulp extirpation has suggested itself to me for this occasion, for at least two specific reasons. First, because of the radical change in the method of procedure whch has been adopted in the past few years, and secondly, because the topic is just now a particularly live one, made so by the more or less discordant notes of warning and of enthusiastic commendation, which are the echoes of the hour.

Lest any one should imagine that it might be my intention to carry him to the realms of a purely scientific discourse in the presentation of this subject, let me at once dispel such a thought, and affirm that the more selfish motive of personal benefit prompts the effort, rather than the expectation of adding new light or particularly original thought to the subject.

And yet, conceding that true progress is to be attained mainly by scientific research and discourse, may we not at the same time contribute to its development by now and then interspersing what some of us are pleased to term " practical" views? I believe we may.

The present popularity of pulp extirpation is doubtless very largely due to the somewhat diversified opinions held by many of our most prominent men.

Any radical departure from the time-trodden paths of successful operative procedure must be productive of just such a condition, for the reason that it will at once appeal particularly to two classes of those who go to make up the whole, each class of which, for the good of the profession be it said, is ever alert and active,—the one eagerly grasping at all things new, and quickly bounding away on the wings of enthusiasm, and the other seeking to restrain such a flight with the bridle of conservatism.

---

[1] Read before the Academy of Stomatology, Philadelphia, February 28, 1905.

Thus the seeming idiosyncrasies of the human mind, portrayed by such widely diversified opinions and experiences as are observed in men engaged in the pursuit of similar lines of effort, such as ours, and particularly of those who are equally and pre-eminently successful, is an interesting study.   And yet, in reality, when we analyze these "seeming idiosyncrasies" we can only deduce that they but emphasize the infallibility of personal equation, for whilst it is true that we all seek knowledge from the same fountain-heads, and that all who are honest and conscientious work to the same end, yet the means employed with success by one would meet only with dismal failure in the hands of another.   This is personal equation, and must enter into the lives and work of all men, else we would soon become mere automata.

With the advent of cocaine and pressure—or so-called " pressure anæsthesia"—for the removal of pulps from teeth, the former procedure seemed to bid fair to be almost completely revolutionized, and hence we now find the operation a source of much variety of opinion and discussion.   On the one hand we hear an enthusiastic cry for the abandonment of a method which has been continuously and successfully employed for half a century and more, and a plea for the universal adoption of the newer and more radical method; on the other hand, we hear in words of caution of the ill-results and failures recorded against this newer procedure.

A perusal of the pages of our recent literature can but confirm this statement, and must excite in those who have not followed the subject closely almost every feeling from surprise to consternation, if there be any intervening.   If this is true,—and I think it quite beyond denial,—should we wonder at disquietude and confusion existing in the minds of that vast majority of the profession, and particularly of the younger men, who look to, and in a large measure depend upon, those who essay to teach and write for their enlightenment, encouragement, and progress?

Or need we marvel at, or ask the occasion for, disquietude or confusion existing in the minds of many concerning this particular subject when we read from a lecture recently delivered by our distinguished friend, Dr. B. Holly Smith, of Baltimore (*Items of Interest,* January, 1905), wherein he says, *literally,* that arsenic for the purpose of devitalizing the pulps of teeth should be relegated to the practices of mediæval dentistry; that its action is positively not limited to the confines of the tooth itself; that when it is applied to the pulp it will go on and result in a destructive process of the tissues contiguous with the end of the root; and in which he then recapitulates by making the broad and sweeping statement that he can prove that every tooth in which arsenic has been sealed for the purpose of devitalizing the pulp will be a source of trouble sooner or later.

If these be facts, is it not a strange coincidence that the profession should only now awaken to a realization of such alarming or dangerous possibilities, after having universally used arsenic since the days of Drs. Greenwood and Spooner in 1837, or thereabouts?

Furthermore, in contradistinction to these and other similar views, we read a paper by Dr. R. Ottolengui, of New York (*Dental Cosmos*, September, 1904), in which is recorded a series of observations and experiences in connection with this newer method,— cocaine and pressure,—the results of which tend to indicate so large a proportion of failures and bad after-effects produced by its employment as to, at least, offer anything but encouragement to those who might otherwise have been influenced by the remarks of the gentlemen previously quoted, to abandon the use of arsenic.

Verily, therefore, the proposition from this view-point needs must appear to be somewhat perplexing, and yet since it becomes necessary to remove pulps, we must, at the present time, at least, either go back to the now ancient and barbarous practice of driving them out with wooden points, resort to the slower process of strangulation and destruction by the use of arsenic, or else adopt the more immediate process of pressure anæsthesia.

While nothing perhaps short of mental aberration would now induce any one to consider the former crude and heroic practice, still it did not serve its purpose, and, in the light of past experience, and of calm, rational judgment is there not virtue in *both* of the latter methods? Personally I indulge in the firm conviction that there *is*, and that each method has its respective sphere of usefulness, and will be found manifestly advantageous in proportion as it may be judiciously selected, and its technique mastered and carefully observed.

As progressive practitioners of a modern science it is our patent duty to study and analyze all methods by which the comfort and convenience of the patient, and in turn of the operator, may be increased or facilitated, and to select and adopt those which in our judgment seem to offer the most favorable opportunities for obtaining the desired results in the case at hand, for, after all, while we may speculate at random, theorize at will, and become " faddists" if we are so inclined, it is nevertheless *results*, pure and simple, that we are after.

That the application of arsenic to the pulps of teeth has caused trouble, and may to-day cause trouble, is indisputable. Still, do not the records of the past, and does not the experience of the present, indicate that such instances are the exceptional rather than the common result?

Notwithstanding the statements previously quoted, nor questioning the sincerity of their author, it is my belief, based entirely upon observation and experience, that more pericemental trouble has resulted from the use of cocaine in the past four or five years than was ever produced by arsenic, and that " lame" teeth are more prevalent to-day, as a result, than they were prior to the introduction of cocaine and pressure for the purpose of removing the pulp.

The troublesome manifestations produced by the use of arsenic may be classified as complex and simplex in character, and the distinction thus drawn would include as complex those wherein pericemental trouble developed and lameness ensued, while those designated as simplex would embrace only that class in which the disturbance is confined to the pulp itself, and hence only of a temporary nature.

In analyzing the cause and effect in the class designated as complex it is but rational to conclude that such physiological disturbances may be attributed to any one of three general sources: first, to the use of too large a quantity of arsenic; second, to allowing it to remain sealed within the tooth for too long a period; or third, to the abnormal enlargement of the foramen. The last condition, however, would include so small a proportion of cases as to make them exceptional, and thus not warrant further consideration, for pericemental trouble would be very likely to ensue from the application of either arsenic or cocaine, because of the difficulty of confining the action of either drug to the pulp itself.

But as regards the former, if one-fiftieth of a grain of arsenic or less be sufficient to destroy the vitality of the pulp, then it is, of course, obvious that the use of a greater quantity simply means that the further absorption of any excess, above the actual requirements, must but increase the action, and in turn the destructive process, and thereby invite trouble beyond the apex.

And further, if twenty-four, or forty-eight, or even seventy-two hours is sufficient time to admit of the absorption of this quantity of arsenic, and of producing a physiological change of the pulp-tissue, then a longer period of time would also only promote a more unlimited action of the drug and the probability of apical disturbance.

Therefore, since the pulp of a tooth is capable of absorbing within itself only a given quantity of arsenic, in proportion as the minimum quantity of the drug is sealed within the tooth and allowed to remain but the minimum period of time will the best results obtain and the percentage of subsequent pericemental troubles decrease; and yet, logical as this may seem, how few practitioners observe it as carefully as might be, or make any distinction, in regard to the quantity used, between a tooth having a large pulp and one with a small one, or between any of the teeth in the denture, or discriminate as to the vital resistance of the various physiological types.

Those troublesome manifestations, which have been classed as being simplex in character, while frequently attributed to the mere presence of arsenic, are doubtless often due to an unwise application, or to faulty technique, and may usually be directly traced to placing the drug in a tooth in which the pulp is already highly inflamed or congested, or to undue pressure produced in sealing the cavity.

Since it is a well-known fact that this drug only acts as a powerful irritant to tissues undergoing any stage of the inflammatory process, it is obvious that its application in these conditions must be preceded by such palliative treatment as will at least temporarily relieve the inflammation and reduce the congestion. Thus, in proportion as the condition of the pulp approaches the normal, will the application of arsenic increase in effectiveness and the susceptibility to its irritating influence be correspondingly decreased.

Furthermore, whenever the physiologically irritating influence of this drug is supplemented by any degree of mechanical irritation. such as may be, and as is so often, produced by undue pressure in sealing the treatment within the tooth, it is manifestly easy to account for the resultant trouble.

In this particular connection Dr. D. D. Smith, of Philadelphia, I believe, has called attention to the fact that arsenic should never be sealed in close proximity with the pulp, and that if the cavity be of such extensive proportions as will prevent an observation of this precaution, it should first be temporarily filled and the application of the arsenic then made by drilling accommodation for it in some other place in the crown more removed from such close proximity, which procedure, I think, is to be highly recommended in many instances.

While it must be conceded that many of the, perhaps, superficially apparent objections to arsenic may be eliminated by a more careful observation of the technique incident to its use, I believe that the primary cause of more subsequent pericemental troubles—and consequently of lame teeth—may be directly attributed to imperfectly filled canals as a result of the employment of such agents as tannic acid for the purpose of shrivelling or shrinking the pulp-tissue prior to its removal, than may be attributed to the possible continuation of the process of destruction resulting from the use of arsenic.

I am well aware of the fact that this practice is recommended, and has been for a long time more or less general, and yet, I believe that its employment only adds to the difficulties encountered in completely removing pulps so treated, and in subsequently thoroughly filling the apices of the canals. In fact, the theory that the "tanning" or "toughening" of the pulp-tissue by the use of a solution of tannic acid and glycerin, or other like agents used for the same purpose, *facilitates its removal* has, like the various theories of pulp mummification, proved to be only a delusion and a fallacy in my hands, and I believe that if pulps *may ever* be removed *en masse* with any degree of facility the procedure may be accomplished with more reasonable certainty immediately after the pulp has been desensitized than at any other time.

And again, and aside from this, there is another very pronounced objection to the use of the glycerite of tannin, to which the attention of the profession has been called. This pertains to the possible discoloration of the tooth which may result, and which in many cases can doubtless be directly attributed to the well-established fact that tannic acid and iron are chemically incompatible, and that when the former is placed in contact with the iron contained in the hæmoglobin, tannate of iron—a black ink—is the resultant compound.

While my former statement might possibly be construed as being an argument in favor of the cocaine and pressure method, and while it is so to a degree, still, irrespective of the possibilities of discoloration subsequently mentioned, the points which I desire to especially emphasize are these: that the pulp should be removed as soon as possible after it has been completely desensitized; that, owing to its fibrous nature, it may be removed *en masse* with greater certainty at this time than at any other; that if it is thus completely removed the opportunities for maintaining asepsis and thoroughly filling the entire canals are materially increased, and that if the canals are thus filled the possibilities of subsequent trouble will be likewise diminished, irrespective of whether arsenic, cocaine, or a combination of both methods be used.

Indeed, a combination of both, followed by *immediate removal*, is preferable to this so-called *shrinking* method, and may often be used to good advantage, for the reason that the hypersensitiveness which sometimes remains after the removal of the arsenic, is usually not sufficiently acute to preclude the further enlargement of the cavity until adequate access for the employment of cocaine and pressure may be obtained; and for the further reason that a more or less thorough mechanical sterilization of the cavity may thus be effected.

And now let us consider this question of sterilization. Undoubtedly a large proportion of the cases recorded by Dr. Ottolengui, and noted by myself and others, in which pericemental trouble followed the use of cocaine by the pressure method, may be attributed to imperfect sterilization of the cavity previous to its application.

This would lead us to agree with Dr. J. P. Buckley, of Chicago, in concluding that the question of cavity sterilization as applied to the use of cocaine in this manner is an important factor, and that whether it be obtained by mechanical or chemical means, it must always obtain.

In the use of arsenic, we usually find after its removal that the dentine is so desensitized as to admit of complete mechanical sterilization by means of the bur, but since such a procedure is rarely possible immediately preceding the application of cocaine by pressure, and since the dentine is usually permeated by micro-organisms and their poisonous biproduct, we must first obtain thorough chemical sterilization, or otherwise force these ptomaines through the tubuli into the pulp, and possibly into the apical tissues, when pressure is applied.

As some of these ptomaines are volatile liquids of an extremely irritating character, if the pressure employed be sufficiently great to force them through the apices and into the apical space, an acute inflammation of these tissues may be established as a direct result of this virulently irritating influence. Or as cocaine is itself a protoplasmic poison, which is admitted by pharmacologists, it may be that many of these disturbances are the direct result of the action and physiological incompatibility of this drug.

Thus as we study how to effectually sterilize the dentine prior to the application of this method; how we may best succeed in forcing our anæsthetic solution, and what it may possibly carry ahead of it only into the pulp-tissue and not into the apical space, and as we learn how to judiciously select our cases, may we employ cocaine and pressure, I think, with a minimum of bad results.

Technique.—Therefore, in my opinion, the successful application of this method demands, first, thorough sterilization of the cavity; secondly, the employment of a sterile solution of cocaine; thirdly, favorable opportunity for the proper application of pressure; fourthly, an observation of the precautions incident to the removal of the pulp and the filling of the canals, and fifthly, a degree of good judgment in the selection of cases.

Sterilization.—Excepting in that class of cases where the natural crown of a tooth which is to be used as an abutment for bridgework is free from caries, and where the extirpation of the pulp may be demanded by the mechanical requirements in connection with the accurate adjustment of an artificial crown, to which this method is most applicable and usually preferable; or, in other words, wherever caries is present, and natural asepsis does not obtain, an absolutely thorough sterilization of the cavity is demanded.

Whilst this may be materially aided by first mechanically excavating the cavity to the fullest possible extent, still, owing to the sensitiveness of the dentine, it may usually be effectually accomplished only by chemical means.

Of the many agents used and recommended for this purpose, the desired results may be obtained to the best advantage, perhaps, by first isolating the tooth with the rubber dam and then flooding the cavity with a 1 in 200 solution of sublamin, or a 1 in 500 solution of bichloride of mercury, preferably the former, after which the excess should be first absorbed with cotton or bibulous paper, and the cavity then thoroughly dehydrated with alcohol.

Cocaine.—As commercially prepared solutions of cocaine are not stable, in order that the second requirement—that of always employing a sterile solution—may obtain to the best advantage, the crystals should be finely pulverized and dissolved with sterilized water in each individual case. While carbolic acid, adrenalin chloride, and other agents are recommended for this purpose, a sterilized water is preferable because of the fact that in the event of being forced through the apex of the tooth—as it is in many cases irrespective of the care used to prevent—less physiological disturbance of the contiguous tissues will be produced.

Ordinary distilled water would, of course, answer the purpose to a degree, but a sterilized or essential oil water is preferable because of thus being absolutely and permanently sterile, and of the probable diminution of troublesome manifestations obtained by its sterility.

Pressure.—As already intimated, no portion of the technique of this procedure is regarded as being of much greater significance than that relating to the proper application of pressure, and as extreme care must be exercised in employing only sufficient pressure to force the solution through the dentine and into the pulp-tissue, I am of the opinion that the various mechanical devices designed for this purpose—in the use of which absolute control of the pressure may not be easily maintained—are therefore dangerous, and that the best results will obtain from the more simple and less heroic methods.

These simpler methods may be employed effectually if means for confining the solution of cocaine within the tooth are observed, and where the shape, location, or proportions of the cavity are not favorable, they may usually be made so either by the employment of matrices or by the use of cement. Indeed, cement will be found indispensable in many classes of cavities, and may be used either to dam up the walls of the cavity, or to previously entirely fill it, subsequently drilling through the filling until the dentine is reached and exposed, through which opening the cocaine and plunger may then be placed and the pressure applied.

It is also my belief that in all instances the pressure should be gentle at first and cautiously increased until a slight response on the part of the patient, which is usually manifested, is noted, when the plunger should be held firmly without increasing or diminishing the pressure for a few moments. After the pain has subsided the pressure may then be gradually increased until no response is observed, which will usually indicate that the cocaine has reached the pulp and that anæsthesia has been effected.

Removal of Pulp.—As soon as anæsthesia is thus indicated an exposure of the pulp should be attempted. If this is not possible, an effort should be made to approach as closely to it as may be done without inflicting pain, and then again resort to further effort with cocaine, until a full and complete exposure may be effected. Ample access should then be secured by enlarging the cavity to the extent of the dimensions of the pulp-chamber, and the pulp immediately removed by mechanical means.

Controlling Hemorrhage.—And now we come to a very important phase of the subject,—the treatment of the more or less copious hemorrhage which usually follows, and the proper time for the filling of the canals.

While adrenalin chloride, hydrogen peroxide, and many other hæmostatic or oxidizing agents are recommended for the control of the hemorrhage and the evacuation of the blood, it is my belief that no effort to control it should be made, that it should be allowed to bleed freely, and that the blood should be evacuated from the canals only by such mechanical means as tepid water or shreds of cotton or bibulous paper twisted on the broach, or by some agent, such as alcohol or chloroform, which will dissolve the blood, for the reason that such a procedure relieves the congestion in the apical area, and is an important factor in preserving the color of the tooth. In this connection every precaution should be taken to remove the blood from the canal and cavity, and not to chemically decompose it within the tooth, as is done when hydrogen peroxide, for instance, is used for this purpose.

Indeed, it is claimed by Dr. Buckley and others that to the use of agents which will oxidize the iron in the hæmoglobin of the blood remaining within the tooth may be attributed to a large extent the subsequent discoloration; and, furthermore, that any discoloration may be avoided by an observation of these precautions.

Filling Canals.—As soon as the hemorrhage may be checked in the manner indicated it is manifestly safe to fill the canals, but unless absolute certainty of their being perfectly dry exists, it is doubtless the best and most conservative practice to seal some healing, antiseptic agent, such as creosote, within them, and defer the filling until a subsequent sitting. This also allows for the natural healing of the disrupted vessels and thereby diminishes the cause and possibilities of the development of pericemental troubles.

Indications and Contraindications.—While, in line with my original argument, the indications for the employment of arsenic are more or less general, yet the same may scarcely be said of this newer method.

Indeed, it must be conceded that the application of cocaine and pressure is particularly contraindicated in at least three general classes of cases: first, in those cases mentioned by Dr. Ottolengui, where the presence of calcific deposits within the tooth retards the penetration of cocaine, and thus precludes or acts as an impediment to the complete anæsthetizing of the pulp; second, that class of cases where the decay is so extensive as to leave the pulp without sufficient protection to withstand the necessary pressure, and yet where it is also not possible to puncture it, at least, perhaps without administering a general anæsthetic; and third, those cases where the remote, unfavorable, or inaccessible location of the cavities, the hypersensitiveness of the dentine, or the physical condition of the patient preclude its use.

In otherwise favorable conditions, however, it will be found most advantageous, and particularly in the extirpation of congested pulps which are giving trouble, and where an exposure may first be obtained, and in teeth the crowns of which are entirely free from or but slightly attacked by caries, and in which the pulps may consequently be more or less normal.

In conclusion, let me summarize by reiterating that both methods possess virtue, and are useful in their place when employed with a proper observation of the prerequisites essential to success, and that, to a very large extent, the selection of the one most applicable to the individual case will be a question the solution of which good judgment alone will dictate.

PREVENTIVE DENTISTRY.[1]

BY C. M. WRIGHT, A.M., D.D.S., CINCINNATI, OHIO.[2]

PREVENTIVE Medicine and Preventive Dentistry are terms of comparatively recent origin, but the prevention of disease has been the foundation principle upon which medicine and dentistry have stood since the earliest times.

The crudest efforts of the primitive dentist to stop decay by driving lead into a hole in a tooth, and the clumsiest attempts on his part to replace lost teeth with ivory, or animals' teeth, or porcelain, must be recognized as operations in preventive dentistry.

Miller's magnificent results in etiology, Bryan's experiments with the systematic application of nitrate of silver, D. D. Smith's repeated and frequent polishing of every exposed surface of every tooth, Michel's analyses of the varying salivary and oral secretions of immunes and the other classes, Black and Johnson's extensions of fillings, Jenkins's artistic creations in porcelain, in short, every individual suggestion from every thinking and working man in the profession of dentistry, discloses the central idea which inspires him. It is the prevention of oral or dental disease.

We have been so busy with actual disease, or disease which is apparent, that we have not given adequate attention to *potential disease*. This must engage our earnest attention for the future.

The coming dentist must operate upon sound teeth and prevent the outbreak of diseases which are lying dormant,—the latent diseases which observation has shown will almost surely appear.

The old preventive dentistry, in which we are all so earnestly engaged, is not to be forgotten, but the modern dentist must, by subtile chemical and surgical means, skilfully and scientifically applied upon sound organs, make these operations unnecessary.

In this field—this field called prophylaxis—the weapons of defence are advanced knowledge of physiology, of etiology and pathology, and of a new therapeutics.

When preventive medicine succeeds in reducing the percentage

---

[1] Read at the Union Meeting in Basel, Switzerland, December 18, 1904.

[2] Professor of Physiology and Pathology in the Ohio College of Dental Surgery.

of deaths from typhoid, small-pox, diphtheria, and tuberculosis,—
I said percentage,—the physician's heart is filled with hope and
joy. He feels the thrill of courage stimulating him to persevere.

The success which has crowned dentistry as a unique profession during its brief existence, or since the establishment of the
first dental school, is so great that we have reason for our faith in
its future in this new field.

Prophylaxis, or active measures for the preservation of the
health and the prevention of disease, presents special opportunities
in dentistry. The necessary manipulations can be readily applied.
The importance of them can be certainly demonstrated. Governments and the heads of schools can be easily convinced of the public utility of them. Its wide-reaching effects on the general health
of citizens can be proved. If properly presented by qualified dentists, oral prophylactic measures can be made so popular that communities will adopt them and be appreciably benefited. Oral
prophylaxis is in line with the most advanced ideas of sanitary
science and preventive special and general medicine. A meeting
like the present, composed of delegates or members of some of the
most important Dental Societies of the civilized world, and meeting in this beautiful city on the Rhine, a city noted for her distinguished medical scientists and practitioners, is, it seems to me, the
·society and place *par excellence* for the inauguration of a new
scientific method. Let a practical method be adopted here to-day,
and the name of dear old Basel will be forever associated with a
reformation in dental practice. I have special personal reasons for
my love of this city and her people, as Dr. Bryan, your president,
and others know. Therefore, permit me to suggest that a committee of one or two resident dentists of Basel be appointed to take the
matter in hand by authority of this society. This committee shall
confer with the sanitary officials of the city, and make arrangements
for the establishment of a class or classes of children selected from
some eleemosynary institution, or from the public schools, and
under the inspection or observation of members of the Sanitary
Board; the object being to demonstrate that by Dr. Bryan's method
of applying the protective solution of nitrate of silver, and Dr. D.
D. Smith's method of fortnightly or monthly polishing of the
teeth, dental caries can be positively prevented—seventy-five to
ninety per cent.

Secondly, that this same method be followed by other committees in other cities in Europe, having delegates now in attendance at this congress.

Medical men recognizing the pathogenetic magnitude of oral sepsis in relation to other contiguous and even remote tissues, will become the most interested spectators of the exposition. This is not an impossible proposition when we think of the astonishing results of enlightened modern prophylactics as applied by the Japanese medical department of her army.

The method of trying to educate school children by lectures, tracts, and popular treatises on physiology and hygiene, as adopted by some European cities in primary schools under government control, has proved and will continue to prove futile. It is not in accordance with modern ideas of education. To the increasing requirements of a heavy curriculum, the addition of lectures on sanitation is like pumping wind into an already over-inflated toy balloon. We can have nothing to expect but the bursting of the balloon and the loss of all our carefully devised labor. Or, as a friend suggests, like the pumping of air into a punctured tire.

By the plan proposed in this paper the simple practical ocular demonstration will so fully illustrate the principle, that children and adults will absorb a knowledge of hygiene which cannot be grasped as a concept by any other plan, and oral prophylaxis will rapidly become a twentieth century necessity.

Reviews of Dental Literature.

In the *British Dental Journal* for September, 1904, is a paper on " Vulcanite Crowns," by E. R. Tebbitt, L.D.S.

These are used for trial crowns, and for the first permanent molars of children between the ages of eight and fourteen, and lower molars which are beyond crowning by the usual methods, as where the root presents a saucer-shaped depression on the gum level, the edges soft and the remaining dentine hard. After preparation of the canals, clear out the general surface of the root with large, coarse burs. If the gum is overhanging, a copper tack with a good supply of gutta-percha will leave a fair field after being in place three days. A gold pin, the projecting end of which has been well flattened, is fitted in the canal, or where the best masticating surface is wanted, and if it is not necessary to avoid the jar use a platinum pin, spread the top with a riveting hammer, and adapt it to take the brunt of the bite. The author has not found a second pin necessary. After the pin is fitted an impression and bite are taken. Cast in Spence metal and mount on an articulator. Remove the pin and oil the root and surrounding gum with any viscid oil. Replace the pin and drop melted wax around it to just cover the root, and if a porcelain facing is to be used it should be fitted; continue to build up to the bite with wax, trimming the edges so that no part of the wax overlaps the gum. Invest, exposing the lingual aspect so as not to disturb either the bite or fit of the crown; as the elasticity of the rubber is of no consequence, but hardness everything, it is well but not necessary to give it two hours in the vulcanizer.

SPENCE metal is composed of sixty parts of sulphide of iron and forty parts of sulphur. The fusing point is 225° F. It is of great value when used as an articulating model in setting up an upper or lower denture, by minimizing the constant attrition of the antagonistic surfaces, which more or less, according to the ability of the mechanic, takes place when teeth of porcelain are brought into repeated contact with very much softer plaster ones. For all models, therefore, to be used solely for antagonizing porcelain teeth during the setting-up process, one will find that Spence metal will not show any signs of wear on the cusps, and that, other things being equal, the case when in the mouth will present the same occlusion as on the articulator.

Used in casting models for metal work, again it has distinct advantages over plaster. Think for a minute of the result of trying an imperfectly fitting gold plate on a plaster model. It is more or less gently rocked to see where it bears heavily, at the same time it rubs an easement for itself where it does not fit; and this process is perhaps repeated after the plate has been swaged once more. with the result that it seems to settle down to reasonable fit. Let the model be of Spence metal, and the least rock is at once apparent, and no amount of persuasive wriggling will wear the model to fit the plate.

It is often difficult to cast a model in Spence metal sufficiently deep to get a reasonably heavy zinc from it. The simplest solution of this difficulty is to cast the Spence metal so as to cover the highest part of the impression material by about a quarter of an inch, then watch for the first signs of setting on the lower edge of the cast, and when the rim has solidified about a quarter of an inch, pour out the remaining molten metal, and the result will be a hollow cast with an inward turned rim. This is now easily filled with plaster and built up to the required height, and the rim will hold the two together quite securely.

For models to be used in fitting a cap crown it has this good point: After fitting the collar to the root, many operators take an impression of the banded tooth with the band in position, and cast the whole in plaster; when the band is removed from the plaster cast, it not infrequently brings with it that part of the model which represents the root, leaving only a fine mark to indicate the correct position. If the impression taken in plaster or composition is oiled and cast in Spence metal, the band may be taken on or off at will, and we may be sure that any slight accidental bend it may get will be corrected when it is next placed on the model.

Like a plaster model, the best result is obtained from a plaster impression; it is nevertheless easily used with other impression materials, ordinary Stent's being very satisfactory, provided reasonable care is taken to pour the metal at the right moment and to direct the stream into some unimportant part of the impression. The Stent should be well chilled before pouring the Spence metal.

For those who did not know the method of manipulating this substance he outlined the way in which it was handled. As bought, it is a grayish-black powder, and is melted in an ordinary enamel saucepan, most conveniently over a Bunsen burner, the flame of which must not be allowed to pass up the sides of the pan, for if it gets on the thin layer of metal adhering to the sides of the pan, the metal will be overheated and give off strong sulphur fumes, and at the same time considerably deteriorate. The impression to be cast is preferably surrounded by one of the " rapid casting cups," and is previously oiled with one of the heavier cycle lubricating oils.

On first applying the heat, when the metal is in powder, it is necessary to stir it until a little of it is melted at the bottom of the pan. The flame is then reduced and the pan shaken over it till the whole forms a very awkward-looking mass, being a kind of stiff black froth. The pan should be now removed from the flame and the contents stirred with a piece of stick. This stirring, with the occasional application of further gentle heat, will reduce the whole into an extremely fluid condition, and when the setting (which begins at the higher parts of the pan) has nearly reached the general level of the liquid portion the metal is poured rapidly, directing the stream on the middle of the back edge of the impression. As soon as set, which takes from one to two minutes, according to the bulk of the metal, the rubber cup is removed.

When casting into a plaster impression it is best to let the whole cool before the plaster is removed, considerably less delicacy being necessary than where plaster is used for both impression and model. If composition has been the impression material, as soon as the rubber cup is detached gentle traction may be exerted on the heel of the composition, when the contained heat of the metal will soften it sufficiently to allow of its removal.

A difficulty, which is only a temporary one, is that when first working on black models after being used to white, the whiter porcelain tooth seems to stand out between its darker neighbors, and the tendency is to set it too far in.

If the material becomes " stodgy," a small addition of sulphur will restore its efficiency.

Comparing Spence metal and plaster, the former is harder, cleaner, takes less time from mouth to finished model, and can be used over and over again.

Spence metal can be procured of C. Ash & Sons.

In the *British Dental Journal* for November there appears a communication by Harry Baldwin, M.R.C.S., L.D.S., entitled " Further Experience of Cement and Amalgam Fillings."

The author advocates a method of filling teeth by lining the cavity with oxyphosphate of zinc, placing amalgam into the cement while still soft, and finishing with an amalgam surface. The points in favor of this method were, that it required a much smaller sacrifice of healthy tooth substance, leaving a stronger tooth less liable to subsequent fracture and necessitating much less pain in excavating. It interposes a non-conducting layer between the sensitive dentine and the metal. Compared with amalgam it does not stain the tooth nor show a nasty color through a thin enamel wall, is more water-tight, and adheres to the cavity.

The author has used this method for a number of patients who presented themselves originally with all or most of their back teeth ragged and ruinous, containing the eroded and abraded remains of phosphate of zinc fillings, presenting everywhere rough edges, spaces into which food crowded, softening edges of exposed dentine, and such an inefficient masticatory mechanism as to be lamentable. These cases now present smooth, well-filled shapes, with restoration of original contours, abolition of irritating spaces, good sound metallic surfaces in contact, and in a condition which may be described as permanent. These cases are very satisfactory, not only because of the improved condition but also because of the extreme simplicity of the means by which the result was secured.

As the beauty of the combination method depends entirely upon a strong and effective adhesion, it is not necessary to emphasize the importance of using materials that are favorable. The best. cement, as far as Dr. Baldwin knows, is "Harvard," and the best amalgam, "Standard" (Eckfeldt & Dubois).

In order to get the best results the amalgam should be packed in a manner not specially inviting shrinkage or change of shape, and the best principle on which to work is that of Bonwill. Bonwill's method consists in forcibly squeezing the amalgam, after packing it in the tooth, with a pad over its whole free surface simultaneously. The pad may be of any soft material, but rolled up thin bibulous paper and india-rubber are the two most generally used. The practical way of effecting this entire compression of the amalgam in the cavity of a tooth is to use a matrix wherever possible, and to squeeze powerfully over the whole free surface of the amalgam with a closely fitted pad. The mercury which is in excess in the amalgam will be forced out, and will escape from under the edges of the pad in fine bright drops, or can be easily scraped away with a spoon excavator on removal of the pad. The greatest care must be taken to pack the amalgam with a fine, almost pointed plugger in the retiring angles between the matrix and the cavity edges, great pressure being used in these positions so as to insure the amalgam being well packed. as dense and as free from surplus mercury as the central portions; otherwise these portions will receive less pressure than the rest, and will absorb surplus mercury from the rest, and so give bad shrinking edges to the filling. The reason for eliminating the surplus mercury is twofold,—first, to make a denser and harder filling; secondly, to prevent change of shape, warpage, in the finished mass.

To understand something of the nature and behavior of amalgam, one should realize that a soft amalgam is in the condition of a sponge containing a quantity of free mercury between its interlacing fibres, just as a sponge contains water in its interspaces.

A good deal of misconception regarding the reason for, and manner of, change of shape in a setting amalgam or amalgam after setting seems still to exist. Authors will be found alluding to the tendency of amalgam to " ball," just as if amalgam were a fluid, like water or mercury, to take a spheroidal shape.

A stiff paste like a setting amalgam has no surface tension and cannot attempt to ball. What happens with a warping amalgam, when that amalgam is of good quality and compounded so as not to shrink or expand, is that, owing to an uneven distribution of the mercury, the mercury is proceeding to redistribute itself more evenly, those parts of the mass which contain less mercury absorbing it from those parts which contain more, and causing an expansion of those parts receiving mercury and a contraction of those parts giving it up. The reason for an amalgam filling, packed merely with steel instruments, containing an uneven distribution of mercury, is simply that the deeper portions are well compressed by the superincumbent layers, and so have had their surplus mercury squeezed out of them, and this surplus has been absorbed by the outer layers. The outermost layer then contains not only its own excess, but a surcharge absorbed from the layers beneath.

Pressure with a steel instrument merely displaces the excess from immediately under the face of the instrument, and the surrounding surface of amalgam simultaneously absorbs it.

It will readily be seen that expression by pressure applied over the whole surface is the best method of getting rid of the surplus, because any method of absorbing it by tin or silver cylinders, unless accompanied or followed by great and well-adapted pressure, will induce shrinkage of the outer part and a porous surface.

BRIEF NOTES ON PYORRHŒA ALVEOLARIS IN INDIA. By Major Andrew Buchanan.

In 1898 the writer observed that many prisoners in one of the large Indian jails were suffering from pyorrhœa. The disease had not been much noticed previously. On inquiry it was found that the disease was more prevalent in those districts where the famine had been most severe. There were two hundred cases in a population of about one thousand.

While it was difficult to get evidence as to its influence on the general health, it was reasonable to suppose that the crowding together of a large number of such cases would have an injurious effect. In a batch of ninety prisoners who had come from one of the districts most affected by the famine, over seventy were suffering from pyorrhœa. The pyorrhœa was cured, and in six weeks there had been an average gain in weight of eight pounds per man.

The improvement in the general condition of these men led one to believe that the curing of the pyorrhœa had considerable influence.

As spongy gums may arise from different causes, he has found the following classification useful:

1. Those due to scurvy, or some form of malnutrition.

2. Those due to mercurialism.

3. Those due to a lack of proper care (with these may be classed those that had scurvy, but in whom the gums had not returned to their normal condition).

4. Those due to loose teeth.

The majority of cases belong to group 3 and are almost all curable.

Treatment.—The tartar was removed and an antiseptic pushed into the pockets with a flat stick. Where the pockets were large they were slit up with a lancet, and powdered sulphate of copper was applied and rubbed into the gums for a few minutes. Where the cases were due to a slight scorbutic condition, antiscorbutic remedies were given at the same time.

It has been found advisable in the Indian jails to examine the gums of all prisoners on admission, remove all tartar and cure pyorrhœa, and then make the prisoners clean their teeth daily, so that if scurvy appears it can be readily detected, as the first signs are those which are seen in the gums.

F. L. B.

PROFESSIONAL EMANCIPATION AND HOW IT MAY BE EFFECTED.[1]
By J. E. Weirick, D.D.S., St. Paul, Minnesota.

It is with a deep sense of appreciation that I am taking advantage of your kind invitation to deliver an address at this meeting. If I had my just deserts, I would be begging at the back

---

[1] Read before the Indiana State Dental Society, June, 1904.

door of your hall for permission to appear here in the rôle of a penitent. That I am, instead, honored with the freedom of the floor and the privileges of a speaker denotes your generous spirit, and is another demonstration of that fine broad character for which Indianapolis and her people have long been famous among those who have enjoyed the boon of your friendship and hospitality. But even *your* indulgence must have been tested in my case. For I plead guilty to having outraged your kindness last year when, after accepting an invitation to attend the annual meeting here, I failed at the last minute and that without warning or advance notice. I know of nothing that has come to me so pleasantly as the renewal of your invitation this year, showing that you had fully forgiven my trespass. I will not try your patience with an explanation of my non-appearance at the last convention, except to say that it was caused by an entirely unexpected professional matter, that pressed on me so urgently I could not get away from St. Paul, though you may rest assured I would have hesitated at no possible sacrifice to fill my engagement with you. Instead, then, of offering a long explanation, I will try to show my appreciation of your forbearance by making my address here as short and sharp and pointed as possible; wasting as little of your time as may be. If you find some of the things I say blunt and undiplomatic and crudely put, please ascribe it to the desire on my part to use as few words as possible. And this request leads naturally to the main idea on which I have taken the liberty to base my address,—that we dentists at our meetings and conventions are entirely too prone to waste our time in bootless talk and impractical action; that we generally come to these gatherings with a bag of wind under one arm and a keg of water under the other; varying the programme only occasionally, by carrying something other than water in the keg.

True, we are no greater sinners in this respect than many of our fellows in the other professions. But there is this difference: They can afford to indulge in a harvest of wind; we cannot. Their status is established; ours is not. They have a professional ancestry; we, as yet, have only a professional progeny. They stand on a solid foundation built for them by their pioneers; we have our foundation still to build, or at least to make solid; and we are not doing it. Instead, we are drifting along in a haphazard way, deceived by the crumbs of recognition thrown us here and there into the belief that we have really arrived; that we are really and broadly ranked with the other learned professions. As a matter of fact, we are not. The more clearly we understand this, the better. For, with such an understanding will come properly directed work, concerted effort, and the measure of achievement that will give us the *substance* of that *high standing;* of which we have now but the *shadow.* At least, I believe that this will be so; that we have but to make clear to ourselves and our associates the ambiguous position we occupy, in order to bring about a condition of affairs that will make any man proud of the fact that he belongs to this profession. Indeed, I believe it only necessary that we wake up to our true situation, to insure our becoming leaders instead of followers in the world's division of medicine and healing. We have but to look back over the history of our progress so far, to make very clear the potential possibilities of our craft. Hampered by the most serious disabilities, disabilities that I will refer to in detail with your permission, we have yet to record the most extraordinary progress. Let us overcome these disabilities, and we will at once take proper rank, and win that professional standing which it must be the aim and desire of every properly constituted man to have for his own.

It is true, undoubtedly, that, even with the progress we are making to-day, we will eventually arrive. The things that we have done demonstrate this clearly enough; but they demonstrate, also, that we are still far from the goal, and that as matters are now moving, it will be a generation, or even two generations, before we can fairly say that our profession is abreast in rank and consideration with the other sections of medical science. And for myself, that rate of progress is too slow. I am not content with the knowledge that the next generation of American dentists, or the one after will come into full recognition. I want this generation to see such a result.

I am tired of seeing the Section on Stomatology of the American Medical Association tagging perpetually at the rear end of the procession. I want to see this section on an equality in the councils of the Association with the sections on ophthalmology, surgery, and the others. I want to see an end to the condescension and the patronizing that are always extended to the practi-

10

tioners in our profession by the members of the older branches
of medicine.

It is unnecessary to point out to any one who has attended
the meetings of the American Medical Association the *humiliating position* that we always occupy. In our personal capacity,
we are well enough. We have nothing to complain of at the social
functions. But when it comes to a voice in the direction of affairs
scientific, we find ourselves barely tolerated.

It is my firm belief that the work we are doing is as important as is the work in any other division of medicine. In numbers we are stronger than any of the other sections. There are
to-day in the United States thirty-five thousand registered dentists. No other division of specialists can show within twenty
thousand of that number. We have made relatively greater progress than any other branch. We have undoubtedly done more to
ameliorate suffering than any equal number of men in the world.
We play a most important part in the physical upbuilding of the
race, by supplying and maintaining sound machinery for the mastication and consequently for the digestion of food. We have
added more to the beauty of the human countenance, during the
few years we have been at work, than have all the other agencies
in the world before us.

Why, then, with such a record, do we still find ourselves at
the foot of the ladder among the professions? The answer is to
be found in ourselves; in the lack of properly directed effort, or
rather in the lack of thoughtful effort. We are started wrong
from the moment we leave college, almost from the moment we
enter college, and somehow we never do seem to get right. The
taint of commercialism is on us from the very beginning, a *small,
pitiful, petty* commercialism. We are yoked at the outset of our
careers to a chariot that carries a company of mercenaries, and
very few of us ever develop sufficient strength to throw off the
yoke. Nor is this to be wondered at in the circumstances.

We all know that the boys who go into dental colleges are,
for the most part, poor. They come from the farms, out of village
stores, out of shops in the large cities, and, in a few instances,
very few, out of colleges, with just about enough money to see
them through the three or four years' course. They are almost
always dependent on their own resources, and where their parents
or relatives are in a position to help, they provide only sufficient

funds to see them through to graduation. From that point the young fellow has his own way to make.

It may very properly be argued that a similar situation prevails in the other professions. But at the point of graduation there is this difference: The young medical student or lawyer goes out under healthy, normal conditions. The young dental student is met at the threshold of his professional life by a band of men, who make it their business to put him at once in a mortgaged condition. I refer, as you no doubt are aware, to the agents of the dental supply houses. Under the present easy-going system, these agents are permitted to mingle freely with the students inside the college walls, to win their friendship and confidence, and to put themselves generally in a position where they may, at graduation, work the young man just as they please. And what is the result? The graduates are tempted into a business deal that leaves them for years, if not throughout their lives, hopelessly in debt. They are beguiled into buying equipment and supplies utterly beyond their means, and far in excess of their necessities. And *there* is laid the foundation of the evil condition that afflicts the entire profession. It is the beginning of the commercial domination that I believe to be the main source of our inability to rise to a level with the other professions. The college authorities, instead of combating this situation, foster it, not because of any selfish or mercenary motive, but because of habit. It has always been so.

The supply people are clever, capable fellows, generally personal friends of the best men in the faculty, and no one dreams of interfering with them. It was the way when I went to college, and it will be the way when the generation still unborn go, unless we get together and put a stop to it, arousing the interest of the college officials, and making clear to them the need for reform. It is hopeless to look for relief to the supply people. With them it is business; and good business. Experience has taught them that it is a perfectly safe proceeding to trust every graduate who may be induced to buy. It is the same scheme that is worked in another form in the mining districts of Pennsylvania, in the plantation districts of the South, and in the milling districts of other States, where the "company store" grants unlimited credit, knowing full well that it has absolute security in the wages to be earned.

In no profession, except ours, does such a situation exist. I can quite conceive of what would happen to any firm, or corporation, or combination, that should attempt systematically to load down the graduate of a medical college with an unnecessary and uncalled for burden of debt, that should attempt to impose upon the inexperience and credulity of young men utterly incapable of judging for themselves of the conditions they will have to face in the working world. But in the dental colleges usage has not alone made this condition a matter of course, but the system has its beginning almost at the outset of the young man's career as a student.

It is my firm belief that the present unsatisfactory standing of the profession is, to a large extent, due to this false start. If the students we send out of our colleges were protected against loading themselves down with a wholly unnecessary outfit, for which they mortgage at least the beginning of their careers, matters would soon right themselves and that taint of commercialism, that to my mind is the greatest curse and the greatest handicap of the profession, would soon disappear.

As it is, the young dentist starts out in life as the bond-slave of the man or combination that has sold him his outfit, and he spends a large part of his professional career in an endeavor to get out of debt. For the most part this is a slow, up-hill struggle. In many instances it is a *hopeless* struggle, and the man begins and ends in debt. In any event, the task hardens the victim and obscures, if it does not wipe out entirely, the humanitarian side of his nature. He looks upon his profession simply as a *money-making* machine, and he sells his services just as the grocer sells sugar and potatoes, and the butcher sells beef.

Only in exceptional cases, and with exceptional men, does a love of the profession survive this situation. For the most part the dentists gradually become merely distributing agents for the supply dealers and manufacturers, bent on getting as large a percentage as possible for their services in this direction. They become tradesmen in spirit, if not in fact, and the pitiful thing is that they must ever remain petty tradesmen, getting nothing like their just due, no matter how mercenary their spirits.

This condition crushes out the broad spirit that should characterize a true representative profession, and that does characterize most professions. The young physician and the young lawyer.

whatever their hardships at the start or throughout life, realize, at least, that they are working for themselves and not for a master who holds a bond on their implements of trade, and who controls every avenue of their activity. This gives them time and inclination to look to higher and better things. *They* are not forever faced with the pecuniary and commercial side of their calling. They find themselves in a profession that is free and untrammelled and not dominated from beginning to the end, from roots to branches, by a commercial oligarchy.

We, who have become hardened to this condition, inured to the atmosphere, may not fully appreciate what an evil effect this commercial despotism has on us. We may not appreciate how far it goes toward making the difference in grade that lies between other professions and ours. But it is only necessary to examine calmly into the facts to arrive at a most convincing conclusion.

I suppose you all know that the great barbers' supply houses and the big breweries have a system that is very much akin to that of the dental supply houses. They find likely men with a little money and fix up for them establishments more or less elaborate, upon which they take a mortgage. And thereafter the barber and the saloon-keeper are simply distributing agents for their masters, just as are the dentists for theirs, unless they have sufficient talent or shrewdness to pay themselves out of their clutches.

I confess that it is rather humiliating to find such a comparison in order. But the facts force it upon us. And, further, the facts show that this situation is by no means confined to the time of graduation, to the time when we enter our profession. So habituated do we become to the domination of the supply men, that we carry them with use in happy comradeship throughout our careers.

In other professions, the men who make and sell the necessary tools, and adjuncts, one meets at their offices or they call at stated intervals to offer and push their wares. But with us they are, at the beginning and at the end, the main thing. At our important conventions the choicest rooms and the most desirable quarters are pre-empted by the supply houses. The agents hobnob with us, and thrust their hospitality upon us, and we are, apparently, glad to have them do so. Can you imagine a medical convention or a lawyers' convention manipulated or controlled by implement and supply men?

I am aware that at the conventions of trade and commercial bodies the manufacturers' displays form one of the most important features. But we are forever boasting that we are far and away above trade and commercialism. We are forever striving for the elevation of our profession and for higher standards of dignity. Yet, wherever we meet in considerable numbers, we are fairly inundated with trade displays. The only difference in this respect between us and the trade convention is that where, for example, the hardware men are confronted with ice-cream freezers, snow-shovels, and patent road-scrapers, and the plumbers' rooms are furnished with the newest styles of sanitary plumbing, we meet chisels, excavators, patent cuspidors, and other cheerful instruments. Mind, I am not finding fault on personal grounds, either with the supply houses or their agents. I know many charming gentlemen and fine fellows in the business, men whom I am glad to meet at all proper times and on all proper occasions, as my friends. Men whom I am glad to have at my home and to whom I am happy to extend hospitality. But I do object to the spirit that it breeds, to the domination of our conventions and our actions by men who, if we asserted ourselves and valued ourselves as do other professions, would be very glad to remain in the background on these occasions when we are supposed to meet for the interchange of experience and opinion. The whole system should be torn up, root and branch, and must be before we can attain to the dignity and standing after which we are all so ardently striving.

A striking manifestation of what we are coming to, or rather what we *have* come to under this system of commercial control, is to be found in our literature. Look the field over, and with one exception you do not find a dental journal that is not controlled by a supply house. And *brazenly* controlled. *No effort* is made at concealment. *There, on the cover of each paper,* you will find calmly set out that it is published by this supply house or that. And the editors are among the best known men in the profession. *This is a condition that is not alone without parallel in the professions, but without parallel in trade.* I have mentioned this peculiarity to a number of friends who are engaged in trade journalism, and without exception they were filled with amazement.

That we should have *not one widely read independent* influential paper of tone, dignity, and national standing, seemed to them an *impossible* situation. Yet, I confess, on me this anomalous condition had never made impress until I began to investigate it. And so, no doubt, it is with you. We have become so habituated to the existing condition, that the possibility of anything better, or different, has probably never suggested itself to us. All the other professions have a number of high-grade independent periodical publications to represent them. So far as I have been able to find, there is no trade *so lowly* that has not its independent mouthpiece. Only the *dental profession* must depend for its periodical literature on "house organs." Probably you do not know what a "house organ" is. It is a technical.term applied in trade to publications issued in the interest of an individual firm or house, and such organs are looked on with scorn by the members of the trade. They have neither weight nor influence, but are frankly advertising devices. In the professions, other than ours, such publications are entirely unknown, or if they exist they have no standing or recognition. Nothing better helps to explain our situation, the backwardness of our professional rank, than the fact that practically all the publications supposedly devoted to our interests, to the promulgation of our science, are controlled by supply houses. *The standing of a profession is determined by its literature.* It was not until the English physicians were represented by the *Lancet* that they obtained recognition as a class. That the dentists of America, in spite of the manifest progress they have made, in spite of the really remarkable achievements that have been theirs, in spite of the fact that they number thirty-five thousand, have so little recognition to-day in the affairs of the American Medical Association is due, no doubt, in large measure to the fact that the physicians have such standard publications as the *Medical Record, American Medicine,* the *Journal of the American Medical Association,* and half a dozen other periodicals to represent them, while we have nothing except house organs that neither merit respect nor obtain it. Imagine the medical profession dependent for its literature upon a publication owned and edited by Johnson & Johnson, or by the owners of Listerine, or by Parke, Davis & Co., or by a jobbing house.

If we had a periodical literature of known independence and high standing, a literature that would command *general respect* and *intelligent attention*, it would serve not only to stimulate the profession as a whole, but it would be certain to develop original research work, in which we are now wofully backward. No important research work has ever been accomplished in any division of science, unless it has had the active good will and co-operation of a considerable body of men. And this can only be brought about by the existence of a medium that is in a position to encourage and promulgate results. No section of medicine stands in greater need of the work of the intelligent investigator than ours. We have many problems to solve. In a dozen different directions we are groping in the dark, proceeding along lines where all is speculation, nothing fact. We know little or nothing of the causes of decay, or the causes of erosion, of the histologic structure of enamel. We need better filling-material. We need substances to take the place of unsightly gold. We need light on the best methods of porcelain inlay. We need instruction and information on a *hundred* different subjects. We need better mechanical appliances, and, *above all*, we need a broader spirit, a spirit that will keep men who *perfect* such processes or appliances from running straight to the patent office with them. Such a broader spirit can be fostered only through a broader literature.

What do you suppose would happen to a physician in good standing who should perfect a new instrument or a new process, and straightway secure a patent that would restrict its use? He would be *pilloried* in *his press*, and treated with *contempt* by his associates. But with us it is a matter of course that a man who finds a new way of doing things should at once take the commercial view and get out of it all he can. Have we not all of us seen reputable dentists buzzing about a convention, buttonholing their fellows to buy this thing or that, which they have just perfected and patented? A pitiful and humiliating sight, truly, but unfortunately a common one.

There is, too, another side to this mercenary, patent-seeking spirit that the present conditions have fostered. This is the way in which the supply combination adapts this professional narrowness to its own uses. Its agents in the field, and its representatives in Washington, watch narrowly for new devices, and anything that promises at all is bought up as soon as the patent rights are perfected, or even before. And then the new device is shelved in order that it may not interfere with the stock designs already on the market. No one knows even remotely how many hundred appliances that would make far better work and easier have been shelved this way, with a consequent arrest of development in the science, and a general lowering of the moral tone.

To overcome this hampering spirit in our ranks will require a strong propaganda, and for this there is only one agency on which we may, with any degree of certainty, rely. That is a sound, far-reaching literature that will preach *higher professional standards* and hold the fraternity *up* to them. Manifestly it is idle to look to the house organ for such work. It could not, even if its editors had the inclination, work against the interests of its owners, as it would have to, in order to do any good along these lines. For such work we must look to *independent publications,* conducted in the interests of the workers in the profession, and *not* in the interest of any supply dealer or manufacturer, no matter how rich or how important.

As the standing of a profession is always determined by the character of its literature, so the rise of the members of the profession, in an ethical and worldly sense, may be distinctly traced in the rise of their periodicals. As I have already pointed out, the physicians of England had neither repute nor standing until the *Lancet* made *both* for them. They were merely leeches and ranked with the barbers.

Railroading, both in England and America, was a trade until the founding of distinctive class publications. Similarly, the electrician was an ordinary handicraftsman, until there appeared in this field papers worthy of the new industry. Then electricity became, as it is to-day, one of the most important and dignified professions in industry. Throughout the field of human endeavor similar progress may be traced. A worthy, dignified literature was always the precursor of a worthy, dignified standing. And it will be so with us. We can have neither hope nor promise of real solidity, we can have neither the high rank nor high reputation we merit, until we put forth publications that shall be untrammelled by commercial interests, and that shall be conducted in the interests of the profession and not in the interests of this house or that.

You may rest assured that until there *are* representative publications that shall record progress, stimulate research, and bring about an interchange of ideas, we will advance, if at all, only at an unsatisfactory pace. Indeed, I am not at all certain that, unless we have such a stimulus, we shall advance at all beyond a certain point; that we shall not be overtaken with dry-rot; that the spirit of dwarfing commercialism which rests on us now, will not eventually cause a retrograde, instead of a forward, movement. As it is now, every step in advance that we have taken has been due to the effort of some energetic, public-spirited individual who has been carried forward by a true love of the profession. Unfortunately, there is not enough of this spirit to warrant our relying on it for general and continued advancement.

At any rate, the time has passed when we *ought* to depend upon *disconnected efforts* here and there. We ought to get together in some manner and through some agency and inaugurate a systematic method of stimulating scientific work. We ought to get the profession farther away from the mechanical and commercial side. We have plenty of men in our ranks who would be only too glad to take up the scientific work so urgently needed, if they were assured practical and substantial encouragement. I can name over a dozen men who have in them the capacity to develop this side of our profession. Like all true scientists they are *impractical* in the business sense. We ought to get behind these men, to establish them in a laboratory of research, and provide them with a publication that would enable them to spread before the profession the results of their work.

Unless we do something of this sort, unless we found a proper literature and arrange for a proper system of original research, we will wake up some morning and find the "pre-eminence of the American dentist" a thing of the past. Even now the foreigners are leading us on the purely scientific side of our work, in the development of those principles and ideas that after all must be the foundation of the profession, as against the mere utilitarian foundation of a trade or industry. On our own part, we have grown to rest too well content upon our superior mechanical ability, oblivious of the fact, apparently, that by neglecting the scientific side of the work, we are pushing *away* from the goal instead of toward it.

The laboratories abroad are going deeply into the questions that we have merely touched on. They are digging to the roots of things. They are creating what must always be the true basis of medical work—they are seeking the *cause* of things for which we simply seek the cure. We are, for the most part, simply meeting the difficulties as we come upon them, and attempt remedying them by mechanical processes, instead of going deeper and preventing the difficulties in the first instance. As the result of such a superficial course, we have already begun to lose standing, so that while our representatives who have gone abroad are accorded a high place as operators, we are scoffed at as scientists, and most of the scientific progress that is made is coming out of European laboratories.

This state of things is to be particularly deplored in view of the fact that our profession has always been shown the greatest consideration by American people and American institutions. The National and the State governments have given us every protection and are prepared to foster our work along any line we may desire to push it. But, instead of taking advantage of this condition, we are puttering, making pretty speeches, developing the purely mechanical side of our work, and doing nothing practical or permanent to develop the scientific or fundamental side.

Let us "cut out" of our meetings some of the long-winded papers that merely kill time and interest. Cut out the rehashes of primary facts that have been drilled into college students, and substitute in their place a measure of new scientific work; something that will be as helpful in the *theory* of dentistry as the clinics are in its *practice*.

In conclusion, I would make these suggestions:

First.—That we institute some organized measure to prevent the exploitation of our students at the outset of their careers by the supply dealers and manufacturers.

Second.—That we keep our meetings and conventions clear of the commercial element.

Third.—That we organize a movement that shall bring about the foundation of an independent literature.

Fourth.—That we organize a systematic movement for original research.

When we accomplish these *four things*, we will have taken a long step toward the emancipation of our profession from those conditions that have kept us behind all the other professions in the upward movement; we will have done that which will insure the up-lifting of our calling toward the high place it ought to occupy; we will have made it clear that we stand for pure ideals, the advance of science, and the eradication of commercialism. Let us but work together in these matters, and we will cast down the last stone in the wall that divides us from equality with the best there is in medicine. This, gentlemen, is what I mean by "Professional Emancipation and how it may be effected."—*Dental Summary.*

ANÆSTHESIA, LOCAL.—The writer describes his method of producing local anæsthesia. He uses B-eucaine, which is far less dangerous than cocaine, while possessing analgesic properties little, if at all, inferior to it, and with the concurrent use of adrenalin for the purpose of securing a retardation of circulation equivalent to constriction of the part, he has removed some of the objections as to the duration of the analgesia, the extent of the area which can be dealt with, and the amount of the toxic drug to be employed. It is necessary to keep within the safe dose of the drug, and to have at our disposal a large enough quantity of the fluid medium to render it possible to spread the analgesic agent over large areas. For ordinary surgical work the following solution is found by the author to answer well: Distilled water, 140 cubic centimetres; B-eucaine, 0.2 grams; sodium chloride, 0.8 grams; 1 in 1000 adrenalin chloride solution, 10 minims. All this quantity of fluid can be used in an ordinary case if necessary, and is quite sufficient for most. Twice as much may be injected without ill results. The duration of the insensibility is secured by the admixture of the adrenalin. Without it sensation is only abolished by eucaine for about fifteen minutes; with it, for from three to four hours. But the analgesia is produced more slowly when adrenalin is employed with the eucaine. It is therefore well before all larger operations to wait some thirty minutes after injection to allow time for the insensibility to become fully developed. After this the effect appears to deepen for a couple of hours. Waiting has another advantage. When eucaine alone is employed the operation must be done at once. The tissues are still in a state of artificial œdema which masks the anatomic details unpleasantly. By adding adrenalin to the eucaine solution and waiting, the artificial œdema has disappeared and details are very clearly seen. Rapid injection is to be avoided; sudden distention of the tissues is disagreeable, if not painful. The fluid should not be used cold nor too hot, for the same reason. All dragging on the parts is to be avoided, lest structures be pulled upon which lie beyond the area of infiltration. The writer has never seen any depressing effects follow the use of

B-eucaine in a long series of operations. A list of operations done under B-eucaine analgesia is appended, and among these are the following: Abdominal sections, hernia operations, amputations, orchidectomy, removal of cyst of thyroid, removal of silver wire from around the patella, operations for fistula in ano, varicose veins, hydrocele, varicocele, etc.—A. E. BARKER (*British Medical Journal*, December 24, 1904.

Reports of Society Meetings.

ACADEMY OF STOMATOLOGY.

A REGULAR meeting of the Academy of Stomatology of Philadelphia was held at its rooms, 1731 Chestnut Street, on the evening of Tuesday, October 25, 1904, the President, Dr. I. N. Broomell, in the chair.

Dr. A. H. Macpherson read a paper entitled "Electrolysis for the Treatment of Peridental Inflammations."

(For Dr. Macpherson's paper, see page 32.)

DISCUSSION.

Dr. Albert P. Brubaker.—The statements made by Dr. Macpherson regarding the treatment of abscesses with the electric current are most interesting and instructive. An explanation of the facts presented is to be found in what is known of the effects of the passage of an electric current through solutions of inorganic salts, organic matter, and upon lower organisms.

With the passage of the electric current through a solution of any inorganic salt, for example, sodium chloride, the salt is decomposed, the chlorine passing to the positive pole, or anode, the sodium passing to the negative pole, or cathode.

If the current is made to flow through a more or less coagulated mass of albumin, it will be found after a short time that the albumin in the neighborhood of the anode is coagulated still more, while in the neighborhood of the cathode it is liquefied. The intermediate portion may or may not be affected, according to the

strength of the current. If the current is made to flow through a
small cell containing low forms of animal life, they will arrange
themselves along certain lines and begin to move toward the negative pole or cathode.

These facts may be utilized in explanation of the facts presented by Dr. Macpherson. Thus an abscess around a tooth, or
elsewhere, is a cavity containing pus, which consists of water,
inorganic salts, albumin, white blood-curpuscles, pus-cells, and
micro-organisms. The tissue overlying the abscess consists largely
of albumin. If the electric current enters the body at any indif-
ferent point—*e.g.*, the hand, the back of the neck, or elsewhere—
through a small electrode, the tissues at that point will be more
or less coagulated. As it leaves through the cathode the tissues
will be liquefied. In the method of treatment advocated by Dr.
Macpherson a small electrode, the cathode, is placed on the outer
surface of the gum overlying the abscess and the current established. On entering the body the current at once diffuses and takes
the lines of least resistance, but as it approaches the cathode the
lines again converge. As it passes through the abscess contents
and the overlying tissues, the inorganic salts are decomposed, pus-
cells and bacteria accumulate in the neighborhood of the cathode,
and the albumin of the overlying tissues is liquefied. The continuous flow of the current soon establishes one or more outlets,
after which the contents of the cavity are discharged on the surface. With this event the swelling, pressure, and pain subside and
repair is initiated. Similar effects are produced, no doubt, in the
walls of the cavity.

In this electrolytic treatment the coagulation which would occur
at the anode is prevented by the use of a large sponge electrode, so
that the current will enter the body through a large area of surface.
It is not the quantity, but the density, of the current which coagu-
lates the tissues, which at this point is not desirable; but at the
cathode, where electrolytic effects are desirable, the electrode should
be small, as in the apparatus employed by Dr. Macpherson. At
this point density of current is required.

· *Mr. F. Geiger.*—I do not think I can add anything to what
Drs. Macpherson and Brubaker have said. I have my battery here
with the various electrodes, and am prepared to give a demonstration
of the work, if we have a patient.

In treating an abscess or a boil that is just forming, if electrodes are properly applied it will bring the pus to the surface in a few moments without any breaking of the skin.

Dr. J. H. Gaskill.—I would like to ask what effect there is on healthy tissue?

Mr. Geiger.—There is no effect at all upon healthy tissue. Where there is pus, if you apply the positive pole to the gum you can drive the pus out into the system if you leave it on long enough. I have taken the pus from one arm to another.

Dr. J. Head.—How do you know you did not draw the pus from other parts of the body?

Mr. Geiger.—In a healthy body an electrode left on all day will not draw inflammation to a point; but if there is pus in the path of the current it will come out at the negative electrode. I can draw pus from one place to another.

Dr. M. H. Cryer.—We employ the same process for tumors, except that we introduce long needles, and if we want to draw out, we use the negative pole; if to drive in, we use the positive.

Dr. Macpherson.—I had a patient who was unable to open his mouth for three days, caused by an impacted lower wisdom-tooth. After the application of electrolysis there was immediate relaxation of the muscles, and there was even more relaxation after a second application. The applications were from fifteen to eighteen minutes' duration, with twenty minutes' interval. The negative pole was placed immediately over the wisdom-tooth and the positive pole at the back of the neck. I also had a patient, a dentist, suffering from an abscess on a left upper bicuspid which she had not been able to make discharge. Pus was discharged upon the application of the electrode by pressure, and on this account the case was not a good one to prove the power of electrolysis. There was, however, relief from the pain, and the swelling decreased. The next day I applied the lancet, and some pus which had accumulated came out. Mr. Geiger said I did not apply the electricity sufficiently long. I never saw an abscess heal so quickly. In two days the gum was in a perfectly normal condition, and now, after two weeks, it remains the same.

Dr. Albert P. Brubaker.—I should like to call the attention of the society to a statement made some years ago, which did not receive very much consideration at the time. It was at the close of a short paper on the causation of dental erosion. It was stated that, as in many cases the mouths of glands on the posterior surface of the upper lip are enlarged, swollen, and discharging an acid fluid, which it is believed is the cause of the erosion, the electric current might be employed for the destruction of these glands and the progress of the erosion checked. The method would be similar to that employed by electro-surgeons for the removal of superfluous hairs. A large electrode, the anode, could be placed on the hand and a needle electrode, the cathode, inserted into the mouth of the gland. In a few minutes the gland structures would be destroyed. If but a dozen of the glands are diseased, it would not be difficult or tedious to destroy them and thus check the further progress of the erosion.

Dr. James Truman.—I am not familiar with this procedure, therefore I can say nothing about it. I was much pleased, however, both in hearing the paper and with Dr. Brubaker's lucid explanation of the process.

Dr. M. I. Schamberg.—We are all very anxious to ascertain just what can be accomplished in dentistry by this new method of treatment. As was said, electrolysis has been practised in medicine for some time, but its mode of application to medicine differs somewhat from the method advocated this evening. I can conceive of the possibility of the destruction of tissue by the production of an electric burn at the point where the negative pole is placed; but to draw pus through the tissues for some distance is a phenomenon with which I am not familiar. It is possible that it may have been done, as is evidenced by a very favorable report of the clinic given by Dr. Macpherson at the State convention this year. I am sorry that I did not see the demonstration, for I have a suspicion that pressure upon the abscessed area caused the pus to exude. This suspicion is somewhat increased by Dr. Macpherson's report of this evening, in which he refers to the case in which he practically admitted that pressure brought the pus through an existing fistula at the first application. It is not unreasonable to suppose that if the fistula existed during the first application, it had not entirely healed when a second application was made. I am taking a sceptical view of this question merely to bring out the truth of the matter. If this method of treatment is to be helpful, we all want to adopt it. If it falls short of doing that which is claimed for it, we naturally want to waste little time with it. I think it is a mistake to allude to electrolysis as a cure for alveolar abscess. It may do as much as the knife will do, and in a neater way, without the aspect of a surgical procedure, but no greater claim should be made than that it will evacuate pus, for when we speak about curing an alveolar abscess by the mere removal of pus we make a big mistake. Many abscesses recur because of the fact that the evacuation of pus is insufficient treatment. If we wish to permanently cure our cases we must remove the cause, and in a large proportion of cases the cause lies in the necrotic end of a root. Most often the surrounding bone is diseased, and unless the débris is removed from the periapical space permanent relief will not be afforded.

I believe it would be a hazardous procedure to cause pus to be passed from one portion of the body to another, if, as is stated by Mr. Geiger, such can be done, for the entire system might thus become infected. This same danger applies to the gum-tissue and alveolus. It puts upon nature a double duty, that of curing the part already affected and the portion through which the pus is made to pass.

It is disappointing not to hear a report of more cases treated, for the few alluded to by the essayist are not, to my mind, sufficiently conclusive. I shall be only too glad to be convinced of the value of this method if it possesses the virtue ascribed to it.

Dr. Gaskill.—I think that Dr. Schamberg's objections in some respects are not very well founded. I have a great deal of faith in the instrument from the results which have been stated. Dr. Schamberg speaks of the possibility of infection by drawing the pus. Whenever pus is evacuated, by whatever means, whether it goes through a cut surface or not, it may cause infection. So, I think that these points are not as well taken as they might have been.

Dr. Macpherson.—My first subject was a patient of my neighbor, Dr. Shoemaker. I made the application, gave him a looking-glass, and had him observe the result. There was over a teaspoonful of pus accumulated at the electrode. That was a year ago, and six months afterwards the part was in perfect condition. He had never had an abscess heal with such satisfactory results. The gentleman who brought the patient to the State meeting had been experimenting with radium and with electricity and he did not believe it was possible to get the results claimed. I was uncertain whether to apply the electrode for pain or for pus. If applied for pain, I would move the electrode; if for pus, I would hold it in

one position. I tried for pus, and the gentleman was absolutely
convinced, and said he thought the result was marvellous. I have
had a number of other cases, and I think I can say there have been
no failures. I have proceeded with great timidity, and would not
have read the paper before the State meeting had I not been
urged by Dr. Broomell. I would like to have made more exact
records of the work, but the apparatus is ready, and I think it is
safe for all to make their own experiments.

Dr. A. N. Gaylord.—If this method is what it appears and is
claimed to be, it is certainly one of vital importance to every one
of us, and the apparatus will find a welcome place in every office.
However, I am a little sceptical, and would very much dislike to
see the opinion of this meeting to go on record as accepting this
method conclusively. Mr. Geiger states that the material which
accumulates at the negative electrode is pus, but admits that his
belief is not substantiated by bacteriological test.

I would like to ask Dr. Macpherson whether, to his knowledge,
any other test has been made except the one which Dr. Broomell
made.

Dr. Broomell.—The chemical test showed about seventy-five
per cent. pus.

Dr. Gaylord.—Dr. Broomell tells me that the case from which
he made a test was one in which there was an open sinus, therefore,
as far as proving anything relative to this method, it is valueless.

The product from a case where it is claimed that pus has been
drawn through the tissues should by all means be given a thorough
test, and not be accepted as pus because it looks like pus. Many
a man has purchased a gold brick because it looked like gold.

I have done a little work in a crude way by adding resistance
to the electro-dental switch-board, and while I was gratified with
the result, feeling that I gave relief to the patient, yet the accumulation around the negative electrode was not to my mind pus. I
believe this product to be the effect of electrolysis on mucus and
saliva.

I witnessed the case of which Dr. Macpherson speaks at the
meeting of the Pennsylvania State Society, in which case he states
that he obtained a teaspoonful of pus. A teaspoonful of pus, if
confined within the bone, would mean a very large necrotic area,
while if it were within the soft tissues, we would naturally look
for considerable swelling. The patient under question had no

apparent swelling, and the history would indicate that his trouble had not passed beyond the stage of pericemental inflammation, and yet it is stated that a teaspoonful of pus was extracted. It looks to me, in this case, as if the accumulation must have been something other than pus, although it had that appearance.

I am by no means trying to cry down this method, but I would like to see the conclusions based on scientific investigation. We should not accept this treatment too readily, and risk becoming the laughing stock of the profession in the future.

Electrolysis has been known to the medical profession for many years, and if it is capable of producing such wonderful results, it seems strange to me that they should not have discovered it ere this.

Dr. Broomell.—They didn't discover anæsthesia.

Dr. Gaylord.—This is very true, but the medical profession has had this apparatus and similar ones manufactured by Mr. Geiger in use for many years, and if it does what he claims for it, it has a much larger field in medicine than in dentistry,—for instance, the venereal specialist in his battle with gonococcus.

Dr. Head.—I think the question is not whether it is true or false pus, whether it looks like mucus or saliva, but, Does this current extract the bacteria from the tissues? The whole thing comes down fundamentally to whether that which is extracted from the tissues contains bacteria. It seems to me the scientific way of deciding that point is to extract the fluid from a place that is supposed to contain pus, and then at once examine it under the microscope. If the bacteria are present I should think they surely would appear under those conditions. The question of whether there are white blood-corpuscles is a minor matter. It is hardly credible that the fluid would be purely in the form of pus. It is more probable that there would be a large admixture of blood-serum.

Dr. Gaylord.—That is my argument. If the product is blood-serum, call it blood-serum; do not call it pus.

Dr. Schamberg.—I would like to ask Dr. Macpherson whether he extracted any material resembling pus from the case in which the patient was suffering from an impacted wisdom-tooth.

Dr. Macpherson.—Yes, a considerable amount of pus. The pus as it adheres to the electrode does not look like the thick pus you get from the lancet; it is much thinner than the ordinary pus.

If not pus, what became of the pus that was causing the abscess and which this treatment relieved most thoroughly?

Dr. Schamberg.—Did you determine whether the patient acquired the use of his jaw through electrical stimulation, which would be possible if tetanic contraction of the muscles prevailed, or was the muscular relaxation due to the actual withdrawal of pus from about the tooth? Was the relief immediate?

Dr. Macpherson.—Yes; as I stated, as soon as the patient was through with the operation, he was on his feet. He said, immediately, " I can open my mouth."

Dr. Schamberg.—If that is the case, I believe the effect was due to electrical stimulation rather than to the withdrawal of pus. Even though pus was removed, it is hardly possible that the muscles would have acquired their normal function so promptly had their rigidity been due to inflammatory action produced by the toxic influence of pyogenic organisms. If a mouth-gag had been applied to the patient's jaw and the muscles exercised thereby, it is a question whether mechanical stimulation would not have acquired for the jaw the same amount of motion as was accomplished by electrical stimulation.

Dr. Macpherson.—In every case in which electrolysis was used the patient felt decidedly better after the operation. The swelling disappeared and the gum resumed its normal feeling to the patient.

Dr. J. C. Curry.—As a matter of history, I would like to say that to my knowledge Dr. Flagg used a method similar to this some ten years ago. He wrote considerably on the subject and gave very interesting demonstrations.

Mr. Geiger.—That was Faradism. This is pure galvanism.

Dr. Schamberg.—Dr. M. L. Rhein has been using the electric method for curing abscess at the apices of teeth. He does it by passing an electrode through the canal. I believe that many cures have been effected by this method. I must admit that I am still sceptical about the possibility of drawing pus through tissues causing the complete evacuation of pus cavities when there is no fistula present.

Dr. Broomell.—There has been sufficient discussion to show that the process has not been absolutely commended at the present time. I am glad that there have been opinions expressed on both sides.

OTTO E. INGLIS,
Editor Academy of Stomatology.

Editorial.

THE "DENTAL REGISTER" AND QUININE.

In the *Dental Register* for January, 1905, there is an editorial of which the following is an abstract. The editor says, as a portion of his criticism, that—

Dr. Joseph Head, in the December *Items*, makes the following statement: after thoroughly cleansing the roots of teeth affected with pyorrhœa, firmly fix the teeth with ligatures or splints and pack the pockets full with quinine sulphate as an antiseptic dressing. The quinine will exclude bacteria and cause the gums to become reattached to the peridental membrane or tooth substance. This is a rather strong statement and one that the pathology of this disease and the pharmacology of the drug will scarcely justify on logical grounds; but Dr. Head quotes Dr. James Truman as the author of the remedy and certifies it from his own clinical experience. We sometimes meet with unexpected therapeutic paradoxes in the clinical use of drugs, which lead us to lose confidence in scientific findings. . . . Quinine may be an ideal remedy for pyorrhœa; but how many patients will submit to such a treatment! The taste of this drug is exceedingly distasteful to almost every one, even when taken in regular form and dosage for systemic impressions. We do not think many patients will be willing to have their gums impregnated with this bitter drug to be gradually dissolved in the mouth fluids and so manifest its bitterness for several hours or perhaps days. The remedy will be worse than the disease, and the dentist who makes use of it ought to be very sure of the loyalty of his patient. Dentists have not as yet reached the sugar-coated stage in therapeutics, and it is possible that their peculiar field is not adapted to that system; but there is too much of the old style use of radical remedies, or it may be thoughtless use of powerful or distasteful drugs."

When the foregoing met the writer's eye, as he was scanning the pages of our esteemed contemporary, it was passed over with many other not over-well-digested paragraphs running through dental literature, but since then this view of the editor of the *Dental Register* has been extensively copied, and with evident approbation, and, to that extent, a loss of "confidence in scientific findings," as the editor expresses it rather sarcastically. This forces the writer to enter a defence of this drug and to meet the implied charge of empiricism contained in the editorial quoted.

The article, in question, is so manifestly the result of prejudice and ignorance as to the therapeutic value of quinine, and all the derivatives of cinchona, that the writer will not attempt to discuss the statements made. They must be left for good or ill, as the reader may choose to interpret them.

It is, however, important that the reasons should be given for the use of this drug, that the sceptical may, at least, be made aware that its therapeutic value in the disease mentioned has been very thoroughly tested, and that for twenty-five years, and yet the writer of this has not reached "the sugar-coated stage" in its use in the treatment of patients.

If our friends of the medical profession were to confine their therapeutics to pleasant-tasted drugs, the methods of treatment would be forced to undergo an entire change. The business of the conscientious practitioner is to endeavor to bring about a restoration to normal conditions, and he is not required to consult the æsthetic tastes of his patients in its accomplishment.

The treatment of pyorrhœa alveolaris is an interesting theme, even though hackneyed, for each individual attempting restorations to health is apparently faithless as to the value of any other method save that which he originated, and he is not, as a rule, quite satisfied with his procedures whether original or adopted. Thus in reviewing the literature of the subject, one is forced to the conclusion that the dental world must still wait expectantly for the man who will be able to satisfy criticism and produce a process of treatment satisfactory to practitioner, teacher, and student. The writer would, therefore, prefer to keep silence and let facts speak for themselves, but he cannot afford to permit a lack of knowledge as to the real therapeutic value of quinine to still further increase present prejudice.

No one, certainly not the writer, has ever claimed quinine as a specific in the disease named. It has been recommended for certain properties believed to be of peculiar value and not common to other drugs. What are these?

1. It acts on broken tissue more kindly than any other antiseptic. It further acts (Binz) to prevent diapedesis of the leucocytes of the blood, and thus, by inhibiting their amœbic action, pus is not, as a rule, produced in the pyorrhœal pockets.

2. It acts as a powerful antiseptic, and will prevent the ingress of pathogenic organism for at least twenty-four hours, thus giving

time for healthy granulations and the eventual filling up of the pockets of normal tissue. It is at the same time absolutely non-irritating.

No claim has ever been made that this agent will alone cure pyorrhœa alveolaris. It is simply one part of the treatment, but by no means the least active in the process of restoration.

The writer has used quinine and the derivatives of cinchona for the reduction of inflammatory conditions of the oral cavity since 1882, and in 1884 called the attention of the American Dental Association to the value of these in the therapeutics of dentistry. For years quinine sulphate has taken a place in the treatment of pyorrhœa alveolaris in the Department of Dentistry, University of Pennsylvania, almost to the exclusion of other drugs for a similar purpose. The writer has tried many old and new drugs as substitutes, including mercurial preparations, but in no one have the results justified hopes and expectations.

During these years there have been treated in this dispensary from fifty to one hundred cases of pyorrhœa during each session, by the method adopted and advocated by the writer, and, as all the pathological cases, of whatever kind, treated by the Senior Class are required to be registered and written out, there is compiled a series of valuable statistics, that fully warrant the assertion that no more thorough clinical experimentation has ever been made of any disease coming under the care of the average practitioner. All cases are not cured, nor will it be possible to accomplish this by any method of local or systemic treatment, for the disease assumes several forms from the simple pericemental inflammation to the senile form (osteomalacia, Talbot). The operator must be able to make a careful differential diagnosis before he assumes the responsibility of treatment. The percentage of success in the clinical work of the department aforesaid has been, in pyorrhœa alveolaris, fully ninety-five per cent., a result quite satisfactory, and, it is thought, not exceeded by other methods of treatment.

The objections to the taste of the drug have no force. It is true, very few patients find it agreeable, but some do, and they all acknowledge it gives them comfort and return for renewal with satisfaction over the *bitter* experience.

The writer has made it the rule of his life not to defend, by lengthy and oft-repeated essays, any proposition which had been originated by him. He has felt satisfied to give it publicity, and there let it rest, confident that sooner or later the truth would find its place. It took twenty years for his views on bleaching teeth to take root as a method of practice in the dental profession, and when the light began to dawn, among the first to discover it was a practitioner in the Middle West, who so fully appreciated the ideas contained in the writer's article in the *American System of Dentistry*, that he took it bodily, placed his name at the top, and read it before one of the societies of that region, and it was published to go down to future generations as the product of John Doe, bleacher. It has taken another twenty years to reach an editorial opposing the use of quinine. There is cause for encouragement.

To satisfy our contemporary, it is hoped, or, in any event, to hasten his enlightenment in this direction, there follows some of the opinions of eminent scientific authorities upon which the use of quinine is based. If, after giving due consideration to these, it is hoped that the editor may conclude that if the so-called "Truman Process" be worthless, it at least has the merit of being founded on eminent authority, and cannot by any twisting of words be classed as a method of practice "worse than the disease."

"It has recently been experimentally proved by Binz, Hallier, Pavesi, and others that one part of the alkaloid (quinine sulphate) in three hundred parts of milk, albuminous solutions, meat, honey, syrup, etc., will keep in check for a long time putrefaction and other fermentations. Professor Binz has shown that this is due to a poisonous influence upon the low forms of life." (United States Dispensatory.)

"Quinia is supposed to control inflammation by its destructive influence on movements of the white corpuscles, and Binz maintains that, after irritating and inflaming the mesentery by the administration of quinia, the white corpuscles are killed and their migration by the tissues is prevented. It is supposed to lower temperature by lessening the ozonizing power of the blood, and thus checking oxidation." (Ringer, "Hand Book of Therapeutics," page 583.)

"As Binz originally noted, quinine when added to freshly drawn blood arrests the amœboid movement of the white cells. Moreover, when applied in very dilute solution to the exposed mesentery of a frog, it suspends, almost immediately, the migration of the leucocytes. This cessation of diapedesis was believed by Binz to be due to poisoning of the corpuscles, but Metschni-koff and his followers attribute it rather to the repelling influence (negative chemotaxis) which quinine, in common with many other substances, exerts upon motile cells." ("Modern Materia Medica and Therapeutics," Stevens.)

"In the blood, quinine arrests the migration of the white corpuscles and checks its amœboid movements; the red cells are rendered less adhesive, and their oxygen-carrying function is impaired. The experiments of Lokoloff upon rabbits show that quinine exerts a favorable influence upon the healing of wounds. Inflammatory degeneration of tissue is notably decreased." ("Materia Medica and Therapeutics," Shoemaker.)

"Binz and his pupils have shown that quinia inhibits or lessens the activity of the white blood-corpuscles, and, indeed, destroys them, or arrests their production; for in cats poisoned by this agent the number of white corpuscles was found to be considerably less than in unpoisoned animals (Scharrenbroich, Martin, Jerusalimsky, Geltowsky). By all the observers just named, by Baxter, who made a series of carefully conducted experiments, and by Cutter, it has been established that quinia inhibits the amœboid movements of the white corpuscles. . . . Quinia has also the power to prevent or arrest the migration of the white corpuscles from the vessels." ("Materia Medica and Therapeutics," Bartholow.)

"The correctness of the original observations of Professor Binz upon the out-wandering of the white blood-corpuscles in the Cohnheim frog must be considered as established, but it is not proved that the failure of the blood-corpuscles to escape from the irritated vessels is due to the arrest of their amœboid movements by the quinine. In a series of experiments Dr. H. A. Hare found that the vessels in the cinchonized frog were much more contracted and had their walls much thicker than in a corresponding frog without quinine. The contraction of the vessels is thought by Dr. Hare to be the result of a direct action exerted by the drug upon the muscular coat of the arterioles. It is certain the alkaloid reduces very markedly the force of the heart. It is, therefore, possible that the quinine prevents the out-wandering by lessening the force which is driving the corpuscles and at the same time increasing the resistance of the capillary walls." ("Therapeutics: Its Principles and Practice," H. C. Wood.)

It would seem unnecessary to multiply authorities further. It must be clearly evident that the consensus of opinion is all in favor of the conclusions of Binz, and it is upon these investigations that the use of the derivatives of cinchona is based. Upon broken tissue quinine acts decidedly.

Before leaving the subject, it may be well to state exactly the place quinine occupies in the treatment of pyorrhœa alveolaris, as understood and practised by the writer. It may also enlighten our critical editor and disabuse his mind of " paradoxes."

Briefly, the treatment starts upon the theory that pyorrhœa alveolaris is based upon local irritation, possibly through calculus and always through pathogenic bacteria, and that this irritation causes active chemotactic influence upon the leucocytes of the blood and consequent free migration of these corpuscles. To meet these conditions the pockets are treated—

1. By free injection of hydrogen dioxide not over three per cent. in strength.

2. Cauterization by sulphuric acid, commercially pure, twenty-five, thirty, or fifty per cent. solution. Action continued from thirty to sixty seconds.

3. Neutralization of acid by a magma of sodium bicarbonate and water, packed in pockets.

4. After free boiling through this action the pockets are freely washed with warm water.

5. Quinine sulphate made in a paste with water, placed in every portion of the pockets and left there for two days.

6. To be followed by a good antiseptic mouth-wash for an indefinite period. The character of this is not so important, but the writer prefers an agent that will be positively inhibiting to pathogenic micro-organisms, beta-naphthol (hydronaphthol) preferred.

This article is not an essay on pyorrhœa alveolaris, hence manipulative details are omitted. The writer is not at all anxious that any one, including our worthy editor, should be convinced of the value of this method of treatment, but he is concerned in an effort to have a much abused agent find a place in the therapeutics of dentistry and be a source of comfort to many suffering patients.

In this connection it may be well to state that McKesson and

Robbins, New York City, have prepared, at the suggestion of Dr. Joseph Head, small delicate wedges of quinine. These are very convenient, and are more readily applied than in the paste form, and should be equally as satisfactory in results.

THE "DENTAL DIGEST" HYSTERICAL.

IN the February issue of the *Dental Digest*, of Chicago, is an editorial entitled "Pretence *versus* Practice," in which the editor abuses the INTERNATIONAL DENTAL JOURNAL and its editor in language unworthy any respectable journal. The reasons for this sudden attack, from a commercial dental journal, are not as yet made clear, but the article is so intrinsically bad that it carries its own condemnation with it. For this reason the writer declines to notice the personal portion of this hysterical outburst.

The reflections made upon the honesty and ethical character of the INTERNATIONAL DENTAL JOURNAL require a definite and positive answer. This journal claims many good friends in the dental profession, who have in the past been equally interested in the so-called Dental Protective Association, and have stood earnestly and persistently by the proprietor of the *Dental Digest* in his strenuous efforts to maintain that Association financially and professionally. That the judgment of these friends may not be warped, it is deemed advisable to notice certain parts of this article. The fact is fully appreciated, however, that a dignified silence is always the best answer to charges that have lost the elements of self-respect.

1. He, the editor of the *Dental Digest*, charges that the INTERNATIONAL DENTAL JOURNAL has made "unwarranted personal attacks" upon his journal and those connected with it. This charge has *no foundation in fact*. This the readers of the INTERNATIONAL can verify by consulting the past volumes. The *Digest* has never been a subject for criticism directly or indirectly.

2. The charge is made that the editor of the INTERNATIONAL DENTAL JOURNAL published a paper written by Dr. Anema, and which was considered to be "the property" of the Pennsylvania State Dental Society. The answer to this must be found in the fact that the editor of the journal named received the paper from

the author with the request that it be published. This was done, the author presumably feeling that he owned the paper. The present writer has not now, nor ever had, any information as to the cash compensation paid Anema for said paper when it, with other matter, passed over to the *Digest* for a consideration.

3. The INTERNATIONAL DENTAL JOURNAL is charged with having published, "without a line of credit," an article entitled "The Pathogeny of Osteomalacia, or Senile Atrophy." It is true that said article found a place upon its pages, having been published in the January issue, 1905. This article was taken from a medical journal sent by direction of the author, and with his consent it was transferred to the department of "Reviews of Dental Literature." The *Dental Digest* was not known in the transaction from beginning to end. The cuts for the illustrations were furnished by the author. The paper was regarded as a very valuable one and eminently worthy of extended circulation.

4. The charge is further made that the editor of the INTERNATIONAL DENTAL JOURNAL has for months sold "*his* space to a professional ad. writer." Those interested can refer to this advertisement in recent numbers. It will be found in a very modest corner of its advertising pages. It is simply an announcement that a writer offers his services in the preparation of advertisements. The professional writer of ads. has become an apparent necessity in the business world of the day, and, while this may be abused, it is neither unethical nor criminal.

The editor of the INTERNATIONAL DENTAL JOURNAL neither owns that periodical, nor has he, *directly or indirectly*, anything to do with the business management, and consequently has no authority in the acceptance or declination of advertisements.

With an apology to our readers for taking up space in allusion to this scurrilous article, we pass from the subject to more congenial matters.

Domestic Correspondence.

NATIONAL ASSOCIATION OF DENTAL EXAMINERS.

To THE EDITOR:

SIR,—In consideration of the conflicting views as to dental educational standards which have existed for some time, the National Association of Dental Examiners, at its annual meeting held at St. Louis, August, 1904, deemed it expedient, and necessary for the upholding of such schools as sought to maintain the standards already published to the world as the minimum that should obtain, to declare what educational standards should be required by the State Boards of Examiners as a criterion of reputability of the schools seeking recognition of their output.

This *ad interim* committee, which is also the Committee on Colleges, was instructed to inform all schools of the action taken, and directed to prepare a recommended list of colleges on the basis of the standards established at that meeting.

Feeling fully the gravity of the duty imposed, this committee has expended much effort in striving to arrive at a basis of fairness to all interests concerned in carrying out its general instructions. The chief requirement established at St. Louis was that of " graduation from an accredited high school or its full equivalent" for admission to the classes of 1905–06.

In several schools and university departments this requirement is already in actual operation, and our committee finds a considerable number of other schools desiring to maintain it. All these, of course, will be placed on the recommended list. There are, however, other schools whose deans assert that to enforce at once this advance requirement would work a serious financial injury to their institutions.

The question of what should constitute a proper length of course for graduation from dental colleges has always been left by the examiners to the colleges themselves, except that, after a school has announced to the public a certain course as necessary to properly fit a student for graduation, if it for private or financial reasons deliberately lowers its requirements in any particular, the question of good faith and reputability of that school becomes at once a matter for adjudication by every board in the country.

We, therefore, acting upon authority of, and *ad interim* representing the National Association of Dental Examiners, which is the advisory body of the various State boards in their official acts, respectfully request that you authorize the Committee on Colleges to place your school on the recommended list of colleges by the acceptance of the following educational requirements for students, —viz.:

For matriculation or registration, " Graduation from an accredited high school or its full equivalent, all examination of credentials and equivalents to be placed in the hands of an acceptable appointee of the State Superintendent of Public Instruction where not otherwise provided for by law," said requirements to be inaugurated not later than the beginning of the school year of *1906–07;* and a college course for graduation optional with you of either four years of seven months each or three years of nine months each, this course requirement to be inaugurated the present year, *1905.*

It is to be expected that schools maintaining these standards will be protected in so doing by the several boards composing the National Association of Dental Examiners.

It is the intention of this Committee to prepare and publish the recommended list of colleges not later than April 1 next, in order to give all schools the earliest opportunity to announce these standards to the public. Therefore information as to your decision is desired as early as possible.

Very respectfully yours,

CHAS. C. CHITTENDEN,
Chairman Committee on Colleges.

Foreign Correspondence.

PERSONAL EXPLANATION.

BERLIN, PARISER PLATZ 7, January 28, 1905.

To THE EDITOR:

SIR,—Upon the occasion of the suicide of Dr. A. H. Sylvester, of this city, an unjust report has been widely published throughout the United States regarding my withdrawal from his practice, which is unfair to me, and in some instances grossly false. Indeed, although I have taken some trouble to collect the American reports, I have yet to find one correct as to the real facts regarding either his life or his death.

In justice to me, Professor W. D. Miller called a meeting of prominent American dentists here, who, after examining the legal papers, published the inclosed statement in the *German Times* of this city. With their consent I forward same to you, and shall feel very grateful to you, if, in the interest of my good name in the profession, you will give it space in your journal.

As my name has been used in all of the American papers that I have seen, I ask you to kindly insert it in the enclosed.

Very truly yours,

GEORGE H. WATSON.

"A PROTEST BY AMERICAN DENTISTS IN BERLIN.

"We, the undersigned American Dentists in Berlin, respectfully present the following urgent protest against a notice in the last number of the German Times (Jan. 16th) in which statements are made which are well calculated to injure the name of a member of the American Colony who is most highly esteemed not only as a skilful practitioner of dentistry but as a man of unwavering integrity of character. Having examined into the business relations of this gentleman with the deceased Dr. Sylvester we are absolutely convinced that he not only most conscientiously and scrupulously lived up to the terms of the contract which existed between him and the deceased, but still more that he evinced a charity in his dealings far beyond that which could have been legally exacted and which has evoked our undivided admiration.

"We herewith express our unreserved confidence in the gentleman in question and our strong disapproval of all attempts to make him in any way responsible for a deplorable event over which he had no control.

"Berlin, Jan. 19th, 1905.

Signed:

W. D. Miller.	Ferd. Foerster.	Charles H. Abbot.
	Geo. O. Webster.	
George Martin.	J. H. Ramsey.	E. Lawley-York.
	George A. Kennedy.	Lee A. Watling.
	E. D. Barrows."	

Current News.

IOWA STATE DENTAL SOCIETY.

THE forty-third annual meeting of the Iowa State Dental Society will be held in Des Moines, May 2, 3, and 4, 1905.

A programme of clinics and papers, promising more than usual interest, will be given. A cordial invitation is extended to the dental profession to attend.

C. W. BRUNER,
Secretary.

CALIFORNIA STATE DENTAL ASSOCIATION.

AT a meeting of the board of trustees of the California State Dental Association, held in San Francisco, February 10, it was unanimously decided to adjourn the State meeting for 1905 in favor of the Lewis and Clarke Dental Congress, to be held at Portland, July 17, 18, 19, and 20, 1905.

JOSEPH LORAN PEASE,
Corresponding Secretary.

PENNSYLVANIA STATE BOARD OF DENTAL EXAMINERS.

THE Board of Dental Examiners of Pennsylvania will conduct examinations simultaneously in Philadelphia and Pittsburg, June 6 to 9, 1905.

Applicants for examination must address

DR. N. C. SCHAEFFER,
Secretary Dental Council.

HARRISBURG, PA.

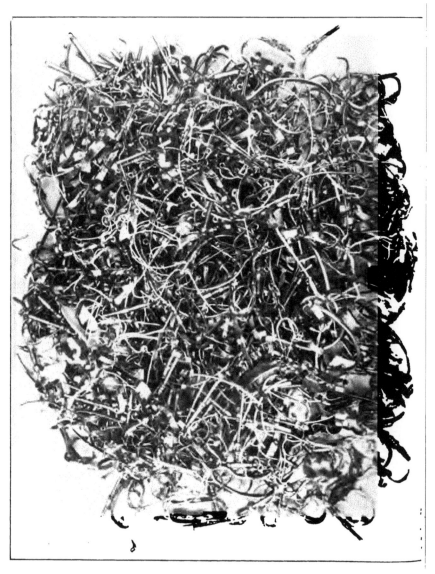

A peep into Dr. Farrar's regulating drawer.

THE

International Dental Journal.

| VOL. XXVI. | MAY, 1905. | No. 5. |

Original Communications.[1]

THE VITAL SIGNIFICANCE OF ORAL DISEASE.[2]

BY DR. G. V. I. BROWN, MILWAUKEE, WIS.

IT is my purpose this evening to use the term vital both in its meaning as being essential and in relation to life, but more especially the latter.

That the work of the oral therapeutist is essential to the health and well-being of the individual goes without saying; that it has a more or less important influence upon pathologic conditions of other parts of the organism, and *vice versa*, is also generally admitted, yet the true relation with regard to vitality is not fully appreciated.

In recent years the great work Talbot has done in the study of auto-intoxication as applied to oral disease and constitutional causes of dental caries has begun to be better understood in its true significance.

Kirk's recognition of certain forms of crystallization in the salivary secretion, and the study of these in association with pathologic expression of disease in other parts, has opened a vast field potent with great possibilities, which we trust may be developed into true science and adopted as a part of diagnosis.

---

[1] The editor and publishers are not responsible for the views of authors f papers published in this department, nor for any claim to novelty, or therwise, that may be made by them. No papers will be received for this epartment that have appeared in any other journal published in the untry.

[2] Read before The New York Institute of Stomatology, January 2, 1905.

It is believed the slides this evening will demonstrate both the value and the absolute necessity of giving full consideration to the vital interrelation between general conditions of health and anatomical construction and the tissues of the mouth in dealing with diseases and deformities thereof, and will be in the nature of a practical demonstration, since all of the illustrations are from cases in my own practice.

The several groups of pictures are introduced to show—

1. Conditions of the blood and visceral organs coincident with disease of the maxillary bones and mucous membrane of the mouth.

2. The value of a recognition of first principles, or the true etiology in the correction of these ills.

3. Extreme nervous affections due to, or at least associated with dental or oral disturbance.

4. Some of the predisposing and exciting causes of malnutrition, local as well as general.

5. The effect of prenatal and postnatal arrest of development upon mouth, nose, and face, and these in turn on the human organism as a whole.

6. The bearing of all this upon longevity.

Necessarily the principles upon which the theoretical structure whereon rests the practical deductions that led to the adoption of the methods of treatment, and results shown, cannot of themselves be new; questions of assimilation, nutritional function, physiologic efficiency of the dental organs as part of the whole digestive system, nerve distribution and its possibilities of reflex action, are matters of common knowledge in an audience such as this, and moreover, have been the theme of so many, and such profuse writing, as to be of little interest so far as general features are concerned.

We are accustomed to be told that affections of the teeth and jaws are frequent causes of remote, or even serious pathologic disturbance, and that it is sometimes difficult or impossible to effect a cure in the face of ill health, be it general or directed to some special organ. But to-night we are brought face to face with death: the screen will show us lesions that no therapeutic or surgical power at present under our command can control. We will pass for the moment beyond that which our usual consideration contemplates, and face actual conditions that are, as a rule, only hinted at or casually referred to by essayists, and look upon real condi-

GROUP I, CASE 1, No. 1.

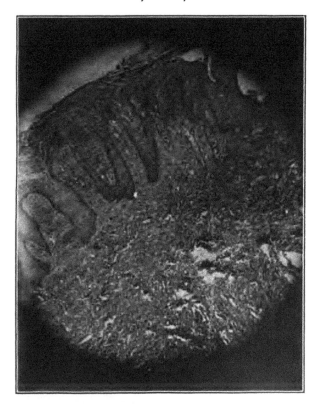

Leukæmia: Section showing necrosis of mucous membrane of the mouth.

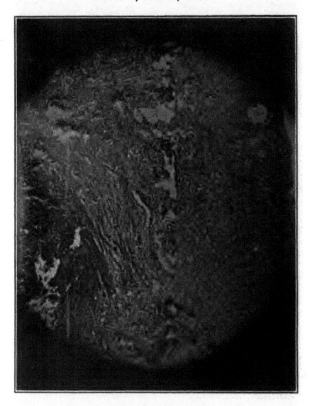

Leukæmia : Deeper section from the mouth of the same patient as No. 1, showing necrosis.

GROUP I, CASE 1, No. 3.

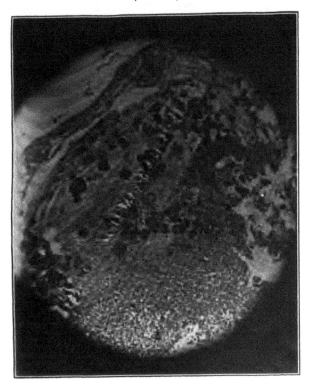

Leukæmia : Another section from mouth of same case as Nos. 1 and 2.

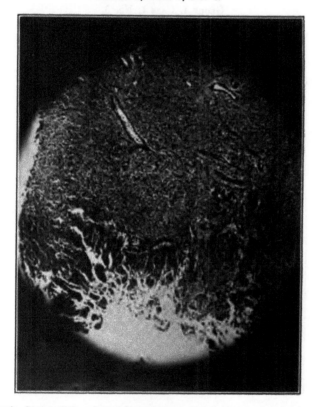

Leukæmia : Section of ulcer of the inner wall of the cæcum, taken from same individual as the preceding numbers.

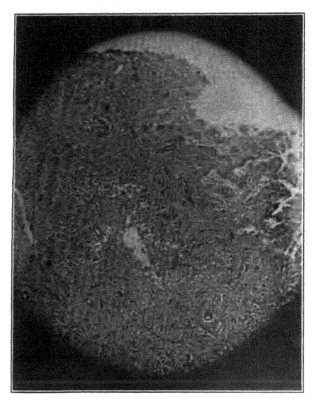

Another section of ulcer of the cæcum from same patient as the foregoing numbers.

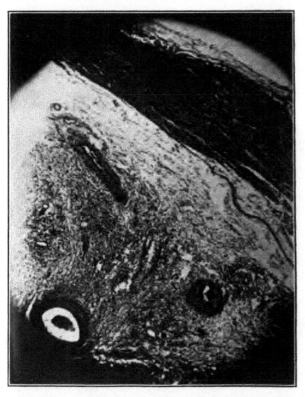

Leukæmia : Section of the same case as the previous numbers, cut through the muscular
coat of the cæcum, showing periarteritis and thrombus.

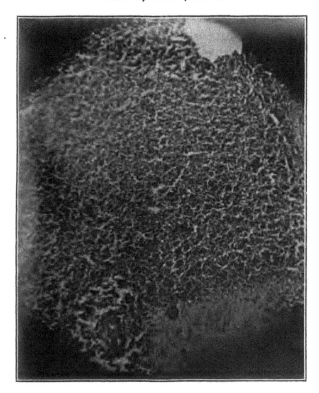

Leukæmia: Section of spleen from same case as Nos. 1 to 7 inclusive.

GROUP I, CASE 1, No. 8.

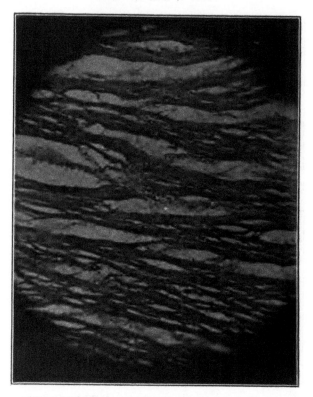

Leukæmia : Section of heart in same case as Nos. 1 to 8 inclusive.

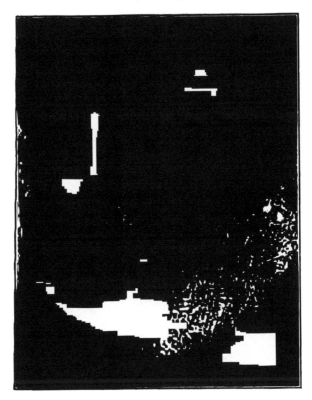

Leukæmia: Section of lung in same case as preceding numbers.

GROUP I, CASE 1, No. 10.

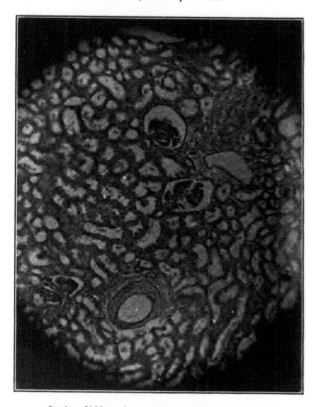

Section of kidneys in same case as preceding numbers.

tions which I believe have not before been shown with absolute certainty of detail in the definite manner we shall undertake to view them for our present purpose, and yet which, notwithstanding the infrequency of actual demonstration, are everywhere about us in one form or another, to be seen if only their diagnosis were better understood.

GROUP I.—Case 1, concerning which we have eleven slides, was a workman fifty-four years of age, married, of good habits and family history, so far as could be learned, with several healthy appearing children. I was called to see him by the family physician under whose care he had been for about two weeks, during which time he had been confined to the house. He gave a further history of some months of ill-health, but able to work.

Anæmic appearance was marked, but, having formerly been of rugged constitution, he was able to get out of bed and go about the house without assistance. Examination of the mouth disclosed interstitial gingivitis chiefly on lingual side of upper incisors. General condition of gums and buccal mucous membrane foul, and tongue heavily coated.

The patient was immediately removed to the hospital, and every effort made to build up the depleted system. Alcohol baths, beef peptonoids, bone-marrow, and other nourishing agents were prescribed, and these supplemented with hypodermic administration of strychnine, normal salt solution per rectum and directly into the tissues, etc.

The blood-count was as follows:

Name.	Norma.	Conditon Present.
Red corpuscles	5,000,000	1,704,640 1,500,000, August 10
Hæmoglobin	100 per cent.	45 per cent. 30 per cent.
Corpuscle index	1 per cent.	1.3 per cent.
White cells	7,000	93,100 105,000, August 10
Polymorphonuclear neutrophiles	70 per cent.	8 per cent.
Small lymphocytes	8 per cent.	28 per cent.
Large lymphocytes	20 per cent.	60 per cent.
Remnants of leucocytes	¼ per cent.	6 per cent.
Megaloblasts	0	1 to each 100 leucocytes
Normoblasts	0	1 to each 100 leucocyte count

Bacteriologic examination of the lesion showed staphylococcic infection.

Temperature ranged from 100° to 102°, with pulse indicative of increasing muscular weakness, both ranging higher toward the last.

Mental faculties were clear until about forty-eight hours before death, which occurred about ten days after I first saw him.

Operation was attempted for the purpose of removing the necrotic tissue that rapidly increased toward the end. An opening was made through the palate into the nares, but it was found to be dead in every direction as far as it seemed advisable to remove it. Gangrene of the soft tissues was so rapid that black masses were removed at each dressing several times daily.

The essentially interesting feature of this case to us at this time is the lesson taught by the blood-count, which indicates leukæmia and microscopic sections of the tissues of the mouth at the seat of the oral affection, and of the important visceral organs, each of which shows practically the same areas of inflammation. By continuity of tissue or direct infection one might expect this to be the case with different portions of the intestinal tract, but the kidneys, liver, heart, and spleen are also more or less involved.

With this striking clinical picture in mind one can no longer question the bearing that conditions of the blood must have upon all of these organs in their common relation, nor can we fail to understand how functional disturbance of any one of them can produce a corresponding effect upon some one or more of the others.

Applying this then to the treatment of less grave mouth diseases, we find at once an answer to much confusing discussion with regard to pyorrhœa alveolaris, dento-alveolar abscess, tooth-pulps, etc.

And finally, to apply directly another feature of the subject, we may in this light realize more keenly the vital importance of a fuller and more far-reaching diagnosis in many apparently simple lesions of the mouth.

Having had one similar previous case in which from an inflammatory area in the vicinity of the third molar noma developed, and death resulted in about the same length of time, I was able to differentiate the condition from ulcerative stomatitis, or pyorrhœa alveolaris, each of which the oral appearance somewhat resembled.

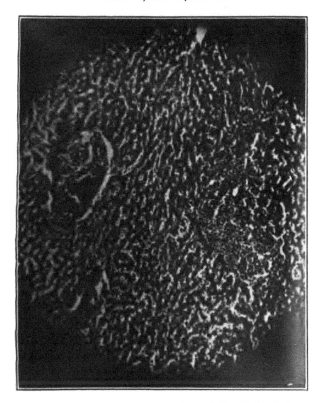

Leukæmia : Section of liver, same patient as in Nos. 1 to 9 inclusive.

GROUP I, CASE 2, No. 12.

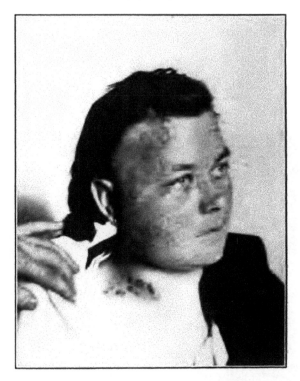

Picture of a young woman showing fistulous opening in region of clavicle, cheek, and angle
of the eye. The whole intervening space was one vast abscess.

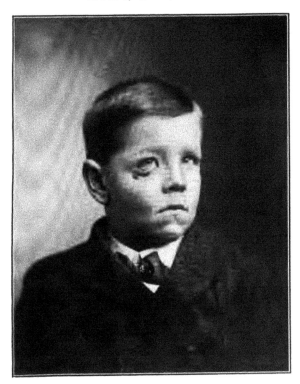

Boy of seven years, extensive necrosis, involving almost entire right superior maxillary, and malar bones. Rapid recovery after removal of sequestra.

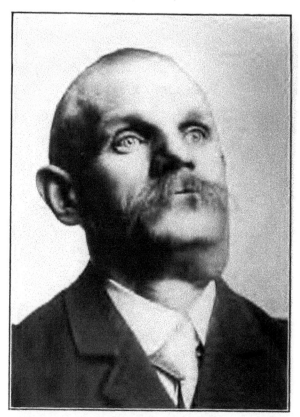

Dermoid cyst of neck.

GROUP II, CASE 1, NO. 15.

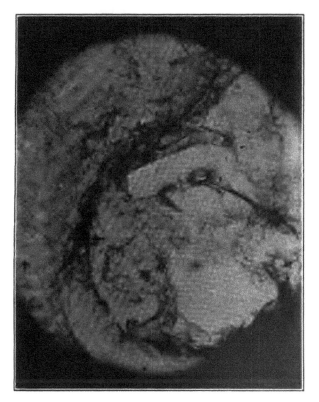

Section of outer wall of dermoid cyst shown in No. 14.

GROUP II, CASE 2, No. 16.

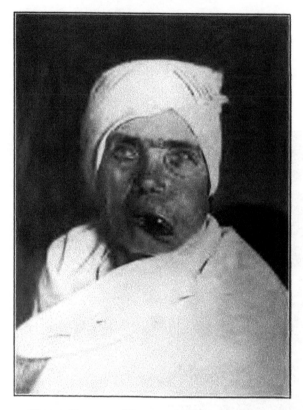

Woman with sarcoma of the antrum involving entire palate.

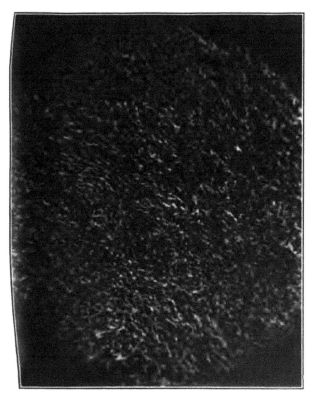

Section of sarcoma taken from patient shown in No. 16, near point of origin. Shows spindle cells.

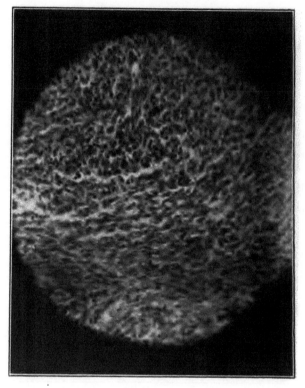

Section of same growth as in Nos. 16 and 17. Taken from a portion of later development.
Increasing malignancy demonstrated by increase of round cells.

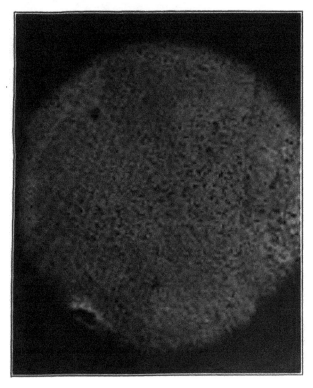

Section of melanotic sarcoma with characteristic pigmentation. Showing the final and hopeless stage of the case illustrated in Nos. 16, 17, and 18.

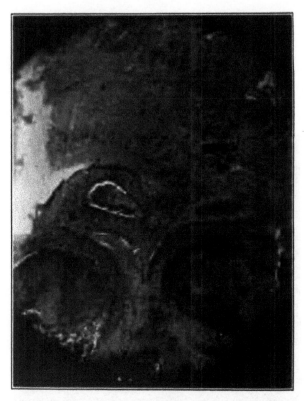

Carcinoma of maxillary sinus, involving also other portions of superior maxillary bones.
Section taken from growth removed from woman seventy years old.

In neither of these cases was there at any time a noticeable quantity of pus. Germicidal agents were absolutely ineffective in effort to check the tissue destructive process, and yet in both we found staphylococcus, not streptococcus as expected.

In contradistinction it is of interest to note the next feature, No. 12, as showing a vast destruction of tissue by pus from a simple dento-alveolar abscess, with profuse discharge for months, yet with record of complete recovery. No. 13 is in this class.

Group II., relating to benign and malignant growths, gives us additional food for reflection.

No. 14 is a picture of a dermoid cyst of the neck. Its history was a little confusing because of an attempted removal some years before, and what appeared to be a recurrence, but microscopic examination of the tumor after removal, and the microscopic section shown in No. 15, proved this to be a mistake, as the original operator could not have reached the growth itself at all.

No. 16 is a woman with a sarcoma. The history of the case seems to show originally a benign disease of the antrum neglected for years, but during the last few months a progressive increase of malignancy set in that was absolutely beyond surgical control. The progressive increase in malignancy may be seen in No. 18. No. 17, an older portion of the growth, reveals spindle-cell sarcoma.

Nos. 17, 18, and 19, spindle- and round-cell, an intermediate section, while the newest area of the growth gives us pigmentation of melanosarcoma, a hopelessly fatal condition owing to delay that I trust in the near future may come to be considered inexcusable.

No. 20 is a slide taken from a growth removed from one of my patients now in the hospital. She is sixty-three years of age, and has always heretofore enjoyed excellent health; family history good, and grown-up children seem to be healthy.

Chronic disease of the maxillary sinus through neglect and imperfect diagnosis, for the physician laughed at the suggestion of a serious disease, and several minor operations performed before she was referred to me, had finally resolved itself into carcinoma as the section indicates; and although extensive removal of tissue was made involving to a considerable extent both maxillæ and the vomer, with prescription for X-ray treatment, the prognosis is most unfavorable, the likelihood of recurrence being very great.

Bringing these demonstrations of ill-omen directly to bear upon practice, we conclude that no chronic inflammatory condition, how-

ever simple and harmless it may appear, should be allowed to
continue without treatment; no source of long-continued irritation
be left uncorrected even though of slight annoyance, and every suspicious growth or lesion concerning which the operator is in doubt
should be promptly referred to some one whose constant familiarity
in practice enables him to decide as to its true character.

No. 21 comes between the last preceding group and the one to
follow, and in its two most important aspects refer to each. The
tooth shown occupies a position in the skull in which it has been
photographed, much like one found in the case of a patient of
seventy-one years of age who had worn a full upper denture without knowledge of its presence, under operation for a suspicious-
looking growth having its beginning in this region, which upon
later examination proved to be malignant, and finally caused her
death.

It is also similarly situated to one found in the jaw of a patient who was a chronic sufferer from excruciating trifacial pain
for a period of seven years, and had become almost a mental as
well as a physical wreck in consequence. With the picture before us
we can readily understand why almost every known method of treatment which he had tried failed to give relief, but we should also
keep in mind the fact that Cryer, Price, and other X-ray investigators have demonstrated that malposed, unerupted teeth are much
more common than we formerly supposed; therefore these two
classes of very serious affections need constant watchful care to
guard against.

Group III. introduces a number of patients with characteristic
nervous affections, all having a noticeable similarity of appearance.
yet each one quite different, some of them diametrically opposite
in character.

No. 22 represents a patient in one of the spasms of pain which
he suffered at intervals of from one to two minutes for a period
of five years. Correction of occlusion, the removal of a tooth-pulp,
and a slight operation upon one of the branches of the submaxillary branch of the fifth nerve left him as shown in No. 23, free
from pain. Observation for some two or more years after operation has confirmed the correctness of the diagnosis of these simple
etiologic features.

Another patient suffered attacks of pain at intervals of a few
minutes, and at times seconds, for twenty-five years.

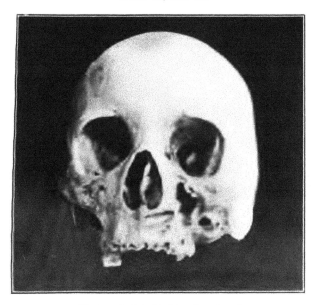

Photograph of skull with malposed tooth.

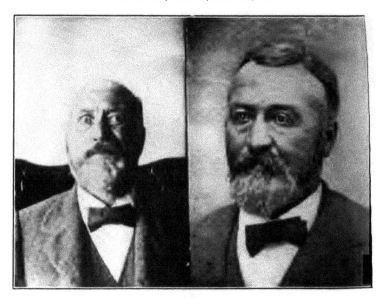

Tic douloureux.

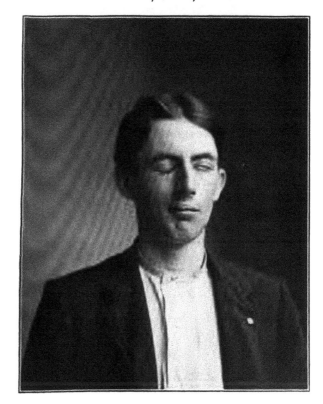

Facial paralysis: Making effort to close both eyelids.

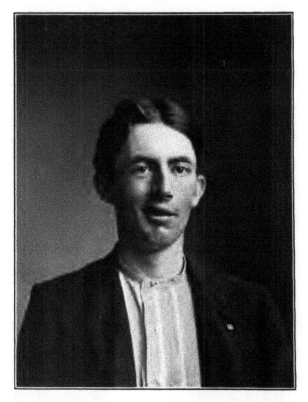

Facial paralysis: Same patient as shown in No. 24, trying to smile.

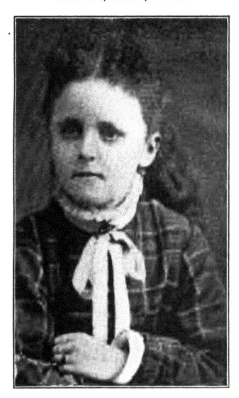

Young girl at about six years of age. Asymmetrical features, an indication of future trouble.

Single harelip showing characteristic deformity.

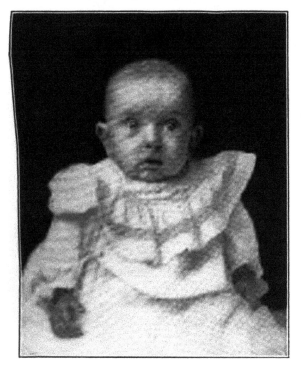

Same baby as shown in No. 27, after operation. Unequal development, flat ala, and deviation of nasal cartilage corrected.

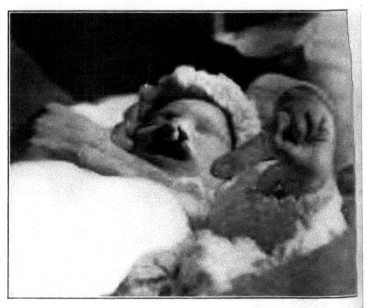

Double harelip and cleft palate. Shows usual distortion of features.

GROUP V, CASE 2, No. 30.

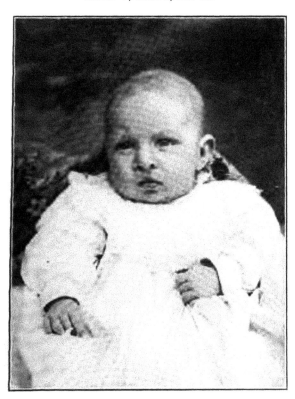

Baby shown in No. 29. After readjustment of deformed parts and operation for closure of lip fissure.

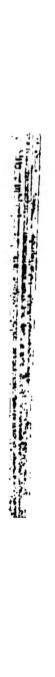

Her family history revealed that several near relatives were affected by some neurosis, and she herself was a typical neurotic; but notwithstanding all this, resection of the inferior dental nerve and an operation for relief of a chronic mucous engorgement of the maxillary sinus gave much permanent benefit and entire relief from pain for a short period of time, with hopeful prospects of a complete cure.

Nos. 24 and 25 show a case of unilateral facial paralysis. Operation for a chronic necrotic condition of the lower jaw upon the affected side removed that diseased condition and gave a slight immediate relief to the paralysis, but his death some weeks later indicated that the true cause of his symptoms was central in character, though we have no post-mortem evidence of the nature of the brain lesion.

Surely one need have no stronger evidence than this mute testimony to bring a realization of the value of great care and discrimination in diagnosis, and of the home truth that in our special field, where the all powerful and wonderful fifth nerve presides, no etiologic factor is so small that it may with impunity be overlooked, and results are often out of all proportion to their causes when even the simplest may be vital in its importance.

GROUP IV.—No. 26 by illustration opens a field rapidly growing as the line of our horizon widens, with a central focal point at which the dentist, the oculist, the rhinologist, the surgeon, and the practitioners of general medicine meet in common interest.

Other slides shown were pictures of an individual at different periods of her life, the last one being at thirty years of age, after face, nose, and mouth have been corrected. These photographs have, I believe, been instrumental in accomplishing much good, having been shown and described by Dr. Nelson M. Black, of Milwaukee, with whom I co-operated in the treatment, and by myself before a number of medical and dental societies during the past few years, and bringing as they do such a striking record of almost total deafness, neurasthenia with mental derangement, a history of a sanitarium and the care of a keeper, followed by improvement of hearing, disappearance of neurotic symptoms, thirty pounds increase in flesh, with restoration to normal health, and finally marriage, which could not have been practicable under former conditions, all by widening of the dental arch and through it the

maxillæ correction of occlusion, and treatment of the nose and
middle ear, made possible by these simple providences.

I do not know who first tried to apply direct pressure to widen
the dental arch by separation of the maxillary bones at the median
suture. I have done it for more than ten years, and doubtless
many others have, but I do believe that the first definite work of
that character done for the specific purpose of assisting the cure
of nasal, aural, and nervous affections systematically carried to a
successful issue was done by Dr. Black and myself, and reported
to the National Dental and other associations. I make this statement not for myself, but in justice to Dr. Black, as it is only to
be expected that as the work assumes its full importance in the
eyes of the profession there will be many claimants.

Doubtless your own Dr. Bogue builded better than he knew when
he began his good fight for the presentation of the first molar. It
lies at the very heart of this question, for arrest of development
must be prenatal or postnatal. If the individual be normal, it is
little less than a crime to deprive him of his birthright by giving
opportunity for an artificial interference with developmental processes, and the first molar is the very key to facial and maxillary
growth, erupting as it does at a stage of life so important as to
be termed a period of stress, and, held accountable by Kierman
for epilepsy and like affections in many cases, its importance cannot be questioned. If, on the other hand, through degenerate
heredity, malnutrition, or other cause, the child be born into the
world with a tendency to insufficient bone development, it is even
more incumbent upon us to assist the necessarily crowded dental
organs to assume a proper position through aiding the proper adjustment of those bones upon which the natural form of every
facial feature depends, because in almost every such individual
there is a neurotic tendency. Such a child as is here shown should
be known at once as one that would require early treatment to
avoid the future trouble that the history of her case describes.

All of the remaining pictures, which there is not time to describe in detail, have been treated by operation with the foregoing principles in mind, the chief effort being to restore the
deformed parts to their normal relations, for, after all, cleft palate
and harelip are only greater deformities due primarily to much
the same causes as the lesser deformities of dental irregularity.
and the same rules apply, for where forcible crushing of the bones

for closure of palates in early infancy has been resorted to, this deformity in later life is often very great.

In closing I would say, let no one forget that without a full dental arch there can seldom or never be a perfect nose, nor can the associated sinuses be normal. With constriction or obstruction of the nares, there cannot be a healthful nose and throat; there must be hypertrophies and chronic thickening of the nasal mucous membrane, deviated nasal septa, spurs, atrophic, and hypertrophic rhinitis must be a natural result.

To the growing individual this means imperfect oxygenation, susceptibility to colds, throat trouble, diphtheria, lungs only partially developed, impaired resistance to pneumonia, and to that dread disease recently called the real cause of race suicide, tuberculosis, an unstable nervous system, impaired or perverted brain development.

In a final word, the sum of all this deducted from the normal record of longevity and the balance is that which it lies within our province to try to increase.

PLASTER OF PARIS.[1]

BY WM. H. GELSTON, D.D.S.

Plaster of Paris, so named because of the situation of the original beds under the city of Paris, is an anhydrous calcium sulphate, which before being calcined is a hydrated sulphate of lime, which is undoubtedly derived from the precipitation of gypsum by evaporation from its solution in circumscribed basins of salt water, like the Dead Sea and Great Salt Lake. Gypsum is also usually associated with greater or less quantities of the salts which are found in sea-water,—namely, the chlorides of sodium, calcium, magnesium, the sulphate of soda, etc. Of all the solid matter contained in sea-water, gypsum is the least soluble, and, therefore, is the first precipitated.

In the carboniferous age evaporating pans where salt water precipitated its solid content existed in Nova Scotia, Michigan,

---

[1] Read before the Southern Dental Society of New Jersey, December 21, 1904.

Virginia, and Arizona. The samples I pass you were taken from the Province of New Brunswick on the Bay of Fundy, where the finest gypsum is quarried to-day. These are all practically pure, containing about ninety-nine per cent. sulphate of lime; they came from various veins or strata in the quarry, and my object in exhibiting them is to show how a sulphate of lime can vary. Being soluble in water it is not infrequent that a pond or lake is to be found in the vicinity of plaster quarries, in the bottom of which is a deposit of sulphate of lime in crystals. The late Professor Cope, of the Academy of Natural Sciences of Philadelphia, contended that the marl-beds of New Jersey, extending from, say, near old White Horse (Berlin) toward Perth Amboy, contained more or less sulphate of lime, and after an exhaustive search he succeeded in finding a number of beautiful and perfectly formed crystals, some of which are deposited in the Academy of Natural Sciences of Philadelphia as convincing proof of his theory, and one of which I have much pleasure in submitting for your examination. I also have one taken from the original beds under the city of Paris. These have been kindly loaned me by Mr. French. And possibly it might not be out of place to state that I am indebted to Mr. French (the president of the College of Pharmacy and senior member of the firm of Samuel H. French & Co., who manufacture almost the entire output of plaster for the dental profession) for his time and courtesies extended in giving samples and statistics that so materially aided in my presentation of this paper.

Gypsum is not only an indispensable article in the form of plaster, but is used extensively by the two most famous breweries of Dublin and London, tons being annually dumped into their wells, wherein lies the success of these famous brews.

Let us spend just a moment at the factory. Gypsum as quarried is thrown into large breakers, which crush it into pieces varying in size from a small pea to a large chestnut. This in turn is carried by conveyors to mills that grind it to an exceedingly fine powder; this powder is conveyed to kettles, where it is calcined, or, to use a commercial term, and one that is familiar to all calciners, where it is " boiled." These kettles have a capacity of about one hundred barrels each. The surplus moisture is thrown off, which causes the plaster to have the appearance of boiling, bubbles forming on the top during the process and breaking and emitting steam. This boiling process causes a material expansion, owing to the generation of steam. After the moisture has all been driven off, the plaster rapidly settles, and to a novice it would almost appear as though the bottom of the kettle had dropped out, but in reality it is simply returning to its original bulk in minute crystal formations. At this stage the heat is not only continued, but is increased so as to break the small crystals and drive off the water of crystallization. After this has been accomplished the calcining process is completed. It is scarcely necessary to say that in calcining plaster it requires a technical knowledge only attained by long experience.

I have given you simply an outline of the calcining process, and it is, of course, to be understood that, in addition to this process in making dental plaster, there are mechanical and technical processes used which have been kept as a manufacturing secret and which is possessed by but few. In other words, the processes by which the setting of plaster is hastened or retarded for the use of the profession is a manufacturing secret.

I will state, in addition to my remarks on calcining plaster, that, from information which I have, I am convinced that the mechanical processes used in the production of dental plaster absolutely prevent any variation in quality in a batch of from nine hundred to twelve hundred barrels. In other words, if one barrel is wrongly manufactured, it must necessarily follow that from nine hundred to twelve hundred barrels are in the same condition, and this would be detected, as each batch is thoroughly tested before leaving the factory.

The dental plaster as manufactured by Samuel H. French & Co. is in three varieties,—impression, setting in from three to five minutes; dental, in from eight to ten minutes; slow-setting, in from thirty to forty minutes. This firm also manufactures an exceedingly slow-setting plaster, which, however, they do not produce for the use of the profession, but for that of the arts.

We will now take up, if you please, the textile strength and different forms of plaster relative to the amount of expansion. The textile strength of plaster is as follows: Twenty-four hour mix, one hundred and fifty-three pounds to the square inch; seven day mix, two hundred and eighty-four pounds to the square inch; twenty-eight day mix, two hundred and ninety-four pounds to the square inch; six months mix, three hundred and fifteen pounds to the square inch; one year mix, three hundred and seventy-two pounds to the square inch.

EXPANSION.

In all these experiments careful relative measurements and temperature of plaster and water were taken before mixing; afterwards, time of stirring, setting, and expansion.

Impression plaster, seven months old, expanded as high as one-sixteenth of an inch, while new expanded $^1/_{136}$.

The expansion of impression plaster with boiled water and boiled lime-water was exactly the same,—$^1/_{100}$.

A saturated solution of plaster of Paris in boiled water before mixing, expansion, $^1/_{200}$.

Impression plaster, boiled water and salt, expansion $^1/_{136}$.

Impression plaster mixed very thin expanded $^1/_{136}$.

Impression plaster with boiled snow expanded $^1/_{136}$.

Impression plaster with cold hydrant water 38° expanded $^1/_{200}$.

Impression plaster with melted snow at 38°, no expansion in twenty hours.

Impression plaster with melted snow at 38°, stirred thirty seconds instead of five, expansion $^1/_{100}$.

Dental plaster in the experiments was about the same as impression.

Slow-setting plaster and boiled water, expansion $^1/_{300}$, after forty-eight hours $^1/_{200}$.

Sixty-minute or gelatin plaster with boiled water, expansion none in three days, after thirty days, expansion $^1/_{200}$.

From the results of these experiments the following might be suggested: Plaster should not be purchased in quantities sufficient to become old before using, as old plaster expands more than new. It should be kept well covered and away from dampness as much as possible. Mr. French states that complaints are confined principally to fall and spring, which seems due to the fact that the heavy rains of both seasons infiltrate the water with foreign matter. Use at least boiled water for impressions and models. Less expansion with a thin mix than with a thick one. Rain water preferable to hydrant. Water at about 36° lessens expansion. Allow the plaster to slack in water rather than long stirring, which latter promotes expansion. Less expansion in slow-setting plaster than either dental or impression plaster. Always use sixty-minute plaster where possible for models. A model will remain harder during the process of vulcanizing if not vulcanized the same day as poured. The steam should be blown off as soon as the case is vulcanized, and the flask cooled to prevent disintegration of the plaster. Subjecting impression plaster to different temperatures of heat, care being taken not to scorch it, produces a slower setting plaster, and if carried to a high degree a plaster can be produced that will require eighty-five minutes to harden with no expansion in twenty-four hours.

After these and many more experiments the subject would seem to be more expansive than the plaster itself, which has as many eccentricities as a bucking broncho, and I know whereof I speak, for I have been " up against" both. But possibly it might be a little more accurate if I used the statement of Mr. French, that " it is as peculiar as individuals." And if you will stop to consider the individual as you meet him day after day in the office, you will all agree some are harder to manage than a broncho.

DISCUSSION.

Dr. Chas. Tuttle claimed that he secured very good results in mixing plaster for models by using boiled water. No reason was given why this should be preferred to the unboiled water.

Dr. J. B. McCullough, gave his method (previously published in the INTERNATIONAL DENTAL JOURNAL) of overcoming the expansion of plaster, by the use of a solution of lime-water, made from water and lime boiled for fifteen minutes; then mixed with the plaster.

Dr. W. W. Crate stated that his method of use, after mixing plaster, was to prepare the plate from the model, as soon as possible for vulcanization.

Dr. Gelston.—In answer to Dr. McCullough, I do not consider his tests with glass tubes accurate or conclusive. I used glass tubes with some of my first experiments with ordinary hydrant water, and some of them cracked while others did not; this being the case, I found it necessary to abandon that method for a more accurate measurement. By actual measurement, I received no better results from boiled lime water than from boiled water. But you will notice from some of the experiments that I mentioned, where I did receive ' better results than from either boiled water or lime water.

DR. J. N. FARRAR'S APPLIANCES.

BY THE EDITOR.

THERE has frequently been a doubt expressed by some dentists, and even some specialists in orthodontia, that the great variety of appliances illustrated by this author are not really practical, or, in other words, had not been made use of in actual cases. In order to settle this question the writer had the pleasure of examining a large collection of these mechanisms, probably several hundred, with names and dates attached, constituting a remarkable exhibit not only in number, but in ingenuity in preparation. The value of this mass, which by no means includes all his mechanisms, lies not only in the fact that all are of 18-carat gold, but have decided interest in showing the very great development he has made in this special line of work. All of Dr. Farrar's mechanisms show great scientific merit in accuracy and ease of action.

It was thought that an exhibit of this kind would not only be instructive, but of interest to all skilful workers in this specialty, as well as settling all disputed questions as to the fact of their great practical use as regulating appliances at rest. Every one here represented has been used and proved by most successful results, in easy management and least discomfort to patient. The exhibit is unique in that it is probably the first that was ever offered to any dental periodical, similarily illustrated.

The frontispiece represents a tangled mass taken from Dr. Farrar's regulating drawers without any attempt at orderly arrangement, but still sufficiently indicative of their character and the use to which they had been applied. The photographs from which these illustrations were made are the first this author has ever presented in his various publications, as he has preferred to illustrate, by "working line plans," all articles in his papers and in his volumes, written upon Orthodontia, which are familiar to all readers of dental literature. His idea is that photography is not equal, as a clear guide, to line drawings for the use of students in mechanics. The common opinion is entertained that photographs represent nothing but the truth, but it is recognized by artists that the effect of photography by varied posings and "foreshortenings," and by "pencilling the negative" in illustrating machinery, architecture, and the human face, can bring about as numerous changes and untruthful results as the padding and coloring of actors upon the

FIG. 1.

Fig. 8.

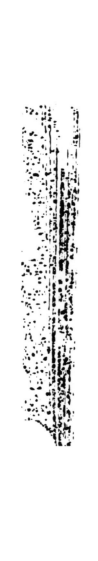

theatrical stage can effect. The modern illustrations often seen in periodicals bear out this view. But the "half-tones," while recognized as by no means perfect, have served, and will doubtless continue to serve, as an aid in the illustration of practical papers, as photographs and line drawings of houses are mutual helps in architecture.

Reviews of Dental Literature.

HIGHEST ORTHODONTIA. 1. FACIAL BEAUTY; 2. DENTAL ANTAGONISM. By John Nutting Farrar, M.D., D.D.S., New York City.[1]

MR. PRESIDENT, LADIES, AND MEMBERS OF THE ALUMNI OF THE NEW YORK COLLEGE OF DENTISTRY,—My subject this evening will be "facial beauty" and "dental antagonism." In other words, I shall speak upon that which I regard should be the highest desideratum in operations for the correction of irregular teeth.

The question is, should mastication of food, without much regard to facial beauty, be the main aim, or should it be, efficient mastication of food with special regard to improvement of facial beauty? For many years my systematic, earnest efforts have by tongue and pen been the pointing out of the steps that have been taken from the early ideas to the present time, the gradual but not regular progress of the art and science of dentistry, especially in the branch for correction of irregularities of natural teeth; showing at the same time a glimpse into its future, for I believe there is yet a great deal to be done before the best results will be accomplished from education along this line.

The question of extraction would naturally come in here for discussion, but as I have already somewhat exhaustively treated this branch of the subject in Chapters LXV., LXVI., LXVII., pp. 681 to 711, in my Volume I., upon "The Irregularities of the Teeth and their Correction," I shall only again incidentally refer to the subject in this lecture. The subject of my lecture, "Facial Beauty *versus* Dental Antagonism," is no new phase of my teaching,

[1] Lecture delivered before the New York Dental College Alumni, January 18, 1905.

either orally or in print; my present object shall be to reach out into broader and loftier branches upon the subject of correction of irregular teeth, pointing out some of the errors of the retrogressive teachings, which I believe if followed will be the entering wedge to the destruction of our highest and noblest branch of dentistry.

Theory of perfection in the correction of irregularities of the teeth, and theory of perfection in treatment in general medicine, are written upon quite similar lines; both are to serve simply as general guides in practice. *There is no one best rule* for all cases. The vicissitudes of circumstances, conditions, and environments must be considered, or results may be unsatisfactory. This variation may be partly illustrated by the difference between hospital practice and family practice, whether it be in medicine or dentistry. Many things that can be forced in hospital practice cannot be forced in family practice, "*subject*" in one, "*independent personality*" in the other; a treatment in the former case that may be satisfactory to the patient, may not be satisfactory to the patient in the latter. Again, the matter of idiosyncrasy, diathesis, mental characteristics, as well as financial and social circumstances, should be taken into consideration. Some heads of families have proper ideas of their own; such persons are not always easily induced to change their views; especially is this true if opposed by illogical presentations.

It is often said that clear knowledge of anatomy is important to the physician and the general surgeon in order to enable him to be thoroughly efficient; but this is no more true of physicians and surgeons than that clear knowledge of anatomy and dental etiology (in which proper antagonism is a factor) is important to the dentist. While the general surgeon needs clear knowledge of the relative position of the muscles, nerves, and blood-vessels, and their relation to the osseous frame, so does a regulator of teeth need clear knowledge of the relations of the different parts of each jaw and the relation of the jaw-bones to the other bones of the head; nor is this equipment of education sufficient without a clear knowledge of anatomy of the soft tissues, and knowledge, in addition, of physiology, and the changes that may take place from physiological conditions to pathological conditions of the tissues during operations.

The regulator of teeth thus prepared will meet more easily the difficulties that may result from operations. But as important as all this knowledge, together with a knowledge of the development of the teeth, and their proper antagonism may be, it ·would not be sufficient to constitute a first-class education (for a regulator), without an equally clear knowledge of the laws of mechanics, in order to take advantage of the above-mentioned knowledge. Furthermore the dentist should understand the rules of proportion, of the different parts of the human face and head, as formulated by recognized great sculptors and painters, and also a knowledge of the differences between the several classes of human faces.

As there are several types of human faces and' heads, and as there are as many types of bones of the heads, each head having its own form of jaw-bones, an effort to establish, in this enlightened age (regarding knowledge of the evolutionary laws), a geometrically formed typical human jaw, from one selected from many, that will constitute an *Adamic type for the whole human race,* may seem strange; but it does not seem strange that artists should attempt to classify beautiful human forms. But while all the classes of the most beautiful forms, as a whole, may be counted by less than the digits of two hands, the different classes of the human head would be greater in number, and the number of forms of heads that might be classified would not be equal to the classes of the various shades of beautiful faces belonging to those heads. For illustration, the heads may be classed, 1, the round or bullet form; 2, the square head; 3, the vertically long but broad head; 4, the long but thin head; 5, the oval head; 6, the egg form, with the smaller end down; and 7, the egg form, with the larger end down (varieties of the oval). Then there is the face with a Greek nose, the Roman nose, the hawkbill nose, the pug nose, the African nose, the ape nose, etc. Then there are the noses of the more beautiful forms of faces; noses the size and form of which harmonize with the other facial features, eyes, mouth, chin, and lips. Then there are the faces beautiful in form, but cold and forbidding; and those that are not so beautiful in form, but otherwise charmingly beautiful by intellectual scintillations shown in the expression through an animated face.

There are so many phases of my subject I cannot, in the limited time of this evening, go over all, and if I repeat, and apparently recross some tracks of my argument, it will be only to fasten the essential points in your memories. In dentistry much is said of

dental antagonism, because much of success depends upon proper
knowledge of the subject. In nature we find that dental antagonism is similar, but not at all uniform. But perfection, though rare,
is sometimes found, and, rare as it is, the *perfect* should serve as a
general guide, but not an absolute guide.

In the winter of 1864–65, Professor J. H. McQuillen gave a
course of " special lectures" upon the subject which he denominated
" Harmony of Antagonism." It was my good fortune to hear the
entire course of these remarkable lectures upon the importance of
proper antagonism. Not only was the " interlocking" or " break-
joint" association of teeth shown, but the line of actual contact in
normal occlusion of the two arches was clearly illustrated. Other
persons have since that time treated in print the same subject, but
none have presented it more clearly and interestingly than did
McQuillen.

While abnormal antagonism of the teeth is often the result of
inherited differences between the size of the jaw and the size of the
teeth of the parents (immediate and remote), extraction of deciduous teeth at the wrong time and the wearing away of adult teeth by
use, causing them to unduly press and slide upon each other, are
also causes of irregularities. Then, again, that class which is
denominated protruding teeth (generally the upper anterior teeth)
may or may not be the result of dental antagonism.

Protruding upper teeth may be caused by inheritance or by
thumb- and finger-sucking; but my experience teaches me that by
far the majority of cases are caused by too long lower anterior
teeth and too short side teeth; the latter being largely caused by
the sag in the sides of the lower alveolar ridge; altogether causing
too much pressure upon the posterior walls of the anterior upper
teeth. But some of the major cases may be apparent only, caused
by too short lower jaw, and others are indirectly the result of
" mouth-breathing," caused by nasal obstruction, that tempt the
jaws to remain apart most of the time in order to breathe easily,
leaving the buccal muscles to act with undue power upon the side
teeth, narrowing the arch and pushing the anterior teeth forward.
Where mouth-breathing is continuous, and the size of the teeth and
the size of the dental arches do not harmonize, and the teeth are
also jumbled, the arches, that thereby become too narrow, may
require widening. But if the patient's head is narrow (from side
to side), the degree of widening should be carefully considered;

especially is this so if the greatest improvement of the face is to be accomplished.

While there is *no one* best rule for regulating all cases, there is generally *one best way* of accomplishing the highest result *in a given case.* The highest aim in this branch of dentistry should be to accomplish not only the greatest possible degree of beauty in facial form, but also an improvement in mental expression, through the form. Movers of teeth there may be many, but moulders of the face, to the highest possible benefit, there are not so many. Those of the latter class may be regarded as the true artists in this kind of mobile surgery.

While efficient antagonism contributes largely to proper mastication, and such mastication contributes to proper digestion, that may lead to healthy complexion; *proper food* and *regular habits* have quite as much to do with it. While the regulator should give great attention to antagonism, he may fail in public and in professional estimation to have the reputation of mastership if he does not also give the greater attention to improvement in facial beauty.

To understand how to bring about *efficient* antagonism of the teeth it is not only important to enable proper correction, but it is also necessary to prevent recurrences of irregularities when once corrected.—*Items of Interest.*

(To be continued.)

ACTINOMYCOSIS OF THE MOUTH AND FACE, WITH THE REPORT OF TEN CASES. By Thomas H. Kellock, M.A., F.R.C.S., etc.

MR. PRESIDENT AND GENTLEMEN,—It was with a good deal of pleasure that I acceded to a request that I should bring before your Society some of the cases of actinomycosis which it has been my fortune to meet with recently in the out-patient department at the Middlesex Hospital, and I am glad to have been able to secure the attendance here this evening of a few patients suffering from this affection in the regions about the mouth, who serve, I hope, to illustrate fairly well the affection in different stages, and also the points connected with the clinical aspect of the disease, to which I would like to call attention. Whether it is that this affection is rapidly becoming more common, or that interest in the subject has caused me to make more careful investigations in probable cases, and thereby recognize it more frequently, I am not sure; one or the other of these must have happened, for otherwise it would seem strange that relatively so many cases of what has generally been looked upon as a rare affection should have occurred in one out-patient department, and that not an exceptionally large one. As I shall presently hope to show, the confirmation of the diagnosis is not by any means always an easy matter, and this fact may account for many cases having been overlooked. On the other hand, it is difficult to understand what became of such cases as those I am showing, if they were not subjected to the treatment which, as far as we are aware, is the only one that has the effect of arresting or curing the disease, which is generally a progressive one, and one that shows little tendency toward spontaneous cure; it is curious, too, as going to show that the affection is more common than formerly, that there should have appeared in quite a recent number of the *Lancet* (October 29. 1904), the reports of three cases of this kind, calling forth from the editor an able leading article on the subject.

It is easily within my memory when actinomycosis was included with such rare affections as hydatid disease and filaria sanguinis, and hardly given a place when discussing the differential diagnosis of tumors and abscesses about the face, jaws, or other parts of the body. The occurrence, however, of so many cases among the out-patients has compelled me to include it in my teaching as a disease that is by no means rare at the present time, and I think its importance, both from the point of view of the patient and of the surgeon, justifies this.

I may, perhaps, be allowed to call attention to a few points in connection with the pathology of this affection. The name actinomycosis was given it with the idea that the fungus, which is the specific cause, could be recognized, microscopically, by its "starred" or "ray-like" appearance. We now know that there are several varieties of fungus or streptothrix that can act as the cause,—fungi which are found in twisted masses of mycelium, and only really visible when suitably stained, the peculiar ray formation being due to refraction of light around particularly disposed masses of these. This it is important to remember, for in attempting to make a diagnosis it is often only an unstained specimen of pus or granulation tissue that is for the moment available, and it by no means follows that this ray formation will be seen in all cases, and one has often failed to find it in cases in which subsequent staining has demonstrated the presence of a streptothrix. Another important point to bear in mind in this connection is that this ray formation may be broken up, and the evidence of it visible in the unstained specimen looking like minute elongated fragments of glass scattered about among the pus cells, and I have once or twice been able to recognize these in specimens where the ray formation was not seen. The difficulty of recognizing the affection from an unstained specimen of the discharge is greatly increased in cases where acute suppuration has supervened; in these cases difficulty is often also experienced even after staining, and I have known one or two cases of this sort where it was only after repeated examination of the pus that streptothrix was found to be stained. This same difficulty is, we know, experienced in demonstrating in similar cases the bacillus of tuberculosis, an organism to which it would seem these streptothrices have in many respects a very close resemblance.

The filaments of these streptothrices stain well by Gram's method, becoming of a red-blue color; they vary somewhat in size and arrangement, but are alike in their twistings and convolutions and in the way in which they stain by this method. The fungus was formerly supposed to flourish ,almost exclusively on straw or hay, and, as you will remember, the chewing of them by man or beast was looked upon as the usual mode of its entry into the body; the occurrrence, however, of this affection among people of many and varied occupations and modes of life, even as instanced by the cases I am showing to-night, seems to indicate that the organism has, at the present time at any rate, a much wider distribution than was formerly supposed.

To turn now to the clinical aspect of the affection, which must be that of chief interest to us as dental or general surgeons, it is fair, I think, to state that experience shows that, in by far the larger number of cases, the organism enters the body by means of the respiratory or alimentary tracts; isolated cases of its infection directly into the skin or subcutaneous tissues have been reported, just as in the case of tuberculosis, but these may be regarded as more or less rarities, and it is in the respiratory and alimentary tracts and in the organs which have a direct communication with them, that we find, at any rate, the primary infection.

With the affection as it is found in the lower parts of the alimentary and respiratory tracts such as the liver, vermiform appendix, pelvis, or lungs, we are not at present concerned, but

I should like to draw attention to one peculiarity of this affection as seen in the lungs, for it illustrates well what is seen in other parts of the body,—namely, its disposition to ignore anatomical boundaries, and spread beyond the limits of the organ primarily infected. It affects the lungs primarily in much the same way as does tuberculosis, but, unlike the latter, it has a great tendency not only to induce adhesions between the lung and the chest wall, but to invade the latter, and an actinomycotic affection of the lungs is often only recognized as such when it has produced an abscess pointing on the surface of the chest. This property is also seen in other organs, such as the salivary glands. Tuberculous affections, as a rule, are easily restrained, as it were, by such anatomical structures as fasciæ, synovial and serous membranes, and in this respect actinomycosis differs from them and more nearly approaches what is seen in malignant growths and tertiary syphilitic manifestations.

The organism having entered the mouth, carried in probably on some article of food or substance that is held in the mouth and chewed, there seem to be several ways in which it may find a resting-place where it may increase and multiply. It is doubtful if it ever affects a healthy, unbroken surface. Case 1, reported below, where the disease occurred in the substance of the tongue, may be an instance of this, but it is there quite easy to suppose a slight previous lesion, possibly only microscopic. Then there are those cases which we were formerly taught to consider the most common, namely, those in which the jaw is the part affected, the organism entering at a breach in the surface round a tooth, carious or otherwise, it matters not, so long as there is an open wound in the gum surrounding it. In its growth in this situation—always it seems in the *lower* jaw—it cultivates under the periosteum, and produces an abscess which generally, if not always, finds its way to the surface on the outside.

When this abscess bursts, or is opened, a track is formed leading down to a patch of bare bone of varying size. I say bare bone, in distinction to dead bone, because I think if these cases are actively treated it does not at all follow that any of the bone exposed by the lifting up of its periosteum by this affection need necessarily perish. If, however, the condition persists for some time, and especially if the surface of bone is exposed to a septic infection in

'

causing inconvenience when by infiltration they impair the function of muscles or other structures. One or more soft spots appear in the indurated area, and between these projecting soft spots the skin at the normal level appears to be drawn in, so giving rise to rather a typical appearance. If left alone these soft spots open spontaneously, and if several do so the swelling assumes a sort of honeycomb appearance. If they are incised, one is often almost disappointed at the very small quantity of pus that escapes compared with what one had expected from the size of the swelling. These soft spots do not, as a rule, communicate directly with each other, and thus several incisions may be required.

In the pus that escapes there can often be recognized the small, particularly spherical masses characteristic of the affection, sometimes bright yellow,—sulphur grains, as they have been called,—sometimes a dull yellowish-white, and sometimes again—an important fact to remember—very small and quite colorless. In the latter case they may be recognized by allowing some of the pus to flow slowly down the side of a test-tube, and in a good light the minute elevations caused by the colorless masses adhering to the glass can be seen.

If, as sometimes happens, when there is an open communication between the seat of the disease and the exterior of the body or the cavity of the mouth, acute suppuration is added, the case takes on a very different aspect, and the diagnosis becomes much more difficult; the patient is often very ill, suffering from all the effects of an ordinary septic abscess, and it is more than likely that the true nature of the affection will be overlooked until, the usual means having been adopted for the treatment of the acute abscess, the persistence of sinuses and the characteristic discharge from them give a clue as to the original cause of the trouble.

As to the treatment of this affection little has to be said, for it is simple; we cannot but look upon it as a communicable disease, and, therefore, prevention of its spread to other persons ought always to be in our minds; when once it is manifest, the proper course of treatment seems to be locally to incise the softened spots freely and scrape away all that is possible of the affected tissues, and generally to treat the patient with large doses of iodide of potassium, commencing with such a dose as fifteen grains three times a day, and increasing this rapidly till he is taking from fifty to sixty grains three or even four times in the twenty-four hours. It has been my custom to add a moderate quantity of arsenic, such as three or four minims of liquor arsenicalis; in the first instance, this was done to try and prevent the skin lesions which the large quantity of iodide might cause, but I cannot help thinking it has some effect on the disease itself. The prognosis under such treatment, at any rate when the affection occurs about the mouth or face, is certainly good, although it may need to be carried out continuously for a considerable time, and it is rather remarkable how comparatively little disfigurement or scarring results if the disease be eventually eradicated.

It only remains for me now to describe the specimens and cases I have to show. The former comprise—

1. Unstained specimens of pus, showing microscopically the characteristic " ray" formation.

2. Specimens showing microscopically a streptothrix stained by Gram's method.

3. Test-tube with pus containing characteristic yellowish-white granules.

4. Culture tube.

Before reading the notes of the patients who are in attendance this evening, I should like to narrate, briefly, those of two or three who have been under my care, but whom I could not bring this evening for various reasons. [The report of cases is omitted.]— *Transactions of the Odontological Society of Great Britain.*

A Brief Review of the Prevailing Theories of Immunity. —It is generally believed that the prevailing theories of immunity are extremely difficult to understand. This is due mainly to the fact that new technical terms have had to be introduced in order to avoid explanatory sentences each time a particular constituent is referred to. As each investigator has interpreted the functions of these various constituents in his own special way, he has deemed it necessary to rename the whole series, so that each substance actually found is now the bearer of many distinguishing appellations, to say nothing of the substances hypothetically introduced in the processes, and also given various names. Bereft of these obscuring features, the three prevailing theories, however, lose their complexity in a great measure.

Metchnikoff's Phagocyte Theory.—Metchnikoff, who began his investigations in 1865, terms " phagocyte" any cell capable of incorporating bacteria and of destroying them by a process of digestion. Haeckel (1862) saw leucocytes ingest indigo; Recklinghausen (1863) noted that pus-cells ingulfed cinnabar grains; Cohnheim (1867) saw leucocytes plunge their pseudopodia through vascular stomata and thus leave the vessels to become pus-cells. Even Metchnikoff's antagonists have recognized that the leprosy bacillus, the gonococcus, and other micro-organisms are always found in cells, while he has himself shown that they can ingest living anthrax bacilli. These organisms, having conquered the cells, passed out into the hanging drop, multiplied therein, and proved virulent on inoculation. As observed by Cantacuzène, anthrax bacilli injected in a vein of a rabbit's ear are destroyed in seven minutes in the liver, in eight minutes in the lungs, and in one hour in the spleen. The organisms that escape from one cell are seized by others, but if their multiplication is excessive they overpower the phagocytic leucocytes and invade the blood-stream.

Various observers, Pfeiffer, Büchner, and others, having demonstrated that the blood-serum and other body-fluids were likewise bactericidal, Metchnikoff ascribed this fact to the disintegration of phagocytes, the properties of these cells being thus imparted to the serum. As shown by Bordet and other French investigators, this property is due to two constituents of the plasma. The one (the specific immune body) circulates in the plasma, according to Metchnikoff, and resists a temperature as high as 100° C. The other, or "cytase," thought to be derived from disintegrated phagocytes, is destroyed by heating to 55° or 56° C. thirty minutes, and is considered by him as belonging to the category of trypsins.

Bulloch, in his review of the bacteriological side of the question of immunity for the section on pathology at the recent meeting of the British Medical Association, states that "thousands of facts point to the conclusion that our leucocytic-forming tissues are our great defensive organs against parasitic invasions," but that "the mystery is how the microbes are destroyed."

Büchner's Alexins, or the Humoral Theory.—The view that the serum is endowed with bactericidal powers has been ably defended by Pfeiffer, von Fodor, Nuttall, and others. Their labors led to a doctrine of which the late Professor Hans Büchner was the main exponent. Both he and Hankin isolated substances which they termed "alexins," and to these bodies they ascribed the power to confer immunity. They were also thought by Büchner to be derived from leucocytes (oxyphil) and kindred cells. Laschtscenko having isolated them from living leucocytes, the bactericidal action was thought by Büchner to be due to a proteolytic enzyme, similar to the ordinary digestive ferments. The "alexins" were found to lose their bactericidal power, however, when exposed thirty minutes to a temperature of 55° C.

Büchner recognized Metchnikoff's doctrine only to a certain extent, the phagocytes being considered by him as mere scavengers capable of removing from the blood various substances foreign to it, including bacteria weakened by the alexins. The cells were deemed incapable, however, of carrying on an active warfare against pathogenic micro-organisms in general. Grüber was also led by a large number of experiments to conclude that the actual destruction of bacteria in all animals, "whether actively or passively immunized," was due to Büchner's alexins, and that these alexins were "general protective substances entirely without specific action." According to Grüber, the bacterial cell walls were first made adhesive by the blood's agglutinins and thus became vulnerable to the destructive action of the alexins.

Büchner's alexins were soon found deficient in many particulars, but the many valuable paths his labors and those of pupils have opened have been utilized in the elaboration of other hypotheses.

Ehrlich's Side Chain Theory.—This theory, advanced by Ehrlich in 1897, aimed to harmonize the results so far reached in the study of natural and artificial immunity and particularly the formation and mode of action of the immunizing constituents of the blood-serum. Reduced to its simplest expression, Ehrlich's theory is, on the whole, not a complex one, and is based on recognized biological and chemical principles.

The body being composed of colonies of cells which differ from one another in their functional attributes, nerve-cells, muscle-cells, gland-cells, etc., we speak of the specific action of drugs, because each kind of cell has a special affinity for certain drugs. Thus, the cerebrospinal motor cells have affinity for strychnine, the cardiac muscle-cells for digitalis, the sweat and salivary gland-cells for jaborandi, etc. Now, toxins differ in no way from remedies in this particular; they also are specific owing to their cellular affinities, toxins being also taken up by specific cells. This specific action of toxins represents the foundation upon which Ehrlich's theory is poised.

The theory itself is based upon the mechanism of cell-nutrition in its relations to the mode of production of specific antitoxins, or bactericidal and antitoxic sera.

The complexity of cellular protoplasm is well known to biologists. Ehrlich assumes that each cell contains an active central nucleus (*leistungs Kern*) and of groups of molecules, or "side chains." These outer, or extranuclear, groups constitute a cardinal feature of the entire scheme, since each of them has for its function to receive (hence the term *receptor* given it by Ehrlich) the molecules of food-stuffs which perpetuate the cell's existence. These molecules Ehrlich terms *haptophores* (ἅπτειν, to touch; φερειν, to bring) owing to their identity as extrinsic carriers. A cell's nutrition is thus carried on through the affinity its "receptors," or "side chains," have for its haptophores.

Unfortunately, the receptors do not combine with these nutrient substances only; their affinity extends to substances which are, in a measure, their chemical analogues and which may include harmful bodies. Thus, a poison, a toxin, or a venom may contain the same elements and the same number of them as a nutrient molecule, or haptophore, the only difference between the latter and the pathogenic molecule being a different arrangement of their respective atoms (isomerism). The formula of turpentine, for instance, is $C_{10}H_{16}$, while that of oil of lemons is also $C_{10}H_{16}$; and yet their properties are quite dissimilar. The same may be said of ethyl formate, methyl acetate, and propionic acid, all of which have a molecular weight of 74, and the same formula,—*i.e.*, $C_3H_6O_2$. This makes it possible for a cell to take up (combined with its nutrient haptophores any number of isomeric non-nutritious bodies, and when one of these happens to be a toxic—thus forming what Ehrlich terms a *toxo*phore—the latter combines with the cell and, if sufficiently active qualitatively and quantitatively, may act destructively upon it.

If the toxic is not sufficiently active to destroy the cell or inhibit its functions, the latter seeks not only to rid itself of the poison, but also to protect itself against further aggressions from this poison and its isomers. Intoxication being due to a toxin, for instance, the toxin group of the haptophoric molecule attaches itself to the receptors and then reacts actively upon the cell proper. The receptors themselves being destroyed, the cell (in keeping with Weigert's theory of overproduction) not only replaces them by reproduction, but the process is so active that many more receptors are created than are required by the cell itself, and they accumulate in the blood and lymph. A very prominent feature of Ehrlich's theory appears in this connection,—viz., these surplus receptors preserve their affinity for their specific haptophores and therefore for any isomeric toxin that may combine with it. The receptors thus become the cell's protectors, since they capture, as it were, and hold the toxin before it can at all reach the cell proper, thus immunizing the latter against the poison. Diphtheria toxin, for instance, by exciting the cells for which it has specific affinity, causes these cells to liberate receptors in large quantities; these, by at once combining with the rest of the toxin in the blood-stream, curtail its morbid effects. *Antitoxin,* according to Ehrlich, owes its curative properties to the receptors (side chains) it contains.

The element of specificity, so evident in all immunizing processes, is easily explained by Ehrlich's conception. As the different cell-colonies constitute clearly defined and autonomous groups, each of which reacts under the influence of poisons which affect none of the other groups, a poison can only cause the production of one kind of receptors, and these receptors injected into another animal can only neutralize that one poison and its isomers. Again, the body being only vulnerable to the toxins with which its cells' haptophores can combine, it follows that Ehrlich's theory covers all diseases caused by toxins and the processes through which the body acquires immunity against them.

The destruction of the more solid pathogenic agents such as bacteria, yeast-cells, worn-out blood-cells, tissue débris, and other cellular structures require the aid of additional factors,—*i.e.,* cell "poisoning" or "killing" agents, which Ehrlich has termed *cytotoxins* or *lysins.* These bodies, according to Ehrlich, not only appear in the blood when useless (and therefore harmful) cellular materials are to be dissolved, but each body is essentially specific as a solvent. Thus, when blood-cells are to be destroyed, there appear in the blood-plasma *hæmo*lysins; when muscle-cells, *myo*lysins; when nerve-cells, *neuro*lysins; when kidney-cells, *nephro*toxins, etc. Each of these is active only in the case of one particular kind of cell and in that of no other. Bacteria, introduced into the circulation, also provoke the elaboration of specific antibodies, *bacterio*lysins, and blood-plasma containing one of these is active only upon the bacillus which, injected into animals, caused its appearance in the blood. Serum obtained by injecting the typhoid bacillus, for instance, will destroy typhoid germs, but it will not dissolve the diphtheria bacillus or any other germ.

Two bodies or substances have been shown experimentally to be necessary in the process, in addition to the cellular material acted upon. One of these bodies is not affected by exposure to relatively high temperatures and has been termed *immune body* by Ehrlich, while the other, the *complement*, is destroyed when kept at a temperature of 55° C. thirty minutes. The immune body's rôle is to attach itself to the cells or bacteria to be dissolved and to act as a link (hence the name *amboceptor* also given it by Erhlich) between them and the complement, the latter having no affinity for the cellular elements. The complement being endowed, according to Ehrlich, with digestive powers, it is thus brought into contact with the cells and these are dissolved.

But how is the marked specificity witnessed in the destruction of these bacteria and other cellular *detritus* accounted for in this process? Ehrlich ascribes it exclusively to the immune body. Thus, if cholera bacilli be introduced into an animal the immune body that will appear in the serum obtained from that animal will attach itself to cholera bacilli only. This is because the combining group of the immune body thus obtained will fit only that particular species of micro-organism as a key does its lock. And this applies to all kinds of bacteria and cellular elements to be disposed of in the body fluids: they represent as many different locks, each of which requires its own particular key. Briefly, while the complement is the solvent, it cannot act upon bacteria or other cellular elements without being linked to them by one of the *great many* immune bodies which, according to Ehrlich and Morgenroth, may occur in the blood-serum.—*Editorial in Monthly Cyclopædia of Practical Medicine.*

COMPRESSED AIR IN DENTISTRY. By George Zederbaum, D.D.S., Charlotte, Michigan.[1]

IT is my purpose to bring before you the many advantageous uses of compressed air in the practice of dentistry.

We shall first consider the apparatus necessary to obtain and maintain a certain pressure of compressed air. In my opinion, the

---

[1] Read before the Michigan Dental Association, June 28, 1904.

best apparatus is the one described and illustrated by Dr. H. C. Register, of Philadelphia, in the April number of the *Dental Brief*, and on exhibition here with Sibley's goods. It consists of a small pump which operates by being connected by a pulley to an electric motor. When the motor is set in motion, the pump compresses the atmospheric air into a storage tank which, by means of an air-gauge, accurately registers the pressure of air stored. From the storage tank leads the outlet pipe, guarded by a suitable valve. Unfortunately the use of this outfit is limited to those who are located where a street electric current is obtainable. The other apparatus, and the one we all can have, is the one depending upon the water-supply, and this is available in almost all towns. No very high pressure is necessary. Here we have an "air pump which is attached to the city water-supply pipe, and which keeps a desired pressure of air in the storage tank automatically." A very small pump, such as I just described, will maintain from thirty to forty pounds pressure of air for a very long period. The manufacturers of these pumps claim that only one pound of pressure is lost by friction, that is, your compressed-air tank, when kept full, will *register* just one pound less than your water supply registers. The temperature of air so obtained is about 25° F. higher than that of *the* water at the same time. Either apparatus described may be had for some twenty-five or thirty dollars. They occupy but very *little* room, and in case of water-motor and tank, these can be stored in the cellar and air piped up to the most convenient point.

There are many other apparatuses on the market, some with hand- and others with foot-pumps, but I would have the same objections to these that I would have to a common rubber bulb atomizer, —namely, insufficient capacity and insufficient pressure of air for prolonged use. So much for the apparatus.

That compressed air is becoming more and more a necessity for us, and not merely a luxury, as many may suggest, one has to look into some of our valuable dental publications. There are quite a few of the thinking practitioners considering the installation of compressed-air outfits in their offices. It is only the other day that I read an advertisement in one of the dental journals of a modern dental office for sale; everything complete, electric engine, lathe, compressed-air outfit, etc. This is my sentiment exactly. No office is complete and up to date in every sense of the word without its compressed-air supply. Now let us consider the many varied uses

for this air. I will suggest only those that I have had experience
with during the last two years. There may be many more advantageous uses for it, but I leave them for others to demonstrate. All
I wish is to show its value to us whether it be for the laboratory,
for the operating-room, or for the extracting-room.

Preparing and filling of sensitive cavities with plastic filling-
materials becomes an easy task when the cavity is thoroughly dry;
a stream of compressed air will dry the cavity and will enable the
operator to do better and quicker work. Let us take a large buccal
cavity in a lower molar, involving, say, middle and gingival thirds
occluso-gingivally and the middle-third mesio-distally. These, we
will all agree, are by no means easy to fill as they should be filled,
especially so in cases where one has to do it without the use of
rubber dam. Such submarine fillings are never satisfactory. A
current of air applied for the period of two minutes will, in most
mouths, entirely dry the seat of operation, and after the filling is
inserted it will require some effort on the part of the patient to
bring about the normal moisture.

In preparing any and all cavities, we are obliged to stop frequently and blow out the chips obscuring the point of operation,
and not infrequently do our patients complain of heat generated by
a rapidly revolving bur. Let us take a very small rubber tube, the
diameter of the opening of which need not be over one-thirty-second
of an inch, and wire it around the engine cable down to the point
of the hand-piece; now turn on your air-pressure and go ahead
with the drilling. The current of the air will not only keep the
point of operation in constant sight and free from chips, but will
also prevent the bur from heating and thereby will, necessarily,
lessen pain and duration of operation. Nowadays we are after
modes and means calculated toward lessening degree and amount
of pain, and toward doing work with expedition, and for this purpose alone the compressed air is a desirable feature. Should it be
desired to heat the air before it reaches the cavity, that is also easily
accomplished, for all that is necessary is for us to state our needs
and wants and there are many ingenious minds among us to devise
such instruments and accessories as may be needed and are not yet
in the market.

In taking impressions and bites in wax or gutta-percha, or in
various modelling compounds requiring heat for their plasticity,
all one has to do after their introduction into the mouth is to turn

on the compressed air and cool off the mass in a minute. You will have a sharper impression or bite as the result, and the patient will not get tired out and spoil the impression by involuntarily closing the mouth or changing the relative position of the jaws in case of bite. Again, you are saving time, and the trouble of preparing another " hot cake" is obviated.

In treatments of empyema of the maxillary sinuses, or of a wound after a root incision, or of any other injury about the mouth, where the parts to be treated are remote from sight and easy reach of the operator, and where a thorough medication is required, whether it be of a liquid or of a powder nature, here again the best mode of application is easily solved. If it be a liquid, a pointed atomizer point will, by means of gentle but steady pressure of air, do the work more effectively than when applied by old methods. If it be some powder medicament, I would use a glass pipette into which I gather a few pinches of this powder; the free end of this pipette is attached to the air valve and the opposite end is inserted just at the opening of the ' wound. Then in the language of ko-dakers, " you touch the button, and it does the rest." The powder so applied will be distributed all over the wound more uniformly; the deepest portions being reached will quickly stimulate healthy granulations. These deepest portions, as a rule, are slighted, owing to inaccessibility of the parts; but here the force can be exerted as the case may require; there is no danger of the powder so distributed coming back into the operator's face, as in the case of a clown in Barnum's circus, who, upon being instructed to give some pulverized medicament to a sick donkey, made a large cardboard pipe and filled it with the prescribed powder. Then upon inserting one end of the pipe into the donkey's mouth and the other end into his own, he took a long breath preparatory to blowing the powder into the donkey's mouth, but the donkey's olfactory nerve became tickled and he blew first! It is needless to say that the attempted operation was not a success. Had the clown used the compressed-air outfit all would have gone well.

In treating pyorrhœa in all its varieties and stages, and in many diseases of the pericementum, one saves much time and effects a permanent cure considerably quicker by the use of a compressed-air atomizer and treating the diseased parts directly by daily spraying with proper medicaments. Marshall, in his work on " Operative Dentistry," suggests the use of atomizers for this purpose.

12

Here again the compressed-air apparatus enables one to send uninterrupted streams as strong or as weak as the case in hand may demand into the deep tissues, down into pus-pockets where it is most needed.

To deodorize malodorous mouths before commencing an operation is a desirable feature beyond dispute; here again comes handy the valuable and efficient use of compressed-air.

While touching upon deodorization, I wish to remark that not infrequently our operating-rooms have peculiar "dental odors" about them. Iodoform, carbolic acid, creosote, oils of cassia, cloves, and other essential oils and highly volatile substances, all added to the office, in the mind of many sensitive patients, still more repugnancy than they already have from fear. It is my habit to spray the room with a weak solution of spirits of lavender; fumigate, so to speak, the entire breadth and length of the operating-room. Compressed air does this admirably, and the room smells sweet and fresh and the air is by far more agreeable.

How many bridges and crowns have to be reset in our practice, and all because, in the majority of cases, they were put on while saliva was running freely in and about the abutments? With a steady compressed-air current I can dry up the mouth so that a bridge or a crown can be set under absolutely dry conditions, thereby assuring their stability.

Have you a long soldering job? Here also take your compressed-air hose and attach to it your blow-pipe, and the absolute ease with which the soldering can be done is surprising. Furthermore, no checking of porcelain is apt to occur when the heat, as in this case, is steadily applied.

After giving nitrous oxide or any other general anæsthetic, the patient is brought to quickly by application of a strong force of compressed-air directed squarely toward his face.

Very often patients faint at extraction; compressed air, applied as above, revives them at once.

The use of local anæsthetics by means of injections with the hypodermic needle is objectionable to many patients; still they will not object if you "freeze the gums" by the local abstraction of heat, directing finely divided streams of ether or rhigolene or other such remedy by means of the compressed-air apparatus. Here also it is by far more effective than atomizers operated by hand or foot bellows. The stream is steady, and consequently less of the drug is used and the required numbness is obtained in much less time.

After extracting, I often check the hæmorrhage by spraying into the alveoli some suitable styptic; here again I use the compressed-air outfit.

The problem of interesting the children, while doing some painful operation for them, is a hard one; I often let the child help me by holding the compressed-air valve and keeping the cavity blown out. They like the idea of helping you, their mind is away from the seat of trouble, and you accomplish better and quicker work with but an occasional involuntary flinch from them.

No doubt there are many and many more useful ways of utilizing the compressed air, once it be installed in our offices. They become apparent as one uses the apparatus and becomes acquainted with it. When I first commenced to use it, I applied it only where I wanted to prepare a difficult cavity without the use of the rubber dam. Since then, all the other various uses I have mentioned followed naturally, each in its respective turn. I know that but very few have ever used compressed air; many have never thought of it. I wish all would try it and become convinced, and, as I have said before, add more to the already numerous enough list of advantageous uses of compressed air in dentistry to commend its intrinsic value.—*Dental Register.*

Reports of Society Meetings.

THE NEW YORK INSTITUTE OF STOMATOLOGY.

A MEETING of the Institute was held at the offices of Drs. Kimball and Parker, No. 27 West Thirty-eighth Street, New York, on Tuesday evening, January 2, 1905, the President, Dr. C. O. Kimball, in the chair.

The minutes of the last meeting were read and approved.

Dr. H. W. Gillett presented a useful appliance for the purpose f holding the gum back for cervical work, and also some appliances for holding the rubber dam for the same kind of cavities.

Dr. G. V. I. Brown, of Milwaukee, read a paper entitled "The Vital Significance of Oral Disease."

(For Dr. Brown's paper, see page 281.)

DISCUSSION.

Dr. H. L. Wheeler.—In the first case mentioned by Dr. Brown he spoke of a necrotic condition, the patient dying of a general breaking up of the tissues. I would like to ask the essayist what the real lesion here was.

Dr. Brown.—It would be difficult to give an exact name to the trouble. Although the tissues were necrotic, there were no pus corpuscles. It was not in the nature of a malignant growth.

Dr. Wheeler.—A point that has been impressed upon my mind is that there seems to be a borderland uncultivated by any one, between where the physician or surgeon leaves off and where the dentist begins and as a result the patient is apt to suffer serious inconvenience if not grave dangers. I think, as a profession, we ought to pay more attention to these things that Dr. Brown has come here to show us to-night, and it has also sometimes seemed to me that physicians ought to pay more attention to the conditions of the mouth. I have myself, within a short space of time, had two cases where I was called in by a physician, and in each case a specialist had apparently been completely baffled. One case was thought to be antrum trouble, and was so treated without success. I found upon examination that it was an alveolar abscess, together with a curious condition of pain between the lateral and the bicuspid on the same side. There was a constant flow of pus coming from a sinus in the mucous membrane, back as far as the molars. From the history of the case this had been going on for a year or two, at intervals. The patient had been going to a nose and throat specialist constantly during that time. Another case came in recently with a bad swelling of the face, with a bright flush about the eye, together with a slight swelling and trouble in the mucous membrane of the mouth. It was an abscess on the palatal root of the first molar.

Dr. Leo. Green.—I should like to hear from Dr. Brown a little further regarding the case of noma.

Dr. Brown.—The case was referred to me by a physician, he having treated the patient for a week or two. When I first saw him the temperature was 104°, with an occasional rise to 105°, and it was only with a great amount of care that I was able to keep the temperature down. The original point of trouble appeared to be back of the third lower molar on the right side. The discharge was inky black and the tissue that died was black. An area very quickly formed in the cheek, and rapidly sloughed through. It was my custom, at each dressing, three or four times a day, to wipe off or remove with instruments the dead tissue, but the adjoining healthy tissue kept dying so rapidly that in two or three hours gangrenous masses again formed. The patient finally died in about ten days, being perfectly clear mentally until the last forty-eight hours. His last stage was marked by expectoration of red blood, the condition having extended into the lungs. There was no history of infection. The man was a laborer, and had apparently been in good health previously. There was, so far as I could find out, no history of syphilis, and the symptoms did not resemble syphilis in any way.

Dr. C. F. Allan.—The subjects dealt with this evening by the essayist are of very great importance to us in our work, in that they prove to us the correctness of our recent theories regarding the extraction of teeth. The essayist has shown us that the malformation of one or both jaws, whether caused by the extraction of a tooth or from other causes, affects the whole physical condition of the face and that a defective nasal septum or diseased nasal sinuses can sometimes be effectively treated by a widening of the upper arch. It is evident from this that, in performing these operations of expanding the arches, we are not only benefiting the patient in so far as their teeth are concerned, but we are also helping their breathing apparatus and benefiting the general conditions dependent upon free nasal passages and an abundant supply of oxygen. Care of these patients in early life would eliminate many of the nasal cases that come to the surgeon later on.

Dr. Bogue, who is not with us to-night, but to whom Dr. Brown has paid tribute, has for several years been paying close attention to the mouths of his very young patients, and he has asked many of us to send him models of such cases. He feels that there is a great advantage in the early correction of these deformities of the jaws, and it would now seem from Dr. Brown's paper that this early correction would greatly benefit some of the unfortunate conditions just described.

Dr. Gillett.—There are two points upon which I wish to say a word,—first, with regard to our duty toward those of our profession who have achieved the skill needful to such results as those shown us by Dr. Brown in the partially occupied field to which Dr. Wheeler has referred; if we cannot be active in this field we may at least direct the attention of the younger men toward it.

My second point pertains to the frequent neglect by practitioners of the chronic inflammations of the mouth and their sequelæ,—in particular, chronic alveolar abscess. It is not an uncommon thing to be told that some dentist has advised against "meddling" with such conditions. Such advice I believe to be malpractice, and that practitioners giving it should be held legally responsible for the ill results which frequently follow.

Dr. J. B. Locherty.—I would like to ask Dr. Brown at what age he operates in these cases of cleft palate.

Dr. Brown.—That depends entirely on the individual case. Always, if possible, before the child begins to speak; certainly before the speech changes from baby-talk to the talk of a grown person. I always attempt to build the child up as thoroughly as possible before operation.

The President.—In widening the arch in these cases, do you use a plate, or is it done by direct pressure upon the bones?

Dr. Brown.—I use an appliance attached to the teeth, where there are teeth, and a screw attached quite close to the gingival margin. I apply the force as rapidly as required, thus making direct pressure. The appliance does not attach to the central incisors. They are left free; therefore separation in this region is an indication of widening of the median suture. I sometimes have to spread the lower arch also, although it frequently follows the upper in course of development without immediate operative assistance.

Dr. Allan.—It has been stated that unless the central incisors are spread there can be no spreading of the bone.

Dr. Brown.—I do not see how that can be possible. Certainly I have accomplished this result without attaching my appliance to the central incisors.

The President.—In a case of cleft palate, the child being strong and the case favorable, how early would you operate?

Dr. Brown.—I doubt if any child ought to be considered strong enough for such an operation without danger earlier than one and one-half or two years of age. My preference would be older than this, yet at a sufficiently early age to prevent the fixation of incorrect speech habits. Naturally the conditions that modify and govern the surgeon's decisions as to time of operation in each individual case vary very greatly. Differences of health, ability to take nourishment, possibility of good post-operative care, and other important considerations have to be taken into account. Sometimes infants are brought long distances, with expectation of immediate operation, and we find that there may never be such opportunity for the child again, and so it becomes imperative to do the best that may be under the circumstances, but, if given a choice, there can be no question of the fact that more perfect results, both from a cosmetic point of view and that of capability of speech mechanism, can be obtained with less danger to the child by careful pre-operative care and treatment, and choosing the time for operation with full understanding of the benefit of willing co-operation in the post-operative treatment, which of course is impossible with very young infants.

The President.—I want to say just a word in regard to a case that came to my knowledge several years ago, relating to the border-line between the profession of the physician and the dentist. It is that of a lady nearly fifty years of age, who during an interval between her annual visits developed a sore on the outside of her face over the lower bicuspid. There was no trouble in the bicuspids nor the first two molars; the third molar, though only partially developed, was apparently in a healthy condition. I could find no connection between the little open sore and the wisdom-tooth. Her physician assured her that it was merely a local trouble, and had nothing whatever to do with the teeth. After it had gone on for a year or more I became convinced that that third molar had something to do with it, and had it removed, finding it dead. Even then I could find no connection between it and the sore, though the latter subsequently healed. In this case I had an instinctive feeling that that wisdom-tooth had something to do with this condition, and the physician was equally sure of his position that it had not.

I mention this to show that there are cases that defy the closest observation, and times when it is difficult to make a correct diagnosis of what seems to be a simple case.

In behalf of the society, I wish to thank Dr. Brown for his paper this evening, and, while regretting the absence of those men who were to have discussed the paper, we perhaps have had a

greater advantage in the opportunity of questioning him than had
the paper been discussed by outside parties not so interested in the
dental aspect.

A vote of thanks was extended to Dr. Brown.

Adjourned.

FRED. L. BOGUE, M.D., D.D.S.,

Editor The New York Institute of Stomatology.

ACADEMY OF STOMATOLOGY.

A REGULAR meeting of the Academy of Stomatology of Philadelphia was held at its rooms, 1731 Chestnut Street, on the evening of Tuesday, November 22, 1904, the President, Dr. I. N.
Broomell, in the chair.

A paper was read by Dr. M. I. Schamberg, of Philadelphia, entitled " The Etiology, Pathology, and Treatment of Troublesome
Tooth Sockets."

(For Dr. Schamberg's paper, see page 217.)

DISCUSSION.

Dr. H. B. Hickman.—I would like to recall a case which I reported here some time ago, and which has relation to this paper.
The case was one in which it was necessary to remove the lower
right second bicuspid to relieve pain, even after the tooth had been
opened through the apical foramen and left open. I found the
root-canal had been filled for ten years. The tooth was extracted
by a specialist who was very careful, both before and after the
operation, in the use of antiseptics. On the day following the
extraction the pain was very severe, and worse when the patient was
lying down. Cocaine, morphia, and sulphate of zinc were tried, but
carbolic acid alone gave relief. Osteomyelitis developed, and the
patient died as the result of this troublesome tooth socket.

Dr. James Truman.—I have not heard any paper in recent
years that has impressed me more than this paper of Dr. Schamberg; not that we have in it anything especially new, and I do not
presume that he gives it with that idea, but it is the first time I
have ever heard a paper that really took the whole matter in hand
and gave us an intelligent conception of the duty of the dentist.

I do not know that I have any criticism to make, except perhaps with reference to his statement of the necessity to remove a tooth. If we are to remove all teeth that are in a diseased condition, I am fearful that we will not keep any when an alveolar abscess, so-called, has developed, for not one of those teeth could be considered healthy. All have a large amount of necrotic tissue at the apex or apices of roots and are liable to produce the so-called gum-boil at any time. I would not want to extract all those teeth.

Upon the whole, I do not quite agree with his view that it is best in the first instance to use hydrogen dioxide. Hydrogen dioxide is, in my opinion, not the harmless agent it has been supposed to be, and by injecting it into tooth sockets there is a possibility of producing trouble. I have seen cases in the clinics in which serious conditions have resulted.

I would like to ask Dr. Schamberg what he would do in a case of abscess when he allows the coagulum to fill up and the patient thereafter suffers intensely from pain of extraction. I do not think it is a good thing to have that coagulum remain without treatment. It seems to me that the socket should be curetted out and antisepticized. I think that spraying with hydronaphthol is more irritating than with phenol sodique. Why the latter should be objectionable in a tooth socket when it is so advantageous in other directions I do not understand. In a general way I think I am in harmony with the treatment given to tooth sockets.

I agree thoroughly with his concluding sentence,—that a man who undertakes to extract teeth and does not make his hands and instruments thoroughly sterile, and does not make the mouth sterile subsequently, does not understand his professional duty to his patient.

Dr. M. H. Cryer.—I am much pleased, and came in from the country purposely to hear Dr. Schamberg's paper.

I would not care to recommend the use of hydrogen dioxide in tooth sockets after extraction, especially in the lower jaw, as the cancellated tissue is so open that when the medicament comes in contact with either pus or blood, oxygen is freely liberated with almost an explosive effect, so that it may force septic matter, if it be present, into the cancellated tissue. Dr. Woodward has just reminded me of a patient that was referred to me for treatment. A diseased lower second bicuspid having an abscess around the root had been extracted; the necrotic socket was treated with hydrogen dioxide for some time, and when I made an examination I could pass an ordinary silver probe from the enlarged tooth socket to the angle of the jaw, and forward to near the symphysis. My opinion is that the internal portion of the bone had been destroyed by the hydrogen dioxide in combination with pyogenic organisms. As soon as this medicament was discontinued and other treatment instituted, the patient had relief, and finally the space was filled with new tissue through granulation.

Hydrogen dioxide is not used by the surgeon as in former years, especially in deep-seated wounds. It is useful in surface wounds, however, when carefully applied, and I have no doubt that, with the care and judgment Dr. Schamberg would give, a tooth socket could be wiped out with hydrogen dioxide upon a piece of cotton.

Dr. William H. Trueman.—There is food for thought in the paper read. There can be no question but that some cases of alveolar abscess are to some patients a serious menace, because cases are on record where they have been followed by serious consequences. So it is with various other diseases usually considered trivial, especially if they are not properly treated. There is no doubt but that in some cases the teeth had better be extracted. We should not, however, consider alone the *possibility* of serious injury, but the *probability*. The danger from alveolar abscess is, under ordinary circumstances, exceedingly slight. I have had six teeth in my own mouth which have abscessed now and again; first one and then another causes me considerable pain and inconvenience, notwithstanding, I have no fear of serious consequences, and would suffer a great deal rather than have them extracted. One case in my experience made a strong impression upon my mind: A gentleman came to me early in my practice with a central incisor badly abscessed. It had been treated unsuccessfully by several dentists. There was a copious discharge of foul-smelling pus from a fistula far back of the roof of the mouth, near the termination of the hard palate, and another through the gum over the apex of the root, and it seemed to be a hopeless case. It was a front tooth, and, as I did not care to spoil his good looks, I attempted treatment. This was successful in so far that in a short time the discharge became very little, and instead of pus was simply a serum. This has continued for about thirty years. Although the fistula on the roof of the mouth seems to have closed, he can now, by making pressure upon the roof of his mouth with his tongue, cause a little serum to ooze out through the fistula on the gum over the root. The gentleman may have taken a very serious risk in retaining that tooth, but the risk has not materialized. Deciding these questions calls for great care and judgment. It is a very serious matter to deprive a patient of a tooth that may be useful, especially one that must be replaced by a substitute.

Another case I recall is of a gentleman who had a badly diseased bicuspid. It had caused an abscess, and around the fistula the tissues had enlarged until they formed a tumor the size of a large marble. He told me it had been in much the same condition several years. I told him it should be removed promptly, but he treated the advice lightly, and said he would have it done at some convenient time. I wrote him a long letter that evening, drawing a very vivid picture of the possibilities if it were left in. I heard nothing from him for about a year, when I again examined his mouth. The tooth was still there, its surroundings quite normal, and there was nothing to show that it had been abscessed, and he assured me it had had no treatment whatever. Had he followed my advice he would have lost a useful tooth. We have to remember the peculiarities of individuals. Some people are susceptible to certain poisons; others are not. We meet with a very few cases, comparatively, that seem to point the moral now and again brought to our notice. These possibilities demand serious consideration; at the same time we must bear in mind not the possibility only, but also the probability.

Dr. Louis Jack.—I have very little to say beyond what has already been said by Dr. Schamberg. I have found from a large experience with hydronaphthol, 1 in 300 parts, that it is entirely non-irritating.

With reference to abscess of the lower third molar, there is danger that the pus will not find its way through the external side, and is inclined to pass inward on account of the less resistance in this direction; therefore such cases require the closest attention. I remember at one time being called upon by a prominent clergyman for an inflamed third molar, which I ordered out. He replied that he would not have it removed. Subsequently I was called to see the patient, who was dangerously ill on account of the condition of the throat. I stated that the tooth should be immediately removed, as I was afraid pus had already begun to burrow into the hyoid tissues. The physician asked me to delay twenty-four hours, but I felt that by so doing the patient's life would be in danger, and my counsel was carried out. The patient was in bed for several weeks in consequence of the pyæmic condition already existing.

I remember a similar case of a patient in the upper part of the city. The patient died. The physician's diagnosis had been malignant quinsy. The post-mortem revealed excessive infiltration at the base of the tongue; even the hyoid bone was infiltrated with pus.

For the relief of pain in a dry socket following extraction I have found most satisfactory a suppository composed of orthoform, vaseline, and oxide of zinc. The pain of a dry socket I consider more severe than almost any other form of toothache, and it is continuous.

When a patient is sent to me immediately after extraction of a tooth, my usual practice is to spray the parts either with acetanilide or with the normal aqueous solution of hydronaphthol.

Dr. P. B. McCullough.—It does not always happen that postoperative treatment, other than that which can be done at the doctor's office, can be carried out. This is true in the majority of cases. It is useless, therefore, to recommend a thing, however valuable, if it cannot be practised. To that end, I have for a number of years prescribed salt, advising the patient to rinse the mouth frequently with a strong salt solution. Salt does not seem to be regarded as possessing very much antiseptic property, and I have not seen any reference to it, except in a newspaper article stating that sugar and salt were mild antiseptics.

With reference to the use of hydrogen dioxide, I have observed the use of this followed by washing with a dilute solution of carbolic acid. To my inquiry why one antiseptic should be followed by another, it was stated that the moment hydrogen dioxide decomposed it ceased to have any beneficial effect, and that, in order to remove what remained of its decomposition, it was to be followed by the use of an unchangeable antiseptic.

Dr. Schamberg (closing).—It is not unusual to read in the dental journals from month to month accounts of fatal cases following tooth-extraction. Some of these are directly traceable to negligence, others are undoubtedly due to predisposing conditions of the patient.

Regarding the case referred to by Dr. Hickman, there is some question in my mind whether death was due to osteomyelitis, or whether the affection of the tooth socket was a result of the lowered state of the patient's vitality. The eruption upon the man's body may have been of septic origin, but in the absence of an autopsy it cannot be positively stated that death resulted from the jaw lesion. It is unusual for a tooth socket to give such serious trouble when the tooth is removed without difficulty and with aseptic precautions, there being no pronounced local disturbance and the patient being otherwise in good health.

Believe me, I do not encourage the removal of troublesome teeth because I make extraction a specialty. The point I wish to bring out is that there is an ultra conservatism at the present time which says, "Keep a tooth as long as you can." Teeth so retained are often a menace to health and barriers to proper mastication. I therefore believe that such teeth, unless promptly cured, should be removed. I also believe that a properly adjusted artificial tooth will render better service than an irritable tooth which interferes with mastication.

I agree with Dr. William Trueman that many people keep uncured abscessed teeth in their mouths for many years. I believe that such people make a great mistake. Dr. Trueman has said that we should consider the *probability* of trouble rather than its *possibility*. If that were the case, there would be some question as to whether it were wise for us to drink unboiled Schuylkill water, for many people who drink Schuylkill water as it comes from the spiggot never get typhoid fever. A proportion, however, who indulge in this indiscretion do acquire that disease, and the practice is, therefore, considered a hazardous one. By similar reasoning it becomes hazardous to retain uncured teeth the pus of which is likely to be absorbed in the mouth or gastro-intestinal tract.

I might mention, with the permission of one of our fellow-members present, the influence of an alveolar abscess upon his wife's general health. The abscess was of fifteen years' duration upon an upper lateral incisor tooth. It had persisted during that long period in spite of treatment directed through the canal of the tooth and conducted by several of our prominent dental practitioners. The doctor brought his wife to me for root amputation because he felt that the abscess had something to do with his wife's impaired health. The operation resulted not alone in a cure of the abscess, but in a marked improvement in the patient's health. This was evidently due to the complete elimination of the septic area surrounding the necrotic end of the root. I believe there are many patients who consult their physician for the treatment of systemic disorders which could more readily be eradicated by the dentist. Some patients suffer from gastro-intestinal disturbances and other constitutional ailments due to the absorption of pus generated in the mouth.

Dr. Jack spoke of the removal of third molars. These teeth are, as a rule, troublesome before, during, and after extraction. I had a patient sent to me recently with Ludwig's angina, there being so much swelling of the throat that the patient almost suffocated. The removal of a crowded wisdom-tooth promptly relieved the patient. This is but one of many conditions which may follow the prolonged retention of bothersome wisdom-teeth. Suppuration around these teeth is not so often due to putrescent pulps as to pus-pockets formed by overlapping gum tissue.

The suppository recommended by Dr. Jack is a very good one. My method of relieving painful sockets is to dip tampons of cotton into campho phenique, then into powdered orthoform, and thence into the socket. These are to remain for twenty-four hours and then renewed.

Dr. McCullough referred to the impracticability of poor people following the post-operative treatment outlined by me. I supply most of my patients with small bottles of mouth-washes to be used after extraction. The manufacturers of these preparations are glad to supply the profession with samples for distribution among their patients. When I learn that a patient has no mouth-wash at home, I supply him with one which is to be renewed at the drug store when exhausted.

The suggestion of Dr. McCullough, to follow the use of hydrogen dioxide by some other antiseptic, is a good one. This is my invariable practice.

Dr. Cryer's objection to peroxide of hydrogen I can only too readily agree with. I realize that a great deal of harm can be done by the injudicious use of this agent.

In speaking to Dr. Daland of the patient who suffered from boils as a result of an abscessed tooth, he expressed himself as being confident of the fact that pus lurking in the oral cavity and gaining access to the system, either by ingestion or absorption, is a factor to be taken into consideration when studying the etiology of furunculosis.

OTTO E. INGLIS,
Editor Academy of Stomatology.

Editorial.

WHITHER ARE WE DRIFTING?

THE business man at certain periods takes account of his affairs and bases his future prospects on his present standing and upon the general tendencies of the world at large and carefully measures the possibilities. The professional man has a similar duty and must follow these well-understood business principles, and adapt them not wholly to financial success, but to that broader life that should be part of his professional heritage and which is part of his duty to cherish.

Dentistry, it seems to the writer, is passing through a phase of experiences that may end in its advantage, or it may result in serious loss. Are we standing upon the brink of a commercial maëlstrom, dashing and whirling, inviting to eventual destruction? or are the unpleasant signs manifest but the distant wind clouds stirring the waters and presaging the storm, destined to clear the atmosphere and restore to more healthful surroundings?

The indications in the dental world point to a condition far from satisfactory. It seems as though we are drifting more and more away from the spirit which actuates and which is the soul of all professions. The commercial taint, the sordid influence of wealth, hoped for or attained, has entered our ranks to an extent that promises to undermine the very foundations of our professional life. The evidences of this are everywhere. The poison is so insidious that few realize the hold it has taken upon the many that in part compose the twenty-five thousand engaged in the practice of dentistry. This large body would probably treat with scorn the charge, made individually, that they were not professional, or that they were dragging down dentistry again into the mire from which it has been painfully and laboriously exhumed. Yet it must be recognized that the spirit of gain is rapidly demoralizing the dental practitioners of this country.

The signs of this are manifest in various directions, but perhaps more notably in the character of certain articles prepared to be read before societies. These are more devoted to the consideration of *fees,* and the writers, and those who take part in the discussions, grow argumentative in regard to the importance of establishing a trust or its equivalent. They are not satisfied with the fees obtained in their several localities. Comparisons are made between those received for dental operations and those recognized as legitimate in medicine and law. It must be acknowledged that remuneration for services rendered is not up to the professional standard, nor in accordance with the standard dentistry should occupy as one of the most important branches of the healing art. The matter has, however, a deeper bearing than is usually recognized in papers, and the remedy is not to be found in binding resolutions or trusts built upon these.

The men who thus eloquently portray their financial losses apparently lose sight of the fact that the tendency of which they complain is the result of non-professional practices, of which the papers alluded to are, in part, a painful exhibit. The man who respects himself and his profession will arrange the charges for service with a due regard to his own higher interests and to the honor of the profession of which he is a member. Who ever hears of a medical practitioner rushing into print and complaining that he finds it impossible to convince his patients that he has not overcharged them, and asking his *confrères* to establish a fee bill that all practising medicine must maintain? The thought of money in connection with professional service is, to that extent, a lowering of the standard of the calling. The time was when the honorarium was left to the patient and to the feelings of gratitude and extent of the purse. It was held to be undignified to present a bill, and patients resented such a departure from professional methods. This feeling still prevails in many communities. The influence of money is too powerful in our modern life to admit a higher standard than will develop into professional procedures, but it nevertheless remains true that those who think constantly of the fees at the end of the work are, to that degree, upon a lower level, and will, increasingly, drop still farther in that self-respect so necessary to loftier aspirations.

Individuals may not be so much to blame for this condition of mind, for they have notable examples furnished them by all the dental organizations of this country. When they see the majority of these dental societies, from the International Dental Congress to the National, State, and local associations, offering their proceedings to the highest bidder, they naturally feel that if the ethics of the representative organizations permit this, the individuals composing the rank and file should work in the same way and for the same end. A few societies are endeavoring to change, by precept and example, this ignoble practice, and if there is to come a better state of things, it must be through their unselfish work. The prospect is, however, not encouraging. The competition between the so-called trade journals for the proceedings of the several dental bodies in this country has become intense; indeed, it promises to reach the proportions of a professional scandal. Every effort is being made to influence societies. Their cupidity is appealed to in the saving of large annual fees to the individual members, as the expense of publishing the transactions will fall upon the successful trade periodical that, in this way, becomes the organ of the society, and this fact, it may be, is paraded on the cover of the journal. The societies so advertised may not regard this of any consequence, but some others look upon it as a badge of dishonor, not to the journal, but one which no professional body imbued with the highest ethical standard should permit.

It is a matter of surprise that the dental profession has been willing to thus weaken its position, and, to that extent, has made it impossible to call it a body worthy the professional name. When the dental organizations cease from this humiliating traffic, an example will be set that will do more to establish a higher grade of thought and practice than any long dissertations on ethics could hope to accomplish.

The National Dental Association has had the question before it for several years, of establishing a journal for the publication of its own proceedings. At the next annual meeting this matter will again come before that body, and it is hoped that it will find a way to meet this demand. A journal once established will force by example the subordinate societies to accept this as the organ for the publication of their proceedings, and in this way, and in no other, will the best thought of the dental profession find a proper and dignified presentation.

The true professional man has no quarrel with the trade that furnishes him with his needed supplies. These are a necessary adjunct to all the professions. The clergyman must have his publications for reference, the lawyer his books, the medical man his medical supplies and his instruments, and the dentist could not practise his work without them. The writer is not in full agreement with the able and incisive article by Dr. J. E. Weirick, of St. Paul, and transferred to the pages of the April number of this journal. He condemns societies for permitting trade exhibits at their meetings. While this has frequently been a detriment to the work of the organization, by offering a counter-attraction, it must be conceded to be an important part of dental education. The occasional abuse of a good thing is not a sufficient cause for total condemnation. Medical associations have the same thing, but they seem able to manage this better than dental societies, and find less interference with the work of their meetings.

It is in the details of professional life that we must exercise the greatest care. It is in those things that many regard as minor matters that this moral disease finds its best culture field. The practitioner who makes out his bill with every item spread out before his patient has no reason to expect that patient to have a very exalted idea of his professional standing. By this act he allies himself with the tradesman and mechanic. He should charge " for professional services," and not descend to undignified particulars.

We are, as a profession, apparently drifting into the stream that runs to the ocean of selfish accumulations. The hope of the future lies in an educated class of young men trained to a better standard of thought and practice. These must carry dentistry out and beyond its present unsatisfactory conditions. If this hope finds no fulfilment, then, indeed, will the end justify the statement of some. —that dentistry is simply a mechanical calling, without culture and without a dignified self-respect.

CORRECTION.

ON page 263 of the April number, in the report of the discussion of the Academy of Stomatology, Dr. M. H. Cryer is arranged as one of the speakers. This is an error, as he desires it understood that he took no part in the discussion.

Bibliography.

ORAL PATHOLOGY AND THERAPEUTICS. A Systematic Presentation
of the Subject from the Stand-Point of Modern Therapeutics.
With One Hundred and Sixteen Illustrations. By ELGIN
MAWHINNEY, D.D.S., Chicago, Professor of Special Pathol-
ogy, Materia Medica, and Therapeutics. Northwestern Uni-
versity Dental School, etc. The Consolidated Dental
Manufacturing Company, New York, N. Y.; Claudius Ash
& Sons (Limited), London, England, 1905.

The author says in the Preface, "This volume is presented
with the hope that it may furnish at least a rational scientific basis
for the management of many oral diseases." The reader will
naturally conclude from this that the book will satisfy all reasonable demands, and will prove a satisfactory arrangement of dental
pathological subjects, embracing etiology and treatment. That
this is not accomplished on its pages will be made evident as the
reader proceeds with his examination.

The author seems to deem any leading up to the main subject
as unnecessary; and he therefore opens at once in Chapter I. with
" Dental Caries." The history of this important subject is confined to just one-half page, and to that extent fails to be even
an outline of the work of the past two centuries. He then follows
this meagre sketch with " Recent Theories," and devotes exactly
five lines to Miller. In view of the fact that the world of dentistry
recognizes Miller as having given not only the most thorough
scientific elucidation of the subject, but the final óne in regard
to the origin of this disease, this unsatisfactory paragraph leaves a
very bad impression on the mind of the reader.

This very objectionable method of treating important matters,
not apparently interesting to the author, seems to be part of the
plan of the volume, for it is found, to a greater or less extent, in
the majority of the chapters.

Chapter III. seems to have been taken without revision from
one of the author's lectures, and even for that its style might be
greatly improved for the benefit of the rising dental generation.

Quotation from a portion of two pages will best illustrate this, leaving the reader to draw his own conclusions. " When you get into practice here are some of the things you must consider. First, the personnel of the dentist. You must have a professional air about you. You want to recognize the fact that our calling is something more than trade; that it is a profession; there is a dignity about it, a professional air. Kind in manner and speech, and, as some one has said, ' Keep your voice low !' There is a whole lot in that." This may be all very good advice to a body of careless students, but wholly inappropriate, as well as that which follows, in a work on dental pathology.

The intelligent reader, after trying to peruse these pages, will be inclined to lay down the book and let it pass out of sight as a mass of words in exceeding bad taste, but this hasty opinion would hardly do the author full justice, for there are some good things stored within its pages.

The following is the author's idea, in part, at least, of " Systemic Medication :" " Morphine is one of the alkaloids of opium, and the one most·used. For purposes of alleviating pain it is without a rival. It is given in doses of one-eighth grain an hour before the operation and another fifteen minutes before. I never tell my patients what they are taking when they take morphine, because so many have a prejudice against it."

The following will interest the critical reader. The author has described a case of " Calcific Degeneration of the Pulp," and then proceeds : " Well, he was an individual who wouldn't bear much work with his teeth. He was one of those individuals who didn't believe much in having much done with his teeth, anyway. and consequently had neglected them until he had lost a number of his molars. He decided on his own hook when one couldn't find the cause of the trouble that he would have a certain one out." The following statement seems even remarkable for Chicago: " In all acute suppuration we have a decided rise in temperature, as I have stated, 101, 102, 103, 104, 105, or even 106 occasionally from an acute alveolar abscess." While death has resulted from an alveolar abscess, it is exceedingly rare, and the ordinary abscess of the peridental membrane will rarely raise the temperature above 103°.

Except in certain special cases, where he is very profuse in his credits, he does not seem to consider this trifling courtesy of much

moment. In his usual breezy way he will take up one method and
give his ideas with a freedom peculiarly characteristic. In the
chapter devoted to bleaching discolored teeth this is prominent.
Credit is, of course, not given to the author of the chlorine method,
nor is this described properly.

On page 166 the author classes the reviewer with those who
entertain the theory that the so-called serumal calculus is the
"result of the presence in the system of unusual quantities of
urates and uric acid." If he will kindly drop the name of Truman
from the list in future editions, it will be appreciated, as the owner
of the name mentioned entertains quite opposite views.

There are some good common-sense ideas expressed on the
pages of this book, and in one chapter, on "Infection, Instrument Sterilization, and Germicides," the work is so much superior
to the rest of the production that it is difficult to realize it is from
the same pen.

The book will not add much to our knowledge of pathological
conditions, and in its present form is not altogether creditible to
the judgment of the author; but if he will eliminate in the next
edition much of the *talk* and confine it to practical teaching, he
may make a book worthy the study of the practitioner and student.

Miscellany.

DR. ENDELMAN ON STOMATITIS.—A careful and intelligent consideration of the several factors involved in the complicated problem of nutrition with the consequent effect upon the body's defensive forces at once points out the etiological solution of nearly
all inflammatory conditions of the oral mucous membrane. These
inflammations of the lining membrane of the mouth I have divided
into two classes,—those entirely localized to the areas of the oral
cavity and those in which the lowering of the vital powers of the
oral tissues brought about by some constitutional disorder has rendered it possible for the exciting factor (the bacteria then present
in the mouth) to exercise its pathogenic influence.

The localized type of buccal inflammation I have named stomatitis simplex, and that in which a constitutional disorder acts as
the predisposing cause, stomatitis complex.

Under the heading of stomatitis simplex I can include only those cases in which the inflammatory disorder is the immediate consequence of localized irritation, such as salivary deposits, carious cavities, rough edges of broken-down teeth, ill-fitting appliances intended for substitutes for the lost natural organs, also prolonged contact of the mucous membrane with substances of extreme temperatures, chemicals, tobacco smoke, etc. By the term stomatitis complex, I refer to all inflammations of the buccal mucous membrane in which the predisposing cause, an existing constitutional pathological error, has so modified the tissues of the mouth as to favor the growth and action of the microbic exciting cause. Here I include aphthous stomatitis, tuberculous stomatitis, ulcerative stomatitis, gangrenous stomatitis, mercurial stomatitis, syphilitic stomatitis, with stomatitis occurring in the course of the eruptive fevers. The so-called erythematous and catarrhal stomatitis may be considered as the primary stages of oral disturbances which if not eradicated at once may degenerate into either one of the above mentioned types of buccal and gingival inflammations.—*Dental Cosmos.*

———

BUSINESS AND PROFESSION.—A business, in its essence, consists in buying and selling—buying in the cheapest, and selling in the dearest, market.

A profession, in its essence, consists in accomplishing the end toward which special skill and special training is directed.

Take one or two simple examples. Merchants, shopkeepers, stock-brokers, are business men, whose main object it is to make as large a turnover as possible; that is to say, all their energies are primarily directed toward the making of profits and the acquisition of wealth. On the other hand, a student of science, an artist, or a physician, these are professional men, who, though they obtain a livelihood by means of their work, are compelled by the very nature of their work to put their work first, and the remuneration they receive for it second. The scientific man, if he is worthy of the name, must make his observations, his investigations, his experiments, his first consideration; the artist, he who is possessed of the creative faculty, if he has any real gift or inspiration, cannot help putting first his picture, his statue, his poem, his sonata; and so also the physician, whose work consists in the application of the healing art—he, unless he is prepared to forfeit the name of professional man, unless he is prepared to prostitute his calling by making it a mere shekel-grinding machine—he must ever direct his energies in the first instance to the healing of sickness, to grappling with disease and death. In other words, he must make his patients' well-being his first consideration. And he must do this, not from a quixotic notion that there is anything derogatory in accepting remuneration for services rendered, but he must do it simply because unless he puts his patients' interests first he will find that the quality of his work will suffer. If a physician makes his pocket, rather than his patient, his first consideration, it is as certain that his work will deteriorate as it is certain that the earth goes round the sun. For if he assumes the unprofessional attitude of the business man who looks first to the profit that is to be made, you will find inevitably that his judgment becomes warped, his knowledge becomes perverted, the edge of his skill becomes dulled and blunted, and he will constantly be taking an easier way than the right way for dealing with his cases, in order to save himself time and trouble and expense. Why is this? Simply because the interests of a man's pocket and the interests of his patients so frequently clash—they are not infrequently diametrically opposed; and so, unless he resolutely keeps before him his patients' welfare as his first, his prime concern, he cannot escape the temptation continually besetting the path of the practitioner to let " second best" stand in the place of " best," and to value a well-filled purse more than the satisfaction that is to be found in rendering faithful service.—L. MATHESON, L.D.S., *Dental Record*, England.

DR. RUDEL'S DETACHABLE WEDGE SEPARATOR.—The object of this apparatus is to facilitate placing the separating wedge in position. It is provided with eight steel wedges, any one of which may be forced between the teeth by screw pressure, after which the apparatus is removed, leaving the wedge in position. Each wedge is provided with a perforation through which a wire may be passed to prevent its slipping back after the pressure is released, and also with a shoulder over which the apparatus may be hooked to facilitate its removal. There seems to be no provision to prevent the wedge pressing unduly into the soft tissues.

DENTAL EXAMINING GLASS (designed by Dr. W. H. Williamson).—This is a lens of one-inch focus enclosed in a round metal tube to prevent as much as possible the breath clouding its surface; it may be stood on either end, and is fitted with studs to prevent its rolling when laid down. It overcomes some objections to the usual watchmaker's lens.

AN EVERTED RIM TUMBLER (designed by Dr. W. A. Hunt).— This is an ordinary tumbler with the edge or rim everted or turned outward; it is said that when so shaped the tumbler comes far more easily to the lips, and is more convenient for feeble patients, or those just recovering from an anæsthetic.

TULLOCH'S ALLOY AND MERCURY MEASURES are intended as a ready means of measuring the amount of alloy and of mercury to be used in mixing for amalgam. The mechanism of the device is not described in the advertisement; as the price is high, it is probably complicated.

FOUNTAIN SPITTOON.—C. J. Plucknett & Co., 28–37 Poland Street, London, W., offer a fountain spittoon to be attached to the wall by a swinging bracket. This has the advantage that all water and waste attachments are made at the wall line, and that it can be swung entirely clear of the chair. The writer used one somewhat similar for years with satisfaction. While the device advertised uses a flexible tube for the waste, the construction may be simplified by making the waste-pipe of the spittoon form the pivot of the bracket, connecting with the drain by a ground joint.

AN AUTOMATIC CYLINDER, for ethyl chloride, graduated on its side, and provided with a stop-cock operated by a gentle pressure with one finger, to secure accuracy of dosage and ease of administration.

Current News.

NATIONAL ASSOCIATION OF DENTAL FACULTIES.

THE annual meeting of the National Association of Dental Faculties will be held at Buffalo, commencing at two P.M. on Thursday, July 27, 1905. The Executive Committee will meet at ten A.M. same day. Special business to come before the National Association of Dental Faculties is the consideration of the proposed revision of the Constitution and By-Laws.

H. B. TILESTON,
Chairman Executive Committee.
JOHN I. HART,
Secretary Executive Committee.

NATIONAL DENTAL ASSOCIATION.

THE ninth annual session of the National Dental Association will be held in Buffalo, N. Y., July 25 to 28, 1905, inclusive.

The Hotel Iroquois has been selected by the Local Committee of Arrangements as head-quarters, where all general sessions of the Association and of the sections will be held. The clinics will be held at the rooms of the Dental Department, University of Buffalo.

Rates at the Hotel Iroquois are: Single room, per day, $1.50, $2.00, and $2.50; rooms for two persons, $3.00 and $4.00; single rooms with bath, $3.00 and $3.50; rooms with bath for two persons, $5.00, $6.00, $7.00, and $7.50; all rooms on the European plan.

The usual railroad rate of one and one-third fare for the round trip, certificate plan, has been arranged for by the Executive Committee.

All pay full fare going, taking the proper certificate therefor from the ticket agent, which, when properly viséd at the meeting, entitles the holder to return for one-third the regular rate.

Tickets going may be purchased from July 20 to 26, and are good returning to and including August 2.

Both the general officers and those of the sections have been working hard to provide an interesting and instructive programme, and a large attendance is expected.

A. H. Peck,
Recording Secretary.

92 State Street, Chicago, Ill.

NATIONAL DENTAL ASSOCIATION CLINIC.

The National Dental Association will meet at Buffalo, N. Y., commencing July 25, 1905. It is the desire of the president and chairman of the Clinic Section to hold the best clinic in the history of the society. The clinics will be held Wednesday and Thursday, July 26 and 27, in the Buffalo Dental College, where there is every facility for making practical operations, as well as ample room for all those wishing to give table clinics. Forty dental operations will be made each day, and there is room for holding three hundred table clinics. Those interested can apply to

Dr. S. W. Bowles, 1315 New York Avenue, Washington, Chairman for District of Columbia, Delaware, and New Jersey.

Dr. E. C. Blasdell, 1 Pleasant Street, Portsmouth, N. H., Chairman for Maine, New Hampshire, and Vermont.

Dr. F. W. Gethro, 31 Washington Street, Chicago, Chairman for Illinois and Wisconsin.

Dr. L. L. Barber, Spitzer Building, Toledo, Ohio, Chairman for Ohio and Indiana.

Dr. S. Eschelman, 421 Franklin Street, Buffalo, N. Y., or Dr. R. Murray, 715 Elmwood Avenue, Buffalo, N. Y., Chairmen for New York and Ontario, Canada.

Dr. M. F. Finley, 1928 First Street, Washington, D. C., Chairman for District of Columbia, Virginia, and West Virginia.

Dr. T. P. Hinman, 22 South Broad Street, Atlanta, Ga., Chairman for Georgia, North Carolina, South Carolina, Florida, Alabama, Mississippi, Tennessee, Louisiana, and Texas.

Dr. H. B. McFadden, 3505 Hamilton Street, Philadelphia, Pa., Chairman for Pennsylvania.

Dr. G. E. Savage, 518 Main Street, Worcester, Mass., Chairman for Massachusetts, Connecticut, and Rhode Island.

Dr. S. H. Voyles, 3201 Washington Avenue, St. Louis, Mo., Chairman for Missouri, Arkansas, Kansas, and Nebraska.

Those having new instruments, appliances, etc., are cordially invited to display them. Communicate with your State Chairman, or with

E. K. WEDELSTAEDT,
Secretary Clinic Section.
204 NEW YORK LIFE BUILDING, ST. PAUL, MINN.

AMERICAN MEDICAL ASSOCIATION, SECTION ON STOMATOLOGY.

THE next meeting of the American Medical Association will be held in Portland, Ore., July 11 to 14, 1905. The programme for the Section on Stomatology is as follows:

1. Chairman's Address. Vida A. Latham, Chicago.

2. "The Causes and the Treatment of the Mouth Manifestations of Certain Metabolic Disorders." Alfred C. Croftan, Chicago.

3. "The Oral Manifestations of Diabetes Mellitus." Herman Prinz, St. Louis, Mo.

4. "The Urine and Saliva in So-called Pyorrhœa Alveolaris." Wm. J. Lederer, New York City.

5. "Further Researches in the Treatment of Interstitial Gingivitis." Eugene S. Talbot, Chicago.

6. "Excretion of Toxic Products into the Mouth, with Relation to Local Infection." Fenton B. Turck, Chicago.

7. "The Relations of Dentistry to General Medicine." Samuel Hopkins, Boston, Mass.

8. "A Common Ground for Medicine and Dentistry." Frank L. Platt, San Francisco.

9. "The Physician as a Dentist." Calvin W. Knowles, San Francisco.

10. "The Physician's Duty to the Child from a Dental Stand-Point." Alice M. Steeves, Boston, Mass.

11. "Dentistry of To-morrow." H. P. Carlton, San Francisco.

12. " What will probably be the Dental Educational Standard for the Coming Decade?" C. C. Chittenden, Madison, Wis.

13. " Fatal Oral Pathologic Conditions." G. V. I. Brown, Milwaukee, Wis.

14. " Surgical Bacteriology of the Mouth." A. H. Levings, Milwaukee, Wis.

15. " Surgical Aspects of Disturbed Dentition of the Third Molar." M. L. Rhein, New York City, N. Y.

16. " The Treatment of Suppurative Affections of the Face and Neck emanating from the Mouth." M. I. Schamberg, Philadelphia.

17. " The Medical Relations of Certain Conditions of the Mouth." L. Duncan Bulkley, New York City.

18. " Some Effects of Inebriety on the Teeth and Jaws." T. D. Crothers, Hartford, Conn.

19. " The Ossification of the Lower Jaw." Edward Fawcett, Bristol, England.

20. " Ankylostomiasis and Tongue Pigment." T. M. Russell Leonard, Grenada, British West India.

21. " Notes on Tooth Genesis in Man." H. W. Marett Tims, London, England.

22. " The Etiology of Tooth Corrugations." G. Lenox Curtis, New York City.

23. " To what Extent are Teeth necessary to the Human Being?" M. H. Fletcher, Cincinnati, Ohio.

24. " Anæsthesia by Ethyl Chloride and Similar Agents." H. C. Miller, Portland, Ore.

25. " The Röntgen Rays in Dentistry." M. Kassabian, Philadelphia.

The programme is entirely scientific. All dentists are invited to be present and take part in the discussions. Those wishing to become members may do so by filling out blanks furnished by the Association, signed by the President and Secretary of State or local dental or medical society, enclosing five dollars, and sending to the Secretary of the Section on Stomatology for his signature. This also includes the *Journal of the American Medical Association* for one year.

VIDA A. LATHAM, *Chairman.*
EUGENE S. TALBOT, *Secretary.*

NEW JERSEY STATE DENTAL SOCIETY.

THE thirty-fifth annual meeting of the New Jersey State Dental Society will be held in the Auditorium, Asbury Park, N. J., commencing July 19, and continuing until July 22, 1905. Headquarters at Hotel Columbia. Rates for one person in room, $3.50; two persons in room, $3.00. Meeting commences promptly at ten A.M. on the 19th. The various committees have been successful in securing eminent practitioners for papers of present interest. Some fifty clinicians in the most modern up-to-date dentistry, and the space in the large Auditorium almost entirely filled with all the newest appliances to practise dentistry.

Friday evening will be devoted to the social side, with a smoker, including a collation and entertainment to the guests, exhibitors, and members. Cut out now the week of July 17, and meet with us.

Seven hundred and fifty-six dentists were registered last July. Make it a thousand this year.

CHARLES A. MEEKER,
Secretary.

MINNESOTA STATE BOARD OF DENTAL EXAMINERS.

THE Minnesota State Board of Dental Examiners will hold a special examination, June 5, 6, and 7, 1905, at the Dental Department of the State University.

The Secretary will be at the Dental Department on the afternoon of June 3 to receive applications. All applications must be in by five P.M. of that date. Application blanks will be furnished upon request, by the Secretary.

F. S. JAMES,
WINONA, MINN.　　　　　　　　　　　　　　　　　*Secretary.*

NORTHERN OHIO DENTAL ASSOCIATION.

THE forty-sixth annual meeting of the Northern Ohio Dental Association will be held June 6, 7, and 8, 1905, at Gray's Armory, Cleveland, Ohio.

This is not only one of the oldest, but is one of the best-attended, meetings in the country. This year the programme is one of unusual strength and interest. The leading subjects for consideration are—

1. Humanitarian Methods.
2. Mistakes.
3. Prophylaxis.

Under the first is considered "High Pressure Anæsthesia," by Dr. C. G. Myers, of Cleveland; and "High Pressure Anæsthesia as compared with other Pain Preventing Methods," by Dr. D. H. Zeigler, of Cleveland.

Essays under the second group include "Mistakes of the Country Dentists," by Dr. R. D. Wallace, Scio, Ohio, "Mistakes of the City Dentists," by Dr. F. J. Spargur, Cleveland, Ohio, and "Mistakes in Ethics," by Professor S. H. Guilford, of Philadelphia, Pa.

The third includes the Essays, "Two Sources of Tooth Life and their Relative Importance," by Dr. D. D. Smith, of Philadelphia, Pa., and "Diseases of the Peridental Membrane and Treatment," by Dr. J. V. Stahl, of Wooster, Ohio.

The Essayists and those who open discussion upon the various papers have been selected for their particular fitness to handle subjects assigned to them.

Under "Mistakes in Ethics," Dr. Guilford will point out. as only he can, some mistakes that are being made by the profession in the relation of its members to each other, together with the mistakes made in treatment of patients and the public. Great good is expected to result from the presentation of this paper and the discussions that follow. Many false impressions have existed in the past and still exist as to the duties we owe to each other, our patients, and the public, and it is expected that the three papers on mistakes will do much to correct this.

Dr. Smith's paper bears upon that all important subject. prophylaxis. He will bring with him a patient showing results accomplished by his method of procedure. He will illuminate his paper with models and instruments.

Throughout the entire programme much attention will be given to the study of Humanitarian Methods (methods which make it possible to perform dental operations free from pain).

The two papers, "Application of High Pressure Anæsthesia," and "High Pressure Anæsthesia as compared with other Pain Preventing Methods," and the discussions to follow, will set forth all that is known of importance in this connection.

There will be about fifty clinics selected and arranged to give the knowledge-seeking dentists the best post-graduate course that can possibly be obtained in a three days' meeting. One session will be devoted to the study of manufacturers' exhibits. The exhibits this year are to be one of the interesting features of the meeting, and the committee has been promised one of the largest exhibits shown in the country.

All communications pertaining to clinics or exhibits should be addressed to the Corresponding Secretary, Dr. W. G. Ebersole, 800 Schofield Building, Cleveland, Ohio.

Special rate of a fare and a third have been granted on the certificate plan by the Central Passenger Association.

The Committee extend a most cordial invitation to the members of the profession to attend.

W. G. EBERSOLE,
GEO. H. WILSON,
VARNEY E. BARNES,
Executive Committee.

MISSOURI DENTAL ASSOCIATION.

THE Missouri State Dental Association will meet in the city of St. Louis, May 24, 25, and 26, 1905.

An excellent programme of papers and clinics is being prepared, and all ethical members of the profession are cordially invited to attend.

SAM T. BASSETT,
Corresponding Secretary.

OKLAHOMA DENTAL ASSOCIATION.

THE fifteenth annual meeting of the Oklahoma Dental Association will be held in Oklahoma City, commencing at eight P.M., May 15, and continuing until the evening of the 17th. Indications are for a large and enthusiastic meeting. The profession is cordially invited to attend.

C. L. WHITE, D.D.S.,
OKLAHOMA CITY, OKLA.
Secretary.

LEBANON VALLEY DENTAL ASSOCIATION.

THE thirtieth annual meeting of the Lebanon Valley Dental Association will be held at Pottstown, Pa., May 16 and 17, 1905.

Meetings, clinics, and exhibits will be held in the "Auditorium," a commodious and well-lighted hall, giving excellent opportunity for exhibits. For space, write the chairman of the Executive Committee,

C. R. SCHOLL.

READING, PA.

SOUTH DAKOTA STATE BOARD OF DENTAL EXAMINERS.

THE next meeting of the South Dakota State Board of Dental Examiners will be held at Mitchell, S. D., July 11, beginning at 1.30 P.M. All candidates will be required to do practical work in both operative and prosthetic dentistry, and should bring all instruments and materials necessary to do the same. Vulcanizer, lathe, and swaging appliances will be furnished by the board. Application, together with fee of ten dollars must positively be in the hands of the Secretary before July 7.

G. W. COLLINS.

"F. D. I." INTERNATIONAL DENTAL FEDERATION.

THE next annual meeting of the Executive Council of the Fédération Dentaire Internationale will convene in Hanover, Germany, August 7, 1905, immediately following the annual meeting of the Central-Verein Deutscher Zahnarzte. Announcement of the programme for the meeting and the projected work for the Federation during the present period will shortly be made through the dental journals and through the official bulletin of the Federation.

EDWARD C. KIRK,
Secretary-General.

THE

International Dental Journal.

VOL. XXVI.   JUNE, 1905.   No. 6.

Original Communications.[1]

SOME RECENT OBSERVATIONS IN METABOLISM AND THEIR IMPORTANCE IN DENTISTRY.[2]

BY SAMUEL A. HOPKINS, M.D., D.D.S., BOSTON, MASS.

IN order to simplify the study of metabolism it is necessary to refresh our memories with a brief reference to protoplasm and some of its properties.

The human body, as you know, is made up of various tissues which enter into the construction of the different organs of the body. We have nerve, muscular, epithelium, connective, and other tissues, each of which has its particular protoplasmic cell, differing in some slight characteristics from cells of the other tissues.

In the complicated structure of the human organism, it is difficult to study the individual cell. We have, however, in the amœba, a low form of protozoan life existing in every stagnant pool, an excellent example of a single protoplasmic cell without tissues and without organs, which has as complete a life cycle as has the complex organism which we call the human body. The amœba receives nutrition; it converts it into energy; it throws

---

[1] The editor and publishers are not responsible for the views of authors of papers published in this department, nor for any claim to novelty, or otherwise, that may be made by them. No papers will be received for this department that have appeared in any other journal published in the country.

[2] Read before The New York Institute of Stomatology, February 7, 1905.

off waste and reproduces itself, and this is life. Weismann tells us that "no amœba ever lost an ancestor by death," the parent cell merely dividing to produce two children.

The tissues of our body are made up, as I said, of these protoplasmic cells, which are receiving nutrition, converting it into energy, and getting rid of the waste.

Protoplasm is an albuminoid substance, which has no recognized histological structure of its own, yet builds up every animal and vegetable tissue. It consists of nitrogen, oxygen, carbon, and hydrogen, and a trace of sulphur in ever changeable and unstable chemical combinations.

Not to go into the recently advanced theory of electrons, it may be said that the shiftings of the molecular combinations of protoplasm produce every expression of life. The poet's dream, the artist's picture, the musician's symphony, and the knock-down blow of the prize-fighter are expressions of the ever-shifting molecular combinations of protoplasm. I have said that protoplasm was an albuminoid substance, and it is evident, therefore, that the protoplasmic cells of the body must depend upon nitrogenous food for their maintenance and activity. The proteids are the nitrogenous food substances which act as tissue-builders and furnish nutrition for the protoplasmic cells. These proteids also produce heat, especially when the carbohydrates and fats are insufficient for the purpose. They vary greatly in their solubility and in their products of decomposition.

Abdelhulden gives the following list of nitrogenous substances which have been split from the proteid molecule which they go to form: glycocol, alanin, amidovalerianic acid, leucine, phrnylalinin, glutamic acid, asparaginic acid, cystein, lysin, aginin, histidin, and others. Buchner has shown that many of these have negative chemotaxis.

Vaughan and Novy, in their excellent work on "Cellular Toxines," have pointed out the fact that many of these substances are toxines capable of great activity. This must be borne in mind, because upon these numerous products of decomposition depend some of the most serious consequences of excessive proteid metabolism. Harrington gives us examples of proteid substances: gluten flour, egg-albumin, blood-fibrin, and casein. In a general way eggs and meat have a large proportion of nitrogen, and are among our favorite forms of proteid food.

Carbohydrates may be looked upon as energy producers, and this energy, converted into heat, is measured by what we know as calories,—a calorie being the amount of heat necessary to raise one kilogram of water one degree centigrade. Fats assist in maintaining the body heat.

It is evident that before the food which we eat finds expression in the work which we do or the thoughts that we think, an infinite variety of chemical changes must take place; and metabolism may be said to be the sum of the chemical changes which take place within the body or within the cells, by which protoplasm is changed to perform special functions.

The building up of the cell we speak of as anabolism, and its breaking down as catabolism. The complete process is metabolism. The protoplasmic cell, in its absorption of nutrition, has the power of differentiation; that is to say, as the blood-stream, laden with nutrition suitable for the various needs of the body, passes through the various tissues, the muscle-cell will seize from the blood-stream that kind of nourishment which is suitable for the maintenance of muscle tissue; while the nerve-cell, ignoring the elements of muscle tissue, will seize and appropriate that which is essential for its particular needs; and so on, through all the tissues. But the presence in the blood-stream of appropriate nutritive material is not the only requirement for proper nutrition. Tired cells will not take up the nutrition presented; cells deprived of oxygen will not convert nutritive material into energy, and cells which do not receive proper exercise cannot throw off waste. And we have presented to us the necessity for normal rest, fresh air, and exercise. The inhibitive action of toxines and of diseases upon the metabolic changes in tissue-cells is very great indeed. Moreover, what I might designate as the electro-vital action of the trophic nerves, while undoubtedly dependent upon cell activity for its power, at the same time furnishes energy to the tissue-cells. You may have the arteries, veins, and capillaries of a given part in perfect condition, and filled with the best possible nutrition, and yet, if you cut off that mysterious vital energy furnished by the trophic nerves, life ceases and the part withers.

Physical chemistry, through the remarkable experiments of Professor Loeb, of California, and others, working in this field, has shown that chemistry of living matter does not differ essentially from the chemistry of inanimate objects, although the chemistry of the body is carried on at a comparatively low temperature.

It would only obstruct the easy comprehension of metabolism to dwell on the nature of the enzymes developed in the body, but it is known that these play an important part in cytology, and their action as catalyzers will doubtless explain many of the changes that go on in the tissues.

Traube discovered that every living cell behaves as if surrounded by a surface film which does not possess equal permeability for water and the substances which may be dissolved in it.

Osmotic pressure can be measured, and the study of this subject and of surface tension has led to the deduction that every particle of protoplasm which is surrounded by watery liquid has on its surface a thin film of oil. Overton has shown that herein lies the explanation of the action of alcohol, ether, chloroform, and similar substances. These have a high degree of solubility in fats, and therefore diffuse most easily in the living cells.

We know that the brain- and nerve-cells are abundantly supplied with fat, and this furnishes a possible explanation of the anæsthetic effects of the substances mentioned.

Speck has shown that when the pressure of oxygen in the air falls below one-third of its normal value, mental activity is soon impaired and consciousness is lost.

Now, before taking up the matter of food and its conversion into nutrition to meet the requirements of the human machine, I wish to express my belief, founded on a reasonably careful observation of followers of *diet systems*, that any one pursuing such a system long enough will end with chronic indigestion, just as surely as the man who follows a system in gambling will end in bankruptcy. The fruit and nut crank, the cereal crank who poultices his stomach three times a day with a mush poultice, the beef-steak and mutton glutton, are in the same danger as the quick-lunch pie fiend, or the dependent on alcoholic stimulants. A reasonable combination of all these foods might make a very appropriate dietary, but a " food hobby," except as once in a thousand times it might meet some pathological requirement, will surely overthrow its victim sooner or later.

While I am far from advocating the system of prolonged mastication introduced by Mr. Horace Fletcher, I am only too glad to pay him a fitting tribute for work which he has done in calling the attention of scientific men and the general public to the possible advantages of a smaller amount of food and a thorough mastication of that which is taken. His explanations do not bear the stamp of scientific accuracy, and his methods are extravagant and difficult to harmonize with the exigencies of our daily life, but he has compelled the attention of scientific men and led to important research work.

There is, I believe, grave danger in the Fletcher method, and instances have been lately recorded where the concentration of mind on the mastication of food and its digestion in the excessive and seemingly ridiculous manner pursued by Mr. Fletcher has led to nervous difficulties in swallowing and to severe indigestion, while the attempt to jump suddenly from a liberal diet to the minimum quantity suggested by him has led to hyperacidity of the stomach and loss of contractile power in the intestines. There is always grave danger in a too rapid change of our habits of life, but much good may come of an intelligent and reasonable attention to the almost lost art of mastication.

We, as dentists, ought to be especially grateful to any one who arouses an interest in this subject. Our respect for our work and the recognition of its importance by other people, as well as our usefulness to mankind, rests chiefly upon establishing the importance of mastication and salivary digestion.

Setting aside for the moment the subject of mastication, the interest of physiologists in Mr. Fletcher was due to the fact that here was a man in unusually good health, having extraordinary bodily energy and a clear active mind, who was subsisting on a much lower daily intake of proteid food than that which had hitherto been supposed to be essential to the maintenance of health; while at the same time, the carbohydrates, as indicated by the number of heat calories, were also considerably below the amount usually considered necessary.

Professor Chittenden, of the Sheffield Scientific School of Yale University, whose book on ' Physiological Economy in Nutrition" is a most important and fascinating one, had Mr. Fletcher under his observation for several months in the winter of 1902–03, and, among other things, asked him to go into the Yale gymnasium and undertake the work which the men in training for the crew were doing. To his surprise, he found that Mr. Fletcher, who was about thirty years older than any of the students, not only went through the arduous exercises of the men in training, but showed less fatigue and exhaustion than did the students.

Some of this work is embodied in an article in the *Popular Science Monthly* for June, 1903. That which appealed to the scientist was not so much the value of prolonged mastication,—which seemed especially to interest Mr. Fletcher,—but the possibility of complete and satisfactory nutrition of the body on an amount of proteid food less than one-half that which had for generations been thought essential to proper nutrition.

The standard established by Carl Voit, of Munich, has been accepted for many years. According to this standard, an adult man, weighing from seventy to seventy-five kilos (equal to about one hundred and fifty-four to one hundred and sixty-five pounds) and doing moderate work, requires one hundred and eighteen grams of proteid, or albuminous food, fifty-six grams of fat, and five hundred grams of carbohydrates, having in all a fuel value of three thousand calories.

To mark the contrast, I will say that Mr. Fletcher, at the time he was under the observation of Professor Chittenden, was taking daily an average of 44.9 grams of proteid matter, thirty-eight grams of fat, and two hundred and fifty-three grams of carbohydrates, with a fuel value of only sixteen hundred and six calories.

If, now, it could be shown that the small amount of nitrogenous food taken by Fletcher was nearer a normal standard than that established by Voit, it would mean an enormous economy in actual dollars and a great economy to the body, which is of no less importance. It is obvious that the strain on the human machine in using and disposing of excessive proteid matter must be very great indeed.

I may as well explain that carbohydrates are oxidized into carbonic acid and water, and except that these carbohydrates may cause an increase of fat which may be uncomfortable, and that they may in some cases give rise to forms of indigestion, they can do no particular harm even in excess, while the proteid foods, which are the builders of the tissues and play the most important part in cell metabolism, differ greatly, as I have said before, in their products of decomposition, many of which are undoubtedly poisonous. These products, absorbed by the intestinal wall and passing through the system in the blood-stream, are capable of seriously interfering with the functional activity of the various organs of the body, while they undoubtedly bear an important part in rendering the individual less resistant to disease.

Biliousness is a very common disturbance which may be attributed to excessive nitrogenous products. The secretions of glands are frequently altered by the poisonous products of decomposing proteids, and it has been well established that the glands which furnish the secretions for digestion are among those frequently affected. Professor Chittenden points out very clearly that the elimination of excessive amounts of these crystalline nitrogenous bodies through the kidneys places upon these organs an unnecessary burden which is liable to endanger their integrity and may result in serious injury and early impairment of function.

With these facts before him, Professor Chittenden thought it wise to ignore the suggestions made by Mr. Fletcher as to the importance of excessive mastication, because he did not wish to have too many factors to complicate his experiments. The sole object in Professor Chittenden's work was, by observations covering a long period of time and made upon different groups of men, to establish if possible a correct standard of food for the human race. It is probable, however, that the interest which had been aroused by Mr. Fletcher did lead, during these experiments, to much greater care in the mastication of food than is ordinarily used at our tables under the circumstances that usually surround us. I may say at once that in all the diets of the different groups of men experimented upon there was no attempt at restricting the kind of food. Everything imaginable entered into their bills of fare: they had coffee and sugar and fruit and cereals and starchy foods and meats, and everything that one could possibly suggest. In fact, everything was done to avoid monotony of diet. In all cases the reduction of their food was gradual. In all cases the appetite was fully satisfied. There was, of course, a tendency to reduce the quantity of meat and eggs taken, because in that way it was easier to cut down the proteids, but the diet was by no means a vegetable diet.

I can only make a brief reference to these experiments, and go on to the conclusions which seem to have a direct bearing upon our work.

The first experiment was with a group of five men who were university professors and instructors, and who took comparatively little exercise, but, on the other hand, were doing important brain-work all the time. There was great variation in age and weight. In these five cases, during the period they were under observation, there was an average excretion of less than eight grams of nitrogen, and the fuel value averaged rather less than two thousand five hundred calories, while the body weight was maintained with slight variations, as was also the nitrogen equilibrium.

You will notice that the extent of proteid metabolism is accurately determined by the nitrogen found in the urine and fæces. A proteid intake of one hundred and eighteen grams would require an excretion of sixteen grams of nitrogen. You will readily see that rather less than one-half the amount of proteid food indicated by the Voit standard was taken, while at the same time the carbohydrates were not increased. A nitrogen equilibrium briefly means that the nitrogenous food eaten should equal the amount of nitrogen excreted. If the nitrogen excreted is greater than the amount taken into the system, it would mean that the tissues were being unduly drained; but if, on the other hand, the excretion is less than the intake, it may be assumed that the system is storing up nitrogen.

These five men, during the period of from six to eight months' experimentation, expressed themselves as feeling unusually well and as having increased capacity for work, and at the end of the experiment they were unwilling to go back to their former dietary. It was impossible, as it was with the other groups of men which I will speak of later, to determine whether their power of resistance to disease was lowered by this diet, because unfortunately they all remained in perfect health. It seems, therefore, that Professor Chittenden has successfully demonstrated that a professional man may practise a physiological economy in proteid food equal to at least one-half the amount called for by the usually accepted dietary standards.

As a matter of practice, the Voit and similar dietary standards answer pretty closely to the amount which the average man consumes. From the reduction mentioned, we may reasonably expect improvement and not impairment in health, with greater capacity for work, greater resistance to fatigue, and probably to disease also.

The next group of men consisted of a detachment of thirteen from the United States Army Hospital Corps, and in their selection particular attention was paid to getting as great a variety of types as possible. In age they ranged from twenty-one to forty-three.

They weighed from fifty-two to seventy-one kilos, and they were showing at the beginning of the experiment an excretion of nitrogen equal to sixteen grams, indicating that they had been averaging an amount of proteid food at least equal to the Carl Voit standard. During the six months following they were doing daily work in the gymnasium, and besides this they had daily drill, setting-up exercises, and other light tasks; that is to say, they were in vigorous exercise. At the end of the six months' period, they were eating less than one-half the nitrogenous food called for by the usual standard, with a fuel value considerably less than the three thousand calories supposed to be necessary. These men were in better physical and mental condition in every way than at the beginning of the experiments.

So much for the soldiers. Admitting all the benefits that were derived from gymnasium work and a regular life, no one can doubt that their mental and physical improvement was due in some measure to the cutting-down of nitrogenous food.

It is also shown by these experiments that the fuel value of accepted standards is probably higher than it need be. It is, however, easier to maintain the nitrogen equilibrium if the fuel value is kept up to a reasonably high point. For the following reason I spoke in the beginning of proteids as tissue-builders and carbohydrates as energy producers, furnishing the fuel for the body. If the carbohydrates fall below the necessary requirements, the proteids will be called upon to furnish heat, and the cells will, therefore, be called upon to give up some of their nitrogen.

The next group to be experimented with consisted of eight university athletes. These were men, unlike the soldiers, in fine bodily condition, and they were exercising their brains in their studies. They were in training, and were taking an enormous amount of proteid food, since it is one of the old beliefs that athletes must be fed on a rich meat diet. Before the experiment some of these men were taking in proteids far in excess of the Voit standard. It might naturally be expected that these men would be intelligently interested in the experiments, and would give their hearty co-operation to Professor Chittenden and his work, and this proved to be the case. At the conclusion of the experiment they were excreting an average of 8.81 grams of nitrogen, corresponding to fifty-five grams of proteid metabolized, instead of double the amount which they were taking when the tests were begun. Although they all had been in training for some time before the beginning of the tests, and were supposed to be in perfect physical condition, yet every man showed improvement in his muscular power in his ability to perform his athletic feats. One man gained two championships, and another won points in track athletics for the first time, on his restricted diet.

Boils and indigestion, so common to the ordinary athlete in training, were unknown, and the capacity for mental work was well maintained.

From these experiments it is fair to deduce that a man either in athletic training or leading a professional life may with safety and, allowing for personal idiosyncrasies, with marked benefit reduce his nitrogenous food to one-half the amount which we usually take. Aside from the money-saving, which is a matter of domestic economy of great importance but not within the scope of this talk, the economy to the body in not having to care for and dispose of an unnecessary amount of food must be very great.

In nearly all the cases upon which Professor Chittenden experimented the amount of uric acid was greatly diminished. This has a direct and exceedingly important bearing upon our treatment of pyorrhœa alveolaris, and I am sorry there is not time to discuss that aspect of the question. To us, as dentists, it is enough to know that faulty metabolism leads to disease. Waste proteid matter creates injurious products of decomposition, which, taken up by the blood, are liable to produce deleterious effect upon all the tissues, including the brain and nerve-centres.

Those of us who wish to take advantage of the benefits to be derived from a reduction in the proteid food we eat, and wish to utilize this knowledge for the benefit of our patients, find ourselves deprived of the wise supervision of such a man as Professor Chittenden, and must look elsewhere for a guide to lead us to this desirable end. Such a guide we may discover in the proper mastication of all food and in reasonable common sense. It must be remembered that all changes in established habits must be made slowly, and that no departure from a generous and varied diet is at all necessary. Overconsumption of food generally comes from rapid eating. It is exceedingly difficult to eat too much if the meal be eaten slowly and each mouthful of food be thoroughly masticated. The appetite is satisfied before the danger point is reached.

It is well-nigh impossible to eat any considerable amount of very rich or highly spiced or indigestible food if you thoroughly masticate each mouthful. Try it with any rich food, and see how many mouthfuls will satisfy your appetite if they are eaten slowly, carefully masticated, and incorporated with the saliva.

(1) Thorough mastication invariably leads to the desire for simple foods.

(2) Mastication promotes the flow of saliva and accomplishes much in the digestion of starchy foods. We had grown into the habit of thinking that salivary digestion accomplished but little, and until the recent work of Dr. Cannon, of the Harvard Medical School, I think physiologists were somewhat inclined to take this view.

About the time that these experiments were being carried on by Professor Chittenden, Dr. Cannon, Assistant Professor in Physiology in the Harvard Medical School, was conducting a series of experiments which seem to throw additional light on one phase of the subject which had not been embraced in Professor Chittenden's work.

Dr. Cannon mixed with the food of cats subnitrate of bismuth, and then proceeded to study the processes of digestion with the assistance of the X-ray, the bismuth making a very satisfactory picture on the fluorescent screen. His methods are most ingenious, and his work most accurate and valuable.

We have long been accustomed to think that if starchy food escaped digestion in the mouth, there were digestive fluids that it would encounter in the intestines that would do the work of digestion. Indeed, it was felt that salivary digestion could not amount to much, because it was erroneously thought to be checked by the acid juices of the stomach. Dr. Cannon showed that while the pyloric end of the stomach had marked peristaltic movement, the cardiac end did not move in this manner. He also found that food particles taken into the stomach remained sometimes for as long a period as an hour and a half in the cardiac portion of the stomach before they became mixed with the acid digestive fluids. It was demonstrated that if food by mastication was thoroughly mixed with the saliva, the salivary digestion thus begun would continue for as long a period as one hour and a half at least after the food had been swallowed, and the vital importance of mastication of starchy foods was established.

Besides the digestion of starchy foods, (3) mastication comminutes the proteid food so that it presents a larger surface to be acted upon by the gastric juices, and relieves the stomach of unnecessary and exhausting labor. (4) It also reduces the danger of ulcers and carcinoma of the stomach to a minimum. Cannon has pointed out that ulcers of the stomach and carcinoma, which occur at the pyloric end, that end being known as the ulcer region, are caused by the rubbing over the delicate mucous membrane of that portion of the stomach of unmasticated lumps of food. They are forced down against the pyloric valve by this peristaltic motion, and then, as the intestine refuses to accept the food in such condition, are thrown back by the closing of the value, and are rubbed backward and forward until ulceration and, in some cases, carcinoma result.

At about the same time, or perhaps slightly previous to this, the medical profession, especially the surgical side of it, had begun to associate ulcers of the stomach with poor teeth, and to-day the medical profession is, by its clinical observation, ready to confirm Dr. Cannon's deduction that unmasticated portions of food produce these lesions at the pyloric end of the stomach.

I have already pointed out to this society on a previous occasion the fact that thorough mastication is the best preservative of teeth against carious action, and I will say further that I have rarely seen an instance of general and rapid carious action in the mouth of an individual who ate slowly and thoroughly masticated his food.

Whether this results from the surface polish given to the teeth or to the brushing off of the bacteria, which are destroyed by the acids of the stomach, or to improved mouth secretions as a result of the healthy stimulus given to the glands, or whether it may be due to an increase in the resistant power of the teeth themselves, the result is the same,—(5) mastication prevents decay. (6) Mastication also prevents disease. I do not speak now of the diseases of the stomach which have their origin in nervous haste or in taxing the stomach with large quantities of unprepared food, but of diseases of specific bacterial origin. We know that nearly all bacteria which produce disease find their entrance into the body by way of the mouth. I have pointed out in a previous paper that pathogenic organisms resting in unclean mouths not only multiply rapidly, but have their virulence increased, and I referred to the pneumococcus as one especially influenced by environment. It seems a far cry from mastication to pneumonia, but it is probably true that the destruction of bacteria by the acid secretions of the stomach goes far to limit disease. This was ably demonstrated by Koch many years ago in the study of the cholera bacillus, and it has been since shown that prolonged mastication, particularly of hard substances, goes far to free the mouth of bacteria. Bacteria are most numerous in the mouth before eating and fewest just after a meal, and the thorough cleansing of the mouth by vigorous mastication must assist in the removal of pathogenic bacteria.

Added to this is the fact that bacteria do not pass through healthy epithelial tissue, but irritated, inflamed, or diseased epithelial tissue lends itself readily to the passage of bacteria, and this latter condition of the alimentary tract may easily be brought about by improper feeding.

(7) The exercise of mastication, besides producing healthy glandular secretions, insures an active and healthy circulation of blood through the tissues of mouth and adjacent parts. It promotes the flow of lymph and secures the healthy nutrition of the teeth themselves.

If this be so in adult life, what must it mean in childhood? The development of the bones of the face and of the teeth, the development of the muscles, and the health of the soft tissues must be very greatly affected by the influence which exercise or its lack affords. There are many serious students of this subject who believe that contracted jaws and accompanying irregularities, adenoid growths, and other diseases of the soft tissues, as well as weakness of the teeth themselves, are largely due to the lack of mastication which our present method of feeding children involves.

I think I have said enough to demonstrate the importance of mastication, but it is interesting to see how, from different points of view, the same conclusions may be arrived at.

In the first place was Mr. Fletcher, who insisted on excessive mastication, and thought that because of excessive mastication smaller amounts of food were needed; then Professor Chittenden, who has demonstrated, without particular attention being given to mastication, that smaller amounts of food are required than we had supposed; then Dr. Cannon's excellent work, showing the danger, from another point of view, of swallowing unmasticated food and the possibilities of salivary digestion if the food was thoroughly masticated; and then the clinical evidence provided by the medical profession of the results of bolting our food.

I should like to include in this paper something of Professor Pawlow's work on nervous and psychological influences of digestion, but I have already taken too much of your time.

In conclusion, I think it will be admitted that in the conservation of the organs of mastication we as dentists have a life work second in importance to no other, and as these truths which I have brought to your attention become more and more recognized, the respect and admiration of the world for our profession will be greater than ever before. It is by the conscientious study of these problems that we make ourselves worthy of the respect and confidence which the public reposes in us.

CONDITIONS OF FAILURE.[1]

BY E. K. WEDELSTAEDT, ST. PAUL, MINN.

MR. PRESIDENT AND GENTLEMEN,—These pictures are made from casts of a condition of failure, which I have obtained for your consideration. If you will compare the conditions represented in the pictures with those you can find existing in the casts, you will observe that the artist has painted an accurate reproduction of the faulty environment which originally surrounded the mesial and distal surfaces of that lower right second bicuspid and the adjacent first molar. If you will examine the cast containing the two gold fillings, you will see to what an extent recurrence of decay has destroyed that portion of the distal surface of the second bicuspid which lies to the buccal of the gold filling. It was not possible to show the cavity of decay that existed to the buccal of the gold filling which had been placed in the mesial surface of the molar. One of the casts, however, very fully illus-

---

[1] Read before the Academy of Stomatology, Philadelphia, December, 9, 1904.

trates this, and gives us an excellent idea of the size of the cavities after the fillings had been removed. The size of the cavities, however, can be compared with the size of the gold fillings. In making this comparison you can obtain a very good idea of the differences which existed in the size of the cavities before and after the fillings had been removed.

In September, 1903, the young man from whom I obtained the impressions from which these casts were made consulted me regarding the condition of that lower right first molar. He complained of the loss of an amalgam filling which had occupied part of the disto-occlusal surface. He was to leave the city in the evening, but wished some kind of temporary operation made. The cavity was filled with cement, and in September, 1904, he returned and made an appointment to have a somewhat different operation made. The first step toward making this operation was to obtain separation, for the contact point between the molars was at the gingival margin. The Perry separator was adjusted and the teeth lifted apart, the cavity and space filled with gutta-percha, an appointment made to make the operation, and the patient dismissed for the time being. He returned, per appointment, and after preparing the cavity I decided that a gold crown would be the best thing for the tooth. If you will examine any of the casts, you will observe that the first molar contains outlines of fillings in the occlusal, buccal, lingual, and mesial surfaces. The filling in the buccal surface was of unusual size, and that portion of the crown to the occlusal of the filling did not have the appearance of being very strong. Besides this, I found a cavity of decay to the buccal of the gold filling that had been placed in the mesial surface, which made it necessary to remove that filling. In consulting with the patient, however, I found that he wished both cavities filled. The cavity in the disto-occlusal surface called for a very extensive operation, and on account of the condition of the tooth just spoken of I was unwilling to make the operation with gold. An amalgam filling was therefore made in the cavity in the disto-occlusal surface, as is illustrated in Figs. 2 and 5. A week later the amalgam filling was polished, and then an impression of the parts was taken. Thereafter several impressions were taken. The casts from the impressions are herewith presented for your examination.

I next turned my attention to the faulty conditions existing in

the mesial surface of the molar and the distal surf
adjacent bicuspid. (You will observe from the illust
well as the conditions existing in the casts, that the orig
tor had a penchant for placing his point of contact at tl
margin. In fact, I may as well tell you now that the
of affairs exists among fillings in the teeth which ar
other parts of this young man's mouth. Evidently l
dentist is not making a comprehensive study of the
with which he deals.) The separator was adjusted and
moved until there was ample space between that molar ar
in which to operate and make fillings which would restor
to a condition of normality. While the separator was st
the fillings were removed and the cavities, as well as
filled with pink base gutta-percha. (The filling in
occlusal surface of the bicuspid was loose.) Prior to
the separator a piece of gutta-percha was placed between
and bicuspid, and then an impression taken. After the
was obtained the gutta-percha was removed, the separato
space obtained, and the fillings removed and placed in t
in the impression with the gutta-percha. The casts are j
came from the impressions. They have not been trim:
cavity of decay in the distal surface of that bicuspid w
It is precisely as it came from the impression. If yo
amine Cast 4, you will observe there are still some re
the modelling compound left in the interproximal spac
the bicuspid and molar. A week or ten days after spac
obtained between the molar and bicuspid the young ɪ
per appointment, and I at once took an impression
gutta-percha *in situ.* On removing the impression
percha was removed and placed in the impression. T
I obtained the casts containing the cavities. The cav
mesio-occlusal surface of the molar was first filled, an
the cavity in the disto-occlusal surface of the bicuspid
On completion of the operations another impression ɪ
Two views have been made of each of the occlusal surfac
reason that it is not possible to shade with gold paint
this, I was very desirous that this particular case be
understood.

For a number of years I have been asking the memt
profession that they study with some care the causes whi

the failure of dental operations. From time to time I have illustrated my remarks with pictures similar to these which are before us. I feel that some good has resulted, and at the present time a few men are thinking along these lines with perhaps more thought than they have previously given this subject. Considerable work of this kind is being done by the men living in the Northwest. Perhaps fifty or sixty men are now taking impressions, and some of these men have a collection of casts of many conditions of failure. My own collection contains about a thousand casts; it may be a trifle more or less. There must also be two hundred or more of just such pictures as I have here, which are used to illustrate the conditions I may speak of, in an effort to interest other practitioners in this work. In talking to these men I say, Observe the conditions as they exist between this second bicuspid and first molar. You all certainly know that decay in the teeth of the young begins at or near the point of contact. After decay has progressed for a while the break in the continuity of the arch causes the teeth to move more closely together. As the teeth move together the interproximal space is constantly being narrowed. If decay is allowed to progress and no attention be given it, the interproximal space is very often entirely obliterated. The teeth contact from the gingival margin to the occlusal surface. Very frequently there is not a point of contact, but a contacted surface. This is an abnormal condition, and before any permanent filling is made in those cavities the teeth should be returned to their normal positions. Notice the point of contact between the first and second molars. The contact there is just below the occlusal surface. There is neither a lingual nor a buccal embrasure between the second bicuspid and first molar. Observe the embrasures here between the first and second molars. Perhaps both the conditions are better illustrated here in Diagram 3. Why was not the disto-lingual portion of that filling in the second bicuspid properly trimmed? A careful examination of the fillings in the casts seems to prove that the man used a rotary disk in the dental engine. With this rotary disk he could not trim the filling to form and give it a proper contour, provided he ran the disk between the fillings from the occlusal surface to the gingival margin. Examine the cast of this condition. Look for a moment at the filling in the disto-occlusal surface of that second bicuspid. The gold extends just to the disto-bucco-occlusal angle. From the disto-bucco-occlusal angle the filling begins to slope toward the lingual. The farther the filling extends gingivally, the greater is the slope toward the lingual. Thus, there is left on the distal surface of that tooth a very faulty condition. This condition we speak of as a condition which invites caries. I have observed, wherever this condition is made or left on any surface of a tooth, sooner or later we have a cavity of decay beside the filling. Such conditions invite disease. Food is wedged in the space between the fillings; it is held there and undergoes changes in its composition, fermentation takes place, an acid is produced, and naturally disease ensues. I have observed that decay naturally follows where such faulty conditions have been left. The man who made these operations evidently overlooked the object in filling teeth. Of this object I have spoken a great many times, and it is, or should be, to take the abnormal conditions as they come to us and return the parts to as near a condition of normality as lies in our power. The original operator in this case did not restore conditions to what is known as normal. I speak thus plainly for the reason that there is always a space at the gum line between teeth which are normal and which are normally situated. In a number of skulls which I have examined I find that the space at the gum line between the lower second bicuspid and first molar is about 1.7 millimetres. In measuring this space as I find it to exist between the same teeth in the mouths of some of my patients, I find that 1.7 millimetres closely approximates the measurement which I have obtained of this space among the teeth in skulls. I find, however, that the space which is in this plaster-of-Paris cast, between the teeth just spoken of, measures 1.8 millimetres, but I do not think that that makes any difference. You can take the condition as it exists between this second bicuspid and molar, in Diagram 3, and compare it with the condition as it exists between the same teeth in Diagram 6.[1] In Diagram 3 you have the abnormal condition pictured, and in Diagram 6 you have the normal condition pictured. At the same time you can make a comparison of the condition as it exists upon the occlusal surface between those two gold fillings, as they are pictured in Diagram 2, with the same condition as it is pictured in Diagram 6. In Diagram 2 you have no point of contact between the fillings. The lingual and buccal embrasures are too

---

[1] Diagrams not furnished for illustration.—ED.

narrow for the purpose for which they are intended. Compare the size and shape of the lingual and buccal embrasures as they are pictured in Diagram 6 with those in Diagram 3. In Diagram 6 you have a point of contact; you have a proper contour given the fillings, consequently the interproximal space is properly contoured. In Diagram 6 we do not have any condition pictured which invites disease. In Diagram 3 you can readily see what we have. The pictures of these conditions speak for themselves. Let us turn once more to Diagram 3. The reason that we did not have any inflammation of the gum between the second bicuspid and first molar is this: The gold filling in the mesial surface of this molar was flattened linguo-buccally from the occlusal surface, gingivally to and including the gingivo-cavo-surface angle of the cavity. From the looks of both the tooth and filling, the entire mesial surface of this molar is flat. But if you will observe the condition of the gingival third of the distal surface of this second bicuspid, you will find that the operator did not pass his rotary disk to the gingival of the middle third. As a consequence, the molar moved mesially and the point of contact was practically between the gingival margins. If, however, the operator had run his disk completely through this space, so that he would have cut away the gingival margin on the distal surface of that second bicuspid, the chances are that the gum septum between the second bicuspid and molar would have been a mass of disease.

For somewhat over twenty-five years I have kept a very careful record of every dental operation which I have made. During this time a number of families have been my patients. I have, therefore, been in a position to observe what the results are where gold fillings, like these pictured in Diagram 2, have been made. Not only have I observed that recurrence of decay always takes place among similarly made operations, which I myself may have made, but it has been my observation that failure of just such operations takes place where they have been made by other men in the profession. To illustrate this a little further, permit me to say that I am a member of the G. V. Black Dental Club of St. Paul. For almost ten years the members of this Club have been carrying on a sort of continuous post-graduate work. Many of the men in this organization are also obtaining casts of the conditions of failure, and they frequently bring these casts to our meetings. A number of our men have made many casts of just such failures as I have here illustrated for your consideration. Now, the membership of the Black Club is scattered over these three Northwestern States. I am, therefore, in a position to state that the conditions of failure that I have here illustrated are not confined to any special locality, among any special set of operators, or among any special set of patients, for all our men find just one thing,—that these conditions of failure always take place where an opportunity is made or left for disease to obtain a foothold. It sometimes seems to me that altogether too many men stumble and fall regarding what constitutes an "opportunity." If we could but firmly establish our ideas regarding what *opportunity* means, and eradicate all opportunities for the recurrence of caries, there would be no necessity for any more essays on "Conditions of Failure of Dental Operations."

Where a man has a dozen casts of conditions which fully illustrate a failure of some dental operations, and he also has casts which illustrate the correction of the conditions, that man is in a position to obtain much independent knowledge, provided he studies the different conditions before him in an intelligent as well as a comprehensive manner. By taking one of the casts illustrating a failure, and obtaining an expression of opinion from four or five other men regarding the cause of that failure, he is greatly benefited by comparing the expressed ideas of others with those he may have of the causes which led to that condition. By this means he can very greatly increase his sphere of usefulness by taking advantage of the knowledge he obtains and in future avoiding the making or leaving of just such faulty conditions as may have led to the failure which he has a copy of. To the student, to the men possessed of a receptive mind, or to any person who wishes to learn, I know of nothing which so materially assists and so greatly aids in a person's advancement as having a collection of just such casts as I have presented for your consideration.

The various elements which enter into and which directly lead to failure are daily being better, as well as more fully, understood through a comprehensive study of the many conditions which lead to failure of dental operations. Among a few men this special work has been reduced to a science. These men have given up much time to a study of conditions which lead to failure. Before many years this special part of our work will be reduced to a system, and these faulty conditions will be as fully understood by all intelligent men as they are to-day by the few who are earnestly striving to do the best which can be done. Teachers will also take up this matter and give instruction regarding it, so that those leaving institutions of learning will be in a position to understand and cope with the conditions which experience has taught are pitfalls, and, therefore, to be avoided. I am of the opinion that the great advance which has been made by some of the men who are living in the Northwest can be traced directly to a continual study of such faulty conditions as are illustrated in these casts. I know of no other method which so fully brings the facts right home to men, thus making a lasting impression, as does this method of having, in plaster-of-Paris casts, copies of conditions of failure.

I thank you very sincerely for honoring me with an invitation to express my views to the members of your society. If I have interested you in this subject, then I have done all that mortal can do.

GOLD PLATES HAVING TEETH ATTACHED WITH VULCANITE.[1]

BY F. J. M'LAREN, NEW YORK, N. Y.

ONE of the most useful dentures we have is the gold plate having the teeth attached with vulcanite. With all its advantages there is one great drawback,—namely, the necessity under ordinary circumstances of removing the rubber attachment if for any reason we are obliged to solder with gold, as when there is a fracture of the gold, or, in partial cases, if the addition of an isolated tooth or an extra clasp is required.

This not only involves a great amount of labor, but is always a source of dissatisfaction to the patient, because, in spite of every precaution, it is impossible to replace the teeth precisely as they were and to which the patient was accustomed.

In consequence I have found it necessary to devise certain methods of overcoming the difficulty, and believing that these are not ordinarily practised, I will endeavor to explain them. For instance, a case which frequently presents is one where an incisor has to be replaced, the plate being one having the bicuspids and

---

[1] Read before The New York Institute of Stomatology, February 7, 1905.

molars attached with vulcanite. The usual impression is taken
with the plate in the mouth, and after pouring the model the
selected tooth is backed and placed in position; a tail-piece is
now fitted from the tooth reaching to and overlapping the plate.
The tooth and tail-piece, being properly adjusted, are removed
from the plate invested and soldered together. The tooth with
the tail-piece soldered to it is now placed on the model and attached to the plate with hard wax. An investment is now made
with which it is possible to have one portion of the plate cold,
thereby protecting the rubber, and another part red hot to facilitate
soldering. The investment is made in the following manner; first
adapt pieces of iron to that portion of the plate under the rubber
attachment; then use one or two large iron bars about the size of
the ridge and extending about two inches back of the plate. If the
bars do not come in sufficient contact with the plate, fill in the
space between the gold and the bars with small nails, binding them
all together with fine iron wire. Invest in plaster and asbestos,
mainly asbestos. Make the investment in three sections separated from one another, one on either side protected by the metal,
the third isolated from the plate but connected with the other
two by means of small bent wires, leaving bare the portion to be
soldered.

Place the case on a retort frame, exposing the isolated tooth
to the heat of a Bunsen burner, being careful not to permit
the heat to touch the part protecting the rubber. While the
tooth is being heated use a bulb syringe to drop a little cold water
on the side investments. This will allow the front tooth to become red for soldering, while the main plate will be perfectly
cold. When the tooth becomes red transfer the investment to a
soldering pan and have an assistant apply water constantly to
the side investments and iron bars while the heat from the blow-
pipe is concentrated on the point to be soldered. Apply the heat
rapidly, and do not for a moment allow the plate to become cold
until soldering is completed.

When a plate has been split, reinforce with a thin piece of
gold held in place by means of small clamps made of thin iron
wire or other material, and place 18-carat filings between the
piece of gold and the main plate.

For applying a clasp close to the vulcanite, it may be necessary
to cut away part of the rubber in order to get a sufficient thick-

ness of non-conducting material, usually asbestos cloth, and where the clasp is very close to the rubber there may be danger of scorching, but the trouble of replacing a small surface of vulcanite is slight as compared with taking off the teeth and disturbing the articulation. Too much stress cannot be placed upon the advisability of using a concentrated flame, and while, as a rule, I use the ordinary foot-power blow-pipe, in many instances it will be found necessary to attach a cylinder of nitrous oxide gas to the air-tube of the blow-pipe. This gives an intense concentrated heat to the point of soldering.

I have successfully used the foregoing methods for several years, and hope that I have been able to make myself clear, as these suggestions may help to eliminate one of the many annoyances in the existence of a busy dentist.

THE RELATION OF THOROUGH MOUTH TREATMENT OF FOOD TO THE AFFECTIONS OF THE TEETH.[1]

BY DR. HORACE L. HOWE, BOSTON, MASS.

THAT the teeth and adjoining tissue are influenced by the general health is a fact long known to science.

Every truth has its corollary.

Thus the general health of the individual is, to a certain extent, influenced by the teeth; in that they are essential for the proper mouth treatment of food, which goes to build up tissue upon which every faculty of mind and body is dependent.

We cannot ignore the function of any part of the body, or any faculty of the mind, without impairing, to a degree, the total capacity of body or mind.

Every part is dependent, to some extent, upon other parts, and has its relation to the whole.

If we attend to the voluntary part of nutrition, or the stage of digestion before the food goes to the stomach, nature will perform the involutary part to perfection.

---

[1] Read before the Harvard Odontological Society, April 20, 1905.

It is my object to-night not to give an extended account of the affections of the teeth, but simply to agitate the subject of nutrition as related to the teeth.

To do this best I will refer to a book written by Mr. Horace Fletcher, and called "The A, B, and Z of Our Own Nutrition."

Mr. Fletcher is startling the medical world with his discoveries regarding right living, and is devoting his life and means in telling the world of his deductions.

That he has searched out the cause of diseases arising from perverted nutrition is acknowledged and accepted by the most eminent physiologists in this country and in Europe.

To show the appreciation of Mr. Fletcher's discoveries by the medical profession, I will quote the following from a letter written him by Dr. J. H. Kellogg, of the Battle Creek Sanitarium, who says, "It is a remarkable spectacle that these great men, these learned professors and scientists and army medical men, should be co-operating so enthusiastically with a layman to learn the true philosophy of life, but it has always been so. The great discoveries have not been made by great scientists and great doctors, but by men whose minds were above the bias of prescribed education, and who were able to learn from the great book of nature."

Mr. Fletcher's discovery is as simple as many great discoveries are, and is this: That we should chew our food until it becomes practically liquefied and of alkaline reaction, by means of our saliva.

In criticism, some say that Mr. Fletcher places too much importance upon the function of mastication, and that some people are troubled with hypochlorhydria or too little hydrochloric acid in the stomach.

For a moment let us consider the process of nutrition. All our food is acid in a varying degree. Our saliva neutral,—but alkaline when we masticate,—our gastric juice acid, and so on, alternating with the other digestive fluids. We understand by Anstie's well-known law—*i.e.*, "glands exciting alkaline fluids are stimulated by the presence of acids"—and the reverse—"glands exciting acid fluids are stimulated by the presence of alkalines"— that the natural stimulus for the gastric glands would be alkalines; that is, the food, after it has been made alkaline by the saliva. If we swallow our food without sufficient chewing, the gastric glands are thus deprived of their natural stimulus, which perhaps may account for the state of hypochlorhydria.

Is it surprising that our stomachs become sour, as the expression is, and rebel, and assimilation and metabolism is affected, when we swallow our food (artificially acid, possibly) without proper mastication? The expression of this rebellion may be slight and soon overcome, but if the abuse goes on disease is sure to follow.

In my own case severe headaches were the forms in which nature showed the result of my neglect. These have been completely eradicated by strict attention to the mouth-treatment of my food.

Let us trace the process of digestion from infancy. Naturally the child is nourished by the human milk, which is normally alkaline in reaction. This is taken directly into the stomach. Thus the gastric glands have their natural stimulus,—*i.e.*, alkaline milk. As the temporary teeth erupt, the salivary glands develop. As the child is given food, the least acid foods first (cow's milk, eggs, crackers, etc.), the salivary glands become equal to the task of converting them into an alkaline solution. If the task be too great, then the trouble begins.

We have all noticed that those who are troubled by pyorrhœa alveolaris have the so-called "general uric acid diathesis," and are also troubled with pains in the joints of the extremities, or gout, rheumatism, constipation, etc.

Dr. Michaels, of Paris, in his very scientific treatise upon saliva, says, "The reaction of the blood to the ordinary agents (litmus, for example) is normally alkaline, but if we study the distribution of acids and bases of the *blood plasma*, we see that the reaction is really acid (Gautrelet, Drouin, Hugorenq), and this acidity is increased and the blood may become decidedly acid by the accumulations of acid waste products, which are not eliminated; the *secretions* and *excretions* becoming then of acid reaction."

This would lead us to believe that the serumal deposits upon the teeth, in cases of alveolar pyorrhœa are salts or urates from the blood, produced by the overacid condition of the system.

The attachments of the teeth to the alveoli are now recognized as true joints. Why is it not reasonable to suppose that deposits might be formed in these joints from the same cause as in the joints of the extremities?

Furthermore, it has been my observation that children who are troubled with sour stomachs and bilious attacks are apt to have present the rapid, soft, white caries so destructive to teeth.

Are not these diseases of the teeth, both caries and pyorrhœa alveolaris, brought on by the absence of the normal amount of alkaline saliva, locally in the mouth and systemically by the absence of nature's neutralizing fluid in the stomach? Tests that I have made seem to bear out this theory.

Since becoming especially interested in this subject I have tested my own saliva and that of many of my patients for acidity. There are many factors that vary the reaction, as we can see by Dr. Michaels's observation. It seems to be normally neutral, but becomes alkaline with the muscular movements of chewing, whether food be present or whether we chew but rubber. It is less alkaline in the morning after sleeping; the muscles of the tongue and jaws being then at rest. It has been observed that it becomes acid after extreme bodily fatigue. In my own case, when I do not feel well my saliva is decidedly acid.

We all know of Gladstone's health, and of his invariable rule of chewing thirty-two times before he swallowed his food.

The remedy for these difficulties that I have pointed out seems to be had in chewing thoroughly the food that we take, thus using Nature's method of neutralizing the system.

However, "reason has but little show against intrenched habit," hence it requires some strength of mind to overcome habit in order to give our food thorough mouth treatment.

It is true that people live, perhaps in good health, without paying particular attention to the voluntary part of digestion; if such be the case, however, the balance is maintained by getting rid of the excess of acids, by perspiration, or by living upon the least acid foods, as eggs, milk, etc. For instance, the Japanese, who live chiefly upon a diet of fish, rice, and other vegetables, are particularly healthy and energetic.

Those who have become vegetarians in this country notice a great improvement in general health and also in the health of the teeth and gums.

The influence of natural living upon the development and condition of the teeth is nicely shown by Dr. Campbell, of London, England. He divides the evolutionary career of man into five stages.

1. The anthropoid stage; with raw vegetable and animal food. Carious teeth were then unknown.

2. The pre-cooking stage, or the stage before the human race used fire for cooking. No caries of the teeth present.

3. The pre-agricultural period, to which period the aboriginal Australians and Bushman still belong and are available for study, with dental caries rare, and chiefly met in the third molars.

4. The early agricultural age, with dental caries more frequent.

5. The late agricultural period, or the time in which we of to-day live.

The chief characteristic of the food of to-day is its extreme softness, due to agriculture and cooking; therefore it requires little mastication. Because of the physiological law, "that the use of a part tends to stimulate its growth and development, and disuse to lack of development and atrophy," the teeth and jaws are less developed and more diseased to-day than in the previous ages.

In this same way Dr. Campbell very aptly places the cause of *adenoids and resulting evils, among them irregular teeth, to insufficient stimulation of the blood in the jaws from lack of exercise of the muscles of mastication.*

In studying the skulls of the early Indians, Hawaiians, and Peruvians at the Peabody Museum, I have noticed the comparative absence of caries and irregularity about the teeth. The greater number have good, sound teeth, much worn, but no *distal occlusion* which accompanies adenoids and undeveloped jaws.

The Ancients used to blame their stomachs for all their ills. Possibly the blame was justly placed, and the word hypochondriac (stomach region) and its modifications may rightly express the truth.

The real influence that lack of thorough mouth-treatment of food and perverted nutrition has upon all diseases, both mental and physical, is fast being made clear by the great scientists of the medical profession. For instance, Dr. Haig, the well-known expert on diet, points out that laziness, stupidity, alcoholism, and other effects that are much against the poor are largely due to excessive meat eating, and estimates that in seventy-five per cent. of the cases of insanity, cancer, debility, and degeneration generally, improper food and habits of eating are to blame for the patients' condition."

Medical history reveals the fact that the greatest physicians have used medicines only to soothe or alleviate suffering. They tried to impress their patients with the importance of proper feeding, exercising, fresh air, etc., whereas the small ones of the profession have used medicine with the idea of curing, and have neglected and overlooked the natural means. As every faculty of the mind and body grows strong only through exercise, so do the teeth grow strong only by exercise.

If we can impress our patients with the importance of the thorough mouth-treatment of food as related to general health, and likewise to the health of the teeth, we can perform for them no greater service.

No one has better opportunity for studying the cause and effect of the abnormal conditions of the saliva than we, whose daily work consists so largely in restoring to usefulness the delicate and highly sensitive dental organs, that are constantly bathed in this very interesting fluid.

I realize that this short paper does not do the subject justice; but if the facts that I have tried to bring out should but stimulate any one to further investigation, the object of this paper will have been fulfilled.

DENTAL EDUCATION FROM THE VIEW OF EXPERIENCE.[1]

BY JAMES TRUMAN, D.D.S., LL.D., PHILADELPHIA.

THE following propositions are, in the opinion of the writer, fundamental to a proper realization of ideals in education.

1. A decided mental tendency, in the individual, in one direction.

2. This established, training must be to develop these mental tendencies.

3. Dental education, to be effective, must, therefore, be developed from these original tendencies; if these are in the direction of its complex character, practical and theoretical.

---

[1] Read at the Fourth International Dental Congress, St. Louis, August 29 to September 3, 1904.

4. In this education the *practical* must *precede* the theoretical.

Considering these propositions *seriatim* it must be conceded that the mental tendencies of the individual are primarily the most important for the educator to consider. The study of the mental inclinations of youth belongs not alone to the teacher, but is part of the important relations held by parents and guardians. The latter may regard this a difficult problem to solve, belonging more properly to the specialist in psychological manifestations. To reason thus is a fatal error, and one so often made that it has become a very serious evil, forcing young minds in wrong directions and wrecking innumerable lives in vain attempts to acquire, to them, useless knowledge.

The general idea prevalent—not alone among parents, but as a part of the general educational thought—is that education, to be of value, must run along hard and fast lines, and that without variation, to meet these special tendencies; in other words, the child is placed, as it were, in a straight-jacket from the time of entering school until the period at which the diploma is reached. This may be the A.B. of the high school, or this degree in Arts of our universities or colleges. Is it any wonder that the student whose tastes run counter to all this should regard with aversion this iron-clad method? The average teacher, however, holds that all that is necessary to draw out the best in the individual is to force the undeveloped being through the universal educational mill. It is immaterial to this teacher whether the student is to become a mechanic, an architect, a minister, a lawyer, a doctor, a dentist, or a journalist; in fact, any of the varied and useful occupations that go to make up what we term civilization. To merely name this variety stamps the preliminary work, as usually given, as the weak point in the school training of America. They have a far better idea of education in some parts of Continental Europe, in that the training is in the direction of the future work of the student, but, while this is an advance, it takes but a limited account of the mental tendencies of the individual. It is true that a thorough classical education is of untold value to any individual, and, other things being equal, may give power and marked advantage over his less fortunate competitor in the race of life; but this will depend so much on natural tendencies and the subsequent use made of these, that no one can wisely prophesy the future of the individual.

Two prominent and very recent illustrations in this country
serve to give point to this by no means original idea. One, a
graduate in arts from one of the leading colleges of the country,
found his acquirements of no practical value in the active world.
His training, good as it was for certain purposes, furnished nothing
that would enable him to reach a position consonant with his tastes
and necessities. His learning failed to meet the demands of his
daily needs, and, nothing else offering, he bravely accepted the
humble position of a laborer on a railway. The result was that
step by step he advanced from this to the position of motorman on
an electric street-car. From this, the presidency, at an early age,
of the system of street railways in the largest city of the country
was the natural result of untiring efforts and original mental
training in other directions.

The other began with no such education; in fact, his scholastic
training was below the average. He started as brakeman on a
railroad, and from that, through all grades, became eventually
many times a millionaire, a United States Senator, and has
recently been nominated for the position of Vice-President of the
United States by one of the great political parties of this country.
The conclusion to be derived from these examples, not at all
uncommon, is that the first demonstrates the power of a liberal
education when started in the direction of the natural bent of
mind in the individual; and the second, that defects in education
may be overcome by mental force concentrated on one object.

If, then, it be true that a mental tendency in the individual is
all important and must be sought for, when found it becomes of
vital importance that the training should be in the direction of
these natural tastes. The problem becomes complicated when the
individual exhibits no special proclivities, but seems willing to
drift along with the world's current. General laws are not for
these, however, and the only test for this very large class of young
persons is to prove their capacity in some one or more directions.
When, however, the tendency is marked, every effort should be
made to begin the individual's career properly. If this is in the
direction of mechanics, no mistake will be made if during the
impressible period of youth the muscles are placed in training in
schools especially devoted to this work. This experience will be
of inestimable value should the youth subsequently prefer the

literary training necessary to become a doctor of medicine, minister, or lawyer. Especially will this apply to the surgeon.

Dental education, then, to be effective must be based on an early investigation of the mental tendencies, and these being discovered, the direction which education must take is then plain. Dentistry is a complex study. It begins with the practical and ends with the theoretical, or should so end. From what has already been stated, the necessity for early muscular training in mechanics must be apparent. No other course is left open. Every added year lost in this cultivation is just one year of less ability to overcome mechanical problems.

The idea is often taught, and as often combated, that the theoretical must precede the practical; in other words, the individual must have a special training before he is supposed to be fitted to begin his work in dentistry. The Association of Faculties says the applicant for the degree of Doctor of Dental Surgery must first show, on matriculating, a certificate of entrance to the third year of a high school. Nothing is said as to the character of the training given in the high school. Our universities demand a fixed standard, easily understood, and very much higher than the ordinary routine of studies. What is the result? Our dental colleges are inundated with educated young men, who have been sent by those in authority over them to master a calling, a prerequisite to success in which is, at least, a taste for mechanical work. Nothing in their previous studies leads to a knowledge of this bent of mind, and the results, therefore, are not always satisfactory.

To decide this question of fitness for the proposed study, the practical must precede the theoretical, and any other course, as far as dentistry is concerned, is simply a great wrong perpetrated in the name of higher education. No greater mistake can be made than to place a youth in a medical college as preliminary to his dental training. The time may come, indeed, is fast coming, if not already here in some institutions, of carrying the studies of medicine and dentistry *pari-passu*. This will doubtless lead to the M.D. degree, but a much longer period of probation than the present four years of training will be required to secure separately either of the degrees of M.D. or D.D.S. The experience of dental educators has been, and this has been confirmed in the writer's life work, that the individual who has passed from the higher schools into those of medicine, and then essays the study of dentistry, fails, with few exceptions, in reaching a high degree of skill. The evidences of the truth of this are among the most painful of the writer's experiences as a teacher in dentistry, and this alone would lead him to enter an earnest protest against this, to him, fatal error in the future proposed education of dentists.

There has been a general impression that the higher preliminary education, if it did not increase ability in the two practical branches of dentistry, would, at least, enable the student to hold his own and, in other respects, make him more valuable in the community. This view is partially borne out by the averages taken in the Dental Department of the University of Pennsylvania. The following table illustrates the average standing of the several classes in Prosthetics and Operative Dentistry from the period when the Department accepted students upon a grammar-school certificate to the time when a high-school diploma was required.

Certificate.	Mechanical Dentistry.	Operative Dentistry.
Grammar school	76.22	84.82
First year high school	81.19	85.91
Second year high school	83.13	80.97
Diploma, high school	75.47	86.54

While averages are somewhat misleading, yet, so far as this goes, as the result in one school, it may be taken as an indication that the boy from the grammar schools stands an equal chance with the boy with a high school diploma in mastering the practical work of dentistry, but it is very evident that the higher education has not improved the high school boy's ability in meeting the difficulties of the practical over the one of the lower. It, however, does show that the higher preliminary training enables the one who has it to hold his own in the realms of the practical and will give him an immense advantage in acquiring the collateral branches peculiar to medicine.

In conclusion, dental education must be first based on mental tendencies, and, these proved, then the education should begin with manual training work. It is immaterial where this is secured. From this the practical side of dentistry, the prosthetic, must be conquered. This will furnish the foundation for the operative branch, and these two constitute the necessary practical for the attainment of success in the future professional life work of the individual. It must, however, never be forgotten that the old age of manual dexterity begins with maturity, and skill, to be of value and permanent, must be acquired while the mind and the hands are in the impressive period of youth.

THE FIRST DENTAL WORK PUBLISHED IN THE UNITED STATES.

BY WILLIAM H. TRUEMAN, D.D.S., PHILADELPHIA.

DENTAL bibliographers assign to a little pamphlet now before me the credit of being the first dental work published in the United States, and to its author, the credit of being the first of a long line of American contributors to dental literature, whose combined work has done much to advance and ennoble the science. It is entitled:

A

TREATISE

on the

HUMAN TEETH,

concisely explaining their structure,

and the cause of

DISEASE AND DECAY:

To which is added,

The most beneficial and effectual method of

treating all disorders incident to the

teeth and gums; with directions for

their judicious extraction, and

proper mode of preservation:

interspersed with observations interesting to, and

worthy the attention of every individual.

BY R. C. SKINNER,

Surgeon Dentist

New-York

Printed by Johnson and Stryker, No. 29 Gold-Street,

For the Author.

- - - - o - - - -

1801

Copy-Right secured

14

It is a pamphlet of twenty-six octavo pages, written, as were many like publications before and since, as an advertisement of its author. Inasmuch as they contain much information the public should know, and have undoubtedly been the means of bringing to the notice of many the resources of dental science for arresting dental disorders and repairing the injury they have done, such works are commendable. Although, strictly speaking, an advertisement, this little work is well within recognized ethical lines; subsequent American writers have no cause to be ashamed of this initial work, nor of its author, so far as this work is concerned, as the father of American dental literature.

This work is exceedingly rare, a brief *résumé* of its contents may, on that account, be of interest.

The author, in his preface, says,—

"Whatever are the merits or defects of this little production, the importance of the subject treated of, as respects every individual, it is presumed, will not be denied. The author has endeavored to combine perspicuity with utility, concisely explaining the causes of disease and decay of the human teeth, their remedies, and only sure and certain method of preservation, etc., etc. The eminent writers on these interesting subjects are too voluminous and expensive to obtain general circulation. The humble efforts of the author of this little tract obviates that difficulty. It is put into the hands of the public for the inconsiderable sum of thirty cents."

His brief descriptions of the structure of the teeth, of the eruption of teeth; of their disorders and the general causes of dental decay; of the alveoli or sockets; of scurvy in the gums; of abscesses in the sockets or gums; of the tartar and septic acid; and directions for extracting teeth, are in accord with accepted ideas current at the time he wrote.

His advice to parents and guardians of children regarding the teeth of those under their charge, while brief, is to the point. He speaks of the distress which frequently accompanies the eruption of the wisdom-teeth, owing to want of room in the jaws, which he says, "must be borne a considerable time, or the tooth extracted to obtain ease." He strongly advises "lacerating or cutting the gum down to the teeth," to relieve the disorders attending difficult dentition of infants, and combats the idea that the resulting cicatrix will later occasion a more difficult eruption of the teeth. He concludes his admonitions enforcing the importance of cleanliness of the teeth and their surroundings in the following words: " It is an established principle from time immemorial, among the ancients as well as moderns, that *cleanliness contributes to health.* If this theory is admitted (which it is presumed no person will deny), it incontestably proves that its application to the teeth and gums, as constituent parts of the body, is as necessary as to the face, hands, feet, or trunk." Caries, he says, "may arise from either internal or external causes and may be divided into soft and dry." This was accepted theory at that time. He further says, "In all cases where a decay is perceptible, the rotten part should be thoroughly and judiciously removed, and the cavity perfectly and solidly filled with gold-, silver-, or lead-foil, prepared for that purpose. If the decay has penetrated to the nerve of the tooth, and pain ensues, it must nevertheless be thoroughly removed, the nerve effectually destroyed, and the cavity filled as before mentioned, or the tooth extracted; otherwise acid and saline particles will enter the hole or cavity of the tooth originally filled with the nerve or cord, wound its membranes, and probably produce an abscess in the socket and gum."

Diseases, he says, "sometimes arise in the sockets when the teeth are perfectly sound; these proceed either from a constitutional cause, or a natural effect taking place prematurely. The former may be removed by proper corrective prescriptions, frequent scarifying, or bleeding the gums, and externally applying antiscorbutic and astringent medicines. The latter is seldom, perhaps never, cured. It generally occasions a total loss of the teeth contiguous to the diseased part. This disease begins by a wasting of the alveolar processes at the edges of the socket, which gradually proceeds to the bottom; the gum loses its connection with the alveolar process and the neck of the tooth, assumes a livid appearance, and continually discharges pus from the diseased surfaces; the teeth affected at length become extremely loose, and at last drop out."

Tartar he divides into three varieties,—"the yellow, the black and the green. The two former are nearly similar in their consistence and effects; the latter is chemically denominated the septic acid. . . . The green tartar (or septic acid) is materially different from the yellow and black, both in its appearance and effects upon the teeth; this substance never forms a concretion. It first appears as a green stain upon that part of the teeth next the gum, where the enamel is very thin, gradually increasing (unless checked by art) until it nearly covers the anterior part of the incisors, canines and small molars of the maxillary superior. The collection of this substance upon the large molars is partial in proportion to what is frequently found upon the teeth before mentioned." This green tartar he credits with being rapidly destructive to the enamel of the teeth, and credits its origin to a putrefactive decomposition of food and other débris which collects about the teeth, stating that it possesses qualities nearly resembling aqua fortis.

He concludes his treatise with a short chapter upon extracting teeth, and from his directions one would infer that he used forceps for this operation. He strongly advocates saving the teeth. He says, " A tooth with one fang or root, that gives pain from any other cause than an abscess, can easily be cured and rendered serviceable, oftentimes, during a person's life. It would be bad practice to extract a front tooth or stump; because it would remove and destroy the solid base, indispensably necessary for the firm security and masticating use of an artificial tooth, which may be set to very great advantage where there is a solid stump standing."

His kindly disposition is evidenced by the following paragraph:

" Poor people afflicted with complaints in the teeth and gums, will be attended to at the dispensary, hospital, almshouse, or at the house of the operator, No. 64 Fair Street, and relieved *gratis*. A request from any physician or surgeon of this city, or any of the superintendents, trustees, or official visitors of either of those benevolent institutions, will be immediately attended to, and assistance given free of any expense."

This kind offer is duly acknowledged by the Board of Managers of the Dispensary of the City of New York, under date of September 2, 1792.

I infer, from a perusal of the following, that the author did not confine his labors exclusively to dental surgery.

ESTABLISHED FEES.

For setting an artificial eye, nose, or ear,—3 guineas each.

For setting an artificial flexible leg, perfectly to imitate nature in muscular motion—4 guineas each.

For setting a common cork leg—3 guineas.

Transplanting a tooth which grows firm in the head—3 guineas each.

Grafting, or setting human teeth in any way on gold—4 dollars each.

Grafting, or setting human teeth on silver—3 dollars each.

Fixing and setting best artificial teeth, on gold springs or pivots—2 dolls. 50 cents.

Grafting or setting (any way) artificial teeth of second quality—2 dollars each.

Grafting or setting third quality—1 doll. 50 cents.

Grafting or setting fourth quality—1 dollar.

Filing, eradicating caries (or rotten parts), or filling cavity with silver- or lead-foil—50 cents each.

Filling cavity with gold—1 dollar each.

Extracting teeth abroad—1 dollar each.

For extracting teeth at his own house—50 cents each. Children's teeth half price.

Eradicating tartar, and cleaning the teeth, from 1 to 3 dollars each set, in proportion to their situation.

In concluding, he says,—

" R. C. Skinner embraces this opportunity of acknowledging the very great obligation he feels himself under to several medical gentlemen of this city, who have particularly honored him with their patronage. He presents them (and every other person who has either patronized or employed him) the warmest effusions of a grateful heart; a heart that will ever feel, and acknowledge (while its pulsations continue) every obligation and favor, either from individuals or the public."

" The public are further respectfully informed, that in any and every case, where part, or the whole of the teeth are decayed and lost new ones may be substituted or set, even if there is neither tooth nor stump standing in the head, from a single tooth to a complete whole set. Even poor people may enjoy the luxury of possessing a good set of front teeth, as some are set as low as one dollar each.

" New York, June 20, 1801."

Taking it all in all, this unpretentious little pamphlet by Mr. Richard C. Skinner, Surgeon Dentist, of New York, pioneer dental writer of the United States, well holds its own when compared with the best of its class and time.

AN INTERESTING CASE.[1]

BY O. G. L. LEWIS, D.D.S., PHILADELPHIA.

PATIENT, Marie Smith, aged fourteen years. Reported at the clinic April 7, 1904, for treatment of a growth which had developed between the upper central incisors. Growth was about the size of a common chestnut.

History.—Patient has a large birth-mark covering the entire right side of the nose and lip. This was first noticed, when a baby three days old, as a spot on the lip, and has gradually spread and grown until it is now beginning to show at various points on the left side of the nose. The growth for which treatment was desired was first noticed about one year ago as a small swelling. The gums at this time became very sensitive and bled upon the slightest provocation.

Examination.—On examination it was found that the birth-mark extended to the under surface of the lip, and that the gums were also more or less affected. There was found a marked condition of hypertrophy or hyperplasia along the entire free margin from the right lateral in front to the second molar behind. On the left side this condition was also found, but only to a limited degree. The large growth in front was found to be attached to the socket of the right central incisor; owing to its appearance and attachment and undoubted association with the disfigurement of the face it was diagnosed as an angiofibroma.

Treatment.—The teeth were carefully cleansed, considerable serumal tartar being removed from beneath the free margin of the gums. A mouth-wash of glycothymoline, fifty per cent. strength, to be used every two hours alternately with one of phenolsodique, three tablespoonfuls to the glass of water, was ordered. On April 15 the gums on the left side had assumed their normal condition, while a marked improvement was also noticed on the right side. At this sitting it was decided to remove the large tumor by means of strangulation. This was successfully accomplished, and at the next sitting the portions overhanging the lateral and cuspid were removed in the same manner. The rest of the mouth continues to improve slowly under weekly treatment. The gums are firm and

---

[1] Treated in Clinic of Dental Department, University of Pennsylvania.

natural-looking but are still considerably enlarged. Owing to the response that has been given to the treatment, I am inclined to believe that the condition, other than that of the large tumor, is due to hypertrophy and not to hyperplasia, and that the primary cause of the disturbance was the serumal deposits which were removed at the first sitting.

The prognosis for the general condition is favorable except in the case of the tumor between the centrals. If this was of partial or complete periosteal origin, and came from the socket of the tooth, it will undoubtedly return and may result in the subsequent exfoliation or extraction of that organ.

Reviews of Dental Literature.

HIGHEST ORTHODONTIA. 1. FACIAL BEAUTY; 2. DENTAL AN-
TAGONISM. By John Nutting Farrar, M.D., D.D.S., New
York City.[1] (Continued from page 299.)

Irregularity is seldom found in very wide jaws, but is often found in narrow jaws; yet the dental arches may be too wide. I have seen cases of regular teeth where the antagonism had forced the upper halves of the arch so far outward as to cause not only separation of the two halves of the jaw-bone, but also separation of the central incisors. The teeth of some upper and lower arches react so detrimentally upon each other that the arches not only become larger and larger, but the spaces between the teeth become wider and wider.

Both of the dental arches can be widened, but whether both need to be widened depends upon somewhat rare circumstances. It may also be said with considerable degree of truth, that the progress in operations for regulating teeth depends upon the amount of osseous tissue that must be absorbed, bent, or otherwise made to yield before the tooth or teeth to be moved. The conformation of the upper and lower jaws differ widely; so do the corresponding parts of the alveolar ridges differ, and the operations for widening must in a measure differ correspondingly. Before a body of intel-

---

[1] Lecture delivered before the New York Dental College Alumni, January 18, 1905.

ligent professional men like this it may be unnecessary to refer to anatomy of the jaws, but in order to make myself clearly understood, let us review the subject a moment.

While the anterior half of the lower jaw is narrower than the anterior half of the upper, the posterior part of the lower is wider than that of the upper. So do the corresponding parts of the two alveolar ridges that support the teeth also differ. While the inner, or lingual, wall of the upper ridge is much more massive than the outer wall, the entire inner, or lingual, wall of the lower is thin. But while the outer wall of all the upper sockets is thin, it is only the anterior outer half of the lower sockets that is thin. The outer wall of the posterior, or molar region is very thick and massive. Because of the thinness of the outer wall of the upper alveolar ridge, the operation for widening the entire length of the (upper) arch is comparatively easy, and when completed the teeth are easily retained in their new positions, provided they antagonize upon firm lower teeth. In regard to the lower arch, the widening of the anterior part is also comparatively easy, as far back as the molars, but because of the great thickness of the buccal side of the molar region, the widening of this section is very slow and tedious. While the thinness of the upper alveolar ridge permits of its teeth being easily moved outward throughout its length, the formation of the outer rear half of the lower is so massive that it is difficult if possible to bend outward. Indeed, these posterior parts are so thick that, if the teeth are to be moved outward, the work must be mainly done through absorption of the bone. But as the apices of the roots of these molar teeth, may, by leverage force, be liable to protrude through the lingual walls of the sockets, care should be exercised if the attempt be made to widen. While, however, these difficulties are true of the lower outer molar region, the teeth anterior to the molars, because of thinness of these alveolar walls, can be moved easily either way.

There are cases of lower arches that need widening, and should be widened, but they are few compared with the number of upper cases that need widening. But whether the upper arch should be widened by always moving the teeth against the sockets, or widened by opening the median suture (excepting the question of antagonism), is not within the province of this essay upon Beauty *vs.* Antagonism.

It is fortunate that in a great majority of cases the lower molars do not need to be moved, nor is it often necessary to move the side teeth anterior to these molars, unless to even an irregular line. Of the few lower teeth that need moving, most of them are the incisors, cuspids, and the second bicuspids; nor is it often necessary to widen the arch to accomplish the best results, as the extraction of an incisor (generally a central) may be more advisable, if by so doing no space be left; these incisors are so nearly of the same size and form, the loss of one is scarcely noticeable. This operation is especially applicable to cases having narrow heads and faces. In normal cases the outer cusps of the upper side teeth overhang closely the outer surface of the lower. The value of this arrangement for the greater bearing upon the fulcral line, along the lower ridge of the jaw, and less upon the lingual side of the ridge and against the thinner wall of the lower sockets, is apparent to the experienced regulator.

While a lower dental arch that needs widening or enlarging is seldom found, there are many upper arches that do need to be widened or enlarged, or both, in order to antagonize properly with the lower teeth. There are also, as before implied, many lower cases in which it is necessary to move one or two side teeth in order to even the line, and there are many cases where the anterior lower teeth are irregular, and need evening in order to properly round out the contour of the lips; the upper as well as the lower.

The small percentage of cases where the lower arch needs widening is fortunate to both operator and patient, because of the avoidance of difficulty of permanently retaining several moved lower side teeth in place sufficiently long to prevent them from becoming driven out of place by antagonism with the upper; more difficult is this than to permanently fix regulated upper teeth. If the widening of the upper arch to make room for the alignment of jumbled teeth, and secure proper antagonism in a thin face and narrow forehead, would injure facial beauty, it should seldom be attempted. But right here is room for careful judgment of the best kind. Different cases may require corresponding differences in the degree of widening.

There is more glory in one entirely successful operation, than in many partially successful operations. One complete success is a permanent evidence of excellence, while partial successes are standing evidences against the operator. To properly move teeth into their proper places is evidence of merit, but to move teeth so that they will not only permanently stay, but cause great beauty of the face, is *proof* of mastership.

The olden time dentists (able in some directions) did not seem to recognize high merit in correction of irregular teeth. Their principal idea of an operation appeared to lie along the line of "evening the row" of teeth, without much regard to antagonism, and with no idea whatever of the value of artistic moulding of the face, further than would result from simply the alignment of the teeth; even this was not often attempted in difficult cases.

When the teeth were greatly jumbled, overlapped, overcrowded, they thought extraction of some of them (and it did not matter much which tooth or teeth) was the only proper way to make room. It is not necessary to say that this plan without artistic aims, without ability to prognosticate with certainty the results, must have led to more or less incongruity, if not total failure. After the days of Delabarre (1826) and Maury (1828) there came a reaction, and that which was regarded as "normal antagonism," but without much idea of that which constitutes proper antagonism, was looked upon as the panacea for all forms of irregularities. It was not taught that antagonism as generally found in nature, in the human race, was seldom perfect antagonism; that it was so rare that in mixed races as found along the border between different nations, and in the United States, only about one per cent. of all is any way near perfect. The normal antagonism hypothesis, as then regarded, had its career, however. This was followed by the hypothesis that all irregular upper teeth should be evened by widening the arch, disregarding the lower. Then followed the hypothesis of normal antagonism by widening both dental arches, if necessary, to even all the irregular teeth. But while the upper arch was often widened, even beyond the antagonizing line of the lower teeth, but few attempts were made to widen both arches at the same time. This plan of so-called "normal" was followed by the hypothesis of "perfect" antagonism, which is still taught somewhat.

In about 1875 the essayist began to express views that although each plan had some points of value, none of the hypotheses previously in vogue could be regarded as an improvement, *par excellence*, over those advocated in earlier days, and that the question of antagonism really was but the alphabet of the subject of this science and art. I then thought, and still think, and have so taught for many years, that the fundamental steps, and all the way up the ladder of knowledge in this line, the aim of the regulator of teeth should be first the accomplishment of the highest degree of beauty of the patient's face, and, as a rule, whatever is necessary to aid in securing this highest result is legitimate and proper. To maintain this highest facial improvement, it may require nearly perfect antagonism; but if perfect antagonism would injure the accomplishment of the highest degree of facial beauty, the attempt at perfection of antagonism may become questionable. Beauty should be carried as high as possible under the circumstances of the case in hand. The great desideratum is beauty with efficient antagonism; not necessarily perfection of antagonism. In other words, the dentist should accomplish as near perfection of antagonism as possible, consistent with the highest degree of facial beauty. But to bring about all this excellence may require a higher grade of mechanical aid than was advocated in the past (1874–75). To meet this lacking was my object in publishing, free to all, many mechanical inventions in many papers upon the subject in the *Dental Cosmos* and various other journals in America and Europe, and later published in book form.

It may here be proper to mention the evil effects of overwidening the arch. By the term overwidening is meant the unnecessary widening. To overwiden the upper arch, carrying the side teeth beyond and outside of the lower teeth, leaving the upper teeth without proper antagonizing restraint and difficult to be safely retained, is questionable practice. To overwiden the upper arch and, at or near the same time, widen the lower arch to match the upper teeth, places the whole case in a dangerous condition, because it is difficult to safely maintain the antagonism between the two unstable arches, unless harnessed in place by retainers for a long time. I do not refer to the very few cases where the opposing arch creeps along with the one being widened. Some of the worst forms of malantagonism and failures that I ever saw were the results of overwidening the upper arch, followed closely by the widening of the lower arch in the attempt at perfection of antagonism.

The reactive tendency of tooth sockets, together with the various directions of force upon the teeth by the lingual, buccal, and labial muscles during the act of swallowing food, and several times every minute by similar action of these muscles while swallowing saliva, causes a combination of forces upon the loosened teeth that tends to prevent a steady retentive disposition, and then one or several

teeth, being thus left in unstable conditions, will drift back more
or less toward their original places. Nor does the use of retaining
mechanisms, as usually made and applied, suffice to overcome these
evil tendencies, unless worn too long for the best interests of the
tissues of the teeth. If, however, small retaining mechanisms can
be cemented upon the teeth so as to be safely left for a long time,
they may be advisable. The use of large retainers, that must be
worn when both arches are widened at the same time, are generally
dangerous collectors of food débris, consequently should not be used
except upon very intelligent and careful patients, who will be sure
to keep these retainers and the teeth clean. The question of retaining the teeth in place sufficiently long for them to firmly set and
remain so, is sometimes more difficult to answer than the question,
How shall teeth be moved? It is not difficult to move teeth, but
to move them properly, and so that they will stay fixed, is not
always easy, and to regulate teeth so as to mould the face to its
highest possibilities in beauty is still more difficult, and a comparative examination of photographs of a " perfect case," before
and after five years' tests, that shows no change, is not only difficult
but very rare. I will say, however, in regard to the latter phase,
that it is not always the regulator's fault if teeth do not remain
corrected, for after repeated warnings to the patients to return to
the operator to have him watch the cases, generally little or no
attention is given to the generous request. This indifference is not
confined to patients after completion of cases, but is often noticeable in failure to keep appointments during the regulating process.
Punctuality is as necessary in this line of work as in other lines.

When a tooth is moved its firm socket-hold becomes more or less
weakened, and the tooth is easily artificially retained in place, but
when several teeth are moved, and are loose, the difficulty is greater,
especially so if the sockets have a tendency to be loculitic (pyor-
rhœic). When this combination of weaknesses exists, the loose teeth
immediately begin playing back and forth, by force of the muscles
of the cheeks and tongue, which, together with the disturbing
action, from the wrongly inclined bearings of the cusps of the
opposing teeth (in the act of swallowing), renders sufficient permanency for new tissue to form and mature almost impossible. The
old school idea, that antagonism is the highest single phase of
dentistry, has a degree of truth, however, so far as it goes, just as
the alphabet is the basal principle of literary education, but the

alphabet of this subject (antagonism) is only the beginning of the highest education in the science and art of correction of irregularities of the teeth, and the remodelling of the face to the highest possibilities.

The proper relation of the teeth, and the proper form of the teeth, and the proper form of the arches of the thin face and narrow head, are different from the proper relation of the teeth and the form of the arches necessary for the wide face. Not only is the poise of the teeth of the upper and the lower jaw different, but the position of the teeth should be maintained by firm antagonism (not rickety). Again, I find by forty years of experience that by far the larger number of cases of protruding (upper) teeth require the dental arch to be shortened, and do not need to be widened. That while to reverse this act (widening) would weaken facial expressions, and would not lead to the highest degree of beauty of the face, the judicious shortening of the arch does not disturb antagonism the least, and in every way improves the case the most.

(To be continued.)

Reports of Society Meetings.

THE NEW YORK INSTITUTE OF STOMATOLOGY.

A MEETING of the Institute was held at the Chelsea, No. 222 West Twenty-third Street, New York, on Tuesday evening, February 7, 1905, the President, Dr. C. O. Kimball, in the chair.

The minutes of the last meeting were read and approved.

Under commuunications upon theory and practice, Dr. F. J. McLaren described his method of investing a gold plate having teeth attached thereto with vulcanite, so that a crack or any necessary soldering might be done without injuring the attachments.

(For Dr. McLaren's paper, see page 365.)

DISCUSSION.

Dr. F. L. Fossume.—I received a suggestion several years ago from a jeweller, for whom I had to repair a plate. He told me to wrap the parts which I did not wish to heat with tissue-paper soaked in water. I found it worked admirably. If a large crack is to be soldered, the tissue-paper may become dry, and it is well to drip water on it during the process of soldering.

Dr. S. E. Davenport.—I think we are fortunate in having Dr. McLaren present this subject to us to-night, as he is an acknowledged expert in these matters. Most dentists nowadays have little real laboratory knowledge, their work being confined principally to the making of fillings and light soldering as used in crown- and bridge-work, but no doubt we could learn a great deal from jewellers, as the experience of Dr. Fossume would indicate. The method of repairing a cracked gold plate to which the teeth are attached with rubber, by swaging a piece of gold and then soldering in place with pure tin and a soldering iron, has been used by all of us many times, and it makes a very good repair indeed.

Dr. E. A. Bogue.—I can testify that Dr. McLaren can do what he has told us about. I wish he would also tell us his method of using heavy iron wires so as to prevent a gold plate from springing when soldering.

Dr. F. J. McLaren.—We all have various methods of doing the same thing, and no doubt you have other means of accomplishing a like result. What Dr. Bogue refers to is simply embedding heavy wire nails in the investment, bent and conformed to the recess made by the ridge of the plate, in such way as to counteract the shrinkage of the investment when soldering. This is especially valuable in large pieces of bridge-work. Here I lay the wire staples in the impression when the crowns are all in place, so that when the impression is poured there can be no subsequent change of shape. To do this, place a leg of each staple within adjoining crowns, so connecting the different parts of the bridge with iron that no contraction of the plaster can have any effect on it.

Dr. Samuel A. Hopkins, of Boston, read a paper entitled " Some Recent Observations in Metabolism, and their Importance in Dentistry."

" For Dr. Hopkins's paper, see page 345.)

DISCUSSION.

Dr. Mandel.—It seems to be the fashion nowadays to make use of simple things. We hear of " Simple Life" on the lecture platform and in the daily press, and even from Washington. Now Dr. Chittenden suggests simplicity in our food. I view all of these doctrines as more or less dangerous. Dr. Chittenden, in his most admirable series of experiments on various individuals doing different work and in different stations of life, claims to have found that one-half or one-third of the nitrogen ordinarily supposed to be necessary to maintain daily life, is quite sufficient. It has maintained the life of individuals experimented upon, and, according to the report of the surgeon who examined them afterwards, they were in perfect health after the experiment. It is unfortunate, as Dr. Hopkins states in his paper, that none of these individuals were taken with any sickness during the progress of the experimentation, and the question has arisen in my mind, What would be the resisting power of this organism fed on the low nitrogenous diet for a year against infection? I do not believe the power of resistance would be as great as in an individual fed with a richer nitrogenous diet. We require nitrogen for cell formation besides the salines and water, and we must supply these substances in a superfluous amount because the kind of nitrogen found in the food is not all the same and not all available in the cell formation and energy production of the body.

It is possible that a low form of nitrogenous diet might do for a certain class of men, but its general adoption I think would be dangerous. The processes of life are simply the transformation of the energy of our food into mechanical, chemical, and heat energy. You cannot get this energy out of a body unless you put the equivalent amount of energy into it in the form of food. I have in my daily life got to accomplish certain things, and I take my food accordingly. I have made some experiments upon myself, although only for a limited length of time, and I find that I take an average of twenty grams of nitrogen daily. I will be told that I am overfeeding; so far I have had no symptoms of overfeeding. I take this amount unconsciously during eight months of the year when I am actively engaged in teaching; during the other four months of the year the quantity of nitrogen is much lower. Of course, I believe an excessive nitrogenous diet will lead to certain disturbances, mental and physical, but we all differ as to the amount we require.

In regard to the processes of the intestines, we cannot get rid of putrefaction going on there. This is a normal condition, and some physiologists claim that it is a necessity, while there are others who have shown that life can be maintained without any putrefaction. We find that these processes are more or less regulated by circumstances and conditions, and although toxic substances, such as phenol, indol, and skatol, are formed in the intestine, still we know that these toxic bodies, when brought to the liver in the blood, are made inert by a process of synthesis and then excreted. Although the nitrogenous foods are the source of these toxic substances, still the amount of these is not necessarily increased when the proteids of the food are increased.

In regard to the flow of saliva, I would call your attention to the observations made by Pawlow and his school, that it is under the influence of the nervous system and the psychic influence of the food itself. If the saliva is necessary for proper mastication, the condition and appearance of our food must necessarily play an important part. Perhaps a too copious discharge of saliva might dilute the acid of the stomach unduly, and produce a harmful rather than a beneficial result. The saliva has a great influence on the process taking place in the stomach, but the process may be considered more as a preparation for the more active digestive processes in the intestine. This is proved by the fact that life has been maintained in a dog for several years after the stomach has been removed.

In closing, I wish to state again that I would deprecate this cutting down of the amount of daily nitrogen consumed as food, as I think its general practice would lead to serious results.

Dr. W. M. Whitlock.—I wish to thank Dr. Hopkins for bringing these matters before us, and to add my testimony to the value of Mr. Fletcher's book. Four years ago there was read before this society a paper with which I was greatly impressed, and from the hints I then received I practically became a vegetarian. I can say, without reserve, that before this time I had never known what it was to feel well, and since that time I have not known what it is to feel otherwise. That summer I read Mr. Fletcher's book. His teachings seemed so sane and reasonable that I at once put them into practice and carried out the system faithfully for three months. I never enjoyed such health. In general Mr. Fletcher's idea is a very limited diet, but a thorough mastication of everything eaten. There are some few points regarding Mr. Fletcher not mentioned by Dr. Hopkins, but which might be of interest. Mr. Fletcher. before beginning this manner of living, had been refused by life insurance companies. He was a very heavy man, weighing somewhat over two hundred pounds. After walking a block he was entirely out of breath. After continuing this treatment for a short time all this was changed. He speaks of starting out one morning and riding his wheel one hundred miles without any previous training, and experiencing no fatigue whatever. It is by thoroughly masticating every particle of food that he takes in that keeps his tissues in such splendid condition. If I understand correctly, pathologic germs cannot exist in healthy tissue; that if we enjoy perfect health there will be no fermentation in the intestines, and the fæces will be without odor.

I can add to my own experience in this matter the weight of the experience of some of my friends. I had in my office to-day a gentleman to whom I gave Mr. Fletcher's book some months ago. He was then suffering from indigestion, from which physicians failed to give him relief. He told me that since adopting Mr. Fletcher's suggestions he had enjoyed perfect health.

Dr. Kellogg, who has been looking for some years for an absolute consistent vegetarian, has at last been rewarded. There recently visited him a young man who, according to the testimony of his mother, had never eaten meat, eggs, nor butter. At nineteen years of age he had never been sick a day in his life. He lived almost entirely upon potatoes and green vegetables.

I saw in to-day's paper an interesting item illustrating perhaps the value of a vegetarian diet in its sustaining powers. A man made a wager that he could live one year on one dollar. He won this wager, the sum total of his expense account for food for that year being eighty-four cents. He came out of the experiment in better condition than at the beginning of the year, having had an increase in weight. His diet consisted of *nettle soup thickened with cornmeal, and greens of all kinds, for which he foraged in the woods.*

I have two little girls who are brought up consistently on a vegetable diet. They are always well, and their teeth are without a flaw. I have a neighbor who has two little girls of about the same age. Their father believes in beefsteak, and they are brought up on beefsteak. They practically never enjoy good health, and their teeth need constant filling.

We may find another illustration of the value of a vegetable diet in the position which our friends the Japs are at present taking. I understand that their diet is almost wholly vegetable.

Dr. Fossume.—I have not read Mr. Fletcher's book, but I have investigated and studied this subject for many years, and have experimented upon myself considerably, and also in the course of my practice have applied the knowledge so gained to patients in whose mouths there have been unmistakable signs of malnutrition and effete intoxication.

The impression conveyed to me by the essayist is that the eating of nitrogenous foods should be reduced.

My experience has been that people suffer more from an excessive amount of carbohydrates. The function of starch is to produce heat and energy. Starchy foods, as they are prepared to-day, are so soluble as to be readily converted into sugar and assimilated. This, in my opinion, is the frequent cause of overheating, fevers, deficient blood, headaches, neuralgia, pimples, bad complexion, and other kindred troubles. Foods giving bulk and acting more as cleansers, such as salads and greens generally, I believe are of the greatest value. Coffee, tea, and cocoa in most cases interfere with the digestion. They certainly do in my case.

The personal equation is so large in relation to this subject that the individual characteristics and need in each particular instance have to be carefully studied.

Dr. H. L. Wheeler.—I think that personal testimony in these matters is valuable only in so far as it is personal. I have two boys. One won't eat meat; the other will eat anything. The latter is strong and healthy, while the former is delicate and listless. When the theory that chunks of unmasticated food irritating the lining of the stomach, causing sarcoma, was mentioned, I could not help thinking, "How many dogs were ever operated upon for sarcoma?"

I think environment has a great deal to do with diet, not only owing to the fact that certain climates require a certain kind of food, but man has adapted himself in many instances to the food of a certain locality.

Dr. Leo Green.—Personal experience is valuable only as it is personal. The man who lays out a diet for himself and tries to force it upon any other individual seems to be the victim of an idea. In contradiction of Dr. Whitlock's idea of a proper diet, I would like to call attention to the large number of savages who have lived for centuries almost entirely upon a meat diet, yet witness their perfect condition of teeth and splendid physical development.

Referring to the value of mastication which Dr. Hopkins has called attention to in his paper, in the institution with which I am connected I have tried to impress the relation between the health of a feeding infant and the condition of the mother's mouth and teeth; that it is impossible for a mother with defective masticating powers to properly nourish a child.

Dr. E. A. Bogue.—I should like to have heard Dr. Mandel tell us about the Greenlanders who are obliged to eat blubber and fat, and not only the Greenlanders, but all who go into that climate, who must needs partake of the same diet. Dr. Whitlock has alluded to the Japs as practically vegetarians. The soldiers who are at present engaged in the campaign do, I understand, eat meat. The native of India lives almost wholly upon rice. In speaking on this subject with one of this nationality, he called my attention to the elephant and the ox as examples of strength, notwithstanding their vegetable diet. When he was confronted with the lion as an example of the carnivora, his excuse was that while the lion was, indeed, strong, its strength could not be as long sustained as the vegetable-eaters'.

It has always been, for one reason or another, one of my fads to always masticate my food thoroughly, and this idea I have tried to instill into my children, as well as my patients. I have masticated thoroughly pretty much all my life, and have never been sick from digestive maladies. Dr. Hopkins says mastication prevents decay of teeth (Yes), and disease (Yes). Dr. Mandel's suggestion that the abundance of saliva dilutes the juices of the stomach might be answered by the question, How about the liquids and drink that we take into our stomach with our food?

When Dr. Whitlock was telling us about his children that have such perfect teeth, my attention was called to the fact that he has good teeth himself, and perhaps his wife also has good teeth. According to the condition of the child from the first to the fifth year, may be reckoned the condition of the permanent teeth.

Dr. Mandel.—About those Greenlanders. A person going from a temperate climate into the intense cold of the polar regions must be recompensed in some way for the great loss in heat due to the surrounding atmosphere, and usually this is best accomplished by increased quantities of fat.

This question of the Japanese has been raised several times.

Some early observations put the amount of proteid material consumed daily at thirty-eight grammes. In recent observations I find that this amount has been increased to fifty-eight grammes per diem. The reason for this increase is simply that the Japanese are rising in the scale of civilization.

Dr. Hopkins.—I fear that I did not make quite strong enough the dangers of a rapid change in one's food habit. Professor Chittenden's position in the scientific world stands for a great deal, and as his opinion is indorsed by other men of like prominence, far be it from me to make any contention for the soundness of his work. I think it stands for itself. I have only to say that Professor Chittenden has advised caution. I would call particular attention to the fact that in all of his experiments the diet was a mixed one, and that the appetite was in all cases thoroughly satisfied. Regarding mastication, I do not go as far as Mr. Fletcher does by any means; in fact, I called attention to certain dangers in his system. These dangers have been brought out in a recent article in the *New York Medical Record.* I believe, however, that we are in much more danger from overeating than from being insufficiently nourished.

A vote of thanks was extended to both Dr. Hopkins and Dr. Mandel for their valuable contribution.

Adjourned.

FRED. L. BOGUE, M.D., D.D.S.,
Editor The New York Institute of Stomatology.

ACADEMY OF STOMATOLOGY.

A SPECIAL meeting of the Academy of Stomatology of Philadelphia was held at its rooms, 1731 Chestnut Street, on the evening of Friday, December 9, 1904, to hear a paper by Dr. E. K. Wedelstaedt, of St. Paul, Minn., entitled " Conditions of Failure."

(For Dr. Wedelstaedt's paper, see page 358.)

DISCUSSION.

Dr. Edwin T. Darby.—I do not know that there is very much in the paper with which we can differ, and our discussion must therefore be in the way of agreeing with what Dr. Wedelstaedt has said. There is one point which we all ought to practise, and that is, making a study and record of our conditions of failure. The doctor has gone to a great deal of trouble to show just the conditions which exist before and after operations. It is undoubtedly true that many fillings upon proximal surfaces fail just because the condition represented in Fig. 2 is allowed to prevail. He accounts for that space between the teeth by saying that the operator probably passed a revolving disk or sand-paper disk from the occlusal to the gingival border of the filling. An up-to-date dentist who is retaining contour would have too good judgment to do just that thing.

I have frequently seen it done by students, and it has made a beautiful operation a failure. The disk has been run through and a space left in which food becomes impacted. A disk ought never to be passed between the teeth after the contour has been restored.

I was hoping that the doctor would say something about extension for prevention. It is the greatest advance in the way of saving operations that we have had in the last twenty or more years. I accepted this idea with a good deal of reluctance, but I have been carefully observing the conditions which I have found in the mouths of my own patients as well as in the mouths of patients coming from other dentists, and I have found that the weak point is along the gingival or buccal border near the gum, at the cervix or near the cervix, and that by following the plan illustrated in Model No. 5 better results are accomplished than by our old method of limiting the cut. I have become what might be called a rather excessive advocate of cutting the buccal and lingual border. The method not only simplifies the operation, but prolongs its usefulness as a saver of the teeth. I might not have said this ten or twenty years ago, but I am so thoroughly convinced that that is the proper procedure that I have adopted it in my own practice to the exclusion of any other. It does simplify the packing of gold, the finishing of the filling, and the completion of the whole operation.

Dr. M. L. Rhein.—This subject is certainly of great interest to all of us. I more than echo the sentiment of the last speaker upon the value of the extension of cavities in the ultimate salvation of the teeth; but, as I said about two years ago before this Academy, I take decided issue with the statement that it is of recent origin or that it is new within the past twenty-five years. I base my assertion, as on that evening, upon the illustrations in Webb's work on "Operative Dentistry." I can never let an opportunity of this kind pass without giving credit to him and to dentists prior to him for advocating this method of preparation, perhaps not with the scientific exactness so well described by Dr. Black, but with all the essential requirements of the case.

There is no opportunity to-night to take issue with the speaker upon his criticism of failing to produce as far as possible a physiological contact point, but I have never listened to anything, either by word of mouth or writing, of Dr. Wedelstaedt's that I have not become extremely antagonistic to his point of view. He speaks at the close of his address about the few men in the Northwest who are ready to make the filling of teeth scientifically exact. As I understand that, he means that he is going to tell the students and the profession the exact measurements for each cavity, the exact amount of gold that shall be placed in each one, and the exact form of contact point. Now, if such a thing were possible I would at once give up operative dentistry, because there would be no attraction in it for me. It would become too commonplace a matter. To me the attraction of saving the human teeth has been in the variance from the normal physiological type. We do not get teeth to fill with normal occlusion and normal points of contact. A dentist's inventive ability is called into play every time he is called upon to fill a tooth so that it may be preserved. The attraction in the work is that when the operation is completed it differs in some slight or great measure from the one that has preceded it. In the majority of cases coming to your office you cannot make such points of contact as are illustrated here. This is the point which I am anxious to bring out in this discussion. Regarding Model No. 5, showing a double compound filling of mesial, distal, and occlusal surfaces, there is no statement made of the amount of tooth-structure destroyed by caries. I have seen teeth filled in the way here shown as correct utterly unable to withstand the force of mastication. This is to me not a proper criticism to make on what he has shown, because I have no doubt that if that tooth were sufficiently destroyed by caries, Dr. Wedelstaedt would have cut down the cusps of the lingual and buccal sides and replaced them by filling-material, so that they would be protected. It illustrates, however, the main point of my criticism, in showing how unjust it is to judge every man's failures in the scarcely ethical way we have listened to this evening. In some mouths there are such irregularities that it is impossible to separate the teeth as he advocates should be done and get the proper results.

Dr. S. H. Guilford.—This method of separating, contouring, and finishing the fillings as described by Dr. Wedelstaedt has been carried on in this section of the country for a very long while; it has also been regularly taught in the colleges.

A matter of almost equal importance to that of preservation of the teeth is the consideration of comfort to the patient. Patients who have had teeth cut, mutilated, and crowded together have been annoyed beyond measure by the discomfort which they have had to endure. All of us have met with such cases, and have noticed how grateful patients are after those conditions have been changed. I remember distinctly a case referred to me by Dr. Jack many years ago. The patient was a man of thirty, and had travelled abroad a great deal. I found upon examination that he had the full complement of teeth above and below, but that they had been filled and refilled and filled again with various filling-materials. He had in the course of his travels fallen into the hands of many dentists, and his teeth had been cut in such a manner that they pressed flatly against each other. I saw that an enormous amount of work would be necessary, and told him it was a question of his willingness to undergo so much repair. He expressed his willingness to endure anything if satisfactory results could be obtained. He went through the tedious operations without a murmur, and from that day to this he has had entire comfort. I never have done such an amount of work in any one mouth, either before or since. His teeth are good in structure, and having been put into their original form, very little has had to be done from that time to this.

Dr. Wedelstaedt and those associated with him are enthusiasts upon this subject, and we need men of that kind in order to awaken a certain amount of energy in the younger men. Dr. Wedelstaedt is not a college teacher, but he is a teacher, nevertheless, and he and his society are doing good work. I believe that in the near future we shall have a school of operators in the Northwest superior to the same number in the Eastern States. The doctor is doing good work and getting others to do good work, and in that respect it seems to me that he is an ideal teacher. I wish to thank him to-night for his paper, and especially for what he has done in his locality.

Dr. William H. Trueman.—While I have listened with a great
deal of interest to the paper of this evening, and it has been a
pleasure to hear Dr. Wedelstaedt explain his ideas in regard to
the cause of failures and his method of making a permanent record
of the conditions leading to, and resulting from such failures, I am
not much impressed with their value. These plaster models which
he presents may faithfully depict the conditions he observed prior
to taking the impressions from which they have been made, but
without a full history of each particular case they will often be
misleading and unjust to the operators whose work is thus presented for criticism. A few days ago I replaced a filling that would
have made a capital illustration of a failure from the essayist's
stand-point; but when I tell you that a few months ago it was
in excellent order, and that the dentist who inserted it has been in
his grave over thirty years, can you, gentlemen, consider it a failure? I recall another case. The models and the diagrams before
you would serve very well to illustrate it, so nearly are they like
it. It was a flat gold filling in the posterior approximal surface
of an upper second bicuspid. No attempt had been made to
contour or to make a contact point; the bicuspid and molar came
together, making an ideal place for recurring decay according to
present notions. When I first saw it, it had been in place a little
over fifty years, and was in perfect order. A few years later I
found it necessary to patch it with gutta-percha. Now, a model
of that case might have presented some points for criticism, but,
remember, the model tells but one part of the story. In this
case, no matter how accurately the model would have represented
the condition of that filling and its surroundings, it would not
have told you that the patient carried it with her to her grave
over sixty years after Dr. Edward Hudson had inserted it, and
that, permit me to suggest, is important in considering the question whether or not that filling was a failure.

Any filling which has fully performed its office sixty years,
or for thirty years, in many cases ten years, or even five years,
is not to be lightly spoken of. It may not conform to our notions
of what should have been, but who can say that our method
would have done better? We strive for permanent work, but
"permanent" means a very long time. I am strongly impressed
that some methods designed to insure permanency invite destruction. There is no one cause of failure, and no one method of

preventing it. I meet with some dentures I cannot save. Whether the cause is in the teeth, or is due to their surroundings, I cannot tell—I set it down to predestination. Now and again such cases fall into the hands of operators who see my mistakes and try to do better, and not unfrequently the poor patient gets a third denture a few years sooner as the result. Many are born into the world badly handicapped, and many of these will live longer and enjoy life more by gracefully accepting the handicap and making the best of it.

The essayist bases his hope of better results by adopting a method different from that which he contends has invited failure in the cases illustrated, on the presumption that the present theory of dental caries is true. Now, do we know beyond doubt the cause of dental caries? We thought we did a great many years ago, but there has been a continual change. A theory lasts about a generation, it is then discarded for a new one more plausible or more scientific. We can do no more when filling an approximal cavity in a biscuspid, by contouring, by properly placing and shaping the contact point, and by extension for prevention, than to approximately make it as safe from germ intrusion as is a filling upon a buccal or labial surface. A well-placed filling upon a buccal or a labial surface is ideal for perfect technic and perfect cleanliness, and yet, nevertheless, recurring decay at the margins of these fillings is not unknown. Why is it that a slight defect in an approximal gold filling is so disastrous, while a filling of gutta-percha in the same position may be imperfect, unclean, an ideal germ culture bed, and yet perfectly protect the tooth from decay. Gutta-percha is not a germicide. There is one thing that I admire very much in Dr. Miller. He has done a great deal of earnest work in the attempt to solve this perplexing problem. His conclusions have more nearly met observed conditions than have those of his predecessors, and none, perhaps, has been so well qualified to pronounce a positive opinion than he, and yet, I observe, he always stops a little short of being absolutely "sure." The last word has not yet been said. Within a few months the question has been raised whether or not a certain constituent of the saliva may be the real destructive agent, or whether it is merely the pabulum that nourishes tooth-destroying germs. The theory of microbic plaques, that a few years ago was accepted as solving one phase of tooth destruction, is now being abandoned.

Who can tell what will be taught the next generation? What becomes of a practice based upon a false theory?

The study of the cause of failures is very interesting; it is important, and, carried on in the right way, is instructive; but I think we should go very, very, *very* slowly in drawing absolute conclusions, because, in a little while the theory on which we are now working may become a back number; there are many things concerning dental caries that it does not explain.

Dr. M. I. Schamberg.—Extremists in dentistry are necessary to bring out valuable points whereby we may profit. Dr. Rhein has alluded to the extreme lessons taught by Dr. Wedelstaedt, and takes exception to them. We are all familiar with the immense amount of good Dr. Rhein has done by taking a decided stand in regard to pyorrhœa. I believe that we are ready to admit that a similar good will follow the teachings of Dr. Wedelstaedt in reference to conditions of operative failure.

Yesterday I treated a brother of mine for the condition of failure noted in Fig. 3, where the point of contact of two approximal fillings is near the gingival border. He was suffering very much with a second lower molar tooth which had been carefully examined and no defect in the tooth found. Before taking an X-ray picture, which he desired me to do, I passed an explorer down to find whether there was caries beneath either of the approximating fillings. I found that the fillings were in contact at and were overhanging the gingival margins of the two cavities. The V-shaped space in which food became packed during mastication was causing pericemental trouble. Relief was promptly afforded by taking sand-paper strips and smoothing away the lower portion of two fillings until they approximated nearer the occlusal surface of the teeth. I do not offer this as a method for relieving that condition of failure, but wish merely to call attention to the possibility of the production of pericemental inflammation through the improper filling of teeth. In a case sent to me yesterday by Dr. Fogg the patient was suffering with a lower second bicuspid tooth which, being devitalized, was carefully cleansed by Dr. Fogg and put in a healthy condition for filling. In spite of the good treatment the tooth received, it pained as if it were vital and responded to an application of chloride of ethyl. Dr. Fogg had also noticed that upon the gum there was an enlargement indicating the possibility of root exostosis. An X-ray picture which I took showed a marked enlargement of the roots of this and the adjoining teeth. I advised extraction, and, in spite of the fact that the patient was eighty-two years of age, I gave him gas and removed the tooth, and with it came the tooth immediately in front of it.

The specimen which I pass among you is interesting, and shows that the teeth came out together because of their attachment at the apical end, due to the hypercementosed condition of both teeth. The unusual phenomenon in this case was the transmission of the sensitivity of the first bicuspid to the second bicuspid through the attachment at their apices. In a large number of cases I believe the packing of food between teeth to be the cause of pericemental troubles. In my search for other causes for exostosis I find and am willing to accept this as the most frequent etiological factor in the production of this abnormality.

Dr. G. Milliken.—There is little to say in discussion upon this system of Dr. Wedelstaedt. We were always taught it at the University of Pennsylvania, and we have insisted upon the contouring of teeth to a greater or less degree, extending the borders out to the brush line. In the last few years we have been teaching extension for prevention; but as to leaving spaces such as Dr. Wedelstaedt describes, this is foreign to any teaching that I have ever heard at the University of Pennsylvania.

Dr. G. W. Warren.—I shall not attempt to discuss in detail the paper of the evening, the ground having been fully covered by Drs. Darby, Guilford, and Trueman. It is true that the principle set forth in the essay—that in filling teeth they should, as far as possible, be restored to their normal physiological condition—has for many years been taught in our colleges. It is equally true that young practitioners, after graduating and getting away from the guidance of their instructors, fall.into slipshod methods of restoration; hence the necessity for reiterating these basal facts in our literature and societies. I am glad of the opportunity to thank Dr. Wedelstaedt for his essay and for coming so far to present it. Many good things are coming from the Northwest.

I was interested in Dr. Trueman's remarks as to just what operations we might call failures; to my mind the term is a relative one. Shall we consider the filling which has preserved a tooth for ten, fifteen, or twenty years a failure? This calls to mind an incident of practice occurring only a short time ago. An old gentleman called my attention to a filling on the distal surface of a lower bicuspid tooth; upon examination I found it needed a slight repair. The gentleman then said, " I want to tell you that your father placed that filling there thirty-two years ago." Here was an operation which had been serviceable for over thirty years, shall we call it a failure, then, because the tooth breaks down around it?

Dr. Trueman, in his remarks, also alluded to the several theories as to the cause of dental decay which from time to time have been advanced and later shown to be erroneous, and he cautions us not to accept too fully the present Miller theory, lest it, too, in time be disproved. I cannot agree with the doctor on this point, for, as I view it, we are accepting the present germ theory as conclusive, not because Dr. Miller has advanced the theory, but because he has demonstrated that the principal and basal cause of dental decay is the growth of oral bacteria.

Dr. James Truman.—I, unfortunately, was absent when the paper was read, and I hoped that I might receive some information from the discussion concerning the subject of the paper, but though I have listened intently, I can gather nothing from what has been said as to the topic. It may be my fault.

In other respects, I may say that I have a great deal of faith in the Northwest. I am perfectly willing, therefore, to believe that all Dr. Wedelstaedt has said here this evening is right. As I look at those drawings, my mind goes back forty or fifty years to the time when I was but a youth in dentistry, and when I had something to do with teaching operative dentistry, and I must say that, if they represent the present method of filling advocated, it is done exactly as we extended cavities for prevention at that period. I do not see that there is any really great advance. I may be mistaken, however, as I was not here when the paper was read.

Dr. M. L. Rhein.—There is one point which I would like to incorporate in my discussion. In this subject of failures in operative dentistry, as illustrated by the charts here, it struck me that Dr. Wedelstaedt omitted what I consider the most important point of all, and that is the lack of proper specific gravity in the filling-material. I am convinced from my experience of many years that most of the instances of recurrent decay in occluso-approximal cavities is due to the ruin of the filling-material under the stress of mastication caused by the running of the gold rather than from insufficient extension, as described by the disciples of Dr. Wedel-staedt.

So far as I can see, my criticisms of Dr. Wedelstaedt concerning these models were a part of the discussion, and with the exception that I said a word in response to what Dr. Darby said, I confined my remarks entirely to the casts, and spoke entirely to the subject.

Regarding the models, the question is simply one of how you read casts. The actual conditions seen in the patient's mouth, with the history then presented, are much more easily understood than casts which are passed around. The question before us this evening is very similar to that of the radiograph. One man will see one thing, and another man something else.

Dr. Roberts.—I would like to ask Dr. Wedelstaedt how long a filling should last when it has been properly prepared to be a success?

Dr. E. K. Wedelstaedt (closing).—Do good and be kind, is the motto I try to live up to. I came before the members of this society with something which I supposed to be new, something which I do not say is new, but something which I have never seen before, although I have been in the practice of dentistry nearly thirty years. The whole theory of dentistry, from pyorrhœa alveolaris to the spreading of gold, seems to have been discussed, and with the exception of a few who have said kind words, very little has been said upon the subject. I brought you a method for studying conditions of failure. I said nothing whatever of extension for prevention. We know what abnormal conditions are and the necessity for correcting them. All that I said was that teeth should be brought to their normal positions. I shall not, therefore, discuss extension for prevention. I shall not answer anything about specific gravity of gold. I did not come here for this purpose, and I am surprised that a thing of this kind should come up. I do not think that when I come before you with plaster-of-Paris casts of conditions as I have found them that I am dogmatic. I said nothing about Dr. Black. There are the casts, and they tell the truth. I am glad that there is in the dental profession a little band of earnest men who are coming more and more closely together and who study conditions of failure in the same manner in which I have presented them to-night.

Otto E. Inglis,
Editor Academy of Stomatology.

Editorial.

WHAT OF THE HARVEST?

Not the harvest of the fertile fields; not the harvest of souls that our evangelist is seeking to ingather to the fold; not the harvest of gold that the financier hopes to accumulate to make old age a peaceful decline into the valley of silence; not any or all of these, but a harvest of professional power, granaries, not of grain, but of practical skill, stored up for the future welfare of the individual and the world.

We have reached, in the years 1904–05, the close of that session, ending three years, which the dental colleges of this country at St. Louis decided was amply sufficient to make a dentist. The three years have been completed, and before the expiration of the month of June all the dental schools from New England to California will have sent out their quota of senior scholars to battle with the conflicting elements, which are ever waging a war against the new man who ventures to meet their antagonizing influences.

Over this broad land there is a small army of earnest and conscientious teachers in dentistry, who have had to contend between their better natures and the sordid elements that make up the two forces in every individual life, and are now, it is presumed, asking the ever-recurring question, Have I succeeded in imparting a portion of my knowledge and skill to the aspiring youth, that his work may be a credit to himself and to his profession? The man who fails to feel this anxiety as to results at the close of every session seems to the writer to have failed to develop the finer sense of the teacher, a feeling of not having approached his ideal. The individual without an ideal to which he may continually aspire is, from the inception of his work, a failure. Teaching is something more than a mere repetition of the dry bones of facts. It must have within these the spirit of the teacher, to give these life and power, and without this they are dead material incapable of furnishing the pabulum necessary to make the fully developed man.

The spring of 1905 finds us, as teachers of dentistry, face to face with the problem of development. The entire dental teaching world is, and has been for several years, endeavoring to solve the educational problem. The man of one idea has solved this for himself. He may be found on the side of the highest preliminary education possible as a panacea for all our educational woes. Again, he will rest content only in a thorough medical education, and that alone will suffice. Again, the man with one idea will have the whole foundation of dental education based on ability to make a denture thoroughly and artistically. The man of broad ideas has been endeavoring for years to harmonize all of these into one composite whole, in which no one will have a preponderance, but each will be given due weight and in proper order of acquirement. It is a healthy sign of growth, with corresponding vigor, that all over the dental world this question as to the best methods of educating dental students is, and has been, an absorbing topic. The writer is not aware that in any other profession is this regarded with the same interest or of equal importance. It will be a subject of continued interest in the Fédération Dentaire Internationale to meet at Hanover, Germany, in August. It will doubtless have a place in the Councils of the British Dental Association, and naturally should be a leading topic in the Association of Faculties of this country. That there will be unanimity of opinion is not.to be expected. The one idea man prevails in Europe, and the broad man has yet to be developed, to any extent, in this country. Narrow conceptions will continue to prevail just so long as we measure our dental education with the yardstick of finance.

Hundreds of young men will, in the coming weeks, pass out from the dental colleges of this country into the greater world of dentistry, and that after three years of study and practice. Are the teachers satisfied with the result? The mason, the printer, the blacksmith, the carpenter, the jeweller, all require from the novitiate the earnest work of, at least, five years, but dentistry, that combines the science that belongs to and is part of medicine, with the skill equally a part of the mechanician, is supposed to be acquired in three years of from seven to nine months each! The farcical character of this must be plain to the average intellect, and requires no argument to demonstrate its weakness, yet the forces in control in this country have placed the stamp of regularity upon this period of probation, and have forced all the dental colleges in this country to adopt this as the true solution of the educational problem. It was, and will continue to remain, the

Bibliography.

ANÆSTHESIA IN DENTAL SURGERY. By Thomas D. Luke, M.B., F.R.C.S.E., Anæsthetist to the Dental Hospital, the Deaconess Hospital, and Instructor in Anæsthetics to the University Surgical Classes, Royal Infirmary, Edinburgh. With twenty-eight Illustrations. Rebman Company, New York, 1903.

This book, while somewhat too limited in the general treatment of a very important branch of practice, is nevertheless one of the most valuable books in its practical application thus far given the dental profession upon the subject of anæsthesia. The book is dedicated to Dr. John Girdwood, of Edinburgh, to whom the dental profession is indebted for many valuable suggestions and improvements.

While this book has been prepared in Scotland, it has been published in New York, probably a wise move on the part of the author, though seemingly too far away from the home of its production.

The author says of it, " The aim of this little work—which, as far as the author knows, is the first of its nature in the field —has been to pass the various anæsthetics and combinations of them used in operative dentistry, as it were, in review before the reader's eye, with a brief description of the properties of some of them, their method of application, advantages, and disadvantages."

The author's extended experience as an anæsthetist naturally leads the reader to expect the book to be a practical manual upon the subject, and in this the reviewer feels he will not be disappointed. It covers all the at present known anæsthetics and analgesics, and, while the author has aimed at brevity, he has given the readers a very satisfactory and instructive book.

The history of anæsthesia, as presented, does full justice to Dr. Horace Wells and also to Dr. William T. Morton, the original discoverers of anæsthesia by inhalation. He also recognizes the services of Dr. James Young Simpson in introducing chloroform,

15

but it is thought more notice of the discoverers of chloroform should have been given than is to be found, very briefly stated, on the first page.

Much space is properly given to nitrous oxide. The author does not regard the after-effects of this anæsthetic of serious import, for he says, "The after-effects of nitrous oxide are usually exceedingly slight and transient. . . . If at all marked, some impurity of the gas may be suspected or the administration may have been faultily conducted." This is probably true, as a rule, but it must not be forgotten that quite serious after-effects are by no means uncommon, frequently assuming serious physical disturbance of a chronic character. This may have been due to the causes stated, but the assertion requires further proof before acceptance.

"Gas and oxygen" claims attention, but the author does not write enthusiastically in regard to this combination, for he says, "We thus find that, while just double the time is required than when using pure N_2O, the anæsthesia obtained is only half as long again in duration."

The results attained by the combination of gas with ether do not warrant its general use. The narcosis may be prolonged, but this is not required in the ordinary operation of extraction, while responsibility is greatly increased. The author prefers ethyl chloride and ether to the former. "There is less cyanosis, and anæsthesia is more pleasantly and rapidly produced."

Ethyl bromide is regarded "as well worthy of the dental surgeon's attention, but the author does not devote much space to its consideration. He states that with this anæsthetic "the mortality has been estimated at under 1 in 5000."

Ethyl chloride is given extended consideration; in fact, the author felt obliged to revise his text, as the manuscript was practically completed before he had had an opportunity to test its value. The comparison between the anæsthetic periods of nitrous oxide and ethyl chloride are in favor of the latter. "Dr. McCardie finds, on the average: Time of induction, fifty-one seconds; length of anæsthesia, seventy seconds, but in some cases extending to two or two and a half minutes.

"This compares very favorably with nitrous oxide, which, according to Hewitt, requires 55.9 seconds to induce full anæsthesia."

Space will not permit a further following of the author through "Mouth-gags," "Anæsthetics in Special Cases," "Local Anæsthesia," "Management of Prolonged Extraction Cases," all of which are valuable, but are too briefly considered.

The great difficulty with all experts seems to be to fail to drop sufficiently into detail. They seem to lose sight of the necessity of talking to "the lowest man in the class."

The author's long dissertation on "The Place of Chloroform in Dental Surgery" will be far more valuable to English practitioners than to Americans, for chloroform is very rarely used here in dental operations.

The author gives a list of deaths from nitrous oxide, made up to 1901. These amount to seventeen, with thirteen additional in doubt as to the cause. This, if correct, is certainly a remarkable showing in view of the many thousands constantly inhaling nitrous oxide for minor surgical operations.

"Accidents of Anæsthesia" concludes the book.

While the author might with great advantage extend the text in future editions by entering more into detail, it is thought the book, as written, furnishes the best small book yet published upon the subject. The dental profession has had several works published on nitrous oxide in this country, and able articles upon anæsthesia in various dental publications, but this is the only work covering the entire subject prepared by a practical anæsthetist, and it is therefore of peculiar value and will meet the needs of many in general practice.

Miscellany.

An Adjustable Indicator, for accurately measuring small quantities of the more volatile anæsthetics, invented by Mr. Vernon Knowles, consists of a flat metallic bar provided with clips engaging the bottom and the neck of a glass bottle for the purpose of securely holding it in a vertical position against the side of the bottle. Attached to, and moving on this bar, are two small curved arms or wings, controlled by a set-screw. One arm is graduated by means of steps for cubic centimetres, 1 to 5, and the other for the divisions of one dram.

Before administration, one of the wings should be adjusted by means of the set-screw, so that the upper edge of the same is on a level with the fluid. If this precaution be taken, the danger incurred by an "overdose" is entirely eliminated, because, as the anæsthesia proceeds, the administrator has only to glance at the indicator, when he can tell exactly the dose that has been given. Having the graduation marked by steps cut out of the metal, instead of marks made upon its surface, is an excellent idea, they are so much more readily seen.

NEW GRIP GAGS, to keep the mouth open when administering anæsthetics, and which may be used while the face-piece is on, are advertised by Taylor's Dental Depot, 17 Poland Street, London, W. These are very much like a pair of pliers, held open by a ratchet, and provided with pads to rest against the teeth.

Current News.

LEWIS AND CLARK DENTAL CONGRESS.

To the Members of the National Dental Association:

GENTLEMEN,—The Executive Committee of the Lewis and Clark Dental Congress invites the National Dental Association to change its meeting place for this year to Portland, Ore., and its dates to correspond with those of the Congress, combining the two meetings and lengthening, if necessary, the sessions to six days,—July 17 to 22.

If this action is not possible, your attention is called to the opportunity of attending both meetings,—the Lewis and Clark Dental Congress closing July 20, in ample time to allow those who desire to reach Buffalo for the opening day of the National Association.

The dentists of the West are taking a great interest in the Congress, and it is demonstrated that more than one thousand from this section alone will attend.

This fact, together with the class and size of the programme which is being formed, the conveniences of the meeting hall, the interest being displayed by the large manufacturers who will exhibit their goods, and many other things as showing the result of the business-like methods adopted in conducting the work of the Congress, as well as the opportunity offered for an enjoyable and instructive vacation trip to the great West, at rates lower than ever before quoted,—one-half fare or less from all sections of the United States,—warrant the committee in asking that the courtesy of attendance and participation in the Congress be granted by the members of the National Dental Association and dentists generally residing in the Eastern States.

You are assured that this will be appreciated, and you may be confident that if you will attend you will return to your homes after the meeting with a feeling of gratification that you made the trip, saw the most magnificent scenery in the United States, and spent the month of July in a most delightful climate.

All of this will have been accomplished for but a small portion of the expense incident to such a trip at any time in the past, and for an indefinite period in the future.

Membership in the Congress, with or without attendance, will entitle each one to a bound copy of the proceedings.

Will you indicate your intentions concerning the Congress, and if you will participate correspond with the Chairman of Committees?

ARTHUR W. CHANCE,
Secretary.

WHERE THE CONGRESS WILL BE HELD.

The Armory of the Oregon National Guard will be the meeting hall of the Lewis and Clark Dental Congress. It is the largest armory west of Chicago and St. Louis. It is 200 x 200 feet, first story of stone, second of brick, provided with all modern conveniences.

The location is very central—eight squares or blocks from all large hotels, post-office, railroad terminal depot, and active centre of city. (City squares or blocks are two hundred feet in length.)

The Assembly hall, where the general meetings take place, is 60 x 100 and will accommodate one thousand people. The Exhibit hall, where the manufacturers' exhibits and professional clinics take place, is 100 x 200 feet, contains twenty thousand square feet of space, is located on the ground floor, and in the north end of the building, where the daylight facilities are first class.

HOTELS AND ROOMS.

Hotel Portland, European, $2.50 to $3.00 single, $5.00 to $6.00 double; Hotel Imperial, European, $2.00 to $4.00; Hotel Perkins, $2.00 to $4.00. Many other hotels at lower rates.

Private Hotels.—The Eaton, European, $1.50 to $5.00; The Norton, American, $4.00 to $6.00; Elton Court, $3.00 to $5.00 European, $5.00 to $7.00 American; Hobart-Curtis, $3.00 to $7.00 American.

EXPOSITION ACCOMMODATION BUREAU (INC.).

Under the supervision and control of Lewis and Clark Centennial Exposition and Oriental Fair five thousand rooms in private families convenient to the Armory have been secured which are offered at the following rates: $1.25 per day for single room; $2.50 per day for double room occupied by one or by two people. Business address: Goodnough Building, Fifth and Yamhill Streets.

Reservations for any of the above hotels or for rooms of the Accommodation Bureau, made in advance.

FEATURES OF THE PROGRAMME.

The essays at the Lewis and Clark Dental Congress will be by the leading men in the dental and medical professions of the United States and Europe. Essayists are being selected with a view of making this part of the programme unique and original in character. Symposiums on various subjects will be given. There will be no sections in the meeting, all of the essays being delivered before the entire Congress.

During the four days that the Congress will be in session there will be one hundred and fifty professional clinics given by dentists from every part of the world. The clinical programme will be a large feature of the Congress, and clinicians have been secured to demonstrate every operation in the range of our profession, especially the newest and latest methods in both operative and prosthetic work. The clinical programme is receiving additions daily.

There will be fifty or more exhibits, covering fifteen thousand square feet, comprising every variety of dental goods made, and there will be clinical demonstrations by manufacturers of every dental appliance and specialty on the market.

Railroad rates will be low,—$56.00 round trip from Chicago,

$45.00 from Missouri River, St. Paul, Minneapolis, Duluth, and the Superiors, one-half regular fare from territory in the scope of the Lewis and Clark Exposition.

In connection with above rates, Eastern lines have authorized one fare for the round trip from point of origin to Chicago and Missouri River.

The membership ticket, which entitles the holder to all privileges, will be five dollars ($5.00).

NATIONAL DENTAL ASSOCIATION.

THE following programmes will be offered for the consideration of Sections I. and II. in Buffalo, July 25 to 27, 1905:

SECTION I.

"Orthodontia." Dr. Calvin S. Case, Chicago; Dr. C. Edmund Kells, Jr., New Orleans, La.; Dr. V. H. Jackson, New York; Dr. R. Ottolengui, New York.

"Prosthetic Dentistry." Dr. H. H. Johnson, Macon, Ga.; Frederic Freeman, Boston.

"Crown- and Bridge-Work." Dr. W. Storer Howe, Philadelphia.

"The D.D.S. Abroad." Special paper by Dr. R. H. Hofheinz, Rochester, N. Y.

DR. THOMAS P. HINMAN, *Chairman,*
Atlanta, Ga.

DR. J. G. FIFE, *Secretary,*
Dallas, Tex.

SECTION II.

"Gold as a Filling Material." J. V. Conzett, Dubuque, Iowa.

Lantern Lecture: "Pioneer Manipulators of Gold-Foil." B. L. Thorp, St. Louis, Mo.

"Dental Education." Chas. Milton Ford, New York City.

"The Necessity for a Method of preserving the Integrity of the Interproximal Space." W. R. Clack, Clear Lake, Iowa.

"A Few Experiments in Porcelain." Dr. D. O. M. LeCron, St. Louis, Mo.

"A Century of Standard Dental Writings." Dr. D. W. Fellows, Portland, Me.

"Operative Dentistry." Dr. B. Holly Smith, Baltimore, Md.

(To be announced.) Professor Geo. B. Snow, Buffalo, N. Y.; Dr. W. H. K. Moyer, Little Falls, Minn.

"Nomenclature." Dr. D. R. Stubblefield, Nashville, Tenn.

"The Nomenclature of Orthodontia." Dr. S. H. Guilford. Philadelphia.

DR. HOWARD E. ROBERTS, *Chairman,*
Philadelphia, Pa.

DR. C. S. BUTLER, *Secretary.*
Buffalo, N. Y.

SOUTH DAKOTA STATE BOARD OF DENTAL EXAMINERS.

THE next meeting of the South Dakota State Board of Dental Examiners will be held at Mitchell, S. D., July 11, beginning at 1.30 P.M. All candidates will be required to do practical work in both operative and prosthetic dentistry, and should bring all instruments and materials necessary to do the same. Vulcanizer, lathe, and swaging appliances will be furnished by the board. Application, together with fee of ten dollars, must positively be in the hands of the Secretary before July 7.

G. W. COLLINS.

"F. D. I." INTERNATIONAL DENTAL FEDERATION.

THE next annual meeting of the Executive Council of the Fédération Dentaire Internationale will convene in Hanover, Germany, August 7, 1905, immediately following the annual meeting of the Central-Verein Deutscher Zahnarzte. Announcement of the programme for the meeting and the projected work for the Federation during the present period will shortly be made through the dental journals and through the official bulletin of the Federation.

EDWARD C. KIRK,
Secretary-General.

THE

International Dental Journal.

Vol. XXVI.   July, 1905.   No. 7.

Original Communications.[1]

A SYSTEM FOR THE SURGICAL CORRECTION OF HARELIP AND CLEFT PALATE.[2]

BY GEO. V. I. BROWN, A.B., D.D.S., M.D., C.M., MILWAUKEE, WIS.

THE reasons for the existence of any system of surgical treatment, and particularly one applied to the correction of a special class of affections, must be, first, a demand for such service; second, its necessity by reason of the large number of failures and extreme difficulty of accomplishing good results by other methods; third, that it makes possible an enlargement of the field of surgical accomplishment in at least one direction.

The blind, the deaf and dumb, the tuberculous, and the crippled almost everywhere have institutions established for their care. States and communities have recognized the duty of ministering to the comforts and necessities of the afflicted in these

---

[1] The editor and publishers are not responsible for the views of authors of papers published in this department, nor for any claim to novelty, or otherwise, that may be made by them. No papers will be received for this department that have appeared in any other journal published in the country.

[2] Read in the Section on Stomatology of the American Medical Association, at the fifty-fifth annual session, June, 1904. The article has been abbreviated by the omission of part of the illustrations. The entire article appears in the reprints. Copied, by consent, from the Journal of the American Medical Association.

directions. Large sums are annually contributed for the maintenance of such work and the encouragement of scientific investigation to increase the efficiency of its usefulness, but no such
responsibility has been assumed by municipalities, nor has any
notable portion of endowments of charitably inclined wealthy citizens been devoted to the relief of these unfortunate individuals,
half dumb through malformation of their mouths and palates and
doubly cursed by having the deformity and the even greater affliction of mental comprehension of difference from their fellows.
Their harelips, scarred and ill-shaped faces, mark them, through
no fault of their own, as were branded the felons in barbaric times:
speech communion with their fellows is almost wholly forbidden,
and they live ever in the dark shadow of misfortune.

NECESSITY FOR NEW AND SYSTEMATIC METHODS.

To those familiar with the literature and practical features of
this subject it is patent that all methods of treatment, whether prosthetic or surgical, have hitherto failed to be successful in a large
number of cases, and have not been able to meet the demands of
many cases at all.

Numerous methods of operation and most ingenious forms of
obturators have been from time to time suggested by authors, and
adopted by practitioners, with more or less benefit in individual
or special kinds of cases, and yet a systematic classification of the
forms, with particular methods to be employed in the correction
of each variety, showing comprehensive consideration of the distinct requirements that are found to be imperative, seems not to
have received the attention that is due. This the system that I
now present to you in my own name, after years of practical study
in the care of a large number of patients, seeks to accomplish in a
considerable measure.

Its methods are necessarily founded on the ground-work constructed by eminent surgeons who have contributed to literature the
results of their efforts in this direction, beginning probably with
Lemonier, in 1776, as the first to attempt to close palate fissures by
surgical means, followed by Eustache in 1799, von Graefe in 1876,
Roux in 1879, Warren, of Boston, in 1820. Diffenbach, Liston,
Sir William Fergusson,[1] the real author of successful staphylor-

---

[1] International Clinics, 1877.

raphy; Sedilot, Pancoast, William, Garretson, Wolf,[1] Erdman, Billroth,[2] von Langenbeck, Trilet (1889), and a host of great sur-

FIG. 1.

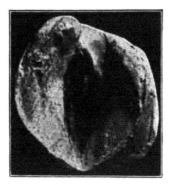

Cast of the mouth of a baby with single harelip, as in Fig. 2, with the characteristic enlarged turbinate.

FIG. 2.

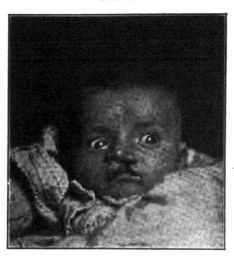

Baby with single harelip. Nose flattened and drawn to one side.

geons, past and present, who, despite great discouragement,—for this work is ever discouraging to surgical procedures when com-

---

[1] Archives of Klinical.

[2] Vienna Medical Presse, 1889.

pared with other fields of operation,—have each lent some share of personal skill and ingenuity to aid the perfection of the operative technic necessary to insure the ultimate success of the work.

ORIGINALITY.

The operation for reduction of the width of the fissure, in combination with the use of the appliance as described, is original with me, and I first performed it in 1897.

The methods of preparatory treatment of infants for the correction of facial deformity in lip cases are, so far as may be judged from careful study of the literature, also original with me.

Various minor steps in the operative technic have been developed from time to time, without previous knowledge of others having introduced them, and are believed to be original.

CLASSIFICATION.

The following is a classification that I have previously reported in other papers, and is designed to cover the important considerations from a surgical point of view:[1]

1. Character: Congenital acquired.
2. Form:
    Fissure in velum palati only (Figs. 32 and 34).
    Fissure of the velum, including part of the hard palate also (Fig. 36).
    Cleft entirely through both hard and soft palates (Fig. 39).
    Median fissure through both hard and soft palates, with bifurcation at the maxillary bone (Fig. 43).
    Double separation divided by the vomer, including the hard palate, with wide fissure almost completely obliterating the velum (Fig. 14).
3. Age:
    At birth or during early infancy (Fig. 1).
    Six months to one year old (Fig. 4).
    Two years old and during the period after deciduous teeth have been erupted, but before their permanent successors have caused them to loosen (Figs. 36 and 39).

---

[1] Brown, George V. I., " Surgical Correction of Malformations and Speech Defects due to or associated with Harelip and Cleft Palate," Jour. A. M. A., 1902. " A System for the Treatment of Harelip and Cleft Palate," Chicago Med. Record, 1903. " Relation and Comparative Merits of Surgery and Prosthesis in the Correction of Harelip and Cleft Palate," Dental Summary, 1903.

Twelve to eighteen years of age, or later years. After permanent teeth have been erupted, but before developmental processes have been completed.

Adults with teeth in upper jaws (Fig. 43).

Adults with edentulous upper jaws (Fig. 18).

FIG. 8.

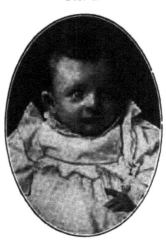

Photograph of same baby shown in Fig 2 after operation, and intended to call attention to the straightness of the nose, equality of shape of alæ, and the fact that the mouth is closed, which indicates that he breathes naturally through the nose.

Either lip or palate may be imperfect without the other being affected, although, as will be noted by study of the illustration, it is common for certain forms of lip and palate deformities to be associated.

Congenital lip deformities are either unilateral (Fig. 2) or bilateral (Figs. 7 and 11). The former may be of first degree, or little more than a notch; of second degree, with a fissure extending completely through both lip and maxillary bones; or of third degree, a wider separation with unilateral protrusion of the intermaxillary bone.

Bilateral or double harelip has usually marked deformity of the vomer with protrusion. To these, unfortunately, must be added the cases that have been imperfectly operated on in early life, which so often call for correction and which, although presenting an infinite variety of imperfections, have nevertheless certain characteristic defects that admit of distinct recognition and may be enumerated as follows: 1. Notch at the labial border. 2. Deflection of the tip of the nose, with deviation of the cartilaginous septum and flatness of the ala on the affected side. 3. Unsightly scars. 4.

FIG. 4.

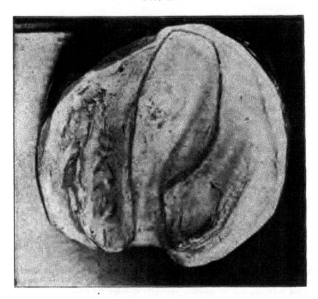

Six months to one year old.

Stenosis of one or both nares. 5. Marked arrest of development due to removal of the intermaxillary portion of jaw.

EARLY OPERATION.

Radical operation for closure of cleft palate in the infant is to be condemned, because the death-rate is unquestionably high. This is true of every serious operation at a period of life when the vital forces are busy adjusting themselves to a new, though natural, environment. The marked change from the direct protection and blood-supply of the uterus to the uncertainties of nourishment and temperature after birth involves a problem fraught with many difficulties of solution, even in the care of normal children. How much greater, then, when the vital forces are sapped by hemorrhage, and the digestive function disturbed by bacterial influences incident to operative procedures in the oral cavity, or wires left in the tissues

FIG. 7.

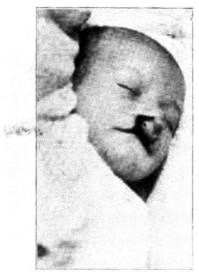

Baby with double harelip and the usual oral, facial, and nasal distortions.

FIG. 8.

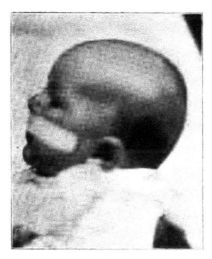

Same baby as in Fig. 7, with parts bound in position after preparatory operation on the vomer and manipulation to replace parts and to bring them into normal position before final operation.

of the mouth and jaws to gather bacteria in spite of antiseptic precautions, as they must and always do under these conditions.

Fig. 9.

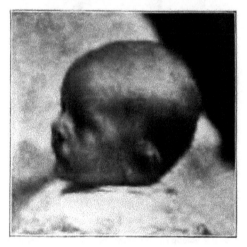

Same baby as in Figs. 7 and 8 and after preparatory operation and treatment, with part ready for closure by final operation.

Fig. 10.

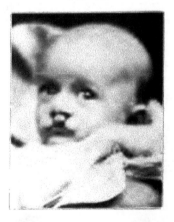

Another view of same baby pictured in Figs. 7 to 9, after treatment, showing that the sides of the fissures remain in contact without sutures, and calling attention to the improvement of the nose. Child is now ready for final operation on lip.

The question of meningitis also becomes a serious consideration when one contemplates the result of crushing the maxillary bones together to approximate the sides of such wide fissures as are found to exist in many cases, because of the correlation of the still unformed semi-cartilaginous bones of the face and head, which share in the effect of compression, and added to this is the danger of infection being carried to the brain through the direct channels of communication.

Fig. 11.

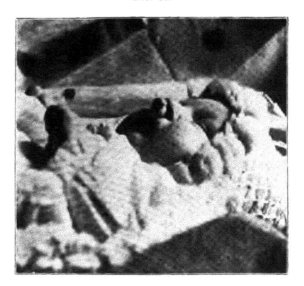

Baby five weeks old, with characteristic deformity of double harelip.

Finally, it may be said that the results of such operations from a cosmetic point of view are certainly not so perfect or pleasing as may be accomplished by other means, and it is, moreover, reasonably certain that the functional possibilities of the palates and mouths thus treated with regard to speech are often not of the best.

Foregoing statements may be better understood and their importance appreciated more fully, also the reasons for methods of treatment described later by a study of the defective operative results illustrated in Figs. 20, 24, 25, 26, 29, and 30, which have been taken from cases in practice, and which may, therefore, be said to be essentially practical.

The excessive unilateral development is a marked and almost

invariable condition in these cases, the more so because arrested development of the opposite side serves to increase this deformity.

The enlarged turbinated, or the appearance of enlargement, which may be noted in each of the pictures and casts, is a very common concomitant, and doubtless is due to a partial unfolding of its curative, in an attempted adjustment to the unusual nasal space occasioned by the fissures.

If, therefore, the sides of the jaws of any such cases are crushed together by immediate closure, as is recommended by some authors, one side of the face will project beyond the other, giving a peaked,

FIG. 18.

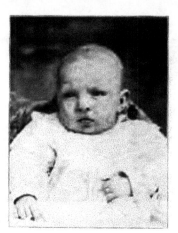

Front view, after operation, of baby shown in Figs. 11 and 12.

extremely unpleasant appearance, that later developments can never hope wholly to overcome.

It must be apparent also that in many instances it is the inferior turbinated bone that must meet in direct line the border of the maxillary portion of the palate on the opposite side, or if not this, then there will be a complete and irreparable permanent stenosis of the naris, on the affected side, at least.

Fig. 26 shows a little boy whose palate was closed in early infancy, and, as may be seen, the breathing is entirely by mouth. There is complete obliteration of one nasal passage, and almost the same condition of the other. The appearance of the face also confirms my statements.

FIG. 14.

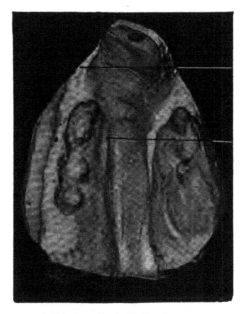

Double separation divided by the vomer.

FIG. 18.

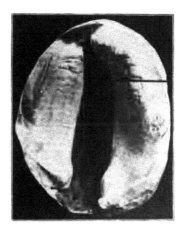

Cast of mouth of young lady shown in Figs. 20, 21, 22, and 23, with cleft extending through both hard and soft palates, the fatal error of extracting all teeth having been made some years before coming to me. Line is drawn where maxillary bone was sawed and fractured to correct unequal maxillary development, with result as shown in Fig. 23.

In these cases the intermaxillary bone is either attached to one side or separated by fissures on both sides. In the former case it projects, as shown in Fig. 2; in the latter, as illustrated by Figs. 7, 11, and 15. Thus an immediate, direct and forcible closing of the fissures would, under both conditions, leave an unsightly protrusion of one side, or the anterior aspect of the mouth and nose, which would be all the more noticeable because of the enforced narrowness.

Fig. 20.

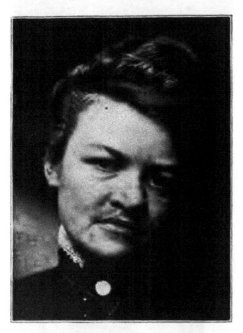

Patient twenty-two years old, the cast of whose mouth is shown in Fig. 18. Although the lip was closed in infancy by a famous surgeon whose skill is beyond criticism, the failure to adjust the maxillary bones resulted, as may be noted, in great nasal and facial deformity. Ala flat and nose almost entirely on one side of the face.

One would expect speech to be facilitated by the fact that when early operation has been performed no opportunity is given to acquire the characteristic defects common to individuals afflicted with imperfect palates, and yet we usually find that this is not the case, owing to insufficient room for the tongue and conditions due to hasty closure of the soft palate, which must of necessity be less perfect than at a later age when more time can safely be given to accurate adjustment of the parts.

The impossibility of preventing infants from crying and straining the muscles of the soft palate, thus endangering the pulling out of stitches, together with the danger to the life of the child, both tend to show that there is real need for other methods.

TREATMENT OF INFANTS.

Provision has been made for all, or, at least, most of the contingencies that arise in the care of these infants. If a child can be

Fig. 21.

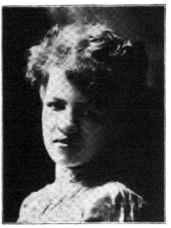

Same view of patient shown in Fig. 20 after lip had been reoperated on, scar tissue removed, and both jaw and nose straightened.

placed under treatment immediately or shortly after birth, when both lip and palate are affected, the method of procedure is as follows :

A day or two is given to allow the infant to become accustomed to its surroundings, if in a hospital, as is best, although not absolutely necessary. The child is weighed and its general condition of health observed, character of fecal passages, etc. If conditions are favorable, strips are then adjusted to prevent the action of the lower jaw from forcing the maxillary bones apart and widening both the palatal fissures and the lip separation. This also brings into play the muscles in such manner as to produce a narrowing effect whenever the little patient laughs or cries; in other words, the forces that ordinarily increase the deformity are now engaged in its reduction, and, in addition thereto, are stretching the lip muscles and skin surfaces on each side, so that in a very short time there will be an abundance of material to bridge across and make a sightly operation, where formerly the supply was perhaps so scant as to make an operation extremely hazardous.

FIG. 22.

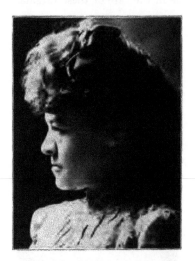

Side view of Fig. 20, to be compared with Fig. 23.

It is necessary that it be trained to eat from a spoon, or dropper. and all habit of sucking should be overcome, if possible, before operation.

Figs. 2 to 16, inclusive. call attention to the practical results of such treatment, and I think all will agree that a few weeks' preparatory care may sometimes be beneficially employed.

AGE FOR PALATE CLOSURE.

The proper time for palate operation depends largely on the physical development and condition of health of the individual. also on training, and subjection to proper control, because the best of health is not only desirable, but imperative, and unless the assistance of the patient can be secured in the way of intelligent co-operation in the post-operative care and treatment, it is most unlikely that good results will be accomplished. Therefore we find

Fig. 23.

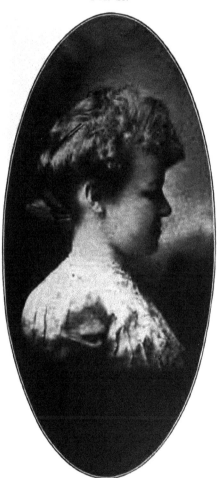

Side view of Fig. 20, showing ala of nose on right side to be the same shape as on the left, as shown in Fig. 22.

that some children can be operated on safely and satisfactorily at a much earlier age than others. Yet it is by all means desirable that no bad speech habits be given time to establish themselves.

Our choice must then come between the years when the deciduous teeth have been fully erupted and before they have become loosened for their permanent successors, and yet, before speech habit has been fully formed. Fortunately the period during which

Fig. 24.

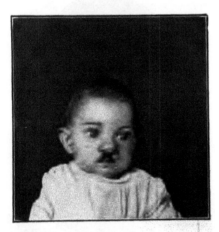

Double harelip.

most children talk " baby talk," as it is called, gives us more or less opportunity to make a satisfactory decision, since during this time the manner and form of speech are not what they will be later, and one change or another is much the same, because correct speech is yet to be acquired in any event.

REDUCTION OF WIDTH OF FISSURE BY THE USE OF AN APPLIANCE.

Having thus determined on the question of time, we next attach an appliance, such as is shown in Fig. 44. No other agent is necessary at this age, as the bones are soft and yielding, so that a slight turn of the little screw two or three times daily is sufficient to materially reduce the width of the fissure and to give the increased angles of the palate surface, which are necessary to make operation simple.

PREPARATORY TREATMENT OF ORAL, NASAL, AND FAUCIAL TISSUES.

During the time of wearing the appliance, daily irrigation with nasal douches of salt water, boric acid, or other mild solutions of like character should be given to correct the diseased condition of the nasal mucous membrane.

This treatment is important in all cases, for whether the patient be young or adult, hypertrophic rhinitis is a natural result of unusual exposure of the nasal and pharyngeal mucous membrane to thermal changes, irritation from mouth bacteria and other irritants.

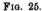

FIG. 25.

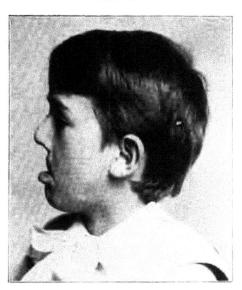

Shows deformed facial appearance, under conditions represented in Fig. 24, after intermaxillary bone has been removed to close double harelip.

Manipulation also should be given when tendency to gag on irritation of the faucial surfaces exists; otherwise, retching or vomiting at the slightest touch will make it almost impracticable to thoroughly cleanse the wound surface of the palate down to the tip of the uvula, as should be done without exciting such disturbances, which might cause destruction of the integrity of the stitches. Proper treatment is of inestimable benefit in these two directions.

TREATMENT AT SIX MONTHS OR OLDER.

· Infants who have reached the age of six months or more sometimes require the assistance of wire passed through the lateral sections of the divided jaw and secured by lead or silver plates, in order that by a slight bending of these wires from day to day a sufficient tension may be produced to bring about a readjustment of the deformed structures.

YOUNG AND ADULT CASES.

The appliance used for attachment to the teeth, and the nut, with threaded metal bar, do not differ materially in young or

FIG. 26.

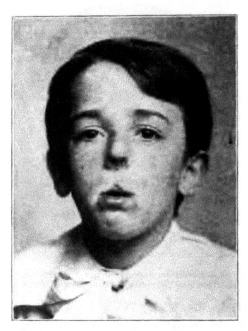

Front view of same boy shown in Fig. 25. His palate was closed in early infancy with what appeared to be a successful operation. The result at seven years old may be seen. Complete stenosis of left naris; right side of nose also absolutely useless for breathing purposes, although probe can be passed through. Disproportionate appearance of upper part of face and head to lower quite apparent, due to arrest of development. Voice shrill, high, and by no means perfect in pronunciation.

adult cases, except that a trifle more strength may often be required for the latter. There is, however, a difference in the manner of application. The yielding quality of the young bones makes it possible, by steadily exerted pressure of the appliance alone, to bring the sides nearer, and thus to reduce the width of the fissure;

at the same time the palatal arch is increased in height and the sides so shaped as to make the angle of their slant more acute; for older patients this is best accomplished by cutting along the external walls of the superior maxillary bones, through the outer plates, particularly at the malar process, and behind the tuberosities. With strong forceps then crush together until a partial fracture

Fɪɢ. 27.

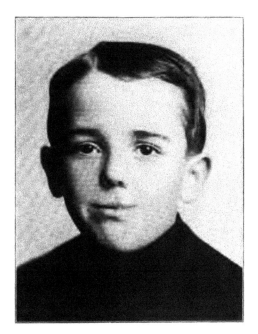

Front view of same boy shown in Figs. 25 and 26, after operation.

makes exact adjustment to proper form an immediate possibility. The appliance, as in Fig. 45, then acts as a splint capable of exerting pressure if needed.

It is most desirable that the anterior or narrower portions of the fissure should be brought into direct contact, sufficiently so, if possible, to allow of freshening not only the soft tissue, but the bony borders as well.

The complete circulation thus secured, after union has taken place, serves to nourish the flaps when the muco-periosteal final operation is performed, and does much to prevent sloughing, which is so much to be dreaded.

IMPROVED FORMS OF NEEDLES.

The curve of each needle should be as exactly fitted to the part of the operation for which it is to be used as possible, be-

Fig. 28.

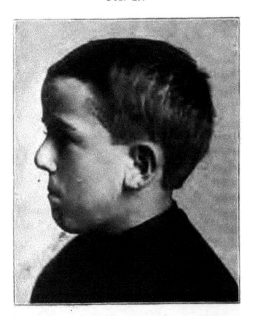

Side view of boy shown in Figs. 25, 26, and 27 after operation and restoration to more natural lines in profile.

cause, in describing the segment of a circle necessary to insert a suture in the anterior portion of the hard palate, where it is high and narrow, and in the posterior portion of the soft palate, where the space is broad and shallow, the requirements are entirely different. This is true also of the intermediate portions of the palate surface. The mucous secretion and hemorrhage make it difficult to see perfectly at all times in the act of catching the point of the needle and to easily secure the suture. Therefore great assistance is rendered if the exact curve of the needle can be so calculated as to enable the operator to know, with some degree of accuracy,

just where the point will reappear on the side opposite the point
of insertion.

Three sizes of needles, after the form of perineum needles,
curved to allow of convenient use at the different angles required
for operations in the mouth, meet the necessities of the situation
very well, but for my own use it is a great advantage, and since I
use both right and left hands in operating, much benefit is derived and the time of operation materially shortened by the use of

Fig. 29.

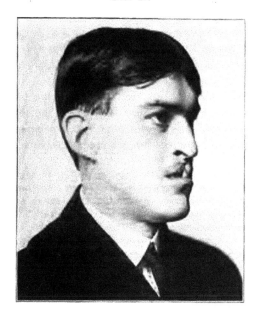

Young man of twenty-two, showing result of early imperfect operation for double harelip.

a set of five pairs of needles (my own design), with opposite curves
(right and left), each pair graded in size from the large one used
in the posterior portion of the soft palate to the smallest, which
are suitable for the extreme anterior portion of the hard palate.
These are threaded with the suture materials before operation, in
order to save time and confusion, and to leave the assistant quite
free to handle sponges and thus reduce to a minimum the troublesome hemorrhage that usually attends operations in this region.

SPEECH RESULTS AND TRAINING.

A system would be but half complete that offered no assistance beyond repair of the imperfect oral instrument and did nothing afterwards to teach the use of it.

Post-operative training must be our final consideration. It is a noticeable fact that individuals who are quite unable to recognize imperfections in the sounds of words, as they pronounce them, detect the difference at once when their own speech records are sounded from a graphophone, the effect being the same as though another person were speaking. To take advantage of this it is advisable to have a record taken before and another immediately after operation, while from time to time, as the training progresses, much encouragement is given by having others taken for comparison. Preferably, the same words should be repeated in order that the test may be exact.

Walter Edward Scripture, in his most valuable work, "The Elements of Experimental Phonetics," makes the following reference to phonographic speech records, which is completely in accord with my practical experience in training these cases:

"When a record is found that speaks clearly, in a natural voice, it can be trusted for what it says, since it cannot say anything more than is on it, and cannot improve its own tracing. The speech represented by a tracing from a record is the speech of the record itself. How nearly this reproduces the original speech can only be determined by comparing it by the ear with the words of the original speaker. By skilful manipulation records can be made whose speech cannot be distinguished from that of a living person, except by their weakness and by the scratching noise due to the friction of the tracing point in the groove."

A study of phonographic records, taken from patients of different ages, temperament, degrees of intelligence, and extent of palate deformity, showed some interesting differences in speech defect.

The facility with which some patients improve in speech after restoration of the palate by operation, and the difficulties that others of the same age and equal mental capacity seem to encounter. as noted by comparison of the phonographic records and casts. indicates very clearly that the extent of the fissure is by no means an exact index to the character of speech defect, there being a somewhat surprising dissimilarity of speech sounds among these patients. Undoubtedly there are certain easily recognizable wrong sounds common to them all, but the inability to speak correctly individual letters, words, and sentences is by no means the same in all cases, even where the palate fissures are quite similar; all of which serves to emphasize the necessity for careful consideration of speech mechanism as absolutely a first essential in the construction of a plan for speech and voice training calculated to give the best results.

Fig. 80.

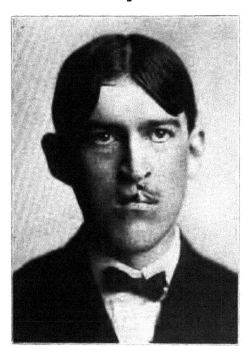

Front view of same case as in Fig. 29.

This, on previous occasions, I have summed up in the following manner:

The first cry of the child is merely a sound caused by reflex action of the muscles, without any guiding influence exerted by the faculty of reason. This is followed by the first efforts of sound to represent intelligent words as objects begin to be recognized, and gradually this is continued and extended until expres-

sion of ideas in speech becomes possible. It will be readily understood that if these efforts have been on normal or correct lines, the
muscular activity necessary to sound-producing must have been
guided by the proper nerve-centres, which will have caused an
increase in the brain development of those centres, and the messages sent from the motor tract to the muscles which are concerned

Fig. 81.

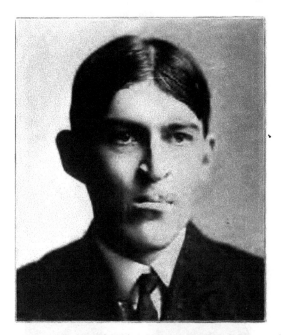

Result in case shown in Figs. 29 and 30 after operation, by which lip, nose, and jaw were
readjusted and scar tissue removed.

in the utterance of words will be in all respects correct, and the
habit of proper speech will have become an established fact. On
the other hand, however, if a deformity has existed from birth, by
reason of which the normal use of certain muscles has been greatly
restricted, and the use of certain other muscles, not commonly used
in the process of word enunciation, has received more stimulation
than would have been the case had there been a perfectly formed
mouth and throat, the results must invariably be an increased development of the nerve-centres which are injurious to speech, with

a faulty development of those that are necessary to perfect speech. This might be termed a habit, but the word habit conveys too restricted an idea of the condition. For example, when the eye, through its retinal image, registers on the brain structures the particular nerve stimulations which in time will become associated with the name of an object, its form record is established by

FIG. 32.

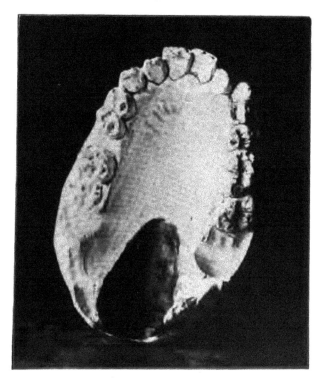

Fissure in velum palati only.

what may be known as the visual memory centres. Precisely also are the somæsthetic areas affected by the tactile sense, and memory of the sense of touch, as well as taste, smell, and other stimuli that may have been excited by or associated with any particular object, and, when the sensorium takes consciousness of this object, the name of which has become known to it, there is required the co-ordination between these different memory centres in order that

the proper message may be sent to the motor centres, through which
certain muscles may be set in motion in the proper manner to
produce the sound which may be clearly recognized as the spoken
name of the object.

It is known that in speech the muscles of the chest, which are
responsible for expiration, the muscles that raise and lower the
larnyx, those that tighten the vocal cords and tip the hyoid bone, as
well as resounding properties due to the nearness of the spinal
column, and the co-operation of the forces that are applied in
raising and lowering the soft palate, the adjustment of the tongue
and proper action of the muscles of the cheeks and lips, are all

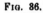

Fig. 36.

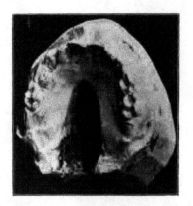

Cast of mouth of child two and one-half years old, with cleft including the velum and parts
of the hard palate.

necessary for the utterance of even a single word. If, therefore,
during the life of the individual, through faulty operation or
adverse action of these agencies, wrong messages have been constantly sent to portions of the brain concerned in making a certain
sound, and if the auditory memory centres have registered, by
the constant hearing, imperfect sounds for specific words, which
accordingly have caused the development of brain structure which
is all active against correct speech, and if there be an insufficient
development of those centres which are needed for perfect speech,
how great becomes the difficulty of giving a speech power to individuals in the face of all these acquired disadvantages.

Kingsley's palatograms (Fig. 47), obtained by coating the

surfaces of thin plates covering the palate surfaces with chalk, in such manner that whenever the tongue touched, in sounding a word or letter, the black surface showed through, are of interest as indicating why certain letters are so troublesome in these cases. It will be noticed by the illustration that points of contact of K and G are post velar, and therefore not only practically impossible without a velum, but almost equally so, unless after operation the soft palate secured be of perfect form and sufficiently flexible, under muscular control, to allow this contact to take place. These, it will be remembered, in support of the accuracy of Kingsley's work, are invariably troublesome sounds. Foster and Reichert, in describing speech under the heads of vowels and consonants, divided into explosives and aspirants, vibratory and resonants, giving in

FIG. 37.

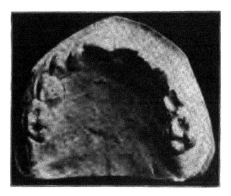

Cast of same patient's mouth as in Fig. 36, after closure by operation.

detail the mechanism of alphabetical sounds, conclude with the following statement, that, from our point of view, is all important:

" On many of the above points, however, there are great differences of opinion, the discussion of which, as well as of other more rare consonantal sounds, would lead us too far away from the purpose of this book. The following tabular statement must therefore be regarded as introduced for convenience only."

Scripture calls attention to the following factors of voice control:

" 1. Reflex tonus: Tonus is a faint muscular contraction due to continuous weak nerve stimulations, easily subject to fatigue, ill health, and other demoralizing conditions, lack of or disarrangement of which causes marked change of voice in both speaking and singing.

" 2. Force of movement: This depends on the amount of stimulus sent to muscles, movements of which include not only those directly involved, but also their antagonists. This requires an excess of effort over what might be expected, but when the innervations are properly co-ordinated this excess is not necessarily large and fatiguing.

" 3. Accuracy of movement: Inaccuracy of movement is a fundamental source of inaccurate and wrong sounds.

FIG. 89.

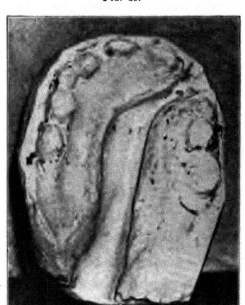

Cast of mouth of boy two and one-half years old. Cleft through hard and soft palates.

" 4. Precision of movement: This refers to regularity and evenness of execution and depends on nervous control.

" 5. Accuracy and precision of co-ordination: This represents the nervous control over simultaneous muscular movements. Some forms of thick speech of alcoholic intoxication and incorrect adjustments during excitement are caused by defective co-ordination in speech effort.

" 6. Quickness of response: This is action of the nervous centres that tends to become automatic. One object in vocal training should be to render speech and song automatic.

"7. Quickness of muscular movement: This depends on both muscular and nervous quickness and must be properly balanced; otherwise, speech appears labored or slurred.

"8. Auditory motor control: The learning of speech sounds consists *largely* in forming connections between motor and auditory sensations.

Fig. 40.

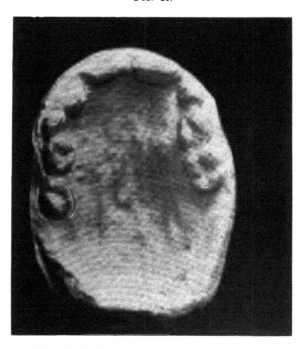

Cast of same mouth as Fig. 39, showing result after operation. Fissure reduced by the use of an appliance and closed by final operation.

"9. Ideomotor control: Sounds occurring simultaneously with sights, *touches*, tastes, smells, emotion, act of will, etc., tend to be connected with them, so that when any one of a complex group occurs again, the others are revived more or less clearly in consciousness. It is in this way that speech movements become associated with printed letters.

"10. General voluntary control: This is subject to changes of nutrition, fatigue, emotion, and general habits, on all of which vocal control must place its dependence."

In my practical training of these cases, I have found that one of the best aids to speech improvement is singing. Even though the sounds be less musical than might be wished, and they often are, vocal lessons, or, in the absence of this, constant use of the voice in chanting sentences, after the manner of intoning church services, will enable the individual to speak reasonably well the particular sentences practised in this manner in a very short time. Combining, as these exercises do, most of the essential points brought out in the foregoing description of speech requirements, it follows that there can be no more beneficial procedure.

Nervousness and over anxiety about rapid improvement in many cases retard progress quite seriously, and must be overcome in so far as possible at the very outset. Such patients are best counselled that improvement must necessarily be slow, and cautioned against making too great effort.

A large majority of these patients are, as might be expected, individuals of extremely unstable nervous organization, and it is of quite frequent occurrence that some of the neuroses common to neurotics occur in the way of speech impediment. Aphasia with regard to certain letters and words, stammering, nervous hurrying, together with letters and sounds, are very often complications that retard progress. Doubtless much confusion in reporting results has occurred through failure to distinguish these affections.

Exactly why interference on the part of any nervous agent that might tend to disturb the rhythm of muscular movement must necessarily disarrange the speech harmony is most beautifully shown by a copy of one of Scripture's plates, which is a reproduction of a photograph of actual sound waves taken during the recital of " Who killed Cock Robin?" (Fig. 48).

PHONOGRAPHIC RECORDS.

The phonographic records show the degree of improvement in speech.

CASE I.—In the case of a girl of fourteen, who had only a fissure in the soft palate, before operation, it was impossible to distinguish speech sounds sufficiently for unaccustomed persons to understand what she said. Therefore, a phonographic record would have been a mere jargon of unintelligible sounds. The fourth grade was as high as she had been able to get in the public schools, because teachers could not understand her. Immediately after operation marked improvement was noted by record. Later records showed remarkable change for the better, and on one or two occasions, after training, she has recited before large audiences, with much clearness and a very good approximation of perfection of sound, verses on which she had been drilled, but in general conversation her progress was not in proportion to that of better educated patients, as was noted in records of other cases. Eagerness in conversation always tended to cause lapses into old speech habits, and in this case, such difficulty was hard to overcome; a difference being apparent if she were allowed to associate for a time with people who themselves spoke incorrectly or carelessly or the reverse.

Fig. 43.

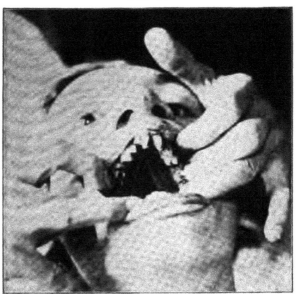

Photograph of mouth of patient with cleft through both hard and soft palates. Casts shown in Figs. 41 and 42 were taken from this patient's mouth.

CASE II.—Another young girl, twenty-two years old, with the same character of fissure, but who had a high school education, could speak much better than the preceding one before operation, the range of her intelligible, even though somewhat nasal, sounds being much less limited. After closure of the cleft, though operative results were quite perfect in both cases, her progress in the line of improvement in conversational sounds was shown by the record to be much more marked.

CASE III.—Patient, mother of a grown-up family, aged thirty-eight. Cleft in soft palate the same as Cases I. and II. She was not well educated, but not ignorant, and of less nervous temperament than the other two. Speech, as might be expected, was better than Case I. and not so good as Case II. Soon after operation, therefore, without training, her record was found to be surprisingly good, due in a considerable measure, no doubt, to freedom from nervousness. Later reports of improvement were much more favorable than was expected, but have not yet been confirmed by record.

CASE IV.—This patient, a girl of sixteen, in whom the fissure was confined to the velum, as in all the preceding cases, was as uneducated as the first patient, but with less natural intelligence. Scarcely a single word in her first record could be understood. Later, and after much training, she was able to recite simple rhymes before large audiences quite well, but she has never acquired good speech. When corrected, she can repeat, after another, sentence by sentence, even most difficult words with little noticeable speech defect.

CASE V.—A girl of twenty-two, who had an acquired fissure of the velum, due to hereditary syphilis, was operated on after preparatory administration of potassium iodide, with successful result, so far as closing the opening was concerned. It was not perfect in the sense that the preceding cases were, because cicatricial contractions, due to previous ulcerative processes, had stiffened the tissue. Notwithstanding the fact that this deformity was acquired at about the age of fourteen, and the patient's education was above the average, there was less improvement after operation than in any of the other cases.

CASE VI.—In contradistinction to these other cases, a little boy of nine years of age, whose congenital cleft in the velum was like that in Case V., with very imperfect speech, was able to improve so rapidly that between the months of May and November defects were so overcome that his school-teacher did not notice unusual difference from other children of the same age.

CASE VII.—A young woman of twenty-two, fairly well educated, with opening in velum palati alone, in whom speech sounds were very bad before operation, was able, by reason of good ear and singing practice, to improve sufficiently to be able to pray and sing alone at Salvation Army meetings within a few months from time of closure. In this case, undoubtedly, religious zeal helped to overcome self-consciousness, together with other mental and nervous hinderances, while constant attendance on the meetings of the army gave the best possible training to the vocal apparatus.

CASE VIII.—A young man of eighteen had a complete cleft of both hard and soft palates. He is a graduate of a high school. Before operation it was almost impossible to understand him, yet, in repeating the alphabet. unusual ability to pronounce each letter was noted, even the G, K, and C being more than ordinarily good. Stammering was the prime cause of his speech difficulty. The record, taken two days after the last stitches were removed, complete union by first intention having taken place throughout. even to the tip of the uvula, showed an almost astonishing result, since his voice from the graphophone, singing the "Holy City," sounded better, perhaps, than many of our own would if a similar record had been taken.

CASE IX.—A young man nineteen years old, with a fair education. had fissures through both hard and soft palates. The first speech record was better than Case VIII., on account of freedom from nervous habit, but ability to make separate sounds was less perfect. He could sing "Rock of Ages" quite well, and showed great speech improvement in later records as a result of two weeks' singing and drill exercise.

CASE X.—A boy of nine, for whom only the preparatory operation has yet been performed, has given us two interesting records. In one he recites the Lord's prayer with an obturator in his mouth, and in the next equally well without it, yet, with cleft through both hard and soft palates, it must be understood he could not have learned to speak so well had he not had the mechanical assistance in the beginning.

CASE XI.—A young woman of twenty-two, highly educated, but with wide cleft through both hard and soft palates, made worse by having had several previous unsuccessful operations, improved so rapidly after the normal form of the palate had been restored by operation that she successfully passed an examination to teach in an Eastern law-school. Although rec-

FIG. 44.

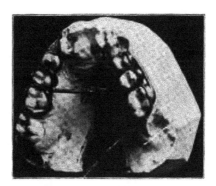

Cast with appliance adjusted as used in the reduction of the width of palate fissure, in cases illustrated in Figs 39 to 43, and all similar others of the same classes.

ords in this case are not complete, the fact that she now holds an important position and daily transacts the telephone business of a large establishment is sufficient proof of her improvement. Undoubtedly, her rare intelligence and persistence have been assisting factors.

CONCLUSIONS.

I have thus presented a number of cases, covering not only different forms of cleft palate deformity, but varying characteristics with the same classes of deformity, due to the several conditions that govern speech habit in these individuals. A large number of other cases of which I have from time to time taken record, under all the various forms and conditions of these patients, confirm the results given in those here cited. All the selections given in these illustrations have been made on the basis of demonstrating distinctive, important differences bearing on operative procedures, and speech results, rather than a multiplication of similar cases, that would involve endless repetition and confuse rather than make the subject clear.

It has been demonstrated that some of these patients, with openings so wide that there appeared to be almost no palate at all, spoke as well or better than others with only a slight velar defect, and individual distinctions have thus been made apparent, from all of which the following conclusions are obvious:

FIG. 46.

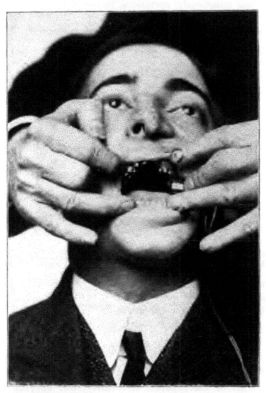

Photograph of patient with palate fissure, as in Fig. 43, after reduction by the use of appliance and final operation, with perfect result throughout the entire extent of both hard and soft palates down to the tip of the uvula.

To get the best results from operations, the palate must be restored in as nearly perfect form as possible. Freedom from scar tissue and from muscular tension sufficient to allow necessary speech movement are essential.

Proper muscular alignment at the point of union greatly facilitates the early usefulness of antagonizing muscles; therefore natural physiologic action is more promptly in evidence.

All these operative conditions are favored by the methods of the system herein described. Individual benefits, assuming that operative results have been perfect or as nearly so as possible, will be governed by patience, earnestness, and application of the patient. Natural intelligence, aided by education, will be manifest in assisting progress. A musical ear (so-called) and ability to note rhythm and time in music are of very great assistance.

FIG. 47.

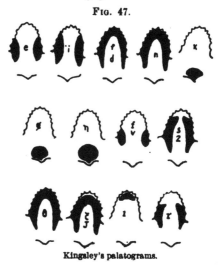

Kingsley's palatograms.

No cleft palate deformity can be so bad that it cannot be corrected by surgical operation, nor need age prevent unless through lack of health on the part of the patient.

It has been my purpose throughout to treat this subject from the broad stand-point of a system to emphasize by precept and illustration the crying need for better treatment of a class of individuals whose misfortunes cannot fail to appeal to every one; to establish an understanding of the necessity for differentiation in the choice of operation and methods of treatment; and, above all, to prove the value of a practical system. Thus matters belonging strictly to surgical technic have been, so far as possible, avoided and left for a future paper, but the post-operative treatment of these patients is so vital to the success of every operation that more than passing notice seems to be imperative.

It is too often taken for granted that more or less sloughing and pus formation must follow extensive mouth operations, and that surgical asepsis is impossible. In a sense, this must be admitted to be true, owing to natural anatomic obstacles to complete sterilization and the constant exposure to infection from so many sources, but, notwithstanding all this, most gratifying results can be secured, and so nearly a true primary union obtained as to make its essential benefit the same even with extensive wound surfaces. With the periosteum stripped from the palate surfaces; incisions reducing circulation to the farthest safe limit; nasal secretions above in contact with raw surface; mouth secretions below, mixed, as often occurs, with gastric regurgitations and vomited matter; only a comparatively thin veil of tissue bridging the space of the palatal separation of the bones and at the velum, exposed to destructive influences at every movement of the tongue or act of swallowing, it goes without saying that only the most rigid adherence to antiseptic surgical care could be effective.

Strong solutions of poisonous, or tissue destructive, germicidal agents are necessarily precluded in the mouth. Dilution in the oral fluids renders otherwise effective solutions of practically no benefit. The histologic character of the nasal, oral, and pharyngeal mucous membrane surfaces render sterilization extremely difficult, and it has been conclusively proved that animal fats, dead mucous cells, and other surface coatings resist even powerful drugs to such an extent as to protect underlying bacteria, while germs on the immediate surface are destroyed. Mechanical cleansing, therefore, is a first necessity, and next to this, frequent use of non-toxic or mild solutions of otherwise injurious germicidal agents. Preparatory preparation of the field of operation consists in scrubbing membranous, dental, and other surfaces, removal or antiseptic care of teeth or roots, and at least temporary stopping of carious tooth cavities. My post-operative sheet-anchor is dioxogen,[1] which gives mechanical cleansing in setting free the dead mucous cells and destroying the resistant nature of the intervening secretions, while at the same time it gives an immediate and powerful effect on bacteria in destroying their vital properties. Dioxogen and 2.5 per cent. carbolic acid should be used alternately once each hour during

---

[1] I use dioxogen because in my experience it has proved the most uniformly free from acid of any of the preparations of H_2O_2, commonly sold as such, and because an impure or a strong acid solution must necessarily be absolutely prohibited when hourly treatments of the mouths of patients, many of whom are infants, is prescribed.

the day, and at least four times at night. These washes are applied with a glass hospital syringe, with force enough to assist in the dislodgement of little particles of débris, but not force enough to be injurious.

In addition to hourly washing, the use of applicators, made in the usual way, of absorbent cotton wrapped on toothpicks, is re-

Fig. 48.

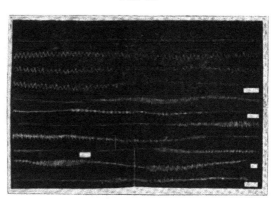

Copy of Scripture's photographs of sound-waves in "Who killed Cock Robin?"

quired from three to four times daily to wipe surfaces that washing alone will not cleanse sufficiently. Almost from the moment of recovery from the anæsthetic, some one of the many oil preparations should be sprayed with a suitable nebulizer through the nasal passages, as well as the mouth, and continued throughout the treatment after each washing.

In dealing with children and infants it is not always possible to follow all these directions, as they sometimes do not submit willingly, and naturally we must therefore do only so much as we safely can, but patience, judgment, and skill on the part of the nurse can do much to overcome such difficulties.[1]

---

[1] Other references which may be consulted are as follows: Le Dentia: La Médecine, June 5, 1890. Ehrmann: Les opérations plastiques sur le palais chez l'enfant, etc., Paris. Taylor: Dublin Journal of Medical Sciences, 1900. Edwin Owen: London Lancet, 1896. Telezit: Tribune Médicale, Paris, 1894. Talbot, Eugene S.: Stigmata of Degeneracy, and The Etiology of Osseous Deformities. Cryer, M. H.: Internal Anatomy of the Face. Fillebrown: Boston Journal of Medicine and Surgery.

A SIMPLE, EFFICIENT CROWN FOR THE POSTERIOR TEETH.

BY ALLISON R. LAWSHE, D.D.S., TRENTON, N. J.

HAVING found much satisfaction from the use of an easily made crown for badly broken down second and third molar teeth, and for first molar teeth not exposed to view, I have thought that others may also find it useful.

Devitalize the pulp, if living, and prepare the root-canal as usual. Grind down the walls, if any remain, half way, and slope to the gum margin. Prepare a well-fitting band of gold, leaving space for cusps, as is usual with all-gold crowns, and make two countersunk holes on the buccal and two on the lingual side. Now coat the inside lower edge of this band with a layer of gutta-percha,

FIG. 1.

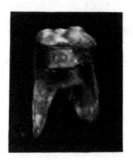

that it may make a perfect fit when pressed to place, and after preparing good, substantial undercuts in the pulp-chamber, or the openings of the root-canals, warm and adjust it, wash the root-stump with alcohol, and carefully and thoroughly pack amalgam into the undercuts and all spaces between stump and band, filling the entire band and building cusps above it. The patient can then be instructed to bite, and the building and carving of the cusps continued until a perfect articulation is secured, when the crown may be considered finished (Fig. 1). A tooth near by should then be washed with chloroform, dried, and a ball of tough gutta-percha fastened thereto to prevent the possibility of damage to the crown by the occluding teeth before the amalgam has set.

Besides being easily made, this crown has the merit of a perfect articulation and comparative ease of adjustment in mouths where an excessive flow of saliva would render the placement of the ordinary gold cap on a thoroughly dried root troublesome and uncertain. It is, moreover, strong and durable.

Reviews of Dental Literature.

HIGHEST ORTHODONTIA. 1. FACIAL BEAUTY; 2. DENTAL ANTAGONISM. By John Nutting Farrar, M.D., D.D.S., New York City.[1] (Continued from page 389.)

HARMONY BETWEEN THE DENTAL ARCHES AND FACIAL FEATURES.

In any of this class of operations, harmony between form and size of the dental arches, and that of the possible future form of the face of the child patient, is of utmost importance; this is necessary in order to accomplish the highest possibilities for the patient's best future personal interests, but this point will not be dwelt upon.

As perfect beauty is inherited or acquired, and all persons are susceptible to beauty, it is natural for all to desire to be as free from deformity as possible, therefore, between the utilitarian aspect (dental antagonism) and beauty of facial features, lies the object sought by all applicants.

Seldom do persons seek the dentist's services purely for the former (mastication of food), but they do often seek it purely for the latter (beauty). Therefore, in the treatment for correction of irregular teeth, the first aim should be to establish a change in their arrangement with the view to cause the highest improvement in the face, not only, as before said, in facial outline, but also in the intellectual expression, shown in and through the facial outline. As Bacon said, " The best part of beauty is that which no picture can express;" this part is the one to which I refer. Incongruity between a too broad dental arch in a narrow face is no less a defect than a too narrow arch in a broad face. Both cause a weakness of intellectual expression. Unless there is harmony between the

---

[1] **Lect**ure delivered before the New York Dental College Alumni, January 18, 1905.

dental arches and the size of the face, as a whole, the accomplishment simply of perfect antagonism cannot be regarded all that is for the patient's good. To so regulate teeth that the moulding will bring out the intellectual scintillations through the smiling wrinkles in the lower half of the face, balancing it with the wrinkles about the eyes, is high art. The former of these results (perfect antagonism) may be accomplished without the latter (beauty). To kill out the intellectual fire by causing a blank face, often gross, and an expression of "all teeth" with the cuspids standing too far apart, stretching the skin so as to kill the finer emotional expressions about the lips, is not evidence of artistic skill.

Harmony between the arrangement of the teeth and the facial features may call for evenly arranged teeth, or it may call for slightly irregular teeth, depending upon the form or contour of the face and head. If the patient has that which is called "high cheek bones" and an aquiline nose, with a corresponding mentality, the teeth should be slightly irregular in order to harmonize. A selfish expression, however, may not necessarily be intensified by inclining the teeth posteriorly, like those of a serpent, nor by leaving the cuspids so long as to cause a ferocious expression. If any deviation is allowed to be made, harshness of expression may be softened somewhat, but not to the extent of causing too much incongruity between the intellectual and the physical, for that would cause an expression of deception. One of the most important aims should be to keep the upper cuspids down as close to the lower teeth as is prudent for proper occlusion of the arches, and not have the six anterior teeth appear like a straight line.

As before implied, to accomplish the highest degree of beauty, and at the same time accomplish perfect antagonism, is not always possible. While perfect antagonism is of great importance, it should not, as elsewhere mentioned, be made at the expense of beauty of facial outline and intellectual expression. To repeat: Every regulator should have high ideas, and always aim upward; high art in the correction of deformities should be the main aim, and should be carried out, as far as possible, but of course no dentist should expect these excellencies in results who does not have some natural artistic gifts and clear knowledge of the ideals known to great artists concerning the proportion of different parts of the human face, and, as before said, know the comparative merits of the several different classes of faces sufficiently to determine at a glance the points that can and the points that cannot be improved by moving the teeth. But to know well the degree to which this knowledge can be best applied in a case, and the degree that circumstances of the patient's health, social position, educational and business environments will permit, must indeed be evidences of sound judgment.

The meaning of the term beauty, of course, may differ with different persons, but the essayist means, by the term beauty, a physical and intellectual harmony of expression that everybody loves to see. In some cases it is not only possible to accomplish this balance, but to stimulate personal confidence, so that it (con-- fidence) will cause an expression of self-reliance that will strengthen and cause an appearance of a balanced mind, free from self-mortification, sometimes engendered by consciousness of personal deformity.

Whether it is right to carry facial beauty in appearance beyond the power of the brain may be questionable, but the essayist thinks that less harm is caused by so doing than by the reverse results, especially in women. The only injury, sometimes noticed, is stimulation of personal pride, into temporary degeneracy called vanity.

THE PHILOSOPHY OF THE AUTHOR'S PLAN VS. THE OLD PLAN.

There are many cases in which the upper arch requires more or less widening in order to establish proper antagonism, but to widen the upper arch beyond the accomplishment of proper antagonism can hardly be regarded as scientific. I shall not attempt, in the limited time here given, to go over the entire field of this question, but shall confine my remarks to the main principles.

In cases of narrow arches, caused by mouth-breathing or by wrong antagonism, or little or no antagonism, it is generally the upper arch that is most at fault. In these cases, the arch tends to narrow more than does the lower. Indeed the lower seldom shows this fault. This is because the position of the upper teeth, by failing to antagonize with the lower teeth (which when properly arranged has greatly to do with keeping the upper in their proper places), go astray by having too much liberty and by pressure of the cheek muscles against them while in the act of swallowing.

The upper teeth depend more upon antagonism with the lower teeth than do the lower depend upon antagonism with the upper. When the upper teeth are thus properly regulated, and the lower are not moved, permanency of the upper teeth is much more easily secured than when the lower teeth also are moved, which leaves them more or less loose. The compactness of the teeth that contribute to make up the lower arch is greater than that which contributes to the maintenance of the upper arch. If a side tooth in the lower arch is lost, this defect in the strength of the arch is proved by the inclining forward of the tooth in rear of the space left by the lost tooth. If a side tooth in the upper arch is lost, the tooth posterior to the space does not tend to incline nearly so far, under similar conditions, as in the lower arch. The tooth anterior to the space may drift posteriorly, but if it does drift, it is generally only slightly.

The stone arch principle is greater in the lower than in the upper arch. In the well-formed lower, all the teeth may be regarded as buttress keys of the arch, while in the upper, even if well formed, the key principle in most cases is weak or nearly wanting. In early adult and in middle life, the upper teeth are mainly held in place by the lower teeth, aided by the cheek muscles. If properly arranged, the lower teeth not only prevent the upper arch from being strongly self-binding, but the (upper) arch needs no key. The teeth of the upper arch, besides being held by the cheek muscles, are prevented from narrowing by the overhanging of the cusps of the lower teeth. Firm upper teeth are held in place by antagonism with the lower teeth. If the lower teeth are loose the antagonism of the upper may or may not be made firmer. If in either arch, however, there are spaces caused by loss of some of the teeth, and the remainder do not lock properly while in antagonism, more or less of them may go astray. As we all know. there are two kinds of antagonism,—cutting antagonism and crushing antagonism. The six front teeth are for the former, while the teeth in the rear of these six are for the latter purpose.

There are two distinct teachings in regard to the treatment of protruding teeth, and also for irregular anterior teeth; both claim improvement through the theory of antagonism. The essayist's plan (since 1864) is founded upon that which he regards as the broad basis of æsthetics, which embraces also efficient antagonism. The other plan is simply to even the teeth of one jaw without much regard (excepting in name) to antagonizing with the teeth of the opposite jaw, and with slight, if any, regard to æsthetics, or the effect of the operation upon the facial features. One is permanent regulation of the teeth of both jaws; the other, the doubtful and almost certain destruction not only of lasting proper antagonism, but injury to facial beauty.

One plan has for its object, first, to beautify the face; second, the accomplishment of permanent efficient antagonism, not necessarily perfect antagonism in all cases, that is firm and strong and not liable to go astray by antagonism. The other plan is to widen the upper arch until all the irregular upper teeth are brought into line, and then leave them, or else widen the lower arch to match, a plan that leaves both arches with little or no support, irresponsible and liable to destroy the equilibrium unless held by artificial retainers.

EXTRACTION.

The treatment of cases of jumbled front teeth or protruding teeth by the essayist's plan, when it is not necessary to widen the upper arch, is to shorten it by extraction of a bicuspid on one, and possibly on both sides, and then to move the teeth anterior to the space posteriorly or diagonally back, along the dental line, and not attempt to widen the arch. The other operation is to shorten the protruding part of the arch by widening it, even if it injures facial expression. By the essayist's plan the operation is not only easier and shorter, but firmness of antagonism is not at all disturbed, and facial expression is improved, not weakened. To extract a first bicuspid and then move the cuspid into the space made, leaves the cuspid in the place of the outer cusps of the extracted first bicuspid. To move the lateral incisor into the place of the cuspid, following this by moving the central, does not disturb antagonism, nor does it in any way injure facial expression, for the lacking of one bicuspid is not noticeable when the line of the upper teeth are properly closed up, because the arch, while it is shortened, leaves none of the weaknesses between the two arches that is caused by over-widening. This plan is natural antagonism, the other is loose artificial antagonism; this one is firm, strong, reliable, generally intensifying facial beauty, while the other scatters and weakens it.

Sometimes it is better to extract a second bicuspid instead of the first, but this depends upon the extent of irregularity to be corrected in the anterior part of the arch.[1]

---

[1] This point may be found explained in Farrar's "Irregularities of the Teeth," vol. i.

Reports of Society Meetings.

THE NEW YORK INSTITUTE OF STOMATOLOGY.

A REGULAR meeting of the Institute was held on Tuesday evening, March 7, 1905, at the Chelsea, No. 222 West Twenty-third Street, New York, the President, Dr. C. O. Kimball, in the chair. The minutes of the last meeting were read and approved.

COMMUNICATIONS ON THEORY AND PRACTICE.

Dr. H. W. Gillett.—I wish to present the cast of a case showing an extra right superior deciduous lateral. The left deciduous central and lateral are missing, and the permanent central on that side is in place. Please notice the worn facet on the anterior edge of the temporary central, showing where the natural tendency is for the child to bring his jaw to rest as a relief from his usual position of posterior occlusion.

Dr. W. M. Dailey.—The case presented by Dr. Gillett is, I think, of unusual importance. I have seen in practice a number of cases of supernumerary deciduous teeth and it has been my opinion for a long time that this condition in almost all cases would cause a malocclusion of the permanent teeth.

It is unfortunate that Dr. Gillett does not show us the lower cast of this case, so that we might see the full results of the malocclusion.

Dr. F. Milton Smith.—I wish to again call to the minds of the society the point brought out by Dr. Howland some time ago concerning the use of the tannate of glycerin rubbed on the necks of teeth to reduce sensitiveness. I use it constantly where I have occasion to polish the sensitive necks of teeth, and I have yet to find a case that cannot be relieved in two or three minutes, so that I can do all the polishing necessary.

The President.—I may speak of the same thing in my own work. A drop of glycerin in a little tray and some crystals of tannic acid rubbed into it. The sensitiveness stays away. There is no stain.

Dr. F. L. Fossume.—I have not had the uniform success with tannate of glycerin that the other two gentlemen have had. Where the teeth have been denuded of the enamel, especially around the necks and in between in the interdental space, and where they are so sensitive that the patient suffers great pain from the slightest irritation, I have found the following treatment to give relief; in fact, I have yet to see the case where it will fail. The rubber dam is to be adjusted on all the teeth to be treated; they are now washed thoroughly with sodium bicarbonate, then dried, and a saturated solution of formalin is applied with cotton pellets and rubbed over the surface with orange-wood sticks until the patient feels no pain. A piece of lintine is to be placed over the patient's nose as a protection against the formaldehyde gas, which is a great irritant to the mucous membrane; in fact, great care must be taken and very small pieces of cotton used. It will also give relief on abraded surfaces on molars. I have used it in very sensitive cavities where the dentine is hard and shiny and where I am sure the pulp is not exposed, my method being to seal it in the cavity for twenty-four hours.

Dr. Gillett.—When formalin was first introduced it was advocated for the devitalization of teeth.

Dr. Fossume.—I have used it a great deal for this purpose, and I can state positively that it is not a devitalizing agent.

Dr. E. A. Bogue.—Years ago there was a mixture put on the market called Naboli. Our friend Dr. Merriam, of Salem, undertook to find out what it contained, and among other things it was found to contain glycerin and tannin. From that a mixture of glycerin, tannin, carbolic acid, alcohol, and atropine was made, and has been used for twenty-five years for sensitive teeth. The glycerin unites directly with the water of the soft part, acting precisely as desiccation would.

Dr. C. F. Allan.—The best way to mix glycerin and tannin is in a hot mortar.

The President.—I will pass around some radiographs sent in by Dr. Tousey, who expresses his regret that he will not be able to be present to discuss Dr. Schamberg's paper.

Dr. Locherty read a letter from the Connecticut State Dental Society, inviting the members of the Institute to attend their meetings to be held April 18 and 19, 1905.

Dr. Morris I. Schamberg, of Philadelphia, gave an interesting address illustrating his remarks with lantern slides. The following are some of the slides he presented:

Several cases of leprosy showing different stages of the disease. One of facial palsy following involvement of the glands of the sub-parotid region, due to an abscessed tooth. A number of slides showing syphilitic lesions of the lips and face; also some of epithelioma to illustrate the differential diagnosis. A case of lupus before and during treatment with X-ray. A case of a fractured jaw broken in two places, treated by the Angle method. Radiograph showing appliance in position. Some radiographs of a case of ankylosis of the jaw in which two operations were performed and from one-quarter to one-half inch of bone was removed from each side; the result was satisfactory. A number of radiographs of impacted third molars in various positions. Radiographs of teeth erupting abnormally. Some radiographs showing roots improperly filled, others of abscesses, and several of root amputation.

Dr. Gillett.—If I had not seen Dr. Schamberg's root amputation clinic a year ago before the District Society I should possibly not have been so anxious to be here to-night. It was one of the prettiest pieces of work that I have ever seen done. I have been waiting for a case of my own to turn up that I might try it myself. I am a little curious to know where so many cases requiring root amputation come from. It would seem to me that quite a large number of these cases might have been handled in other ways. I would like to know how Dr. Schamberg distinguishes between such cases. It would seem that the simple fact of an abscess of long standing is not a sufficient excuse. .

Regarding Dr. Schamberg's work with impacted third molars, I think his statement, that the second molar should never be sacrificed, ought to be widely published. In spite of my decided opinion on this subject, I once had a case where it seemed the only available way. The patient was a chronic invalid, and I did not feel like exposing her to any unnecessary strain. In this case, after the removal of the abscessed second molar I was enabled to clean up the third molar and retain it as the posterior support for a bridge for which the first molar was the main support, using a crown cemented on the first molar with a dowel-pin in a filling in the third molar, according to the method explained by Dr. S. S. Stowell.

It would seem, in extracting a single rooted molar, advisable before removing the crown, as mentioned by Dr. Schamberg, to grasp the whole tooth in the forceps and give it a rotating motion, thus breaking its attachment to the process. This makes the removal of the root easier. I have also found it helpful to split such teeth, taking away, first, the top part, and then lifting out the remainder.

Had I known the course the paper would have taken in relation to impacted wisdom-teeth, I should have been glad to have brought some casts of such a case where I desired to save the patient as much physical suffering as possible. For nearly a year I tried, by means of packing gutta-percha between the second and third molars, to lift the latter tooth up so that I would be enabled to get at it. The results I attained in this way were not very satisfactory. Finally, Dr. Bogue told me of the grass-line wedges, and I set to work with them. In a couple of months I had lifted the molar upward and backward enough so that it could be removed without interfering with the second molar. Grass line is kept by the sporting-goods stores. I found at one store a remnant of a large size that they do not carry in stock generally. They will order any size required.

Dr. Rice.—In Dr. Schamberg's picture of impacted wisdom-teeth I noticed none with the molar tipping forward. They were all slanting away from the second molar. I have recently had experience with a case where the third molar was tilted forward, and, indeed, was actually under the second molar. A general surgeon was to remove the tooth, and I was called and asked to furnish appliances in the way of a dental engine, etc. After the patient had been etherized the surgeon decided that he did not know much about it, and asked me to go ahead and take the tooth out. It was a very embarrassing case. There was considerable swelling, and it was very difficult of access. I attempted to use a right-angle bur, but it was not long enough. With a straight bur I attempted to remove the bone sufficiently to take out the tooth. I made a cross-section, and part of the tooth was extracted. At first there was entire relief, but after a few days there was a return of great pain, which was relieved by packing antikamnia into the socket. I would like to know of a practical method of removing a tooth like this without first removing the second molar.

Dr. E. A. Bogue.—Referring to what Dr. Gillett has said regarding impacted wisdom-teeth, sometimes these impacted teeth can be saved by wedging them backward and causing them gradually to assume an upright position. Sometimes they can be wedged so as to facilitate their extraction. I have in mind such a case. Dr. Hasbrouck had refused to attempt the operation. I was enabled, by means of tape, to wedge the tooth into a sufficiently upright position to be easily taken out. In many cases that I have seen two or three weeks of preliminary wedging would greatly facilitate the extraction of an impacted tooth, without injury to its neighbors.

Dr. Schamberg has shown us a number of cases of root amputation, and the question came up as to the need of such an operation. I think such operations are very important and necessary many times. I have had such a tooth in my own mouth,—a molar that was doing work for ten or twelve years with only the buccal roots. In one case I amputated the apices of central and lateral incisors, and the cuspid and first bicuspid roots. All these teeth were dead and in bad condition, due to an abscess beginning with the cuspid and spreading to the adjoining teeth. The patient had suffered for thirteen years, and was radically cured of a stubborn neuralgia, as he called it, by the operation.

Dr. Schamberg spoke of a splint used by him in a case of fracture of the lower maxilla. I was disappointed that he did not speak of the interdental splint of rubber, because all of this wiring of the teeth together is injurious and I do not believe that it is often necessary. The dentist, knowing the proper occlusion of the teeth, can take an impression, and then, the lower model being broken apart and the teeth replaced in their proper position relative to the upper teeth, an interdental splint can be made on these models that will hold the mandible in position. Dr. Schamberg will forgive me for reminding him of this omission.

I am much pleased at Dr. Schamberg bringing so prominently before us the very great advantages of the X-ray.

Dr. Gillett.—I have seen one case where the third molar was directly over the second molar and the two crowns pointing in exactly opposite directions.

Dr. F. Milton Smith.—I have been exceedingly interested in Dr. Schamberg's talk and the pictures he has shown us. He has greatly impressed us with the benefits of the X-ray in our work. The thought given expression to by Dr. Gillett also impressed me, as to the apparent great number of cases in Dr. Schamberg's practice requiring root amputation. I presume it can be partially accounted for from the fact that he has sent him patients from other dentists. In my own practice I have, in five cases found it necessary to remove the end of an abscessed root. I have found exceedingly few cases that I cannot cure.

Dr. Fossume.—Relative to the extraction of teeth, I wish to make a plea for greater precaution against infection during the operation and also in the after treatment, and if one is called upon to treat such infected sockets, I know of no more reliable and efficacious germicide than permanganate of potassium. Men making a specialty of the extraction of teeth should at least advise the patient to return to their family dentist to have the dressings removed and the wounds looked after. I have had some difficulty in this direction, and can see no excuse for such neglect.

Dr. Gillett.—I would add, " not only after-care, but preliminary care of the mouth before extraction."

I would like to ask Dr. Schamberg if, in amputating the roots of the lower bicuspids and molars, he has any difficulty in avoiding the inferior dental nerve.

Dr. Schamberg.—Regarding the apparent frequency with which I perform the operation of root amputation, I admit that I do perform it with more frequency than most practitioners. I will admit that perhaps in the majority of cases of an abscessed tooth, proper medication and treatment will bring about a complete cure. However, there is a large proportion of cases where this method will only bring about a temporary cure, so to speak, but where, owing to the diseased end of the root and surrounding tissue, it is impossible to effect a complete and permanent cure. In these cases surgical interference is desirable and necessary. For that reason I believe that there are many cases where the operation is indicated, but where it is not performed at the present time. There are many persons going around with gum-boils in their mouths who have been told that they are nothing to bother about. There are many roots that it is practically impossible to fill to the very end, and I always make due allowance for root-canal work. We often feel confident that we have reached the end of the root with our filling, when as a matter of fact the X-ray will show that we have not.

Regarding the root of the wisdom-tooth which pointed in an

opposite direction from those I showed on the screen, no matter how difficult, the root should be removed, as the prognosis is always bad when a root of this kind is left. Of course, sometimes it is a difficult thing to get the mouth open wide enough. Oftentimes it is absolutely necessary to allow the acute inflammation to subside. The socket of a tooth so extracted should always be packed so that it will heal from the bottom up. I use iodoform gauze for this purpose.

I do not find much danger in interfering with the inferior dental nerve, and even if the nerve is severed it will always unite again.

I do not favor interdental splints, as a rule, because they are not applicable to cases where the fracture is far back toward the ramus. If the mouth is opened in these cases the portion of the fracture at the ramus will not assume its proper relation to the body of the inferior maxilla. I see that the case is kept in a clean condition by having the patient come to me every day for an antiseptic spray between the teeth. The nourishment is also taken in like manner between the teeth.

I do not believe that any operation of the mouth, causing the shedding of blood, should be done without first rendering the mouth as far as possible aseptic. I thoroughly approve of the preliminary use of the permanganate of potash, and I follow up the extraction with an antiseptic wash for some time. The patient should always be impressed with the necessity for treatment of the socket. There should be no deception regarding the failure to remove all the roots. It does not hurt the operator's reputation and it may save the patient's health. Of course, the question of extraction becomes more difficult every day, because we do not now take out teeth that are little decayed, but only complicated cases of impaction come to us for extraction.

I thank you, gentlemen, for your kind attention.

Upon motion, a vote of thanks from the society was extended to Dr. Schamberg for his very interesting and valuable talk.

Adjourned.

FRED. L. BOGUE, M.D., D.D.S.,
Editor The New York Institute of Stomatology.

ACADEMY OF STOMATOLOGY.

A REGULAR meeting of the Philadelphia Academy of Stomatology was held at its rooms, 1731 Chestnut Street, on the evening of Tuesday, February 28, 1905, the President, Dr. I. N. Broomell, in the chair. A paper was read by Dr. Hart J. Goslee, of Chicago, entitled " The Rationale of Pulp Extirpation."

(For Dr. Goslee's paper, see page 228.)

DISCUSSION.

Dr. R. Ottolengui, New York City.—There is very little in the paper with which I feel inclined to take any exception, and if you will pardon me I will direct my remarks to the general subject rather than to the paper. It is a remarkable fact how little we know about pulp removal, one of the most important operations the dentist is called upon to perform. There are two methods by which operations become established. Usually we have a period of experimentation followed by a record of what may be called clinical experiences, dental deductions which may be known as clinical facts, and it is only at the very end that the real scientist comes in and sifts these clinical facts in order to find the scientific truth. The paper before us is admitted by the author to be a contribution to the knowledge of clinical facts, a compilation of deductions from experience. A great many dental topics have been made almost a life study by our scientists, but little of real science has been gathered on this question of pulp extirpation. What do we really know about the series of results from this application of arsenic? We tell our patients, many of us, " I am obliged to kill the nerve." As a matter of fact, we do not even try to kill the nerve, but we try with our arsenic to so act upon the pulp as to make removal possible without pain. There is the difference between the assertion and the actual fact. Has it actually been demonstrated beyond scientific argument just why the application of arsenic enables us to remove the pulp without pain? I can scarcely believe it is the action of the arsenic upon the nerve-fibres that allows this, because we have all, perhaps, had experiences in which pulps were painful after many applications of arsenic. I may be wrong, but I think that the general explanation is that the arsenic acts as a constringent of the capillaries.

Just how this constringent effect enables us to painlessly remove the pulps is a question. If we wait until this disorganized tissue separates at the apex, then, of course, we have dead matter which is removed painlessly. Apparently, however, we usually remove that pulp not painlessly, but with less pain, after the application of arsenic than in its normal condition. We are all clamoring for an established mode of procedure. The application of arsenic as a means of painlessly removing pulps has been an established procedure for half a century, with little complaint against the method. Now we have a new method offered, but I call your attention to the fact that the new method is even now, five or ten years after introduction, rather in an empirical state. How much of actual study has been given to the desensitizing of pulp tissue by cocaine pressure? Who of us knows exactly what happens when cocaine is applied to the pulp, and that after the application of the cocaine and of pressure, this tissue can be removed painlessly? Gentlemen, I ask you again, who knows? Who has tried to find out? Here I meet my own dilemma. I have tried to find out, but I have not the histological and chemical knowledge with which to solve the problem, but you have in this scientific centre of research a number of gentlemen who, I think, have the equipment; and if you will pardon my taking the time, I will outline a mode of clinically studying this problem with the hope that Dr. Broomell or Dr. Truman, or one of the many others with you, may take this up. Something more than a year ago I began the microscopic examination of pulps which I removed. I noticed an extreme difference between the pulps treated by arsenic and those by cocaine. It must be remembered that in the pulps treated by arsenic there is a constringence of the capillaries with the compulsory retention of a certain proportion of blood within the capillaries, and the pulp removed is a brilliant red. If you remove the pulp-tissue while the capillaries are still engorged with blood, you leave all the blood that was in the pulp in the canal and bring forth a whitened tissue. By allowing these removed pulps to dry it has seemed to me that I have been able to detect crystals, which I have taken to be crystals of arsenic. In the pulps treated by cocaine I have also seen crystals which are of a different appearance. This should be a question for the scientists, and if it be a fact that we can thus make visible the crystals of the drug used, it should be established.

The next fact to be determined is whether, if we can force

these medicines along the capillary tracts, they will pass beyond the apex. I suggest the following experiments, which I had hoped to have carried out in New York, but for which I have lacked material, having seen but three freshly exposed pulps this winter. My plan was to determine the action of the cocaine or arsenic, and also the presence or absence of bacteria. First, upon exposing the pulp I would collect some of the blood and examine it for the bacteria, and keep it for comparison in the future. Secondly, my plan would be to cocainize this pulp, remove it, and make a slide to be examined under the microscope or by chemical means, to determine whether the cocaine actually passes into the pulp-tissue, and if so, whether it follows the blood tracts. Finally, upon removal of the pulp, collect the first blood, the blood which was originally in the pulp, and discover, if possible, whether the blood contains cocaine or bacteria. This would aid in deciding whether or not we have forced bacteria into the pulp in applying the cocaine. By another series of experiments we might first disinfect or sterilize the cavity, when, if bacteria were found in the blood of the pulp after its removal, we would know that the infection had been in the pulp prior to its removal. If it is possible for an exposed pulp to absorb chemical agents, why should it not suffer from ptomaine poisoning when in contact with caries said to be of bacterial origin? If it be proved that there may be bacteria in the pulp where there is deep-seated caries, and if it be proved that by pressure we can force chemicals and bacteria beyond the apex, we may in this way account for lame teeth after the treatment by cocaine pressure. My final experiment would be to allow all of this first lot of blood to pass away, the canal to be several times washed with sterilized warm fluids, and then to make several examinations of the blood coming from beyond the apex, to determine the presence of bacteria and cocaine. We need the aid of scientific research along these lines to know beyond peradventure just what we are doing. I hope some one may be interested to take up the work.

Dr. F. J. Capon, Toronto.—I feel that I am somewhat under false colors in being placed on the programme to discuss this paper, as I am merely a visitor in your city.

I must congratulate Dr. Goslee on the splendid essay he has presented, and also upon the practical way in which he has set the subject before us.

I may say that I have almost entirely adopted the pressure

anæsthesia method for the extirpation of pulps, either by dealing with the exposed pulps directly, or by way of the dentinal tubules, and find each of them very efficient in their indicated place. One with a busy practice will naturally drift away from the difficult to an easier way of doing an operation, if the results obtained are as satisfactory. I was one of those who in the year 1894 or 1895 paid twenty-five dollars to Dr. Funk, of Chicago, to learn this, a secret method at that time, and I have employed it more or less ever since, and have found it so satisfactory that the arsenical method has been almost cast aside.

In those cases where there is a deposit of dentine in the pulp-chamber I prefer to take the chances with cocaine and pressure rather than with arsenic, but they are often troublesome with either. This again may be said when teeth are badly decayed below the gum margin and an aching and exposed pulp exists. Pressure anæsthesia is then especially indicated as a speedy and safe treatment.

The after-trouble that has been spoken of is not more frequent with immediate extirpation, although a soreness is more liable when bleeding has not followed the removal of the pulp. I must be fortunate with my treatment, as I do not experience the soreness that has been mentioned to-night. When dealing with an anæsthetized live pulp a sterilized broach should be used.

Dr. Emory A. Bryant.—As a usual thing, I am not in the habit of agreeing with a man simply to " pat him on the back," as is a generally observed custom in the discussions of papers read before dental societies, but I must confess that the ideas as expressed by the essayist this evening so closely coincide with my practical experience with pulp extirpation that I am at a loss as to what to say.

I cannot, however, resist the temptation of referring to that part of the paper quoting my friend B. Holly Smith in regard to the ill-effects of the use of arsenic in pulp extirpation upon the tissue as well as the teeth. I doubt very much his ability to prove his assertions, or that any such results have to be contended with by careful operators.

From the paper one would judge that in 1904 Dr. Smith discovered an unknown characteristic property of arsenic in its dental uses, but in referring to a card published to the public in April, 1881, by Dr. Williams Donnally we find the following:

"In treating the natural teeth my object is to preserve every one that time, patience, and modern methods of treatment can save. The use of arsenic in destroying exposed pulps is condemned by the more enlightened of the dental profession, on account of its turning the teeth dark, inducing abscess, and, finally, the loss of the teeth. The pulp, which is the source of life to the tooth, should always be treated, when exposed, with a view to its restoration to health."

Thus, you see, Dr. Smith's discovery was previously published to the world by his friend Dr. Donnally by some twenty-three years, and if it was a fact at that period, it would seem strange that the profession has so long failed to recognize the disastrous effects, and only awake to realization upon the advent of pressure anæsthesia as a substitute.

I was so struck with the force of Dr. Donnally's argument that I published it in an article of my own in the June, 1903, *Items of Interest.*

Pressure anæsthesia is one of the greatest aids to quick work under certain conditions that has been given to the profession. Those conditions are laid down so perfectly by Dr. Goslee that it is useless to further refer to them. Practically speaking, I cannot say that I have had any of the ill effects spoken of. I had the pleasure of seeing, the other day, a patent, taken out seventeen years ago, upon an instrument which is practically the pressure anæsthesia instrument of to-day. My friend used in this phenol sodique, carbolic acid, or alcohol, and, as he stated in a letter which I received from him the other day, he had been using pressure anæsthesia for years and did not know it. He could not remember at what date he commenced the use of cocaine, and in that date I am much interested, inasmuch as there is now before the Patent Office an application for a patent upon the method and process of producing pressure anæsthesia, and unless that application can be antedated by the publication of the fact of the use of pressure anæsthesia previous to the application for a patent, the profession is liable to again have to contend with a state of affairs similar to that it had with the Goodyear Dental Vulcanite Company and the International Tooth Crown Company.

If that patent is once allowed, the profession will have to go into the courts to prove its previous use, and I hope to have the necessary data to place before the Patent-Office in the near future, so that the patent will not be issued. I wish to thank Dr. Goslee for his timely paper, and the members of this society for so patiently listening to me.

Dr. Charles F. Ash, Brooklyn.—I have been much interested in the subject of pulp extirpation. The trouble seems to be not in getting the pulp out, but in the results which ensue in some cases. Eleven years ago there came to my office a case of exposed pulp so intensely hypertrophied that it was impossible for the patient to use that side of the mouth. He had had the tooth treated, but without success. It was exceedingly sensitive, and I made on that occasion my first application of pressure anæsthesia. The thought was original to me then, and I used pressure anæsthesia with cocaine and a piece of unvulcanized rubber with good success. I removed the pulp in not more than fifteen minutes. I treated the root, and the patient returned in a few days, when I put a filling of gutta-percha in the root and of cement in the cavity. That tooth is still doing good service, and has never given any trouble. From that time on I have used pressure anæsthesia in that way. It seems to me that the gist of Dr. Goslee's paper is contained in his statement that success in pulp extirpation lies in the judicious selection of the kind of treatment for a given case. I did not cease using arsenic when I discovered that I could use pressure anæsthesia, nor have I stopped using it to this day. I have found cases in which I was able to successfully use pressure anæsthesia and remove the pulp from two canals, while the other canal was too small for the smallest broach, and in this I have applied arsenic. These are the cases in which a good many fail because they do not carry their efforts far enough. I have not had a case of pressure anæsthesia followed by continued soreness or lameness, as stated by some gentlemen. I have had cases in which there has been a temporary soreness, but I think this has been due to a slight secondary hemorrhage occurring after the effect of the adrenalin chloride had ceased. Until that blood is absorbed there is apt to be soreness.

Dr. Frank Bliven, Worcester, Mass.—I thank you for the invitation to discuss this subject. We all appreciate the paper of Dr. Goslee and the able way in which he has presented it. Dr. Ottolengui has entered into the scientific side of the question and given us his admirable views. We have also listened to other men, and it is a question whether there remains much to be said. Dr. Ottolengui has made a statement relative to the dead matter left in the root. There is no such thing as dead matter. If the matter were dead and left in the root it would be inert and could not possibly cause future trouble. It is live matter left in the root, and it depends upon the character of that life what the result will be. Matter may change indefinitely in its form, but we cannot eliminate it from the universe. It was my pleasure to listen, in New Hampshire, to quite an able paper on this subject and to the discussion upon it. There was an old man there with a great deal of experience, but with little scientific knowledge, and, after all the scientists had got through with the discussion, he rose and said,—I will try to repeat his words as spoken,—"Well, you scientific men know a lot about this killing pulps and taking them out and filling up the canals and performing scientific operations, and getting a big fee for them; but when I commenced practice we did not have time for that sort of thing. All we used to do was to put the arsenic into the tooth, and when we thought the nerve was dead we took out what we could get out and put in cotton and creosote and filled up the cavity, and we did not have any more trouble than you do now." There is a lot of truth in what he said, for they did not have much trouble. But the scientific side is now before the profession, and it calls upon the ablest men we have to solve the problem and ascertain whether we do force what Dr. Ottolengui has called dead matter, or what we call live matter, beyond the apical foramen. I think much depends upon our judgment of the application best suited to the individual case. When we have had long experience with pressure anæsthesia we shall perhaps be able to form better deductions from our results. After all possible scientific light has been brought to bear upon this subject, I still believe that it will depend wholly and entirely upon the condition or personal equation of our patients what the result will be.

Dr. Ottolengui.—I did not say anything about pressing dead matter through the apical foramen. If a pulp treated with arsenic were left in the mouth long, so that it separated from the parts beyond, it might be called dead matter, and therefore its removal would be painless. We know that what we call infection is from something quite alive, since it is capable of reproduction.

Dr. Joseph Head.—Dr. Goslee has referred to the possibility of the dental pulp absorbing the arsenic which might be carried through the tissues. Dr. Flagg in his experiments took a number of dental pulps and, after snipping off the portion that had been touched by the arsenic, applied Marsh's test, and found no arsenic present. He therefore felt that the pulp was not destroyed by arsenic poison, but by a peculiar arsenical impress, which is not understood, except that it caused strangulation of the pulp at the apical foramen.

Dr. Ottolengui brought out the point that we did not have scientific knowledge of the way in which a pulp was affected by the cocaine. We know that when cocaine is injected into the tissues it has a certain well-defined physiological action, and that the cocaine has an effect on the terminals of the nerves. Cocaine almost to a certainty acts on the pulp in this way. By application of the cocaine to the perfectly healthy nerve, and with sufficient pressure to force a little of it into the tissue, the circulation, where there is circulation, in half a minute will give us anæsthesia. We also know that where there are pulp-stones, and where the circulation has been lessened, we have greater difficulty. Pulp anæsthesia as the result of the cocaine injection seems to me a simple problem.

Dr. J. H. Gaskill.—I think we can get as complete anæsthesia of the pulp without the use of cocaine as we can with it. I have frequently produced anæsthesia with carbolic acid, and I question whether it is really the cocaine which produces the anæsthesia.

Dr. G. E. Root.—I believe that we can get pressure anæsthesia when using Schuylkill water as well as when using a solution of cocaine. I believe that it is the pressure which produces anæsthesia as much as the cocaine, and with the use of the arsenic I think the anæsthesia is not so much the result of the action of the arsenic itself as that the arsenic causes a contraction at the apex of the pulp and we have the anæsthesia from the congestion rather than from the arsenic.

Dr. James Truman.—I am particularly gratified to find that one of the younger members of our profession has so far sustained the verdict of fifty or more years, that arsenic is worthy of preservation. We have heard much in recent times and through our journals from those who assert that they no longer use arsenic. and that pressure anæsthesia is the one thing for the present and for the future in the eradication of pulps. I have had some experience with the latter, and I have had some fifty years' experience with the former. I do not understand why it is that men in practice who make use of arsenic condemn it. My only explanation is that the general profession, as a rule, do not understand the action of arsenic and do not fully realize the action of cocaine. The use of arsenic in the past has been largely empirical, and it is empirical to-day. I find the majority using arsenic without any clear idea of the amount that is necessary to destroy the pulp of a single-rooted tooth, and it is no wonder that it frequently is carried beyond the pulp to produce periodontitis. I try to impress upon my students that we must get away from the old method, introduced by Dr. J. D. White, of applying arsenic without any scientific basis.

It was demonstrated by Miller, in his celebrated experiments upon mice, that arsenic was a paralyzer, and all my own clinical experience has equally demonstrated that its effect is to paralyze the sensory nerves, cutting off nutrition. Cocaine does precisely the same thing,—paralyzes the sensory nerves. That has been understood as one of the peculiar properties of this agent, and why should we here to-night hear the question asked, "How does cocaine act?" It is very well known that in the injection hypodermically along the margin of the gums sloughing is frequently produced. The explanation of this may be found in the local disturbance of the vasomotor system, cutting off nutrition. I believe this to be scientifically correct. The pressure method has the same antagonism to meet as arsenic, in that where there has been long continued inflammation we find that arsenic and cocaine are equally antagonized by the congested vessels of the pulp. We have to-day to meet each case separately and judge accordingly. I would not contend that either method is absolute; we may probably never get away from arsenic, and we may find in the future that all the difficulties that have been enumerated by the essayist will be found increasing in proportion as we make use of the so-called pressure anæsthesia.

Dr. Edwin T. Darby.—I think I voice the sentiment of the Academy when I say that it has listened with the greatest pleasure to Dr. Goslee's paper as well as to the discussion which has followed. I thought while Dr. Goslee was reading his paper that if I could write with the same apparent ease that he does, and deliver it with the same grace that he did, that I should write oftener for the Academy.

The point concerning the danger of infecting the pulp and the tissue beyond by forcing septic matter into the pulp-canal was new to me. It may be remembered by some of you that at the meeting of the National Dental Association held at Old Point Comfort, some years ago, before the pressure method of anæsthetizing pulps was introduced, I narrated an experience that I had had in anæsthetizing a pulp by injecting with a syringe a solution of chloroform and carbolic acid. I practised this method for some time with the greatest satisfaction. The first case was that of a lateral incisor which I was preparing for a filling. The cavity was confluent with one on the opposite side, and so frail was the tooth that I broke the crown near the gum. My patient was to sail for Europe the next day, and it gave me no little concern. I took a small hypodermic syringe, and with a canula instead of a needle inserted it into the pulp-chamber (first laying a crystal of carbolic acid upon the pulp to paralyze it). I injected chloroform and carbolic acid into the pulp-canal, and in less than half a minute I had anæsthetized it, and with my brooch took it out, prepared the canal, and put an artificial crown upon the root. I knew nothing then of using cocaine. In a case at the University, where I sought to demonstrate this method, I broke the canula of my syringe, but substituted a pellet of bibulous paper well saturated with carbolic acid and chloroform, put it into the cavity of decay, placed some soft rubber over that, and forced the carbolic acid and chloroform into the pulp and extracted it in less than a minute.

I have heard men say that the anæsthetization can be produced as well with water, chloroform, alcohol, or other fluids as with cocaine. I have not experimented with these, but I do know that by the use of cocaine crystals I have brought about the desired effect. I do not understand what the gentlemen mean by making a solution of cocaine for pressure anæsthesia. My own method is to put the cocaine crystal into the cavity and my rubber immediately upon that, and by the time I am ready to make pressure the moisture from the air and the moisture in the tooth has given me a deliquesced solution of cocaine. The mistake is often made of trying to use a solution of cocaine of insufficient strength. I see no harm in using the crystals direct, even though you use more than enough to anæsthetize several pulps. The chances are that you will not force it beyond the foramen of the tooth.

Dr. Ottolengui.—I desire to make reply to some of the remarks that have been made. I am the one who expressed the view that we know little about the physiological action of cocaine or of arsenic in the pulp. I am glad to have had my attention called to Dr. Miller's paper, but unless Dr. Miller tells us much more than

Dr. Truman has told us, I fail to see how we are any nearer to the facts that I am trying to discover. Dr. Truman says that arsenic paralyzes the nerves. If we say it anæsthetizes the nerves, we know almost as much as when we hear that it paralyzes. The paralysis of the nerve is the making of the nerve inert. If the nerve is inert and ceases to act, the resultant lack of muscular effort which that nerve is supposed to supply is called paralysis. In sensory nerves, if we have inaction we have lack of sensation. We have the condition, but are not told what produces it. Dr. Head has said that just exactly what anæsthesia is we do not know. It would require a great many experiments similar to those of Dr. Flagg to determine this. We believe that the presence of pulp-stones hinders the action or result that we hope to obtain, and I know that in pulps which I removed under cocaine anæsthesia, when the pulp-stones were present there was this appearance of crystals all around the pulp-nodules, with no such appearance beyond these pulp-nodules. This carries out my view that cocaine actually enters the pulp-tissue; if it does not enter the pulp-tissue it cannot be carried beyond. That is a point which has not yet been determined.

I ask any gentleman to show me the expression " pressure anæsthesia" anywhere in our literature before it was used by Dr. W. J. Morton.

Dr. Morton, in a meeting in which cataphoresis was being discussed, stated that he had discovered a new means of producing anæsthesia with cocaine applied under pressure, but the experiment which he reported was not that kind of pressure which we now use,—namely, mechanical pressure. He dissolved the cocaine in guaiacol and ether and applied them under a cover-glass on his arm, and incisions with a lancet could be made on his arm painlessly, from which he gathered the idea that it was the chemical evaporation of the ether which caused a pressure forcing the cocaine into the tissues. Immediately after this a preparation was put upon the market called " Vapocain;" other dentists around the country applied mechanical pressure instead of this method.

I am intensely interested in the statement made by Dr. Ash that he used the unvulcanized rubber and cocaine over ten years ago. If this is correct, pressure anæsthesia was first done by Dr. Ash.

Dr. Ash.—I hope that none of the gentlemen will suppose that I make any claim for priority in the matter of pressure anæsthesia.

Dr. M. I. Schamberg.—It is well that attention be directed to the fact that we are blaming arsenic and cocaine pressure for conditions for which they, in a large proportion of cases, are not responsible. It is also well to remember that the removal of the pulp is a surgical procedure. Whenever a pulp is removed it is to be expected that some reaction will follow the severance of this once vital tissue from the remainder of the body. When arsenic is used, if it passes beyond the end of the tooth it will cause tissue destruction as it does in the pulp-chamber. When cocaine reaches the periapical tissues it temporarily anæsthetizes the tissues with which it comes in contact. It is a question in my mind whether cocaine so used is as likely to cause absolute destruction or permanent harm to the periapical tissues as is arsenic. Patients subjected to the cocaine pressure method occasionally show slight toxic symptoms, proving that the drug may enter the general circulation. The action of the arsenic, however, is purely local. The soreness following pulp extirpation is probably largely due to the traumatism attending this slight surgical procedure. If you remove a gangrenous finger or amputate any part of the body, even though it be not diseased, you must look for a certain amount of inflammatory reaction. You ought, therefore, to expect a certain amount of reaction following the removal of a pulp. It is, however, the permanent after-troubles which are of such serious moment to us when dealing with pulp-canals, and the cause of these, I believe, can readily be appreciated when one examines teeth that are removed with abscesses and other periapical troubles associated with them. In dealing with the pulp we work largely in the dark and without a clear perception of the minuteness, the length, and the tortuosity of the canals we treat. It is not surprising, then, that portions of the pulp remain to undergo putrefaction, and that fillings frequently fail to reach the ends of teeth. I maintain that we are blaming methods for the destruction of the pulp which are good and useful, and are overlooking the more potent etiological factors in the production of lame teeth. Dr. Osler, in his recent address at Johns Hopkins University, shocked the entire world by stating that man's time is up at forty, asserting the comparative uselessness of men above forty and advocating the enforced retirement of all men at sixty. It has occurred to me that Dr. Osler unwisely failed to provide for the chloroforming of the large number of men at twenty who are more worthless than many at sixty.

This principle applies equally well to the teeth of man. Inasmuch as modern dentistry teaches us to conserve the teeth for twenty, forty, or sixty years, we naturally, during these long periods, in consequence of our laudable attempts, encounter many more abscesses and other tooth-disturbances than did the practitioner of old. One of the previous speakers has stated that the old custom was to place arsenic in the tooth, allow it to remain, and upon the first indication of trouble the tooth was removed. Such a tooth, according to their judgment, had lost its field of usefulness. In our present endeavor to make a tooth useful for forty or sixty years we find ourselves occasionally confronted with conditions which could never have existed had the tooth been lost at twenty. In spite of what has been said, if all work upon the pulp and pulp-canal was done under strict surgical antisepsis, much of the trouble that we encounter with devitalized teeth would be averted.

Dr. Goslee (closing).—In the anticipation of my visit to this city, if there was one thing I could have wished for more than another, it would doubtless have been to have heard the expressions that my good friends have made to-night in support of the few things which I have said in my paper, because we in Chicago look up to the profession of Philadelphia with considerable deference, and if I had asked for one special thing more than another it would have been for the approval of Dr. Truman and Dr. Darby. The tribute paid me by Dr. Darby is highly appreciated. From his personal and professional life and from his writings I have received much inspiration.

It is true that we do have trouble in the use of arsenic, as we do in the application of cocaine and pressure. I called attention, however, to the fact that, as a rule, many do not discriminate in the application of arsenic, or between the size of the tooth and of the pulp, and that we often make no discrimination in the physical condition of the patient upon which we operate. I think that this discrimination, however, has to do very largely with the successful application of such an agent as arsenic. I also think, at the same time, that a great many of the bad results which we do have resulting from cocaine and pressure can be averted by previously thoroughly sterilizing the tract so that the likelihood of infecting the tissue in the apical region will be overcome.

I do not know whether the period during which Dr. Funk went about demonstrating the present method of pressure anæsthesia antedates that attributed to Dr. Morton or not. We in Chicago learned to believe that Dr. Funk was probably the first man to introduce the mechanical means now employed. I took up this method as soon as I learned of it, and in my experimental work in the college in the first six months we removed probably ninety per cent. of pulps by this method. We did have much subsequent trouble, and, though only of temporary nature, its use was for this reason almost entirely discontinued for a time. Since then we have begun to again use it more extensively, and in my personal practice I also use it to a large extent and perhaps always shall. I think that success with any method, however, depends largely upon the selection of the proper one for the individual case.

Again let me thank you for the courtesy extended to me.

Upon motion of Dr. Darby, a vote of thanks was extended to Dr. Goslee for his interesting paper.

OTTO E. INGLIS,
Editor Academy of Stomatology.

Editorial.

HASTY CONCLUSIONS.

THE literature of dentistry is replete with crude decisions based on incomplete examinations and equally erroneous deductions from faulty research work. It is not to be expected that the earnest historical writer, ever seeking for corroborative details, will be developed speedily in our young profession. This exactness comes only from matured thinking and generations of experience. It must, however, be regarded as true that dentistry is inclined to run to hasty conclusions more extensively than is warranted even through youthful extravagant expression.

This is largely due, it is thought, to careless habits in writing. The essayist who aims to prepare a paper for a society sits down to the task apparently, in many instances, to develop this from memory and experience. The memory side will be prepared from quotations copied from the last article read on a related subject, and no effort will be made to establish the truth of statements or to correct errors of history. This leads to false records, and false history in dentistry is becoming more and more a source of annoyance, and will result in the future to the great injury of the truly original toilers in the profession. The plagiarist we will probably always have with us, but his first cousin, the careless writer, ought to be eliminated by individual effort. The first is the manifestation of degeneracy, the latter of pure physical inertia.

The writer could multiply instances of this peculiarity, but this does not seem necessary in view of the fact that it is constantly made apparent in books, in articles and in discussions before societies; in fact, wherever the professional mind seeks an outlet for ideas, it apparently has the unfortunate tendency to neglect detailed examination of the history connected with the subject. This frequently is a source of intense mortification to the younger writers, when, after discussing some scientific problem, in which neglect is apparent in giving due acknowledgment to the labor of previous investigators, they are called to account for careless writing by some one more conversant with the facts in dental literature. The first duty of a writer, in assuming to elucidate some obscure problem, is to seek first the literature of the subject. This, in dentistry, is not a far search; perhaps a century and a half might cover it in its entirety, and possibly a half-century the period of greatest activity. When this has been completed the research worker is prepared to enter the arena of disputation fully armed for the conflict. The importance of this care in writing cannot be too frequently or too earnestly impressed on the younger generation of workers, who are enriching the literature of dentistry to-day more than at any previous period of its history. To be correct means labor, but it is a labor that is accompanied with its own great reward.

The editors of our journals have, it is presumed, more trouble with the careless habit of writers in giving proper names without examination than with all other errors combined. A name should never be written without careful verification. The average essayist apparently regards the editor, compositor, and proof-reader as the final arbiters of these difficult matters, evidently forgetting that their neglect very frequently means a serious loss of time for some one to make a lengthy search in order to be exact, for no journal of reputation can afford to exhibit ignorance in this direction. Unless the writer is absolutely assured that his spelling of the name is correct, he has no right to make use of it, to the possible injury of an original worker.

There is another and quite different exhibition of careless thinking, speaking, and writing, in the habit indulged in by some of ascribing to individuals, associations, and institutions statements, conclusions, and practices that do not belong to either. It is the loose method of setting up a man of straw to gain an opportunity to pull it to pieces without much labor. This sort of thing is manifested more frequently in charging dental educational institutions with all sorts of teachings not in harmony with the writer's conception of what constitutes a proper dental standard. The writer has been constantly impressed with this mental tendency in some otherwise very careful and capable writers. They will start out in an article on dental education, basing their conclusions on the knowledge of dental college work and dental college instruction obtained by them during their undergraduate experience ten, fifteen, or even forty years in the past. Upon this moss-grown experience they weave an article upon the curriculum of the present, and assume that the teaching of the dental colleges is not in accord with modern dental thought. The writer of this assumes that there does not exist a single mind capable of sounding the depth or the quality of the dental teaching in this country or any other in the range of civilization. This must be evident without waste of words in argument. The curricula of the various dental schools are given briefly in their annual announcements, but these are merely the skeletons, the soul, so to speak, being left to each individual teacher to fashion as he is prepared for the work. How impossible, then, is it for any outsider to declare that this is taught, or that is not taught, in the schools of dentistry anywhere. The curriculum of any dental college is, therefore, closed to all but the undergraduate of the immediate session in which he is a student. The teaching of each member of a faculty is practically a sealed book to every one of his colleagues. It must be, therefore, clear to all interested that knowledge of dental college teaching is an unwarranted assumption, even by those engaged intimately in the work. The writer would not attempt to express an opinion as to the value of any dental teaching unless he had an opportunity to examine the product. For this State boards of examiners have been provided, and we are obliged to be satisfied with this not very perfect solution of the problem.

The same careless method of thought and writing enters into all the several professional relations. Our moral law makes it a wrong to criticise a brother practitioner, but how many obey the code or hesitate to assume a more or less accurate knowledge of the practice of prominent dental practitioners. This would be amusing were it not a cause of much bad feeling, as it is an evidence of a lack of true professional courtesy. It is assuming to know our neighbor as we suppose we know ourselves, but, as we do not know ourselves, we are naturally ignorant of our neighbor's household.

The advice of the writer would be to those ambitious of entering the ranks of professional authors, to first acquire some degree of exactness in thought and then to make surety doubly sure that all the statements made will present an unassailable basis of truth. Style in writing may come by care and experience; good models may be of value, but they are not essential. Those who aim to acquire style in writing through this channel make a mistake with the result,—stilted composition. True style is individualized, and is an outgrowth of the spiritual nature developed through the refinement of general culture. Crude thinking is analogous to carelessness in the care of the body, for both may eventuate into a habit which, by use, is increasingly developed and is not, as a rule, ever eradicated, but becomes a bar to eventual success in all professional literary work.

Domestic Correspondence.

CORRESPONDENCE ON ORTHODONTIA.

June 6, 1905.

To THE EDITOR:

SIR,—I send you a little bit of a correspondence that has recently passed between one of my most respected fellow-practitioners and myself.

The end is not yet, but it occurs to me that a good many of your readers may be interested in the question raised and in the answer that may perhaps be elicited from any one who knows how to surmount the difficulty mentioned.

I should esteem it a great favor to receive an adequate reply to my question.

Truly yours,

E. A. Bogue.

63 West Forty-eighth Street, New York City.

Dear Doctor,—What do you do in cases of unilateral dislocation of the principal molars?

How do you correct the misplaced teeth without interfering with the others?

Answer: "It is difficult to answer the question regarding unilateral dislocation. I probably do as you do—the best I can—under the varying circumstances.

"Sometimes I have helped matters by using an intermaxillary elastic on one side only; sometimes, perhaps, an extraction might be resorted to."

I wanted so much to talk over with you the actual fundamental principles that underlie orthodontia.

For twenty-three years I have eschewed the extraction of teeth for that purpose.

There has been in that length of time but one exception to this rule in my own practice, and that was a case where a number of teeth had already been lost, and the patient, a young lady, was about thirty years of age.

I have seen one other case (Baker's patient), in which I consented, *at that time*, that extraction was best; but I must be permitted, in the interests of consistency, to claim the right to change my mind when I learn that I have been wrong; and I think I have learned a little every year.

I have lately spent a week in Washington, studying every single one of the children's skulls in the National Museum, and a good many of the adult ones.

I find that when Bonwill's old method of laying out the teeth is followed, there are just enough to go round, no more, no less. That when we get hold of a young patient, especially during the second period of growth (between seven and fourteen), we have occasion, in pretty much all the cases of misplacement of the teeth, to enlarge one or both of the arches.

I did not think this was so universally true until you yourself brought it to my attention.

I find that when we enlarge these arches, especially the upper, we necessarily remove an obstruction that has prevented their proper development. That when this obstruction is removed, nature resumes her work and growth or development begins again; and if permitted or aided, by keeping obstructions out of the way as fast as Nature grows up to them, the whole series of bones lying above and adjacent to the maxillary bone grow up to their normal size.

This enlarges the whole facial region; it enlarges the nasal meatus, the antrum of Highmore, all the sinuses of the ethmoid bone, and straightens the nasal septum, develops the vomer, and provides a normal palatine vault in which the functions of the tongue are freely and easily performed in the enclosure formed by the normal arrangement of all the teeth properly articulating each with the others, according to the arrangement of Nature, which has provided teeth for each individual case exactly adapted to the size of that individual.

The absence, therefore, from whatever cause,—non-eruption, extraction, or accident,—of one single member from the arch completely disarranges, though with more or less grave results, the entire adaptation of the arches to each other. (See page 13 of my paper on Extraction.)

I have laid emphasis upon beginning the work of regulation early, because by that means we can push the completed crowns (by gentle pressure) into their proper places, that the formation of the roots may be completed after they are in place and that the alveolus may form around those roots while these latter are in process of formation.

This, you see, permits all of the teeth to interdigitate or cusp properly; which condition holds them in position, with the assistance of the tongue on one side and the lips and cheeks on the other, through life.

But without this cusping there can be no surety of teeth, moved from one position to another, retaining their new positions.

Yours truly,

E. A. Bogue.

Current News.

LEWIS AND CLARK DENTAL CONGRESS.

FOLLOWING is the programme of the Lewis and Clark Dental Congress, to be held at Portland, Ore., July 17, 18, 19, and 20, 1905:

MORNING.

9 to 12.   Exhibits.

10.00.   Meeting of General Committee.

10.30.   Salutation, Norris R. Cox, Chairman General Committee.

Address of welcome, Harry Lane, M.D., Mayor of Portland.

Response.

Organization and election of officers.

AFTERNOON.

Papers, clinics, exhibits.   To follow on July 17, 18, 19, 20, as arranged later.   Programme to be completed at 5 P.M., July 20.

Evening of July 20, Congress adjourns to "The Trail," Lewis and Clark Fair.

ESSAYS.

(Not complete.)

I. "Pathology."   John Endleman, Philadelphia Pa.   Discussion opened by B. S. Scott, Tacoma, Wash.

II. Symposium on Empyema of the Maxillary Sinus (ten-minute papers):

1. "The Anatomy of the Maxillary Sinus and the Relation of the Superior Teeth to the Sinus."   Dr. James G. Sharp, San Francisco, Cal.

2. "The Etiology and Diagnosis of Empyema of the Maxillary Sinus."   Dr. Frank L. Platt, San Francisco, Cal.

3. "The Surgical Treatment of the Maxillary Sinus."   Dr. John S. Marshall, U.S.A.

Symposium on Fractures of the Mandible (ten-minute papers):

1. "The Anatomy of the Mandible, with Special Reference to the Muscles which control its Movements and the Localities at

which Fractures are most liable to occur." Dr. James G. Sharp, San Francisco, Cal.

2. " The Classification of Fractures of the Mandible, and their Diagnosis." Dr. William A. Bryant, San Francisco, Cal.

3. " The Surgical Treatment of Fractures of the Mandible, Suturing, etc." Dr. John S. Marshall, U.S.A.

4. " The Mechanical Treatment of Fractures of the Mandible. Interdental Splints, External Splints, Fracture Bands, etc." Dr. Charles H. Bowman, San Francisco, Cal.

III. " Why are not All Successful?" Dr. J. C. Hennessy, Reno, Nev. Discussion opened by D. J. Wait, Helena, Mont.

IV. " Mouth Breathing: Its Relation to Orthodontia." (Eighteen lantern slides.) Ray D. Robinson, Los Angeles, Cal. Discussion opened by E. G. Howard, Los Angeles, Cal.

V. " Dental Lesions of Animals—Domestic, Captive, and Wild." (Lantern slides.) William Bebb, Los Angeles, Cal. Discussion opened by Arthur D. Black, Chicago, Ill.

VI. " History of Dentistry." (Lantern slides.) Burton Lee Thorpe, St. Louis, Mo. Discussion opened by Arthur W. Chance, Portland, Ore.

VII. " Accidental Cleft Palates." H. J. Janlusz, New York, N. Y. Discussion opened by J. A. Meyer, Tacoma, Wash.

VIII. " The Status of the Inlay: Gold and Porcelain." C. N. Thompson, Chicago, Ill. Discussion opened by B. F. Eshleman, Tacoma, Wash.

IX. " Interstitial Gingivitis." Eugene S. Talbot, Chicago, Ill. Discussion opened by G. V. I. Brown, Milwaukee, Wis.

X. Ether Spray as an Obtundent." Crittenden Van Wyck, Oakland, Cal. Discussion opened by William A. Bryant, San Francisco, Cal.

XI. " Dental Standards." Clyde Payne, San Francisco, Cal. Discussion opened by William A. Cumming, Portland, Ore.

XII. " Discrimination in the Selection of Filling-Material." C. N. Johnson, Chicago, Ill. Discussion opened by John S. Marshall, San Francisco, Cal.

XIII. Subject not announced. G. V. I. Brown, Milwaukee, Wis. Discussion opened by Eugene S. Talbot, Chicago, Ill.

XIV. " Pulp Technique." M. L. Rhein, New York, N. Y. Discussion opened by C. N. Johnson, Chicago, Ill.

XV. " A Plea for the Left Hand." F. H. Metcalf, Sacramento, Cal. Discussion opened by S. J. Barber, Portland, Ore.

XVI. "The Needs of Reform in Dental Education." D. D. Smith, M.D., D.D.S., Philadelphia, Pa. Discussion opened by ——.

XVII. Not completed.

XVIII. "Local Anæsthesia," or "Dental Education." W. G. Wyckoff, Philadelphia, Pa. Discussion opened by ——.

XIX. "Diagnostic and Therapeutic Uses of X-Rays in Dentistry and Oral Surgery." (With lantern slides.) M. I. Schamberg, Philadelphia, Pa. Discussion opened by

CLINICS AND CLINICIANS.

1. M. L. Rhein, New York, N. Y. "Technique of Pulp Removal and Root-Canal Cleansing, and packing Gold by Means of Electro-Magnetic Mallet."

2. Morris T. Schamberg, Philadelphia, Pa. "Root Amputation *versus* Ablation for the Cure of Chronic Apical Abscesses."

3. C. N. Thompson, Chicago, Ill. "Gold Inlay." Table Clinic: "Porcelain Inlays."

4. G. V. I. Brown, Milwaukee, Wis. Surgical clinic.

5. R. B. Gentle, New York, N. Y. "Cavity Preparation for Porcelain Inlays."

6. Alice M. Steeves, Boston, Mass. "Useful Root-Canal Filling."

7. P. M. Wuillemin, San Francisco, Cal. "Extraction under Nitrous Oxide Anæsthesia."

8. F. R. Sandusky, Nashville, Tenn. "Saddle Bridge-Work. Molars supplied, using all Porcelain Dummies, with Porcelain Crowns for Anchorage."

9. R. C. Brophy, Chicago, Ill. (a) "Porcelain Work without Use of Electricity." (b) "Metalo-Plastic Plate-Work."

10. Ray D. Robinson, Los Angeles, Cal. "Appliances for retaining Teeth after shifting Occlusion."

11. J. M. Yates, Portland, Ore. "Administration of Somnoform."

12. J. L. Pease, Oakland, Cal. Subject to be announced.

13. F. W. Hergert, Seattle, Wash. "Swaging Metal Plates by the Holmes-Palmer Method."

14. O. J. Fruth, St. Louis, Mo. "Raising the Bite by Means of Gold Inlays and Method of making the Same."

15. F. L. Platt, San Francisco, Cal. "Porcelain Inlays in Crown- and Bridge-Work."

16. B. F. Eshelman, Tacoma, Wash. "Something Interesting to Porcelain Workers."

17. C. B. Reynolds, Seattle, Wash. "Use of Cohesive and Non-Cohesive Gold in Molar."

18. J. S. Engs, Oakland, Cal. "Photo-Micrographs."

19. J. S. Baldridge, Wooley, Wash. "The Restoration of an Incisal Angle with High-Fusing Porcelain."

20. H. J. Smith, Genesee, Idaho. "Removal of Deposits and Stains from Teeth of Adults and Children, with Medical Applications Before and After."

21. H. W. Bates, Denver, Col. "Simple Manner of making Dies and Swaging Plates from Plaster Impressions."

22. A. M. Baker, San Jose, Cal. Subject to be announced.

23. G. W. Schwartz, Chicago, Ill. "Removable Bridges."

24. F. K. Ledyard, San Jose, Cal. Subject to be announced.

25. C. L. Rose, Fargo, N. D. "Gold Inlay."

26. J. H. Merritt, Oakland, Cal. "Restoration of Incisal Angle, using Jenkins Porcelain."

27. A. M. Magee, Louisiana, Mo. "Some Difficult Things presenting, and what We will do with Them."

28. W. V. B. Ames, Chicago, Ill. "Adaptation of Entire Artificial Dentures."

29. C. A. Southwell, Boise, Idaho. "Filling Molar-Appro-Mesial Cavity with Gold, using Electric or Automatic Mallet."

30. F. W. Lawrence, St. Louis, Mo. "Something in Porcelain."

31. C. N. Johnson, Chicago, Ill. "Demonstrations of Cavity Preparation on Models." (Table clinic.)

32. R. A. Rawlings, Bismarck, N. D. "Filling Disto-Occlusal Cavity in Upper Bicuspid with Gold."

33. William Bebb, Los Angeles, Cal. "Anatomical Specimens." (Table clinic.)

34. William H. DeFord, Des Moines, Iowa. "Demonstrations on Somnoform."

35. Jessie R. DeFord, Des Moines, Iowa. "Demonstrations of Somnoform."

36. C. S. Irwin, Vancouver, Wash. Table and Chair Clinic, using Tin.

37. E. R. Tait, Oakland, Cal. "Filling Teeth with Plastic Mat Gold."

38. J. W. Nebett, Chicago, Ill. " Showing Method of swaging with Water; also, Filling Matrix with Porcelain in a Manner that will overcome Warping."

39. V. H. Frederick, St. Louis, Mo. " Continuous Gum Work."

40. E. B. Edgers, Seattle, Wash. " Treating Putrescent Pulp-Canals by the Use of Sodium and Potassium Compound and filling immediately."

41. L. P. Haskell, Chicago, Ill. " Continuous Gum Work."

42. A. J. Holmes, New Westminster, B. C. " Simple Method of constructing Richmond Crown."

43. Crittenden Van Wyck, San Francisco, Cal. " Showing Van Wyck Obtunder and Practical Demonstrations with Same."

44. B. F. Eshelman, Tacoma, Wash. " Something Interesting to Porcelain Workers."

45. George N. Wasser, Cleveland, Ohio. " High-Fusing Porcelain Inlay."

46. W. J. Hacking, New Westminster, B. C. " Technique of an Accurate Fitting and Articulated Seamless Crown."

47. H. Russell Hill, Hamilton, Mo. " Open Face Contour Crown-Work."

48. Los Angeles Porcelain Club (seven in number). Seven men will work porcelain—a continuous clinic.

49. W. N. Murray, Minneapolis, Minn. " Gold Inlay."

50. Valentine K. Irjon, New Orleans, La. " A Full Porcelain Bridge without Use of Furnace or Baking" (the Lowque system).

51. A. P. Johnstone, Anderson, S. C. " A New and Original Way of fitting Porcelain Crowns, Incisors, Cuspids, Bicuspids, and Molars, Upper or Lower, to their Respective Roots." (Table clinic.)

52. Fred H. Metcalf, Sacramento, Cal. " Positions at the Chair for Ambidextrous Operator."

53. G. M. Osterberg, Seattle, Wash. " Adaptation of the Davis Crown by baking."

54. G. Maurice Crow, Los Angeles, Cal. " The Use of Porcelain Stains."

55. C. F. Sweet, Minot, N. D. " Gold Fillings in Porcelain Teeth."

56. W. A. Cummings, Portland, Ore. Subject to be announced.

57. J. J. F. McLaughlin, North Adams, Mass. " Rowan's Extra Pliable Gold Rolls and Rolled Gold for Contour Fillings."

58. E. DeWitt R. Garden, Tarrytown, N. Y. "Mineral Plate Work."

59. J. G. Hollingsworth, Kansas City, Mo. "Demonstrating New Reinforcement for Porcelain Crowns." (Table clinic.)

60. Portland Porcelain Club (six in number).

61. D. D. Smith, Philadelphia, Pa. "Exhibition of the Correct Method of filling Front Teeth."

62. N. R. Cox, Portland, Ore. "Somnoform Demonstrations."

63. D. I. Wadsworth, Portland, Ore. "Gold Inlay showing Swaging Device." (Table clinic.)

64. George D. Peters, Portland, Ore. "Removable Crown- and Bridge-Work." (Peeso's method.)

65. John S. Marshall, U.S.A., Presidio, Cal. Surgical Clinic.

66. E. A. Tripp, Salt Lake City, Utah. "Impressions of Cleft Plate and Obturator."

67. Mark Hayter, Dallas, Ore. "Backing Porcelain Facings."

68. J. B. Burns, Payette, Idaho. "Practical Cases of Removable Upper Partial Plate, with Attachments." "Deposits on Teeth, and Effect." (Table clinic.)

69. L. A. Stemmly, Myrtle Point, Ore. (*a*) "Method of backing Facings." (Table demonstration.) (*b*) "Method of placing Fillings in Porcelain Crowns."

70. J. R. Cardwell, Portland, Ore. "Trimming Model for Vacuum Plates."

71. W. N. Murray, Minneapolis, Minn. "Gold Inlay."

72. W. G. Wyckoff, Philadelphia, Pa. "Painless Extraction with Local Antiseptic."

73. E. L. Hutchinson, Honolulu, S. I. "Gold Inlay."

74. F. E. Roach, Chicago, Ill. "A New Fusible Cement."

75. J. S. Kirkwood, Salt Lake City, Utah. "Extraction of Teeth and Live Pulps by Use of Somnoform."

76. Charles W. Day, Vinita, Ind. Ter. "Invisible Attachments for Fixed or Removable Bridges."

77. Frank N. Walgamott, Portland, Ore. "Hypnotism and its Use in Dentistry." (Demonstration.)

78. J. R. Entrikin, Des Moines, Iowa. "The Filling of Root-Canals with other than the Ordinary Chloropercha."

79. R. Siddall, The Dalles, Ore. "Extracting Teeth, showing Use of Elevator."

80. W. F. Mack, Salt Lake City, Utah. "A New Idea in a Porcelain Crown."

81. D. T. Hill, Syracuse, Neb. Dental Crown and Plate Anchor."

82. D. O. M. LeCron, St. Louis, Mo. "Porcelain and its Correct Fusing 'Table.'"

83. H. N. Smith, Seattle, Wash. "Method of making Seam Crowns with Smith's Contour Pliers."

84. S. M. Hampton, Helena, Mont. Gold Filling."

85. D. J. Wait, Helena, Mont. "Use of Vernon's Gold for filling."

86. A. F. Merriman, Oakland, Cal. "Gold Filling."

87. O. D. Ireland, Portland, Ore. "Articulation of Teeth after Bonwill."

88. Dr. Stratford, New York, N. Y. "Somnoform Demonstration."

89. Lelan Otis Green, Chicago, Ill. "Painless Extraction under Influence of the Local Anæsthetic Acestoria."

90. E. W. Dodez, Ft. Wayne, Ind. "The Filling of Root-Canals with Oxpara."

LIST OF EXHIBITORS.

S. S. White Dental Manufacturing Company, Philadelphia, Pa. Ritter Dental Manufacturing Company, Rochester, N. Y. L. D. Caulk Company, Philadelphia, Pa. Gideon Sibley, 1314 Filbert Street, Philadelphia, Pa. Klewe & Co., Portland, Me. Boston Pharmacal Company, San Francisco, Cal. The J. W. Edwards Company, San Francisco, Cal. W. V. B. Ames, 36 Washington Street, Chicago, Ill. Buffalo Dental Manufacturing Company, Buffalo, N. Y. J. W. Ivory, 51 N. Tenth Street, Philadelphia, Pa. Detroit Dental Manufacturing Company, Detroit, Mich. Dr. X. Dodal, 1307 Howard, San Francisco, Cal. Edward Rowan, 831-7 East 163d Street, New York, N. Y. Dr. L. O. Green, 100 State Street, Chicago, Ill. C. H. Pinches, 1181 Broadway, New York, N. Y. Keasby Mattison Company, Ambler, Pa. Hisey Dental Manufacturing Company, St. Louis, Mo. Chicago Dental Specialty Company, Chicago, Ill. The American Cabinet Company, Two Rivers, Wis. The Rasom & Randolph Company, Toledo, Ohio. Lambert Pharmacal Company, St. Louis, Mo. Armour & Co., Chicago, Ill. Kress & Owen Company, Chicago, Ill. A. P. Gould & Co., Canton, Ohio. Dr. J. C. Graft, Newark, N. J. Harvard Dental Manufacturing Company, Canton, Ohio. A. C. Clark & Co., 21 East Randolph Street, Chicago, Ill. Blair Manufacturing Company, Louisville, Ky. Lee S. Smith & Son, 1301-3 Arch Street, Philadelphia, Pa. J. M. Ney & Co., 265 Asylum Street, Hartford, Conn. Dentists' Supply Company, 109 West 42d Street, New York, N. Y. E. DeTrey & Son, Philadelphia, Pa. Electro-Dental Manufacturing Company, 1228 Cherry Street, Philadelphia, Pa. Cleveland Dental Manufacturing Company, Cleveland, Ohio. Horlick Food Company, Racine, Wis. Oakland Chemical Company, New York, N. Y. Hall & Ruckel, New York, N. Y. Victor Electric Company, 56-61 Market Street, Chicago, Ill. Florence Manufacturing Company, Florence, Mass. E. C. Moore & Co., 112 Miami Avenue, Detroit, Mich. B. C. Smith & Son, Pittsburg, Pa. A. J. Watts & Co., 127 East 23d Street, New York, N. Y. Sanitol Chemical Company, St. Louis, Mo. Randall-Faichney & Co., Boston, Mass. Tenax Dental Compound Company, Terra Haute, Ind.

This programme is not complete up to date. The entire programme will be completed by July 1.

Kindly call attention to the location of a sub-station of the Portland Post-Office in the meeting of the Congress. Dentists should have their mail addressed to Lewis & Clark Dental Congress, Armory Oregon National Guard, Portland, Ore.

The social programme of the Congress will be largely of an informal character. The Stomatological Club of Portland has arranged for club-rooms in the Armory Building, the meeting-place of the Congress, where informal social gatherings will take place each day.

The Congress invites its members to participate in all the exhibitions and shows on the Trail of the Lewis & Clark Fair for the final entertainment following the Congress, on the night of July 20.

NATIONAL DENTAL ASSOCIATION, SECTION II.

FOLLOWING is the corrected programme for Section II. of the National Dental Association:

Dr. J. V. Conzett, Dubuque, Iowa, "Gold as a Filling-Material."

Dr. B. L. Thorp, 3666 Olive Street, St. Louis, Lantern Lecture: "Pioneer Manipulators of Gold-Foil."

Dr. Chas. Milton Ford, 523 West One Hundred and Forty-first Street, New York, "Dental Education."

Dr. W. R. Clack, Clear Lake, Iowa, "The Necessity for a Method of preserving the Integrity of the Interproximal Space."

Dr. D. O. M. LeCron, 501 Missouri Trust Building, St. Louis, "A Few Experiments in Porcelain."

Dr. D. W. Fellows, Portland, Me., "A Century of Standard Dental Writings."

Dr. B. Holly Smith, 1007 Madison Avenue, Baltimore, "Operative Dentistry."

Dr. S. H. Guilford, 1631 Walnut Street, Philadelphia, "The Nomenclature of Orthodontia."

Dr. Wm. H. Potter, 16 Arlington Street, Boston, Mass., "The Use of the Summer Vacation in the Education of the Dental Student."

Dr. I. J. Wetherbee, 120 Boylston Street, Boston, Mass., "Tin-and-Gold: Its Possibilities and Uses as a Filling-Material."

Dr. H. E. Roberts, *Chairman,*

Philadelphia, Pa.

Dr. C. S. Butler, *Secretary,*

Buffalo, N. Y.

CLINIC SECTION OF THE NATIONAL DENTAL ASSOCIATION.

The work of the Clinic Section is progressing most favorably. Everything at present indicates that the operative clinic will be the largest that the National Dental Association has ever held. There will be forty operators for both mornings upon which the clinics will be held. The territory from Maine to Utah and from Minnesota to Texas has been very fully covered, and men from almost all of the States in the section named have signified their willingness to be present and operate. The majority of the men of the G. V. Black Dental Club will be present and will operate upon both days. Such well-known Northwestern men as Drs. Searl, Lewis, Clack, Conzett, Beemer, G. D. Moyer, W. H. K.

Moyer, W. D. James, F. S. James, Gallagher, Carlson, Fawcett, etc., will once more operate in a body, as was done at the International Dental Congress.

Dr. T. W. Brophy, of Chicago, has kindly consented to assist and will make a surgical operation. Dr. Brophy's clinics are of such a high order that those interested are certain of seeing something which they will not soon forget.

The well-known Dr. M. E. Smith, of Lynn, Mass., will also make a surgical operation.

Somnoform and narcotile will be very fully demonstrated.

A large number of gentlemen will give table clinics.

At the present writing I feel confident in saying that the best men in the profession will operate at Buffalo on July 26 and 27. A full report has not been received from all the men on the committee, but sufficient data are before me upon which to base the opinion above expressed.

E. K. WEDELSTAEDT,
Secretary Clinic Section.

NEW YORK LIFE BUILDING, ST. PAUL, MINN.

MAINE DENTAL SOCIETY.

THE Fortieth annual meeting of the Maine Dental Society will be held at Portland, Me., July 18, 19, and 20, 1905.

GEORGE E. DOW,
Chairman Executive Committee.

GRADUATES OF THE KANSAS CITY DENTAL COLLEGE.

WILL you kindly forward your address to me, so as to complete a roster of the graduates? Don't take it for granted your address is known.

J. P. ROOT.

DEARDORFF BUILDING, KANSAS CITY, MO.

FARGO DISTRICT DENTAL SOCIETY.

THERE has been organized the Fargo District Dental Society, at Fargo, North Dakota, which meets the third Monday of every month. The following officers were elected:

President, S. J. Hill; Vice-President, H. L. Starling; Secretary, Albert Hallenberg; Treasurer, C. L. Rose.

Executive Committee.—L. C. Davenport, J. L. Graves, F. A. Bricker.

ALBERT HALLENBERG,
Secretary.

SOUTH DAKOTA STATE BOARD OF DENTAL EXAMINERS.

THE next meeting of the South Dakota State Board of Dental Examiners will be held at Mitchell, S. D., July 11, beginning at 1.30 P.M. All candidates will be required to do practical work in both operative and prosthetic dentistry, and should bring all instruments and materials necessary to do the same. Vulcanizer, lathe, and swaging appliances will be furnished by the board. Application, together with fee of ten dollars, must positively be in the hands of the Secretary before July 7.

G. W. COLLINS.

"F. D. I." INTERNATIONAL DENTAL FEDERATION.

THE next annual meeting of the Executive Council of the Fédération Dentaire Internationale will convene in Hanover, Germany, August 7, 1905, immediately following the annual meeting of the Central-Verein Deutscher Zahnarzte. Announcement of the programme for the meeting and the projected work for the Federation during the present period will shortly be made through the dental journals and through the official bulletin of the Federation.

EDWARD C. KIRK,
Secretary-General.

THE

International Dental Journal.

VOL. XXVI.   AUGUST, 1905.   No. 8.

Original Communications.[1]

THE RATIONALE OF THE PORCELAIN INLAY.[2]

BY DR. J. Q. BYRAM, INDIANAPOLIS, IND.

I WISH to express my appreciation of the honor conferred upon me by your society in inviting me to appear as your essayist this evening. I assure you that I feel my incompetency to read a paper on a subject which is not only familiar to you, but one on which several of your members are authority.

It seems quite impossible to add anything of value to the discussion of porcelain inlays; so much has been written on this subject within the last four years. But a repetition of the old enables one to become more familiar with a problem. That there is a growing interest in porcelain as a filling-material is indicated by the number of dentists who are becoming skilful in this branch of dental art. Yet the majority of dentists know little about porcelain, and many believe that the insertion of porcelain inlays is a fad. It is probable that many of the enthusiasts have gone to extremes, and that many articles have been written which deal with the ideal rather than the practical, and that those writers

---

[1] The editor and publishers are not responsible for the views of authors of papers published in this department, nor for any claim to novelty, or otherwise, that may be made by them. No papers will be received for this department that have appeared in any other journal published in the country.

[2] Read before the Academy of Stomatology, Philadelphia, Pa., March 28, 1905.

who have been so fanciful should be classed as visionaries and idealists. But the idealist by his enthusiasm has been an educator to a keener appreciation of artistic dentistry. We need more hobbyists on the subject of porcelain; for had it not been for the enthusiasts, its virtues would not be admitted to the extent that they are to-day.

One of the elements of true dental art consists in disguising the artificiality of the material by which lost tissue or organs are replaced. If the enthusiastic exponents of porcelain inlays, in their desire to conceal their art, have gone beyond reasonable limits in the use of inlays, this enthusiasm has caused many dentists to develop their skill and æsthetic sense to a higher degree, thus enabling them to practise dentistry in a more artistic manner.

Porcelain is now recognized as a meritorious filling-material, and its adoption will come of necessity, if not from choice. It will be but a short time until the dentist who fails to master the technique of constructing porcelain inlays will be relegated to the rear ranks of the profession; for porcelain is the material which should be used in filling most conspicuous cavities.

It is true that, at the present time, the extent of the use of porcelain as a filling-material is dependent on the dentist. Many dentists will be required to develop their æsthetic sense before it can be universally used. Much has been said about educating the public to a higher appreciation of artistic dentistry, but until more dentists are educated along this line we can hardly expect to make much progress in the education of the laity. Paradoxical as it may seem, however, the laity is assisting in educating the profession.

Many dentists are discouraging the use of porcelain, because they are not familiar with its good qualities. Some may have seen a few failures, and because of ignorance of its properties are condemning it. Others, through inexperience and lack of knowledge of the properties of porcelain, have made failures. So they are condemning it.

The construction of porcelain inlays involves four sets of manipulative principles:

1. The preparation of the cavity.
2. The construction of the matrix.
3. The selection, the application, and the fusing of the porcelain.

4. The finishing and setting of the inlay.

Each of these steps involves a series of mechanical principles, and if they are not executed according to these principles, an imperfect filling will be the result. The failure of many inlays may be attributed to lack of detail, for too many beginners attempt the construction of inlays for the mouth before they have mastered the technique.

There is a difference of opinion regarding the preparation of cavities for inlays. Some insist that inlays can be retained in cavities without any retentive form, and that their retention is wholly dependent upon close adaptation and the adhesive properties of the cement. Others believe that cavities should be given as nearly a self-retentive form as it is possible to make, in order to resist the tendency of dislodgement of the filling under stress. They also believe that the cement tends to stay inlays rather than retain them. Those who follow the teachings of the latter will have fewer inlays to reconstruct or reset. Cavities for inlays should be prepared with the same carefulness that should be used in the preparation of cavities for other fillings. The mechanical principles by which inlays are retained must be observed with absolute accuracy, and all cavities should be given a retentive form to resist stress. The cavity must be sufficiently deep to give ample thickness of porcelain, which will insure structural strength and avoid defects in the construction of the inlay. The cavity margins should be formed to avoid unsupported enamel-rods, they should be smooth and in curves or straight lines, avoiding angles whenever possible. There should be no bevel of the enamel margins to give frail edges of porcelain. Two requirements for the proper construction of matrices are accessibility and working space. It is essential that teeth with proximal cavities be separated to insure the proper withdrawal of the matrix and the insertion of the inlay.

THE PREPARATION OF CAVITIES.

Dr. C. N. Thompson [1] suggests that the walls of a labial or a buccal cavity should be at right angles with the curves of the surface (Fig. 1). This causes them to converge slightly toward the pulpal wall. The pulpal wall should be flat and its junction with the other walls should be in curves instead of angles. The cavity

---

[1] Dental Digest, May, 1904.

should be deep enough to afford the best possible anchorage and
to prevent the cement's changing the color of the inlay.

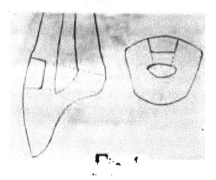

In simple proximal cavities involving both labial and lingual
surfaces the gingival wall should form a right angle with the
pulpal wall. The incisal wall should form a right angle with
the curve of the proximal surface (Fig. 2, A). These walls should

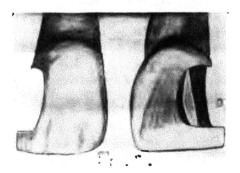

extend far enough to prevent frail margins of porcelain, but care
should be exercised to guard against undue weakness of the incisal angle. The labial and lingual walls should extend far
enough to reach sound enamel, and these margins should unite
with the gingival and the incisal margins in curves. The cavity
should have no undercuts or sharp angles between these walls.
The lingual wall may extend farther than the labial, and a step
may be cut in the middle and gingival thirds (Fig. 2, B), to insure additional retentive resistance.

Because of the variation in proximo-incisal cavities it is almost impossible to outline a conventional form of cavity preparation. Proximo-incisal cavities may be divided into (1) cavities involving but a small portion of the labial and the lingual surfaces, and (2) extensive cavities requiring a step for additional retentive resistance.

THE PREPARATION OF SMALL PROXIMO-INCISAL CAVITIES.

The gingival wall should be flat, but its margins should be concave mesio-distally (Fig. 3, A). The incisal enamel margins

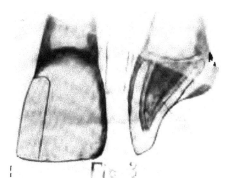

should be extended to avoid frail enamel. Cut a triangular cavity, extending from the gingival to the incisal wall, and having parallel walls, as deep as the pulp will permit (Fig. 3, B). A concavity should be made in the dentine of the incisal wall, after the inlay has been completed, and a groove in the ridge on the inlay (Fig. 3, C), giving it something of a mortise form.

PROXIMO-INCISAL CAVITIES WITH STEPS.

Since the necessity for retentive resistance increases in ratio to the increased width of the inlay, a step should be made in large proximo-incisal cavities to resist the tipping stress. The gingival wall of the cavity should be flat, with its margins concave mesio-distally. The labial and lingual walls should be extended parallel until sound enamel, supported by dentine, is reached. Then a shallow cavity should be cut between the labial and lingual walls (Fig. 4, A). A step should be prepared, involving enough tooth-structure to give a mass of porcelain large enough to withstand the force of mastication.

PREPARATION OF THE STEP.

The step should be cut across the incisal edge, extending from one and one-half to three millimetres; it should be from one to

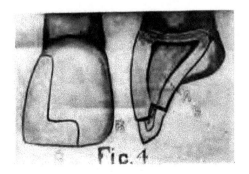

FIG. 4

two millimetres deep on the labial surface, and from one and one-half to three millimetres deep on the lingual. The labial and lingual margins should both form right angles with the gingivo-incisal curves of these surfaces (Fig. 4, B), and they should form

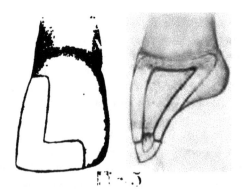

FIG. 5

slight reverse curves with the axial margins of the cavity (Fig. 4, C). A shallow cavity may be cut between the labial and the lingual plates when they are approximately the same length (Fig. 5, A). The lingual plate should be cut almost one-half the thickness of the incisal end if it is extended farther gingivally than the labial plate (Fig. 4, B). It should be so formed that its gingival wall will be at right angles with the concavity of the lingual surface.

A step may also be formed involving only the lingual plate in those teeth with thick incisal edges (Fig. 6, A). It should involve

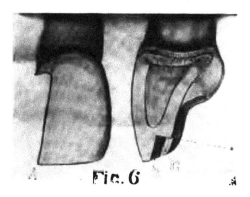

Fig. 6

at least one-half the thickness of the incisal edge, extending from one and one-half to three millimetres gingivally. The gingival wall should form a right angle with the concavity of the lingual surface (Fig. 6, B). A slight groove may extend along the labio-

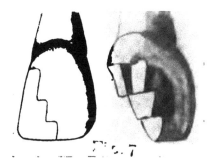

Fig. 7

proximal angle (Fig. 6, C). Dr. J. E. Nyman [1] suggests a method of preparing proximo-incisal cavities by cutting a series of reverse curves as illustrated in Fig. 7. He says, "This irregular outline results in a less conspicuous line of demarcation between the

[1] Dental Summary, January, 1905.

porcelain and the tooth enamel than if the margin were cut in a straight line and obtains the essential right-angle margins."

CAVITIES INVOLVING THE INCISAL EDGE.

Simple cavities are usually caused by malformation. The mesial and distal walls of these should extend gingivally from two to three millimetres, and should slightly diverge toward the incisal edge (Fig. 8, A). They should be slightly grooved between

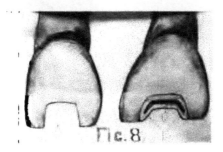

their plates of enamel to resist the lingual stress (Fig. 8, B). The seat should slope toward the centre from the labial and lingual margins (Fig. 8, C).

Cavities involving the entire incisal edge are very rare. The inlay must be retained by pins (Fig. 9) or by a step cut on the lingual surface (Fig. 4, B).

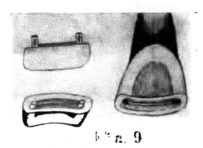

Porcelain is not the safest material for filling small cavities in bicuspids and molars. Their occlusal surfaces present a series of inclined planes, which, when restored with a friable material, lacking in edge strength, cause imperfect fillings in a short time by the breaking down of frail margins. Porcelain should not be used in this class of cavities unless they are in the line of vision. Gold inlays or fillings may be inserted which are just as compatible with the tooth-structure as porcelain.

PREPARATION OF CAVITIES FOR BICUSPIDS AND MOLARS.

The gingival wall should form a right angle with the pulpal wall. The buccal and lingual walls should diverge toward the proximal and occlusal margins. They should be grooved in the dentine occluso-gingivally to form mortices (Fig. 10, A). When

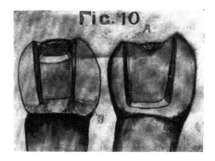

the buccal and lingual surfaces are involved, they should extend far enough to prevent frail margins of porcelain (Fig. 10, B). If a step is required, it should extend wide and deep enough to insure strength to the porcelain.

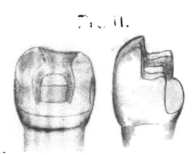

In extensive cases the buccal and lingual cusps should be involved and the cavity margins extended on the buccal surfaces, obliterating to a large degree frail margins of porcelain on the occlusal surface (Fig. 11).

lowish or bluish hue, and blue.. Normal dentine is some shade of yellow, while the enamel seems to be a variety of colors.

The variation of color so often noticeable when an inlay is cemented in place is quite perplexing. The inlay may be a good match when the incidence of light rays is at an angle that will permit of their transmission. But when the angle of incidence is changed, some portion of the inlay may appear a different color. The cement is also a factor in the color problem. If it were transparent, it would not prevent the passage of light rays through the tooth. But when light is incident upon an opaque cement, it is excluded from the dentine, and the color of an opaque body is due to the kind of light it reflects, the remaining colors being wholly or partly absorbed on the surface.

A " shadow" is formed when an inlay is cemented into a cavity with a cement which dimly reflects and partially absorbs the transmitted rays if the incidence of light is at such an angle that unabsorbed rays cannot be transmitted.

Dr. W. T. Reeves, of Chicago, was the first to suggest that inlays should be built in layers, and claims for this method a more translucent inlay, avoidance of the " shadow," and a prevention of the cement's reflecting from beneath. This method of constructing inlays will assist in overcoming these obstacles, but it does not wholly remove them.

Mr. Robert Brewster has produced a white opaque porcelain for lining matrices. He says for it: " It is of a bright reflecting character and dense enough to counteract the absorbing effect of the cement. That portion of the inlay to be in contact with the cement is made of this lining. The matrix is then filled with the regular porcelain. When the light strikes the inlay the transmitted rays are reflected through the inlay, thus preventing the absorption of the light rays by the cement."

In the selection of colors for an inlay, note the variation of color of the natural tooth. There are usually three or more colors or shades of colors in a tooth. The foundation of the inlay, representing the dentine, should be yellow (presuming the tooth is vital), while the overlying colors should approach the color of the enamel in their respective positions. The foundation body should be applied and contoured to replace the dentine. It should be fused, provided it is of a higher fusing porcelain than that used to replace the enamel. Care should be exercised to prevent porcelain-of different colors from mixing when applying them to their respective positions. If the colors are applied separately and biscuited, then a uniform color be applied over the entire mass and properly fused, the colors will be true and the fused porcelain will have a more natural appearance.

The fusing of the porcelain is as exacting as any step in the construction of the inlay. It is difficult to fuse porcelain at a definite degree of heat without some means of measuring it, and many otherwise good inlays are spoiled in the furnace. Variations in the heat of the muffle will cause variations in the shade and strength of the porcelain. Underfused porcelain is of a darker hue and less translucent, while overfused porcelain is lighter. In either case the porcelain is more porous because of the imperfect rearrangement of the molecules. Overfused porcelain, the result of repeated or prolonged contact with its maximum heat, produces an ebulition of the double silicates, and this causes a blistering of the masses and a change of color.

Since the introduction of the dental pyrometer, the fusing of porcelain has been simplified and positive results can be obtained. To Dr. W. A. Price, of Cleveland, Ohio, belongs the credit of placing the first dental pyrometer on the market. The pyrometer designed by Dr. Price depends upon the principle of a thermopile. When certain metals are subjected to heat, an electrical current is generated, the quantity of which depends upon the temperature to which these metals are subjected. Every increase in the temperature causes a corresponding increase in the quantity of current given off by these metals. A small pellet of the metal rhodium is welded to two platinum wires, and one or more of these miniature thermopiles are introduced in the rear of the muffle. When they are heated, a feeble current is generated. As the temperature increases, the quantity of current in a like manner increases, and this is measured by means of a delicate millameter. Hence the amount of current generated is accurately recorded by this delicate instrument.

The pyrometer designed by Mr. N. K. Garhart, of Indianapolis, Ind., depends upon an entirely different principle. He interposes in the current of a low voltage circuit a " Nernst Glower," and measures the quantity of current passing through the " glower" by means of a delicate millameter. The " Nernst Glower" is a peculiar variety of porcelain which is a non-conductor when cold but a conductor when heated. The conductivity of the "glower" is in ratio to the increased temperature of the muffle. The amount of current required for the "glower" is so small in quantity and slight in pressure that the "glower" seems to undergo no change from repeated use. The current is obtained from the street circuit on the shunt plan, and owing to the minute amount required for this purpose, slight fluctuations of the street supply current do not impair the accuracy of the instrument.

Very little finishing of the inlay is required if proper care is exercised in applying the porcelain. All margins of porcelain overhanging the enamel margins should be removed with cuttle-fish disks. In order to insure better adhesion of the porcelain to the cement, that portion of the inlay which is to be inserted into the cavity should be grooved and present a roughened surface. The roughening of the surface is best accomplished by embedding the margins of the inlay in wax, then painting the surface with hydrofluoric acid until it becomes sufficiently roughened. The acid should then be neutralized and the inlay thoroughly cleansed and dried.

The ideal cement for setting inlays should be transparent and very adhesive. But since we are compelled to use an opaque cement, the white is probably the best color to use in setting large proximal inlays. A variety of colors can be obtained from the white cement by the use of pigments without any apparent detrimental effect on the cement. The pigments are useful in coloring the cement the color of the enamel for labial cavities, for the incidence of light on inlays, in cavities on the labial surfaces, is always in such direction that the rays are feebly reflected and partially absorbed by the cement.

In order to obtain the greatest adhesiveness, the cement powder and liquid should be mixed in definite proportions, and they should be thoroughly spatulated. Three grains of powder and two drops of liquid seem to give the proper consistency for Ames's hydraulic cement, while four grains of powder and two drops of liquid seem to give the best results for the Harvard slow-setting cement.

The cavity should be washed with chloroform and dried. A thin film of cement should be placed over the walls and margins of the cavity. The inlay is then forced into position with soft wood or semi-vulcanized rubber; it should be retained in position with wedges or floss tied around it, to allow the cement to crystallize under pressure. After the cement has thoroughly crystallized the surplus is removed and the margins of the inlay are polished with cuttle-fish disks and Arkansas stones.

The fact that inlays are held in position with cement has caused many dentists to doubt the durability of these fillings. The permanency of the cement depends upon the close adaptation of the inlay to the cavity margins, for clinical experience has demonstrated that the dissolution of a thin film of cement between the cavity and the inlay margins is only for a slight depth, leaving the margins sealed to prevent recurrence of decay. The use of porcelain as a filling-material gives to our patients fillings that harmonize with the natural teeth and enables us to perform æsthetic operations in such manner that the nervous strain is lessened upon both patient and dentist.

A REPORT OF AN UNUSUAL CASE OF ORTHO-DONTIA.[1]

BY LAWRENCE W. BAKER, D.M.D., BOSTON, MASS.

I SHALL attempt to interest you, gentlemen, for a short time this evening by showing you a series of lantern slides illustrating what, to me at least, is a very interesting case of orthodontia.

This slide (Fig. 1) shows the two side views of the casts before treatment. No doubt your eye falls at once upon the marked deformity in the relation of the two jaws, which at first glance might be considered due to a protrusion of the upper arch, but on consulting the occlusal landmarks it is found that in reality the deformity is caused largely by a decided recession of the lower jaw. Normally, we know, the point of the lower cuspid occupies the space between the upper cuspid and lateral, and in an ordinary case of " distal occlusion" this point falls between the first bicuspid and cuspid, while in this extreme case this same point occupies the space *one* plane back of the ordinary distal position, or between the two bicuspids. So in simple distal occlusion the jaw recedes one

---

[1] **Read** before the American Academy of Dental Science, April 5, 1905.

occlusal notch, while in this case the lower jaw recedes not one, but two occlusal notches, to which deformity it seems logical to apply the term *double distal.*

Fig. 1.

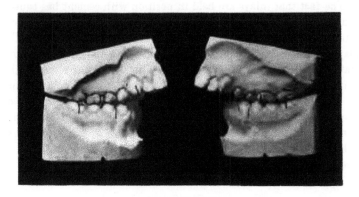

That this malformation caused a great impairment of the function of mastication, as well as a pronounced facial disfigurement. can be judged by studying this illustration. I should have hesitated at the responsibility of treating such a case had I not had great confidence in the possibilities of the " Baker anchorage."

Fig. 2.

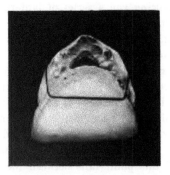

By way of history, I should like to state that when the child came to me the lower sixth-year molars were beyond saving, so at the proper time the bits of roots were removed, allowing the twelfth-year molars to come forward into the places of the missing sixth-year molars, with the result that you see here. The loss of these natural abutments of the arch greatly complicated the treatment of the case.

Fig. 2 shows another view of the deformity. The effects of the extreme distal position of the lower jaw upon its function is here clearly shown,—the ten or twelve anterior teeth were entirely useless for masticating·purposes. It was possible to pass the forefinger between the two arches, even though they were in close apposition, which illustrates their lack of function. This disuse is further indicated by the presence of the cusplets of development, which by use soon wear away.

Fig. 3.

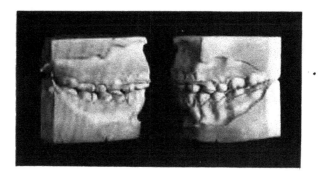

Next (Fig. 3) we have the two side views after treatment. It is clearly seen that the lower jaw has been brought forward to its intended position,—one notch to simple distal and another notch to normal,—greatly improving the facial contour as well as increasing the utility of the entire dental apparatus.

In this case many would have considered extracting in the upper arch necessary; probably the removal of two biscuspids would have been resorted to, or possibly the entire bicuspid region would have been sacrificed. In other words, the upper arch would have been mutilated to correspond with the misplaced lower arch; that is, another deformity would have been created equal to the already existing one. I believe that by keeping the upper arch intact and bringing the receding jaw forward not only were the jaws given full power, but the facial lines were placed in much better balance. Instead of weakening the lower part of the face by moulding it to the weak receding lower jaw, the whole face was strengthened by bringing the chin forward to harmonize with the general facial contour.

In Fig. 4 we see a comparative view of the case. This further illustrates that the jaws and teeth have been brought to their

FIG. 4.

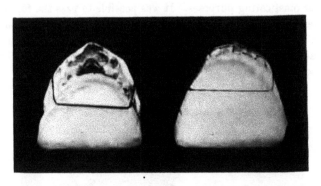

maximum usefulness. This great increase of function is the very secret of the lower jaw remaining in its new position. It was necessary to hold it in its forward position only until the patient unconsciously learned this fact, or until the position became habitual.

This occlusal balance also acts as a perfect natural retainer, the lower arch serving as a form upon which the upper one was moulded, so that later the retainer can be removed without fear of a recurrence of the deformity.

Next we see (Fig. 5) the palatal aspect of the upper arch before and after treatment. Note the great amount of expansion. This expansion was necessary for the proper interlocking of the cusps. for when the lower jaw was brought forward it required a much larger upper jaw than before. The former contracted state was nature's way of compensating for the malposition of the lower arch. The normal placing of this arch required a normal modelling of the upper one. Fig. A shows the contracted condition and B the expanded arch, the difference being indicated by the measurement.

By studying this view it is seen how the lower jaw is locked in its new position. The tendency for it to slip back, even one occlusal notch, to the simple distal position has been prevented, for the utility would be destroyed, there would be no interlocking of the bicuspids and molars, and the cuspids and incisors would have absolutely no antagonism. That the occlusal balance serves as a natural retainer is again clearly shown. The anterior teeth are

FIG. 5.

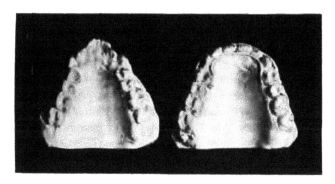

mechanically retained by means of the device indicated in Fig. B. It will be noted that the teeth posterior to the first bicuspid are not included in the retainer; their new position is maintained by the force of occlusion alone. The bringing forward of this arch just compensated for the expansion of the upper, thus a true occlusal balance is established.

Those of you who have followed this description at all carefully must realize that this case is a typical illustration of the carrying out of one of nature's simple laws, a law that is the very foundation of the science of orthodontia,—the law of occlusion: occlusion for utility, occlusion for retention, and occlusion for facial balance.

THE PACKING OF AMALGAM, WITH A REVIEW OF SOME LITERATURE UPON THE SUBJECT.[1]

BY HERBERT LOCKE WHEELER, D.D.S., NEW YORK CITY.

IT is with hesitation that I assume to speak upon the subject of amalgam, because the amount of scientific knowledge we possess upon the subject is so meagre that, though there are pages and

---

[1] Read before the Harvard Odontological Society, Boston, May, 1905.

pages of matter to be found touching upon the subject, the valuable information contained therein seems to be very slight, and
none of them seem to possess the virtue of having obtained scientific data from a series of reported observations upon the behavior
of this material in the mouth for a long period of years.

Considering the effectual quiescence apparently placed upon
further effort in this line of investigation by the series of papers
upon this subject written by Dr. Black, which appeared in the
Dental Cosmos in 1895–96, it is with some trepidation that I now
address this dignified body of *confrères*.   It seems to me that
there is a feeling abroad among many that these papers contained
about all that is knowable upon the subject,—past, present, and
future. For my own part, I am amazed that such a cataract of
words which contain such a mere rivulet of thought should receive
the plaudits of men who seem to have some considerable reputation for discrimination and sense.   Anyway, there seems to have
been a marked temerity in addressing ourselves to this problem.

In order to get at a suitable understanding of what I shall say
concerning the knowledge of the behavior of amalgams in the
mouth and the processes of insertion, I shall quote freely from
various authors who have written upon this subject both here and
abroad.

You are doubtless all so well acquainted with the experiments
of Drs. Bogue and Hitchcock, who were connected with Harvard,
that I shall not dwell much upon their experiments. Of all the
early experiments in this field, it seems to me that Dr. J. Foster
Flagg accomplished the most in introducing this material and
producing known and useful formulæ; also in discovering the
various qualities of amalgams.

This seems to have been to some extent due to his greater independence of action and freedom from association with dental
supply houses. I fancy Dr. Hitchcock made to some extent the
mistake that is apparent in some of Dr. Black's work of giving
too much credence to the statements of interested parties.

The principal properties that it has been desirable to overcome
are shrinkage and the tendency to change form,—called spheroiding by some, and " flow" by others,—and much work has been
expended in trying to find the peculiarities of various combinations of metals that would produce good amalgams and perfect fillings. In this Flagg's work stood out pre-eminently, and he prob-

ably produced as good alloy for filling-material as any of the more modern and more heralded alloys of secret formulæ that have been made possible by these wonderful scientific (?) papers of Dr. Black.

The unfortunate comparison made at the beginning of this series of papers would seem to indicate confusion in the mind of the author as to the difference between operating upon a physical, sensitive, living organism, with its temperamental peculiarities, and upon inanimate wood, stone, and iron, and he does not seem to have observed that a comparison between intermittent force of muscular derivation and steady strain of known weight from the force of gravity hardly constitutes a reasonable analogy. However, this paragraph is quite in keeping with the wilderness of words that one is forced to wander through in order to get what little there is of value in the articles. The remarks upon stress and the necessity for great strength in a filling-material in order to avoid bulging could be more easily accepted if the fillings of various qualities of gutta-percha were not often known to stand up well, even when it has to withstand the force of mastication. If a tooth does not bear upon it harder than upon the other surfaces during repose, much wear will often take place from the grinding process without causing the least particle of bulging. This seems to me pretty good evidence that Professor Black's theory of stress in untenable. Furthermore, how common it is to find amalgam fillings in buccal cavities of molars quite as badly creviced and changed in form as compound fillings upon the approximal and grinding surfaces. Dr. Black says that the past literature upon the subject has in no wise been ignored by him, but this is a vague statement, and a careful reading of the papers would indicate that further reading could have been done by him with considerable advantage.

Mr. Charles Tomes, of England, who is probably not surpassed in the breadth of his learning and the accuracy of his observations by any one in our calling, has remarked that Dr. Black did not quote anybody's researches, as a general rule, and that a fault of his paper was that he stated the whole question *tabula rasa*.

It is not impossible that Dr. Black's notes of thanks for favors received occupied much of his time, for he says, " I wish to thank manufacturers of dental goods for the hearty support they have given me in this work. When it was announced to them that I would undertake an investigation of the physical properties of amalgam, I received within a few weeks about eighty different alloys (apparently it was known to the manufacturers what the investigation was to be long before it was known to the profession). A number of manufacturers have also given me their formulæ, thus enabling me to conduct the investigation on *purely scientific lines.* These formulæ are trade secrets which must be respected." This, then, is the wonderful scientific spirit of these articles, started in the very beginning by giving a first mortgage to the commercial interests. Verily this is giving unselfish service to the dental supply houses.

Professor Flagg described the change that takes place in an amalgam filling after its insertion as bulging, which he attributed to spheroiding, and, according to Dr. St. George Elliott, Dr. J. Smith Dodge first promulgated this theory many years ago,—that is, a tendency of the mercury in the mass to form globules; but this explanation has by no means been proved, and I think is not generally accepted by those who have been investigating. It is, however, worthy of notice that Dr. Flagg stated that this change is more pronounced in alloys composed of metals of more yielding texture, less obdurate in melting, and more deliberate in cooling, and this quality in amalgams is what produces crevicing, sometimes called the " black ditch."

Professor Black describes the same quality, and attributed it to stress. He called this quality " flow," and maintained that an increase in stress is required to continue the " flow" after the area of amalgam had been greatly increased by the flattening of the mass, but that it has to receive pressure slowly, as a silver-tin amalgam is not malleable. It is well to notice that in one of his experiments, in which the formula given is silver, 47.06; tin, 51.76; copper, 0.94; and zinc, 0.24, it was mixed with mercury in a mortar. The mass was divided into various parts, some in which the excess of mercury was removed, and some in which it was not. Of these, the block that showed the least flow was one in which the amalgam had been wrung through muslin to squeeze out the excess of mercury. The filling from this mass was made with mallet force, all the mercury possible being removed in the filling process. The filling which was made in this way showed a flow of about seventeen per cent. in one hour, while some of those in which the excess of mercury was not removed the flow was as high as eighty-nine per cent.

In my estimation, this is far from substantiating Dr. Black's claim that the best way to pack amalgam is with a serrated instrument, avoiding the removal of mercury. On the contrary, it seems to be evident that the chief necessity in obtaining good amalgam fillings is to remove all the mercury possible.

Dr. Black also claims that the strength of the mass depends mostly on the perfect evenness of the distribution of the mercury. He does not seem to have considered that the size and shapes of the crystals which form in the setting process may have an important bearing upon the strength of the filling-materials, and claims that after mercury is mixed with alloy, and evenly distributed, any form of violence weakens the product, as, for instance, the burnishing process after crystallization has commenced. I do not see that he has produced one iota of evidence to prove this.

Mr. Amos Kirby, of England, of whom Dr. Black seems never to have heard, contends that there is a rearrangement of the mercury through the mass of amalgam after the filling is completed, to which rearrangement Mr. Kirby ascribes the warpage, as he chooses to call it, of amalgam fillings, and he has apparently demonstrated with blocks of amalgam that he can prevent their contraction and keep them straight or can make them bend one way or the other, according to the distribution of mercury in the mass. Mr. Tomes has found by the use of the microscope that the setting of an amalgam is a process of crystallization, and that the question of the quantity of the mercury in mixing the amalgam made no material difference in the crystals or rhombs, and he decided that the reason for an amalgam filling having a mat surface, as it were, when fully hardened, although it had been carefully burnished in the filling process, is due to this crystallization. He also discovered that the crystallization takes place so that the crystals or rhombs stand up from all surfaces of the filling in such a way as to make the surface look like pavement epithelium, or, on a minute scale, furry.

He found the size of the crystal to differ greatly in different amalgams. In Welch's amalgam,—tin, 51.52; silver, 48.48,—which Mr. Tomes used in his experiment, the rhombs were one-twelve-hundredth to one-eighteen-hundredth of an inch in diameter and about twice as long as they were wide.

In standard amalgam, made by Eckfelt and Du Bois,—silver,

52; tin, 40.60; gold, 4.40; copper, 3,—they are about half as large, and with an amalgam made of precipitate of silver they are smaller yet. Mr. Tomes thinks that it may be the sprouting of crystals over the surface of amalgam that failed to show expansion by specific gravity tests that may cause the breaking of glass tubes in which they are packed, but he suggests that it is not certain that the crystals do sprout up—it may be that the intermediate portions sink. Mr. Tomes also finds that these crystals are plastic, and suggests that the quality called "flow" by Dr. Black, which he determined by pressing a foreign substance against an amalgam by the pressure of a strong spring was accounted for in this way.

Mr. Tomes further adds, of the so-called flow: "I do not believe that it has, as supposed by Dr. Black, anything to do with the ultimate failure of amalgams, for I doubt if the very intermittent pressure to which they are subjected would bring it about."

Dr. Black speaks of alloys that were cut very fine, as showing a great amount of flow, and speaks of coarse-cut alloy taking up less mercury in mixing than fine cut.

Dr. J. Morgan Howe called attention to this some years before. —January, 1894, *Transactions of the New York Odontological Society*,—but no one seems to have noticed it.

Dr. Black states that the loss in weight in wringing an amalgam in cloth was purely the mercury. This is not indicated by the experiment of Mr. Tomes, who says, speaking of expressed mercury that he pressed from an amalgam mix which he had put under a glass slide for examination by the microscope, "No rhombs appeared, but only foliaceous forms similar to those in which tin crystallizes." From which it appears that tin is carried off by the mercury in the squeezing-out process. Dr. Black shows, in his first paper, experiments with alloys with sixteen different formulæ, and he states immediately under this table that the formula of the alloy controls in a large degree the flow of the amalgam formed. He states, also, that every silver-tin amalgam in the market is, when mixed with a low percentage of mercury, so strong that they will not break down or crush, and yet he assumes that what he is pleased to call the "black ditch" about the margins is caused by the stress of mastication. I have never yet seen an amalgam filling made after the so-called "Black method" with modern alloys that did not show crevicing at the edge. And while stating, as Dr. Black does, that the product of the manufacturers is quite all that is necessary for the profession, he says in his last paper that what the dental profession and the men who supply its members need to know is the conditions of contraction and expansion of amalgam, including the formula of alloy and whatever else may influence. In comparison with this statement I wish to read a letter from Dr. Black to the S. S. White Dental Company, which has been published, and which is hardly in keeping with the statements in these papers.

"CHICAGO, April 16, 19.5.

" MR. C. L. BINGHAM, Chicago:

" DEAR SIR,—Your note of the 7th inst. has remained unanswered for reason that I was out of town. You inquire as to the matter of the advertising of alloys purporting to be made in strict accord with Dr. G. V. Black's formula. I have become aware that some such advertisements were being made use of wrongfully. No one has any such right from me. Furthermore, I have no formula by which a thoroughly reliable alloy can be made by any one. Any one who knows the methods which I have developed, and has made a sufficient study of the metals to enable him to make alloys understandingly, needs no formulæ. Even then he will be unable to make reliable alloys without the special instruments developed, for that purpose; for he will know that uniform alloys cannot be made from any fixed formula. Therefore, any advertisement setting forth that any given alloy is made according to my formula is without authority from me, and is a fraud.

" Certain persons, all of whom you know, are making alloys after the methods which I have developed, they having prepared themselves for so doing by a regular course of study and technical drill and providing themselves with the necessary apparatus.

" Very truly,

" G. V. BLACK."

Dr. Black's contention, that in amalgams which show both contraction and expansion the contraction is in the upper half of the filling and expansion in the lower, is quite in keeping with some of Mr. Kirby's experiments, and also an evidence that the method of packing amalgam filling is important, and the most important part of the process is to remove the mercury to such an extent that the upper surface is as dry, when completed, as the lower.

Dr. Black's position in protecting these wonderful secret formulæ and ignoring the plain ethical demands of his profession, by upholding secret and proprietary formulæ, is only a part of that influence that is commercializing the world to-day to the detriment of the individual, and in so far as he has done this it seems to me he has contributed not to the advancement of our profession, but to its degradation.

And after all of this laborious work done for our kind benefactors, the manufacturers, behold the wonderful result! He concludes that a formula composed of silver, 68.5; tin, 25.5; gold, 5; zinc, 1, has been watched long enough to assure its success.

This statement appeared in December, 1896. When I was in college in 1889–90 the formula for an especially hard contour amalgam which Professor J. Foster Flagg was teaching to his students was silver, 70; tin, 26; gold, 3; zinc, 1. Not much difference in these, is there? And the original formula, of which this was a modification,—silver, 68; tin, 27; gold, 4; zinc, 1,—was brought out by Dr. Flagg in 1884, twelve years before this wonderful discovery.

Now let us consider the approximate formulæ of some of the modern alloys, bearing in mind that they are all heralded as Black's method or formula. These alloys were analyzed by Booth, Garrett, and Blair, of Philadelphia; Fellowship alloy, silver. 67.73; tin, 26.33; copper, 4.71; zinc, 1.23. Rego alloy, silver. 66.54; tin, 28.14; copper, 4.21; zinc, 1.06. Triumph alloy. silver, 66.74; tin, 27.44; copper, 4.24; zinc, 1.42. Twentieth Century. silver. 66.81; tin, 27.32; copper, 4.39; zinc, 1.51. Wonderful, is it not? All of these marvellous, perfect modern, scientific, *à la* G. V. Black dental alloys have succeeded in eliminating the one expensive metal. gold, from their formulæ, and yet raise the price higher than formerly, and are highly commended by their worthy benefactor as furnishing alloys of the "purest of metals."

And this is the practical outcome, as far as dentists are concerned, of the experiments of Professor Black. It is well to place here the words of our British cousin, Mr. Tomes, when we are prone to pat ourselves upon our backs because of our superior knowledge of dentistry. He says, "I believe that an enormous amount of experience in the hands of countless operators has been entirely wasted through our being content to use amalgams, the composition of which is unknown to us. For my own part, since I have been experimenting I have resolved to use no amalgam the composition of which is not known to me, and I think the manufacturers would do well to always publish it on the bottles."

Dr. Black's statement, that alloys cut very fine make a soft. pasty mass, and work smoothly and easily, while those that are

cut coarse make a mass that is not so pasty, and that does not
work so smoothly, is not at all in accordance with the careful
observation of Dr. J. Morgan Howe, given to the New York Odontological Society in the paper before mentioned.

Dr. Howe found, in the coarse filling and the fine filling of the
same batch of any given alloy, using the same quantity of mercury
for mixing each, that the coarse fillings made by far the most
plastic mass, while these same fillings mixed with thirty-three and
one-third per cent. less mercury than the fine gave about the same
plasticity,—so nearly the same that the difference was not dis-
cernible,—and that after several hours the filling made from the
coarse-grain alloy seemed to be much harder. Dr. Howe, after
years of observation of the behavior of fillings in the mouth, has
come to think that the addition of zinc in any quantity to an alloy
for amalgams is probably a disadvantage, and deleterious to the
filling. My own experience in the working of amalgams is that
the more mercury that can be expressed from the mass in the
filling process, the less change is there in the mass after the filling is completed. For my methods in obtaining the desired result I am entirely indebted to Dr. Howe. We do not find that
the formula makes any great difference, so long as there is a
reasonable proportion of desirable metals in the alloy; as, for
instance, we use the same method when we use dentalloy, which is
probably about 72 silver, as when we use the alloy which we have
made up for us by Baker & Co., which is 49 silver, 48 tin, 2 gold,
and 1 platinum. In the first place, the cavity must be a *cul de
sac,* or pocket. If it is a compound cavity it must be made so by
the use of the matrix. The practice of Dr. Howe and myself is
to use a very thin steel band encircling the tooth, soldered together
with soft solder. The first amalgam inserted is comparatively
plastic. In order to increase the dryness of the material we do not
squeeze the amalgam through cloth or anything else; we gradually add filings until the material is so dry that it almost
crumbles. Even then the mercury works to the top, and as it
does we remove the softened mass and add more of the drier
material until the last pellet added is almost a powdery mass. It
is then possible to work a little mercury to the surface, which we
absorb by the addition of precipitate of silver. This last substance
was suggested for this purpose several years ago by Dr. Howe.
Now, when the mass is completely hard (which it will be as soon

as the process of insertion is finished), the matrix is in most cases immediately removed and the filling trimmed by cutting away any surplus with sharp instruments. As crystallization is not yet complete, it is better to polish at another sitting. I have seen fillings put in in this way that had perfect margins ten or twelve years after their insertion, and these fillings have been of different formulæ, which would indicate that with any reasonable formula the chief thing is the careful extraction of the mercury in the packing, and the proper manipulation in inserting.

I have with me to-night some glass tubes which have been filled by me according to the above-described process,—some in January, 1902, and some last week. All have been recently left to lie in a bath of carmine ink, and you can see for yourselves how much leakage has followed.

The unmarked tube, which shows a slight evidence of leakage, was filled in 1902, and is from a sample of " Columbian A" alloy, which it is claimed has sixty per cent. silver.

I. Columbian D alloy: Sixty-seven per cent. silver, made in 1902; no leakage.

II. Bement's alloy: Silver, 49.85; tin, 49.55; zinc, 0.45; gold, 0.15; made in 1902; leaks.

IV. Flagg's submarine: Silver, 60; tin, 33; copper, 7 (according to his later formula); made in 1902; leaks in spots.

V. True dentalloy: Probably over seventy per cent. silver, mixed according to directions; alloy, 9; mercury, 11; gradually added filings until proportion was filings, 12; mercury, 11; made in 1902; no leakage.

VI. True dentalloy made according to directions after method proposed by Dr. Black: Slight leakage at margins; very much softer than the two made by the other method; done May 9, 1905.

VII. An alloy made for Dr. Howe which we use regularly: Silver, 49; tin, 48; gold, 2; platinum, 1; packed by the method I have described by absorbing surplus mercury, by working in more filings, but no precipitated silver used; no leakage; made May 9, 1905.

VIII. Same as No. VII. was made, except precipitated silver added to finally absorb the last mercury that worked to the surface; no leakage; made May 9, 1905.

IX. True dentalloy made by the same process as No. VIII.: no leakage, and much harder than No. VI.

There is an interesting and instructive paper on amalgams by Dr. St. George Elliott in the April *Dental Cosmos,* which shows a shrinkage in all amalgams sooner or later, and he says that he has little hope that a good reliable amalgam will be produced in the immediate future because of the impossibility of getting pure metals in our alloys and the difficulty of getting a proper mixture of the metals in the melting process.

If mechanical tests made outside the mouth were conclusive it might be so, but it is quite probable that what Mr. Fletcher said in 1875 about external experiments being of little value in our clinical experience is quite as true now, and it seems to me that more care in the manipulation of any ordinary amalgam of known formula might at least contribute to much superior work than the rough, unfinished, and slovenly looking fillings of this material that we so often encounter now.

It is unfortunate that I have not had time to look up the work of Drs. Bogue and Hitchcock (*Transactions of the New York Odontological Society,* 1874).

REFERENCES.

Mr. Fletcher: New York Odontological Society Transactions, 1875.
Dr. J. Foster Flagg: Plastics and Plastic Fillings.
New York Odontological Society Transactions, 1878.
Dr. G. V. Black: Dental Cosmos, 1895-96.
Dr. J. Morgan Howe: New York Odontological Society Transactions, 1894.
Mr. Charles Tomes: Transactions of the British Odontological Society, 1894-95, 1895-96.
Mr. George Cunningham and Mr. Baldwin: Transactions of the British Odontological Society, 1895-96.
Dr. St. George Elliott: Dental Cosmos, April, 1905.

CLEANSING TEETH, AS THE SUBJECT APPEARS TO THE WRITER.[1]

BY DR. W. M. WHITLOCK, NEW YORK, N. Y.

I am here to-night, gentlemen, to tell you an old, old story, a story we have heard lately many times; and yet it is one that is always new. In spite of all that has been said and written on the

[1] Read before The New York Institute of Stomatology, April 4, 1905.

subject of dental prophylaxis, and notwithstanding its endless discussion, this fact is brought home to us every day in our practice, that there seems to be a lamentable failure on the part of the profession to grasp its importance, a discrepancy between what we are preaching and what we are practising.

I am afraid we hear too much about the " rapid strides our profession is making;" too many vain-glorious generalizations. It might be well for us to stop occasionally and view ourselves in a candid and unbiassed manner.

Sixty years ago Dr. E. J. Dunning established for himself ideals of dental prophylaxis so high and so perfect that succeeding generations and years have failed to improve upon them one iota. and what is more, Dr. E. J. Dunning and Dr. Dunning's associates lived up to these ideals. These men never had any trouble with pyorrhœa; they did not know what it was, and where these teachings of sixty years ago have been faithfully followed, pyorrhœa has never developed. And so I do not hesitate to say, and this will bear me out, that among all dental operations the operation of the cleansing of the teeth stands first. This is the point I wish to emphasize most of all, that in cleansing our patient's teeth we are doing for them our most skilful work, and giving them the greatest benefit. All this has been proved so many times that it would seem there could be no difference of opinion at least regarding its necessity, yet as a matter of fact our daily observation shows that in the mind of the ordinary dental practitioner the importance of oral prophylaxis ranges all the way from these ideals down to a practical zero, where the cleansing is either not done at all, or is relegated to the unskilled assistant, while his principal is devoting his time to the manufacture of bridges and appliances to hinder rather than facilitate oral cleanliness.

Cleansing is the first operation in two senses: it is the most important, and again it is the first operation to be performed when a patient is placed in our hands for treatment. I invariably make this my rule, never deviating therefrom unless for the relief of actual pain. I feel that this is a duty, first, to myself, that I may work thereafter in wholesome and congenial surroundings, as it were; and secondly, a duty to my patient, as with a mouth free from tartar and stain I am enabled to make a more thorough and accurate examination.

The instruments described are legion; no one can master them all. To the practitioner so many are impracticable; to the student they must be discouraging. Really they are not necessary. Results perfect in every detail can be accomplished with very few. It is the thorough mastery of one or two or a few simple instruments that counts.

The first instrument I take from my cabinet is a simple delicate examining instrument, with a straight shank drawn down to an 18-gauge Brown & Sharp, with a right-angle blade one-sixteenth of an inch long and slightly flattened laterally. I depend upon *this* instrument for locating any tartar, and it can also be used for removing the more yielding deposits, but in conjunction with it I use an instrument of practically the same design, but more heavily constructed for deposits that cannot be removed with the lighter one. In quite difficult cases it is possible with these two instruments to remove the tartar from every surface with great thoroughness. However, I have found it desirable for the posterior surfaces, as, for instance, the posterior surface of the last tooth, to use a double bend instrument flattened anteroposteriorly, carrying a small hook at the extreme end of the anterior face.

These instruments were shown me by Dr. Kimball when I first became associated with him some years ago.

For severe cases where there is considerable alveolar absorption, I have selected from the set of instruments devised by Dr. D. D. Smith a certain few that I have found very efficacious.

These are all the instruments I use for the removal of tartar, no matter how extreme the case may be.

Remembering that every tooth has four surfaces, with my delicate instrument I examine every portion of that tooth, from its morsal edge down to the union of the tooth and gum, recognizing the slightest roughness; if tartar, removing it either with this or the heavier instruments, and if caries, noting it upon my examination blank. Great delicacy and accuracy in handling these instruments should be cultivated to prevent wounding the gum, especially where the tartar is very adherent.

Every surface of every tooth should be thoroughly polished. Generally speaking, I do not believe much can be accomplished by the appliances devised for use in the dental engine. At best only the most accessible surfaces can be reached in this way, and I find it no great task to polish such surfaces along with the more difficult places where it is necessary to use the cedar and orange polishing stick. With these sticks and the orange stick in the porte-polisher, practically every surface can be reached. Some doubtful approximal surfaces can be still further polished by means of floss silk and pumice, or by tucum fibre.

I consider the porte-polisher, devised by Dr. F. M. Smith, the most practical, both on account of its size and because it can be easily cleansed. It may be well to have two or three of these on hand with sticks set in at different angles.

Though I have completed this operation to my satisfaction, I do not consider that my duty ends here. I always devote a certain portion of time to minutely outlining to my patients the best methods for the daily care of the teeth; trying to impress upon them the fact that they have their teeth always; that upon themselves depends the success or failure of my work. What I have done is merely to give them a fresh start, as it were; that the real responsibility must rest with them. Here as elsewhere, "eternal vigilance is the price of safety."

THE IDLE MOMENTS OF BUSY MEN.[1]

BY DR. F. C. BRUSH, NEW YORK, N. Y.

THE thought often comes to young men, How is it that busy men find the time for study, research, preparation of professional papers, devising of instruments and methods, and the kindred other things that we have continual evidence they are doing?

It is really the busiest man that has the most time for varied things, for he is one that has learned to make use of every fleeting moment. He has few idle moments, yet many for rest and recreation, as true rest is not idleness but a change; even a change of thought, not necessarily a decided change of occupation. The developing of a new thought or the pursuit of some investigation is a mental rest and recreation that produces its good result quite as well as the more violent physical exercises which so many deem essential. To obtain the best results from this kind of a mental change, one must, of course, have a great love for one's work and all its details; so much so that it becomes a hobby rather than the

---

[1] Read before The New York Institute of Stomatology, April 4, 1905.

mere daily drudgery which must be pursued for its financial returns. It is the kind of love that takes possession of a man and causes him, when his office hours are drawing to a close, to long for the restful hours of evening, when he may develop some thought or work out some problem that has come to him during the routine work of the day; and then when the evening is waning and another day approaching, to long for the morning, that he may return to the office and put into execution and test the results of the evening's labor.

Some time since I had the good fortune to gain the confidence and friendship of such a man, and with it an opportunity to know him more intimately. As I learned to know and understand him, and to see more of his habits and methods, he became a constant revelation and inspiration to me. I began to understand some-thing of his success, aside from the charm of his personality and intense individuality. Many little traits and habits that at first were inexplicable to me were understood later, and their meaning became clear. In the midst of the proceedings of a meeting I have observed him hastily writing on some scrap of paper the gist of a telling point made by a speaker, a bit of new information or a thought of his own that may have come to him on the subject; later, when he has shown a surprising fund of knowledge on a wide range of subjects, I have realized how a deal of this knowledge has been absorbed and laid away for use at a fitting time. Though knowing him to be a linguist of ability, I was surprised on one occasion to hear him make use of still another language; upon inquiry, he informed me that for some time it had been his habit to have a grammar of this language upon his dresser and to learn a certain number of the words each morning while arranging his toilet.

How many of we younger men would have the courage and tenacity of purpose to undertake a task like that? And yet we sit with idle hands and wonder how they do it—we haven't the time. To be sure, we cannot all be "Bogues," yet how many there are that are idling and complaining they haven't time, who, if they would but apply themselves systematically, would find that measure of success which all are seeking. It is surprising how much time we may find we have, and the things we may accomplish, if we will but get busy and utilize the spare moments.

How can we do this? Well, a good plan is to have a memorandum pad handy by the operating-chair, and when, in the midst of

20

an operation, an idea comes regarding the work in hand, or of an instrument or something that may be arranged to facilitate your work or add to the comfort of the patient, jot it down. These little notes should be filed in a conspicuous place on your desk, and when an opportunity comes, such as a rainy day or a broken appointment, you may turn to them and find at once something you can be doing, instead of sitting around and rummaging your brain in a futile effort to recall that very important thing you were going to do the very first chance you had.

If while reading the journals or engaged in your work a good idea comes to you on the subject, try to write it out and express it in a way to be clearly understood by others who may not be in touch with your own train of thought. Then when your society calls upon you to do your part, you will have something to turn to, and from your notes you may no doubt be enabled to evolve a paper which will be creditable to yourself and of some material help to others. If such prove to be the case, the notes will not have been in vain nor the time wasted.

Another excellent plan is to observe closely the mouths of all patients that come under our care. Not the mere searching out of cavities, that fillings may be inserted and fees obtained, but observing all conditions carefully, that we may study them and compare and reflect.

We labor under the same general disadvantage as does the physician, in that we are called upon to treat the results of pathological conditions rather than normal ones. Rarely is it that we have an opportunity of examining a mouth that is perfectly normal, particularly in regard to the form, shape, and size of the arches, the shape of the teeth, their position in the alveolus, and their relation one with another. Unless we have a clear idea of what the normal is or should be, how can we pass judgment on these abnormal or pathological conditions and feel that the treatment purposed is the best for the case in hand?

Have we gone beyond the study of the best filling-material for some individual tooth, and considered the important part which that tooth plays in the economy of mastication and vocalization, not merely as a crusher of food or as an aid in the enunciation of certain sounds, but as an integral part of the whole machine, that has an essential function to perform in preserving and regulating the harmony of all the other parts? How can we appreciate all this if our attention is continually centred only upon the small part which is our immediate field of operation?

As an aid in studying this broader field, I try, whenever possible, to secure models of mouths that present what we may call unusual conditions, whatever they may be. These models are being filed away for future reference, study, and comparison, and they have proved of inestimable value in diagnosing and prognosing other cases.

It may be permissible in this connection to relate an incident that occurred in my practice a short time ago. A patient, while in the operating-chair, volunteered the information that the young lady accompanying her had beautiful teeth, and had never required the services of a dentist. I stated that if such were the case there must certainly be a good reason for it, and I believed that reason to be that nature had provided her with a practically normal mouth, and I dared say I could describe the general conditions of her mouth, the positions of the teeth, and their relation one to another. The patient became interested, and called her friend into the operating-room. An examination was made, and, to the surprise of the young ladies and my gratification, it was found that my description was essentially correct. This incident made quite an impression on the young ladies, and I feel that there are at least two more people who have a higher appreciation of the importance of saving their teeth and, I trust, of the services that dentistry aims to render.

But—some of you may say—we are busy men, and haven't the time for such things. That no doubt is true, but it is the truly busy man that in his idle moments finds the time for many things.

Reviews of Dental Literature.

HAND STERILIZATION.—In carrying out hand sterilization, mechanical and chemical methods are employed.

(1) *Mechanical.*—Careful use of a stiff nail-brush with soap and hot water removes many bacteria and detaches superficial epidermal cells and grease with contained organisms. The time required and the injurious effect on the hands render it beyond the limit of practicability to produce efficient sterilization by this method alone.

(2) *Chemical.*—Ordinary operating-room methods are to a considerable extent inefficacious in rendering the hands sterile. The fact that cultures of a staphylococcus could be obtained from an inoculated silk thread after thirty minutes in a watery solution of corrosive sublimate (1 in 1000) speaks for the weakness of this popular preparation. Absolute alcohol has but a slight germicidal power, but the diluted fluid (seventy per cent.) has a far greater action than a watery solution of bichloride or biniodide of mercury (1 in 1000) or a saturated solution of permanganate of potash. Prolonged use of alcohol, however, will cause pain, roughen the skin, and may produce eczema.

The writer has held that the ideal cleansing agent must be a solution capable of dissolving fatty matter and of penetrating the epidermis, strongly germicidal, rapid in action, and non-injurious to the skin. After long experimentations the writer suggests the unpurified clove oil as an approach to the ideal. After five minutes' scrubbing with soap and hot water the skin should be dried with a sterile towel and rubbed for one minute with alcohol to remove any remaining moisture. Clove oil is then rubbed into the skin for five minutes and afterwards washed off with alcohol. A slight burning sensation may result, but the skin is not injured. The hands should then be covered with dry sterile rubber gloves. Wet gloves macerate the skin, which may readily yield organisms which have not been destroyed through any undetected hole in the glove. The use of various "hand coatings," wax paraffins, and rubber solutions are not to be recommended, as they are prone to crack and peel off in long operations.—J. C. WEBSTER (*American Journal of Obstetrics*, April, 1905), *Cyclopedia of Practical Medicine.*

RESEARCHES IN HÆMOPHILIA.—The writer had the rare luck to observe four typical cases of hæmophilia and to study the peculiarities of the blood in this strange disorder. According to some, the condition is due to high blood-pressure, but this is improbable, since diseases commonly associated with high blood-pressure, such as chronic nephritis, do not usually run with hæmophilia symptoms. In the author's case, the figures obtained with the Riva-Rocci instrument were normal or below normal. Microscopical examination of the blood showed only a moderate, relative diminution of polynuclear leucocytes, with relative increase of lymphocytes. The absolute number of leucocytes was normal or diminished. In two cases the platelets were also counted repeatedly, but their number was never above normal. The alkalinity of the blood, the dry residue of the serum, the depression of the freezing point, and the amount of fibrin in the blood were not altered. The time of coagulation was estimated most carefully, and it was found that in the intervals between the hemorrhages clotting was much delayed, but normal, or even hastened, during severe bleeding. The following new method was employed: A column of blood, about one centimetre high, is allowed to flow into a capilary pipette one to two millimetres in diameter. An absolutely clean, white strand of horsehair is then passed into the blood, and drawn out a short distance every half to one minute. If the hair has been carefully deprived of all grease, no blood will adhere to it at first, but as soon as coagulation has set in, the withdrawn section will no longer appear white, but red. The rapid clotting during bleeding, despite continued hemorrhage, is probably due to an abnormal quality of the vessel walls. Under normal conditions, the latter probably furnish certain substances necessary for the production of fibrin-ferment (thrombo-kinase) locally at the site of injury, so that a clot will soon obstruct the opening in the vessel. During hemophilia, the torn edges of the vessel do not supply the blood with this substance, hence no local clot forms. The imperfect clotting during the intervals is due to a similar deficiency on the part of the blood-cells and the hæmatopoietic apparatus. Chemical changes in the vessel walls will also explain the occurrence of spontaneous hemorrhages and the reported cases of hæmophilia of single organs (Senator's renal hæmophilia). Very little can be done for the disease, except to improve the general constitution. The local hemorrhages are best controlled with compression, gelatin, and adrenalin, but the latter two drugs should never be injected subcutaneously. It is not likely that the local application of thrombo-kinase will do much good. There is as yet no drug from which good results can be expected on internal administration.—H. SAHLI (*Zeitschrift für klinische Medicin*, Bd. lxv., Nu. 3 und 4; *Medical News*, May 6, 1905), *Cyclopedia of Practical Medicine.*

PAROTID GLAND.—The function of the parotid gland is the subject of a scientific research by the writer, who found that the secretion of the gland varies in amount and quality according to the stimulus given by contact with various substances in the mouth. The amount of secretion of the parotid varies as the square root of the amount of stimulant applied to the mouth. Chewing has much to do with the rapidity of the secretion from the parotid, and the saliva is not only more abundant, but more viscid, when mastication is vigorous and prolonged. When food is chewed on one side, the corresponding parotid gland works more than the opposite gland, while when chewing goes on on both sides both glands work equally. The alkalinity of the saliva is in proportion to the amount of ash therein. As the amount of ash increases, and as the rapidity of the secretion is enhanced, the alkalinity grows more marked. The digestive power of the saliva is proportionate to the amount of organic matter therein. The digestion of starch by the parotid secretion, after it reaches the stomach, is possible in proportion to the alkalinity of the saliva. The action of ptyalin in the stomach is only possible during the beginning and the final stages of digestion. At the acme of gastric digestion, when the free hydrochloric acid is abundant, the action of the saliva is only possible when there are large amounts of highly alkaline saliva in the stomach. The influence of saliva in the digestion of proteids reduces itself to a dilution of the hydrochloric acid of the gastric juice, and in disease makes hypoacidity worse, while it tends to make hyperacidity less severe.—E. A. ZHERBOVSKI (*Roussky Vratch*, March 5, 1905; *New York Medical Journal* and *Philadelphia Medical Journal*, April 29, 1905), *Cyclopedia of Practical Medicine.*

Reports of Society Meetings.

THE NEW YORK INSTITUTE OF STOMATOLOGY.

A MEETING of the Institute was held at the " Chelsea," No. 222 West Twenty-third Street, New York, on Tuesday evening, April 4, 1905, the President, Dr. C. O. Kimball, in the chair.

The minutes of the last meeting were read and approved.

INCIDENTS OF OFFICE PRACTICE.

Dr. H. W. Gillett.—I have here the casts showing the impacted third molar I spoke of at the last meeting. You will note that the first cast shows the tooth lying nearly horizontal with the side of one cusp showing. Packing the angle with gutta-percha, as described by Dr. Allis, served to accomplish little more than to force the gum back. A few weeks' work with grass-line wedge resulted in enough upward and backward movement to make it accessible to the forceps.

The next cast illustrates a means of retaining the rubber dam on partially erupted molars. A 6-gauge seamless German silver band from the orthodontia outfit is quickly filled and cemented on the tooth with rapid setting cement, and the turned edge serves to hold the rubber effectually.

I want to show you Dr. Dwight M. Clapp's "rolling" tooth-brush. Note the small size, the short bristles, and the reverse curve of the handle. These points facilitate getting the brush well under the cheek and tongue, the use of the *ends* of the bristles, which is most important, and the wrist motion essential to the rolling motion which Dr. Clapp prescribes.

I find it helpful to demonstrate in the patient's mouth (with a brush to be given them afterwards) the manner in which I wish them to use the brush. With these brushes my patients are obtaining results in the care of their teeth that surpass all my previous experience. I recommend them to your careful consideration as a most valuable adjunct to prophylaxis. Note particularly the smallest size. It is intended for the baby, but is wonderfully effective for cleaning around regulating apparatus, under bridge-work and tipping molars, and the exposed bifurcations of molar roots. For general use I prefer the smaller adult size in the S. grade.

Dr. D. H. Allis.—Dr. Gillett refers to the use of gutta-percha after a method of mine. This is somewhat ancient history. It was several years ago that I used it in this manner, and experience has taught me something since that time about the use of gutta-percha. However, I have seen very satisfactory results from this method, but it must be persistently followed up. At any rate, I think we would all rather see these cases of impacted wisdom-teeth come to the other man's practice.

The President.—I reported last month the case of a third molar that I am interested in. I have seen the case to-day, and it is progressing favorably. Originally it showed only one cusp above the gum. There was decay in the back of the second molar, which was filled, and also a cavity in the crown of the third molar. This cavity I filled with amalgam, projecting upward in such a way that a wedge could be brought to bear. From time to time I am adding more amalgam and continuing the wedging. I am endeavoring to make the tooth assume a normal position and become useful.

Dr. F. C. Brush.—I frequently have occasion to devise and use little appliances that may be useful to others. One of these is a "reinforced wedge." It consists of a piece of cotton-wood, compressed and shaped in the usual way, with a small hole drilled through it. Through this hole is stretched a thick piece of separating rubber, the principle being that after the wood has fully expanded the rubber will be released and will try to resume its original form, thus continuing the pressure. Such a wedge is very effective for use across wide spaces, especially in orthodontia work, where it may be necessary to regain the space of a missing tooth.

Dr. F. Milton Smith.—I want to pass around a porte-polisher. Dr. Gaylord sent this one to me, and he has recommended for use with it ordinary wooden shoe-pegs. They can be obtained in various sizes.

I also wish to call attention to two little approximal trimmers that have been very useful to me. They are in Ivory's set.

Dr. S. H. McNaughton.—Several years ago it occurred to me, that it might be a good idea to use a combination of Abbey's soft foil and one of the ordinary foils in the same pellet or cylinder, the idea being that Abbey's soft foil is not made cohesive by annealing, while the other foil in the combination is, and that it might have some advantages over an all-cohesive or an all-non-cohesive cylinder. I think it has. In using the combination of the two kinds of foils I use pointed pluggers. In contours where great strength is required it should not be used. It works very much like tinfoil, but it has the cohesive quality. It is particularly useful in starting fillings and in filling against the walls. In compound approximal cavities the occlusal portion should be filled with cohesive gold.

A little point in regard to wedging teeth. A few days ago I had in my chair a little girl who had quite a good-sized cavity in an upper first molar. The adjoining bicuspid was only about one-third erupted, and, suspecting that there might be a cavity in the distal surface of this bicuspid, it was very necessary to wedge, and it seemed as though it would be a troublesome place to wedge. As a sort of starter I excavated the cavity in the molar and filled it about two-thirds full of glutol (a gelatin which has been treated with formaldehyde, and thus made insoluble), and over this packed gutta-percha into the cavity and against the bicuspid. She came back in about a week with the teeth so nicely wedged that I was able to fill the cavity in the bicuspid with gutta-percha without any opening to the occlusal surface.

Dr. LeRoy presented the reprint of a paper, apropos of supernumerary teeth. The paper mentioned some curious instances in different animals, and following this data presented a course of reasoning tending to show that such occurrences were merely anomalous and not examples of reversion.

Dr. F. C. Brush, of New York, read a paper entitled "The Idle Moments of Busy Men."

(For Dr. Brush's paper, see page 528.)

A paper entitled "Cleansing Teeth, as the Subject appears to the Writer," was then presented by Dr. W. M. Whitlock, of New York.

(For Dr. Whitlock's paper, see page 525.)

Dr. C. F. Allan.—I should like to have Dr. Eames, who is with us to-night, tell us about some very beautifully made and delicate cleansing instruments he has recently shown me.

Dr. G. F. Eames.—I admit that I did show some instruments to Dr. Allan, but had no thought that they were of sufficient importance to provoke discussion. Referring to the porte-polisher mentioned, I would say that I have devised a simple way of taking one made from brass tubing of different sizes, by soldering to one end of the larger size, at desirable angles, a short piece of the smaller tubing. This makes a very good porte-polisher. I have fifteen or twenty of them, and have sticks prepared ready for use of the various desirable shapes, so that I can pick them up without the waste of an instant of time.

I suppose the essayist referred to those patients who come to him for the first time when he mentioned "congenial surroundings." Surely his regular patients would not present in this condition. I do not make it my invariable practice to first cleanse the patient's teeth. It is possible that at times other things may be of more importance.

Dr. F. Milton Smith.—It is a constant question with me to know how to get some moments for my own personal use. The days are so full, sometimes far into the night, that a few minutes that actually belong to me are very valuable; any suggestion as to how best to use them is certainly helpful. A suggestion in Dr. Brush's paper that especially recommended itself to me was the having of a memorandum-pad right at one's hand if we don't have some one to jot things down for us. I have found this an exceedingly valuable aid to my memory and a great saving of spare moments.

Regarding the paper of Dr. Whitlock, I did not know that Dr. Whitlock was using a polisher designed by Dr. Smith. His suggestion that cleansing the teeth is the most important operation that we do for our patients, I think I agree with, if the patients would only keep them clean. If they would do this we would be out of business. Regarding the suggestion that he first cleanses the the teeth before anything else, I do not always do this. Never in my practice have I been able to tell beforehand exactly how long it was going to take me to put in a given filling, and for this reason I often remove simply the heavier accumulations at the first sitting. Thereafter the closing minutes of each sitting are used for more careful cleansing and polishing. This obviates the loss of time that is apt to occur by reserving too much time for one filling and not enough for two.

Dr. Allis.—Along the line of Dr. Brush's paper, I think a very good way to keep data of all kinds, whether of articles of interest in different journals or other data, is by the use of an index system; then whenever it is desirable to write upon any given subject all your material is at hand.

Dr. Eames.—I use a regular card index system for this purpose. the same as is used in the public libraries. I use this not only for literature, but for various other purposes.

Dr. C. F. Allan.—I have only one thing to say in regard to the matter at present under discussion, and that is the great advantage it is to every dentist to have a good secretary. I do not mean one who will do what she is told, but one who can look up an article in a magazine, take enough interest in your work to keep track of magazine articles for you, and who is a memory and, in a measure, an intelligence for you. Such a person is invaluable!

Dr. C. D. Cook.—I should like to ask a question referring to a suggestion by Dr. Whitlock, that sixty years ago the dentists of that day cleansed their patients' teeth so carefully as to prevent pyorrhœa alveolaris, as we understand it. Now, I do not know that I understand pyorrhœa as others understand it. I do not know that Dr. Riggs understood the difference between pyorrhœa and that recession of the gums due to a deposit of tartar. I believe that disease caused by tartar to be a very different one from what I conceive to be true pyorrhœa, where two or three teeth in different parts of the mouth may be affected with looseness, with no especial deposits of tartar except in minute quantities about the necks of the teeth. I can look back fifty years,—not very keenly, perhaps,—but I do not remember any such disease as I find nowadays, any more than the physician would find diphtheria, for instance, then as now. At any rate, I think there is a very great difference between the two causes of absorption of the alveolar process due to deposits of tartar and true pyorrhœa.

Dr. H. L. Wheeler.—It might be interesting, in connection with what Dr. Cook has just said, to state that I have recently been examining quite a number of skulls from prehistoric man, and I am satisfied, from my observations thus far, that this destruction of alveolar process apparently has no relation to the amount of calcic deposit from the saliva, and that it is of a systemic character. I have found skulls where there was a large quantity of calcic deposit, with no apparent injury to the process. I have found a great many cases where the teeth have been extracted and there has been no tilting. I doubt if there is any such thing as an ideal perfect mouth. I find in the cliff-dwellers practically perfect teeth. I have never seen in them evidences of caries nor alveolar absorption, yet never in any skull of these people have I found a case where they were in the ideal relations described by Dr. Bogue and Dr. Angle. The first molars are about the same, but anterior to that point they differ radically, and invariably I have found the centrals, upper and lower, standing edge to edge. In the case of the Peruvians, while there is a great amount of calcic deposit, there is no great destruction of bone. I have a theory that these people did not suffer from pyorrhœa because they were obliged to exercise their teeth in masticating hard food substances. If a tooth-brush can be made to do the same work, you will get the same results.

It is all a question of environment. If this is changed, Nature has to go to work by a slow process to adapt herself to the changed conditions. Things are not created perfect and then degenerate. They are all the time adjusting themselves to their environment.

The President.—I should like to say just a word, if I may be permitted to do so, on this subject of pyorrhœa alveolaris. Dr.

Cook has asked a question, and in answer I should like to mention one case that came into my hands some years ago,—that of a
boy sixteen years of age with the history of the loss of teeth from
pyorrhœa alveolaris. He had lost one of the central incisors and
a lower first molar. One of the upper first molars was hanging
by a thread. There was not very much tartar around the teeth.
The question was what to do. I simply followed out this plan that
Dr. Whitlock has spoken of,—a thorough systematic cleansing of
the teeth,—and everything has gone well with the boy since. I
think Dr. Whitlock, in his paper, alluded to a fact which I stated
some years ago. I said then that although I had been practising
twenty-five years, I had seen hardly a single case of pyorrhœa
alveolaris, and I could not understand why, although judging
from the literature on the subject there was apparently so much
of it abroad, I had seen so little of it in my practice. Since then
more cases have come under my observation, but up to that time
I had been working in a practice where it had been the rule to
cleanse the teeth first and regularly. The teeth of these patients
were cleansed at regular intervals, not because there were great
masses of tartar present, but the teeth were searched with these
fine examining instruments, under the gums and on every surface, to detect any microscopical particles of tartar; between
the upper molars as well as the lower incisors, and back of the
last molars; in fact, everywhere. It was a habit of care and
patience that my preceptor had insisted upon for himself, and
it had borne fruit, so that I cannot help but feel that pyorrhœa
alveolaris, as I understand it and have seen it, is a preventable
disease entirely by the very simple method of persistent and faithful cleansing of the teeth in the manner in which Dr. Whitlock
has described. Our friend Dr. D. D. Smith wants to do it every
month, but in my observation there is no hard and fast rule as
to the interval of time. This is a point upon which I should
take issue with Dr. Smith. I have patients whom I can see once
a year and keep their teeth thoroughly in order. I have had
one patient whose teeth I did not clean once in fifteen years. I
really could not find a trace of tartar in that mouth, and there was
no stain even to polish off. It was the only case I have ever seen.
I invariably cleanse the teeth first. The intervals of time to be
allowed to pass to keep a mouth in perfect condition must be governed entirely by each individual case. For certain ones a year

may elapse, while in other cases the patient must be seen every six or four months, or perhaps every month.

Dr. Brush.—Regarding this patient who collected so little deposit, I should like to ask if the arches were in perfect condition.

The President.—I have not seen this patient for fifteen years, but my impression is that there were lost teeth in both arches.

Dr. Brush.—I have noticed that where the arches are unbroken and are normal in shape there is less deposit than where teeth are missing and perhaps others tilted.

Dr. LeRoy.—It has been my experience that the greatest amount of calcic deposit occurs after the teeth have been cleansed; also that the teeth that accumulate tartar most rapidly at the neck are those that are bell-shaped. Such teeth are most subject to pyorrhœa.

Regarding the case mentioned by the president, of the boy sixteen years of age with teeth affected by pyorrhœa, was it not possible that this was a case of salivation due to a mercurial treatment?

Regarding the statements that pyorrhœa did not exist in former times, I have been attending meetings for twenty-five years, and it seemed to be as prevalent then as now.

The President.—I did not mean to say that pyorrhœa was unknown twenty-five years ago, but that owing to the careful work of my predecessors in my own practice it had been eliminated.

Dr. Brush.—In closing the discussion on my paper, there is perhaps but one thing that I might say, and that is, that there was a time when I never used a memorandum of any kind. I prided myself on my memory and ability to carry in my head all the things I needed. Later, an elderly man suggested to me that this was a foolish practice, making a garret of my brain; that the useless lumber should be conveniently stored out of the way, making room for the more important things of the moment.

Dr. Whitlock.—In line with the thoughts already expressed, that pyorrhœa is curable by the simple method of thorough cleansing, I wish to mention one or two cases.

A lady was brought to me by her sister, asking if it was necessary for her to lose all her teeth. I examined them. There did not seem to be many cavities, but the teeth were all loose and in some places there was a good deal of tartar. I was convinced from the appearance of her gums that a great deal of the trouble was due to lack of use, and I asked her, as I always ask patients of this kind, if she did not bolt her food. She admitted that she did. I told her that if she would learn to masticate her food properly I could cure her. I cleansed her teeth thoroughly, taking three hours to do it. She carried out her part faithfully. To-day you would never mistrust that there had ever been anything the matter with her mouth, with the exception that before I saw her she had already had one molar extracted, and I think that tooth could have been saved.

A gentleman had a great deal of trouble when he was a young man. He had had his teeth cleansed regularly, and had had a great many fillings inserted. He told me that a few years ago he started the habit of eating only such foods as he could masticate. He did not eat soup nor ice-cream; in fact, nothing that did not require the use of his teeth. For two years he has not had a filling to be inserted, and, although a smoker, his teeth have not been stained with tobacco.

I have among my patients a young man who bolts his food. Though he brushes his teeth three times daily, it is simply impossible for me or any one else to keep his teeth even in a fairly decent condition. I always impress my patients with the necessity of using their teeth for masticating.

Adjourned.

FRED. L. BOGUE, M.D., D.D.S.,
Editor The New York Institute of Stomatology.

ACADEMY OF STOMATOLOGY.

A REGULAR meeting of the Academy of Stomatology, of Philadelphia, was held at its rooms, 1731 Chestnut Street, on the evening of March 28, 1905, the President Dr. I. N. Broomell, in the chair. A paper entitled "The Rationale of the Porcelain Inlay" was read by Dr. J. Q. Byram, of Indianapolis, Ind.

(For Dr. Byram's paper, see page 497.)

DISCUSSION.

Dr. Joseph Head.—In talking with Dr. Byram this afternoon he told me that he would consider it a personal favor if, as a scientific man who has worked from a scientific basis, I would adversely criticise his paper, and felt that he would rather have the truth than compliments. Any one who has listened to this paper and seen this array of plates knows that, while the work may be improved upon in the future, it is a distinct advance in dentistry. I feel that we should be very glad that Dr. Byram has been with us this evening.

The essayist spoke of the necessity of making a filling so that it will be held in place, not so much by the cement, as by stepping in the cavity, and that the cement will act merely as a stayer of the filling. I have had that belief for a long time, but in the light of some experiments which I have been carrying on since last August, I still believe that we do not at present thoroughly understand the exact value of cement with reference to a thin line and a thick line. We do not understand whether a thin line is stronger than a coarse line, or whether the cement will act as a glue or as a dowel. In my experiments I put the ordinary Harvard cement under a pressure of eight pounds to ¼-inch square between flat glass plates, and found that the thinnest cement line obtainable was 0.0003 of an inch. I made a long series of experiments, which will be published in the *Dental Cosmos.* For the sake of bringing out the point of the paper, I will give the ultimate tests, to show the adhesive strength of inlays. I drilled into ivory a number of cavities of the standard size of one-eighth inch in diameter and three-sixteenths of an inch in depth, and then made ten porcelain fillings to fit the cavities. A plunger could be inserted from underneath. These fillings were cemented in under ordinary thumb-pressure of about four pounds and pressure continued for about a minute. In testing the amount of force required to pull out the fillings, a spring balance was used coated with carbon, and in that way accurate readings were made. Every one of the glazed fillings came out with a pressure of about six ounces. The same fillings, etched and cemented under the same conditions, were removed at an average of about two pounds. I undercut the ivory, and found the pressure went up to about sixteen pounds for the Harvard, and twelve pounds for the Ames. I then undercut the fillings deeply, and set them again, and found that they came out under twenty-five pounds pressure for the Harvard cement, and nineteen pounds for the Ames. My conclusion was that inlays should always be put in so that there are undercuts in the fillings, undercuts in the dentine, and that the porcelain should also be etched.

The color problem is a difficult one. I feel that if we get a good color, a color of cement that approximates the color of the dentine, perhaps a little lighter, in order to overcome the shadow cast by the layer between the light and the porcelain, we will secure a color about as good as it is possible to get.

The filling that Dr. Byram put in to-day in his clinic was a beautiful match, and I am delighted that it was made in layers.

But when I turned the patient around so that the light struck the tooth, at first it looked something like " blue mud." I think the best we can do, so far, is to put in a porcelain filling that from the general point of view from which it is ordinarily seen will look well.

In reference to the use of pyrometers in the baking of porcelain, I think we have to know how to bake porcelain even with this instrument. The time may vary, and this is the important element. While the pyrometers may be a help, the principle is much the same as in studying Latin composition,—the only way to study it is to study it, and the only way to bake porcelain is just to bake it. The mixing of cement liquids in certain proportions to the powder is fine in theory; the only trouble is that in warm weather the liquid will deliquesce and set in varying lengths of time.

Dr. W. A. Capon.—I also would like to thank Dr. Byram for his practical and concise paper, which must be of advantage to all and of particular interest to many. Of course, I do not believe in everything that has been said. I have not made the experiment* outside of the mouth which he has, but I have done a great deal of work within the mouth. I think the plates he has shown us are very beautiful, and some of them very practical. All of them may be practical, but they are not exactly my ideal. It is much the same as in the filling of root-canals; different materials are used, and with apparently the best results. The preparation of cavities in the early days did not bother us much, and yet these fillings are still in the mouth, therefore the cement must have had much to do with their retention. Now that more attention is paid to the preparation of cavities, we should have better results, and I believe we shall have. I think the diagrams Nos. 1, 2, 3, and 4 are all practical. No. 6 I object to on account of the little piece of porcelain extended on the incisal edge. That will break off after a little wear. I had an illustration of this in a clinical case a couple of years ago. I do not see the advantage of such angles as shown in Fig. 7, and think that the graceful lines belonging to porcelain fillings are destroyed by such angles. In preparing such a cavity I do away with them entirely. Fig. 8 is all right, but it is an exceptional cavity.

I ceased using the pins seen in Fig. 9 ten years ago, and substitute the loop of platinum wire, because the ends are kept in position more easily, and they help to retain the cement.

In the making of the matrix, I agree with the essayist that there is only one way to do it, which is to work on the tooth proper. I never seem to get as nice adaptation as on natural enamel, although we hear of some men doing beautiful work by the swaging process.

In reference to the porcelain basal shades, I think it is a splendid idea to follow out the shade of the tooth. I do that and finish with enamels, but I, with others, know the disadvantage of an opaque substance like cement as an attachment.

I do not think that white cements give the best results in point of strength. The cement should be shaded to suit the tooth as nearly as possible. The cavity preparation has a great deal to do with the retention of the inlay and the ultimate results, and almost any good cement will hold a well-made and placed inlay.

Dr. J. H. Gaskill.—I do not see why I should be called upon to discuss this paper, because I am not a specialist nor an enthusiast on the subject of porcelains, but I am interested in some of the results which I have seen, and do some porcelain work. I have been much interested in Dr. Byram's paper, and I think he has taught us a great deal. In his clinic this afternoon he showed by his technic and manipulation his thorough mastery of the art of porcelain inlay work. I could not help feeling, however, that he carried his cutting of tooth-structure to extremes. He made use of the expression, "I cut until I get what I want." Is he justified in getting what he wants? From the cavity which he filled this afternoon he took a gold filling. A comparatively small portion of the tooth was gone from the labial side, but before he was through with it the third of the tooth was sacrificed. His excuse was that the enamel was checked. He did not take into consideration the support which the cement gives the porcelain inlay. I think we see many cases in which, with the lingual surface gone and the labial surface intact, we get æsthetically a better piece of work. You may put an inlay in place, and in certain lights it matches beautifully; in other lights it is very dark. This may be extreme, but it illustrates the condition which we have to meet.

As Dr. Byram stood in a strong light this afternoon and I noticed his teeth, I thought for the moment that he was negligent
of cleansing his mouth. I looked again and found that his teeth
were filled with porcelain inlays. They were beautifully put in,
and the color in most of them was beautiful, but as he stood in
certain lights there was a dark line where the cement had washed
out, giving the appearance of a carelessly kept mouth. In filling
with gold underneath, as a good and experienced operator should
do, a great deal of gold can be kept out of sight, and a better piece
of work will be the result. The cement problem is the one vital
point in inlay work. I agree with Dr. Byram as against Dr.
Capon in the results of the use of white cement. Dr. Head uses the
Harvard cement, which they call white, but it takes a bluish tinge.
The reflection against the whitish cement gives better results.

In the preparation of cavities Dr. Byram has, I think, developed a system which is wonderful as to the shaping of the edges
so that there is a mechanical retention of the inlay, and the cement becomes merely a necessary adjunct, because the force of
stress is in such a direction that the pressure locks the inlay in
position.

I wish to thank Dr. Byram for his paper and for the clinic.

Dr. G. F. Root.—Dr. Byram's technic is certainly fine, but I
believe one has to have the ideal cases in which to use ideal technic.
As a rule, each case presents problems that have to be solved, and
we cannot always use the methods which our theory teaches us
are the best.

I have seen some teeth filled with porcelain which were blue at
the gingival border.

Dr. Chas. R. Turner.—I was impressed with one feature of Dr.
Byram's paper, which indicated that he was dealing with the practical rather than with the ideal. As I looked at the cavities and
heard his description of the technic of filling them, it occurred to
me that they might be cavities in any teeth, and not necessarily
cavities that present themselves under ideal conditions. In order
to get them into the exact shape in which they are presented, what
has been termed " sacrifice of tooth-structure" is necessary, but, inasmuch as the ultimate success of the operation is the point in
view, it is justifiable; in other words it is a sacrifice of tooth-structure for the preservation of the balance of the tooth.

I was also interested in the very scientific attitude taken by the essayist upon the question of color. The backing up of the inlay with a white cement struck me as a good idea.

In conclusion, I wish to compliment the essayist upon the great detail with which he has worked out his technic, and to thank him personally for the presentation in a very succinct and comprehensive form of the general problem of porcelain inlay.

Dr. Roberts.—There has been considerable discussion about the ideal cavity and the inability to find cavities that could be so prepared as to be exactly like the drawings which the essayist has presented. My idea of successful inlay work is for a man to make a cavity ideal and representative without necessarily following any of the exact lines pointed out by the essayist. If he finds that he has a small cavity and one that will not show, he certainly will not sacrifice a great amount of tooth-structure to bring about a cavity similar to that of Fig. 2. He will prepare a cavity so as to save all the tooth-structure he can, and yet get it on ideal lines. If it be a small cavity, he will use gold, while the successful inlay worker will take any cavity and so prepare it that it will in a measure be self-retentive to the filling, the cement simply keeping the porcelain in place, and he does not have to follow any of the ideal shapes here presented. He makes his ideals as he progresses.

I was much interested in the paper, and congratulate the essayist upon the able manner in which it was presented.

Dr. Byram (closing).—I first want to thank you for the kind reception given me. As I remarked to my friend, Dr. Head, if there is any one thing I dislike, it is to read a paper and then have every one " agree with the essayist." I take it as a favor to have criticism.

I take it that we are all striving for knowledge on the subject of inlays. While I am here as your guest, and an enthusiastic inlay worker, I want it distinctly understood that I am but a novice. The more I study the subject, the more I find I do not know. I have received many good suggestions since coming to your city which will be of value to me after my return.

I congratulate Dr. Head upon the thorough manner in which he has been testing cements. I believe that he is doing one of the best works in the subject that could be done. I only wish I could join him in this line of experimental work.

There seems to be a difference of opinion as to what, I mean by constructing inlays in layers. Dr. Head does the work as I do in many cases, with a few modifications. I first select my basal color, which I hope will represent as nearly as possible the color of the dentine. Then I select the color of the enamel in the different locations. If it is brown or yellow in the gingival, then I select enamel of a corresponding color. For the incisal I usually select enamel of a bluish hue. After the colors have been biscuited, I apply a uniform color over the entire mass and fuse.

In writing a paper of this kind it must be taken into consideration that there are many points of interest to the beginners in this work which are not of interest to those who are familiar with the details of porcelain work. I do not do everything just as I have stated in this paper. Those experienced in teaching know that we must teach beginners to do that which they can do when they commence, not what they will do in three or four years. I do not always apply my color as I have said. I can hardly see how any one can construct an inlay extending from the gingival line to the incisal edge and use but one colored porcelain. I have yet to see one tooth in which there are not two and usually three shades of color. By selecting porcelains that more nearly approach the color of the tooth in their respective locations I can do better work. If that is what is called constructing in layers, then I am an advocate of the layer method.

In regard to the pyrometer, I may say that I have never had anything in my porcelain work that has given me the pleasure my pyrometer has, and if I know anything about the fusing of porcelain it has been learned since using this instrument. The pyrometer has assisted me in obtaining accurate results, and it has been instrumental in teaching me how to fuse porcelain. To obtain accurate results, you must fuse under exactly the same conditions.

I find that I get better results in mixing cements by weighing the parts. Changes may have to be made according to the weather.

In reply to Dr. Capon, I would say that pioneers in any line of work have done good service. When I see some of the gold fillings that were inserted forty years ago, I am ashamed of my work. When we think of how these men labored preparing their cavities by hand, and taking hours at it, and when we remember how they mastered the technic of inserting these fillings by hand. I say it makes me feel ashamed when I look at many of our gold fillings. Those who began inlay work fifteen or twenty years ago are in the same position. They did not have the modern improvements, porcelains, furnaces, etc. They had to become skilful at once. Those entering this work to-day are not required to go through such experimental work as were Dr. Capon and Dr. Head, and that is the reason we are not so skilful as those who started years ago.

In reference to the thickness of the incisal edge, there are certain cases in which the edges are thick enough to prepare the cavities according to Fig. 6. It is impossible to use these reverse curves without having more space than with some of the other forms of cavity preparation.

In reply to Dr. Gaskill, I will say that in the preparation of a cavity every man must have his ideal, and while I may not carry out in detail my ideal, I try to work to that as nearly as possible. My ideal is to have the cavity as nearly self-retentive as possible. In regard to cutting, I will say that I do cut. Some ask if the patient will stand it? My reply is, I am the dentist, and if they want me to insert inlays, they must submit to my method of operation. We were taught not to leave frail walls for gold fillings, and I would not have you believe that you may leave frail walls for inlays and expect them to give the best service.

In the case of this afternoon I did not make the excuse that the enamel was checked. The cavity was not prepared in an ideal manner, nor under ideal conditions. It was half-past two when I commenced, and it was three o'clock when we secured an engine, and to have prepared the cavity in an ideal manner and constructed the inlay would have taken until seven o'clock. The case was that of a student, and if the filling comes out it can easily be replaced.

Dr. Capon thinks the matrix lining is good because it is white. I do not understand why he would not use a white cement for the same reason that he uses the matrix lining, because the matrix lining is only next to the cement, and he has the enamel over all. If the white cement is used, there is a white film between the inlay and the tooth. Dr. Capon also feels that the white cement or the yellow has not the strength of the darker ones. I would like to ask Dr. Head if he found this to be so in his tests?

Dr. Head (answering Dr. Byram).—I was much surprised to hear Dr. Capon say what he did. Although I have not gone into the tests as much as I hope to, yet it seemed to me that, since the dark cements are made so by means of foreign pigments, and the light yellow cement is pure oxide of zinc as it is brought from the crucible, the uncolored cement ought to be stronger than, or at least quite as strong as, the dark.

Dr. Byram.—So, I say again that I believe the white cement, or as white as we can get it, is the best cement to use in setting inlays, because we have a cement that has the least power of absorption and the greatest power of reflection of our light rays. For the first few weeks there will be a white line, but in a few weeks it will be just about as brown as if you had used the yellow cement. I will have to offer a word of apology about the inlays in my mouth.

Dr. Gaskill.—I was not questioning the workmanship of those inlays, because they are beautiful and the color is good; but simply meant to say that in certain lights the reflection gives the bluish or opaque appearance which you are bound to get in certain lights.

Dr. Byram.—I have been experimenting with this matrix lining in my mouth, and, like Dr. Capon, I find I shall have to learn to apply my colors again. A busy man, however, has not time to have inlays made for his mouth more than once. I wish to say that I have some inlays of which I am very proud, put in under my direction by one of my associates. They are the first inlays he ever constructed, except two by the Jenkins system made by him last summer.

Dr. Head.—When I spoke of "blue mud," I did not mean to intimate that the filling was not all right, but simply that it followed the law of all these fillings when the light strikes them.

Dr. Byram.—I think Dr. Head's remarks were clear. In my paper I tried to make it plain that when the light shines in certain directions against the fillings we always have that change in color.

I would like to meet those of you who are particularly interested in inlay work to exhibit some inlay burs. I am to meet a representative of the S. S. White Dental Company to-morrow, and your endorsement will assist me in having them place the burs on the market.

I would like to say in conclusion that I appreciate the kindness and honor that have been bestowed upon me by the members of this Academy in inviting me here. Coming as I do from a distant State, practically unknown to you, I assure you that I feel very grateful to you.

OTTO E. INGLIS,
Editor Academy of Stomatology.

Editorial.

HAS THE LECTURE A FUTURE IN EDUCATION?

LECTURES have been from the remote periods of human history the favorite method of imparting information to the aspiring student and in many branches of professional work they have been, until recent years, the principal means of instruction.

The evolution of thought and the gradual unfolding of practical ideas has brought about a sceptical condition of mind in regard to this as a means of successful training, and there has grown in many quarters a revolt against what is regarded as a mediæval method of education, and thought to be unworthy this progressive and practical age.

A writer in the *British Dental Journal* of April 16, N. G. Bennett, ventures upon a philippic against the old practice of imparting information, and styles it the "Comedy of Lectures." Another writer in the present number, W. H. Trueman, quotes, with approbation, the action of Princeton in increasing the number of preceptors to keep in constant touch with students as "guides, advisors, and testers of their learning." The cry is by no means a new one. It has been sounded in the halls of professsional learning these many years, without apparently producing much effect. Sixty-six years ago (1839) Dr. Harris, in organizing the first dental college of the world, when he was refused co-operation by the medical educators of his city, made the first great innovation in professional teaching, and for this he has never received proper credit. He evidently was impressed with the futility of the course of lectures, as a sole means of educating the medical man, prevalent in his day, and in establishing his dental college he started out with the fixed idea that the student must be trained mainly upon the living subject. From that day to the present the dental student expects to secure his practical knowledge in the operative and prosthetic branches through this method. It is not at all probable that Harris appreciated the full extent and far-reaching possibilities of his wise procedure, and could he now witness the almost daily exhibit, in our large dental colleges, of probably a hundred and fifty men working over that many chairs and on patients under personal supervision, and performing delicate operations certain to be required in future practice, he would feel that this was by no means the least important work he did for his profession and for the improvement of general medical instruction.

The method that Harris inaugurated naturally led to an examination of the technical possibilities in teaching, and observant educators were not slow to see the fallacy of depending solely on didactic work. In the medical schools the old lecture system still held, partly through the force of tradition, and more from lack of means and room to establish personal supervision in laboratories adapted for the purpose. It is not many years since the new order came gradually into force, and the importance of the lecture has been greatly lessened. Men, not very old, can remember when chemistry was taught in lectures, when bacteriology was an unknown subject, and histology was regarded very much as a toy to while away an hour among the unknown mysteries of life. Now the graduate in dentistry and medicine would be deprived of a large portion of his professional skill were he suddenly to be bereft of the knowledge obtained in the laboratories devoted to these several subjects.

From working on the living subject to that devoted to technical training seems very much like reversing the natural order, but it was through observing the defects of the method of teaching in dental schools that led the observant mind to regard manual training as a necessary prerequisite, and the technical class-work was the natural result. It is some forty years since the mind of the present writer was forcibly awakened to the necessity of a change in the then existing methods of teaching dentistry. The time then was not ripe for radical measures in this direction, but in an experimental way a section upon histological studies was formed under his personal supervision. The success of this brought about, in after years, in the school with which he was connected, the technic training, and this has spontaneously become an essential part of the curricula of all the dental colleges of this country, and which has increased so much the development of dentistry in this part of the world.

While the value of this practical training cannot be overestimated, it must not be forgotten that the older methods have not,

by any means, became a "comedy" to rouse the laugh of the unthinking. They are still the inspiring life of dental education and
are full of meaning for the future.

Lectures are not to be relegated to the shelves of forgotten
methods of teaching. They have performed a noble work in the
past, and will continue to do it in the future. The part they
must play will be to inspire the soul, that Haeckel says exists in
all created things, and will make the dry body of mere technical
teaching teem with life. The fault of this older method is not in
the process, but in those who attempt to carry it out. To be a
lecturer worthy the subject means three things,—first, to be able
to think on the feet; second, to be thoroughly saturated with the
subject; and third, to *never cease to train for every lecture.*

The series of lectures, as described by the English writer
quoted, causes in the reading a sense of weariness of soul. It is
true, as he writes, thus, "The systematic course of lectures on
text-book subjects is, to a large extent, and for a number of men,
a painful waste of time." Is that lecturing in the best sense?
The man who places a manuscript between himself and his audience raises a barrier that genius may be unable to surmount. On
the other hand, the man who stands before his class fully alive
to the importance of his subject, inspired by practical experience,
with text-books in the dark background, and only referred to, if at
all, to enforce a point, notes confined to a few headings and rarely
referred to,—such a lecture, delivered with earnestness and clear
enunciation, will strike home as no amount of personal talk over
the chair or in the laboratory can possibly effect. The philosophy
of practice can be taught only in this manner. The life of the
subject can be inspired here, and the class will be forced to think,
to reason, and compare. The men never sleep under such a lecturer. They are imbued with the magnetic force of a great inspiration and such lectures live and become a vital energy long
after their deliverance. Lectures have not had their day. They
have come down to us through the centuries, and will continue a
power in the centuries yet to be. How many of us can recall certain lectures of our student days that still continue with us as an
inspiration! They have moulded our thoughts and made our lives
more valuable. Why is it that Dr. Thomas Watson's lectures,
delivered in London, on the "Principles and Practice of Physic,"
some sixty-nine years ago,—1836–37,—are to-day classic in medi-

cine? It is only necessary to read these to secure the answer and, at the same time, to feel the inspiration that that model lecturer infused into them, and which will be felt as long as English medical literature exists.

There is too much of a disposition to consider old things as having lost their usefulness. The world cannot afford to part with anything that once possessed a certain value. It has taken centuries to mould into form the present methods of education, and our duty then is not to destroy but to build anew on this old foundation, combining past and present ideas, renewing the vitality of the present, leading directly to a broader superstructure that may develop, through experience, into better methods for the training of men.

THE NEW YORK INSTITUTE OF STOMATOLOGY— OFFER OF PRIZES.

Upon another page will be found the announcement of The New York Institute of Stomatology, offering two prizes for the best papers submitted on or before March 1, 1906. The first prize will be a gold medal and two hundred and fifty dollars. The second, a gold medal and one hundred dollars.

This generous offer, the first, it is believed, ever emanating from a local society, should receive an equally generous response. The time might profitably be extended, as the working months, so far as this country is concerned, will be practically limited to six, a time too short for serious research work.

This offer should stimulate the scientific mind of the country to compete upon a proper basis. The Fourth International Dental Congress made a somewhat similar offer, with the result that the response from this country was not at all representative, while all the papers from abroad were of a high order of merit. There is ample room for work in unsolved problems in dentistry, and we possess now a large body of educated young men who should make these the subject of careful research, and this is their golden opportunity. Will the response be equal to the occasion?

Bibliography.

NOTES ON DENTAL PORCELAIN. A Practical Treatise especially devoted to the Interests of the Beginner. By V. Walter Gilbert, D.D.S. Over one hundred practical illustrations. The S. S. White Dental Manufacturing Company, Philadelphia; Claudius Ash & Sons, Limited, London, 1905.

History constantly repeats itself, but assumes new forms at every repetition. This is being demonstrated in dentistry at almost every recurring decade. This fact was impressed upon the writer upon taking up Dr. Gilbert's book for review, and his mind reverted to a period when the knowledge of dental porcelain was an absolute necessity for any one attempting the practice of dentistry. Then came a long interregnum in which the knowledge of dental porcelain was confined to the manufacturers of porcelain teeth, and now the eternal cycle of thought has brought the student of dentistry, as well as practitioners, face to face with the fact that he must learn, willingly or unwillingly, the manipulation of porcelain bodies as his fathers did before him.

It is, therefore, very appropriate that a book should have been written by one combining a scientific and practical training in one of the largest dental schools of the country with a very exact knowledge of porcelain through his intimate connection with one of the largest, if not the largest, manufactures of dental porcelain of the world. All the experience accumulated in this house since the days of Stockton have been at the author's command, and that he has made good use of this knowledge is apparent throughout the book.

There has been so much written, of a seemingly partisan character, by those engaged in the modern use of porcelain in practice, that it is not surprising that the novice is in a state of embarrassment as he hears and reads of " high fusing" and " low fusing," until he questions the value of either and naturally fears to attempt this material in any form, or, as the author states it, " The opinion of the high-fusing enthusiast is accepted only to be discarded upon reading or hearing the opinion of the low-fusing enthusiast, and *vice versa.*"

The author, very properly, begins his first chapter on the consideration of "Porcelain: Its Place in Dentistry." Its place is so important that, while dentistry existed prior to the advent of porcelain in tooth forms, it was not dentistry as understood to-day, and the author very forcibly places this before his readers, wherein he imagines the condition if "All the artificial teeth, porcelain bodies, gum enamels, etc., were destroyed and no longer obtainable." Where, indeed, would dentistry be were such to happen? Prosthetic dentistry is dependent upon porcelain. Operative dentistry is becoming more and more subject to its artistic influence, and the world at large is dependent upon it for mastication of food, health, and even length of life.

There is so much to learn regarding porcelains, that it has become a serious question whether the schools will not be forced to go back to the work of the Fathers and teach the entire process. The author expresses the importance of this knowledge when he writes: "Do not make an initial mistake by supposing that any one grade of porcelain may be regarded as a 'cure all' and that it possesses qualities which will meet all dental requirements. . . . A porcelain compound which has been especially prepared to meet the requirements of a full artificial denture will not be entirely satisfactory for the production of a small inlay. A porcelain compound especially prepared to meet the requirements of a small inlay will not be entirely suitable for the production of a full artificial denture." These are wise words, and should be carefully considered by those who rush from an inlay to the making of a crown, or crowns, entirely of porcelain.

The confusion of terms, "High Fusing" and "Low Fusing," which really mean nothing, but which the novice in porcelain work regards as defining a definite quality, places the operator in an embarrassing position. The author attempts to remedy this by defining the meaning which should be placed on these terms. He says, "In order to make the term a little more comprehensive to the student, the generally accepted definition of 'High Fusing' will be modified to read as follows: A porcelain which vitrifies or takes the glaze at a temperature somewhere between the melting point of pure gold and the glazing point of an American-made porcelain tooth;" and "Low Fusing" is applied to "compounds which vitrify or take the glaze at a temperature below the melting point of pure gold."

The author's chapter on "Laboratory experiments" is an exceedingly interesting one, but aside from this it is of very decided practical value. In order to test the "differences in fusing point," ten of the best known products were taken and subjected, in the form of cones of porcelain, to a heat sufficient to glaze. The result demonstrated the effect of heat upon the different bodies, melting absolutely the low-fusing, and proportionately so with the others, eventually leaving one cone to stand up against all the others of the high-fusing series. These experiments are not only novel in character, but demonstrate at a glance the futility of calling all the compounds by one name,—" High Fusing."

Space will not permit following this valuable book through all the chapters. These are written in a captivating style, that holds the reader to the end, at least such was the experience of the reviewer. The author has the faculty of making each operation clear, and the beginner who proposes to enter upon the preparation of porcelain in any of its dental forms will do well to procure this book, and in so doing will be able to work his way through a maze of many difficulties.

In order that our readers may have a general idea of the scope of this book of one hundred and twenty-six pages, the titles of chapters are appended: " Porcelain: Its Place in Dentistry. Dental Porcelains. Laboratory Experiments. Practical Application of Block Bodies. Porcelain Crowns. Porcelain Fillings. Shading Porcelain. Mineral Stains. Furnaces. Fusing Porcelains."

It is a gratification to find one of the younger men connected with dentistry ready to place his acquired knowledge in the hands of those struggling amidst many difficulties in the acquirement of a difficult art, but while it has been written with these principally in view, it will be found a very suggestive production for those older practitioners who may feel themselves well grounded in the work.

MESSRS. LEA BROTHERS & Co. announce a new edition of " Gray's Anatomy," to be published about midsummer, and embodying nearly two years of labor on the part of the editor, J. Chalmers Da Costa, M.D., of Philadelphia, and a corps of special assistants.

Commensurately with the importance of the largest-selling medical work ever published, this new edition will present a revision so thorough and searching that the entire book has been

reset in new type. In addition to the changes necessary to bring
it abreast of the most modern knowledge of its subject, several
important alterations have been made with the view of adapting
it still more closely to present-day teaching methods, and, in fact,
to anticipate the trend of anatomical work and study.

The illustrations have come in for their full share of the general revision, so that at this writing more than four hundred new
and elaborate engravings in black and colors have been prepared.
" Gray" has always been noted for its richness of illustration, but
the new edition far exceeds anything that has hitherto been
attempted.

A MANUAL OF MECHANICAL DENTISTRY AND METALLURGY. By
Geo. W. Warren, A.M., D.D.S., Professor of Clinical Den-
tistry, Pennsylvania College of Dental Surgery; author of
" A Compend of Dental Pathology and Dental Medicine,"
etc. Second edition, revised, with seventy-nine illustrations.
P. Blakiston's Son & Co., Philadelphia.

This work of two hundred and fifty-seven pages has been greatly
improved since the first edition was reviewed in this journal.

All manuals must be in a large degree unsatisfactory to the
one fond of detail, and it may be doubted whether they are of
much real benefit to the student. Their tendency, as a rule, seems
to be to cultivate superficial knowledge at the expense of thoroughness. This the author has tried to avoid, and has measurably
succeeded for the purpose intended,—that of giving a " conservative guide for the student in his study of the subjects considered."
The author says, " It is presented as a convenient every-day working book," and in this sense it can be recommended as a work of
reference in the laboratory.

HENRY'S APPOINTMENT-REGISTER-DAY-BOOK FOR DENTISTS. By
Robert S. Henry, D.D.S., Chattanooga, Tenn.

This appointment-book is one of the most satisfactory of its
kind. It covers every day from January to December, and with
the proper date given on each page. Upon each page at its head
is a diagram of the teeth in each jaw, anterior and posterior, with
abbreviations to designate the various operations, and in addition
Dr. and Cr. columns. The facility with which a record can be

made in it of examinations constitutes its greatest recommendation, but it seems, in other respects, to cover all the requirements of an engagement-book for the daily work of the office.

Domestic Correspondence.

MAKE-UP OF THE DENTAL PROFESSION IN GREAT BRITAIN.

" THE *Dental Register* for 1905 has recently been issued, and shows that at last the number of those holding licenses in Dental Surgery exceeds that of those who appear therein by virtue of being in *bona fide* practice at the passing of the Act. It is true that the *Register* does not tell us exactly how many dentists are in practice, for there are some holding the license who have not subscribed their names. On the other hand, it is probable that many who did register at the passing of the Act are not in active practice, and that some others have definitely retired. The *Register*, however, constitutes the official record published for the General Medical Council, and contains the names of 4734 persons, an increase of fifty-eight over last year. Of these, 2374 held a license in dental surgery from one or other of the four colleges which grant such diplomas; of the rest, 2332 were admitted to the *Register* on the strength of the fact that they were in *bona fide* practice as dentists before the passing of the Dentists' Act of 1878; a few of these, however, held ordinary medical or surgical degrees or diplomas. The balance of the names in the *Register* is made up by three gentlemen admitted thereto as holders of Colonial dental certificates and by twenty-five others who have been granted degrees in dental medicine or dental surgery by recognized universities in the United States of America. Of the holders of these colonial or foreign diplomas, some ten or eleven appear to practise abroad. In regard to those who hold licenses in dental surgery, sixty per cent. of them derive their title from the Royal College of Surgeons of England, eighteen per cent. from that in Ireland, twelve per cent. from that in Edinburgh, and eight per cent. from the Faculty of Physicians and Surgeons of Glasgow. Of the total,

2374, some 280 hold ordinary medical and surgical degrees or diplomas in addition to one in dentistry."

The above, an editorial in the *British Journal of Dental Science* for May 15, 1905, page 458, shows conclusively that the provisions in the dental Act, to that end and the construction placed upon them by the General Medical Council, has proved a gratifying success in building up the home schools; of the two thousand four hundred and two admitted to the *Register* by virtue of an educational qualification, twenty-eight only obtained this qualification abroad. As a result of the encouragement the home schools have thus received, they have vastly improved, they have increased in number, and the well-trained practitioners they have year by year sent out have been a grand uplift to the profession. The profession and the community in Great Britain is now reaping the benefit of the wisely planned dental reform of nearly a generation ago.

W. H. T.

Obituary.

CLARK LA MOTTE GODDARD, A.B., D.D.S., A.M.

CLARK LA MOTTE GODDARD, A.B., D.D.S., A.M., died in San Francisco, March 30, 1905, aged fifty-five years.

" Dr. Goddard was born of American parents, in Beloit, Wis., June 26, 1849, where he spent most of his boyhood days, and he also received his early educational training in the public schools of his native city.

" In 1868 he entered the Beloit College, from which he graduated four years later, receiving the degree of Bachelor of Arts, and in 1875 the degree of Master of Arts was conferred upon him by the same institution.

" At an early age he determined to make dentistry his life's work and began the study of it at first with E. M. Clark, M.D., of Beloit, later matriculating at the Philadelphia College of Dentistry and received therefrom his degree of Doctor of Dental Surgery in 1874.

" He first began practice in Chicago, but soon made up his

mind to locate in San Francisco, arriving here in 1875, where he has been in practice ever since, associating himself first with Dr. J. L. Cogswell, and in 1876 with Dr. H. E. Knox for four years.

"He was constantly active in all associational work, which is shown by the fact that he became a member of the San Francisco Dental Association and the California State Dental Association in 1875, the California State Odontological Society in 1884, and the American Dental Association in 1890. He was initiated into the Delta Sigma Delta Fraternity in 1892; was made an honorary member of the Washington, D. C., Dental Association in 1895, and of the Oregon State Dental Association in 1897; in 1891 he was the president of the San Francisco Dental Association; a year later he was chairman of the Dental Section of the American Medical Association, and in 1898 was president of the Pacific Coast Dental Congress held in Portland, Oregon.

"In addition to the foregoing he has repeatedly been a delegate to the National Association of Dental Faculties, and has been further honored by election and appointment to various other offices in different societies.

"At the time of organizing the Dental Department of the University of California, in 1882, he was appointed by the regents of the University a member of the faculty, giving practically a continuous service since that time, and the longest in the history of the College.

"The various appointments in that direction were successively, Professor of Mechanical Dentistry; Professor of Mechanical Dentistry, Dental Metallurgy, and Orthodontia; Professor of Orthodontia and Dental Metallurgy; Professor of Orthodontia.

"In 1902 he retired from active membership in the faculty, when he was appointed to the honorary position of Emeritus Professor of Orthodontia, but since then he has given a yearly special course in comparative Odontology. During his long experience in teaching he served as dean of the faculty for eight years at different periods.

"He has contributed largely to dental literature, and has presented valuable treatises, some of which have been included in recent text-books and accepted as the best authority on the subjects selected. Among them might be mentioned the chapters in the ' American Text-Book of Prosthetic Dentistry' on the 'Principles of Metal Work and Orthodontia Technic,' and on ' Cast

Dentures of Aluminum and Fusible Alloys;' and in the ' American Text-Book of Operative Dentistry' the chapter on the ' Management of Deciduous Teeth' and another on ' Orthodontia.'

" Dr. Goddard married Miss Emily Louise Bunker, August 13, 1881, and as an issue of this union there are two children, a son and a daughter, all of whom survive him."

We are indebted for the foregoing facts in the life of Dr. Goddard to the *Pacific Dental Gazette*. The announcement of the death of this eminent practitioner came as a serious blow to his many friends in the East. He was probably better known personally than most of our coworkers on the Pacific coast. His valuable contributions to dental literature made his name familiar to those who were not brought in personal contact with him at the various conventions in which he was so frequently an active participant. At the meetings of the Association of Faculties his presence and cultured manner in debate held his audience in many of the stormy sessions of that body and largely aided in producing conviction for the side he advocated. Whether in opposition or in favor of any disputed question, his message always commanded respect.

His death at a comparatively early age is a serious loss, not to the Pacific coast only, but to the larger body throughout the country, for he labored earnestly for the broader professional life based upon a true professional spirit, unfortunately too much lacking in dental circles in this country. His work and example should be a stimulus to higher ideals and more important results.

RESOLUTIONS OF RESPECT TO DR. ELLERY C. YOUNG.

WHEREAS, It has pleased Almighty God to remove from our midst on December 6, 1904, at the age of sixty-one, Ellery C. Young, of Leipzig, court dentist to the Grand Duke of Anhalt, be it

Resolved, That the American Dental Society of Europe has sustained a serious loss in this, the death of one of its oldest members, who was respected in his community for his uprightness and sterling worth, and who was recognized by all as a superior dentist and a worthy colleague.

Resolved, That this resolution be published in the leading dental journals of the United States and a copy be forwarded to the bereaved wife of our friend and colleague, and that this resolution be placed upon record as part of the proceedings of the Society.

WILLIAM A. SPRING,
G. H. WATSON,
W. MITCHELL,
Committee.

Miscellany.

FRENCH DENTAL COLLEGE IN CANADA.—L'École de Chirurgie Dentaire de l'Université de Laval, at Montreal (Canada), is the only dental college in America in which the instruction is given entirely in the French language. Under another name and built upon a different basis, it has taken the place of the French faculty of the Dental College of Quebec. The courses were opened with an increased number of students. The professors are prominent dentists of high standing. They are Drs. Eudore Dubeau, M. Josef Nolin, M. Y. G. A. Gendreau. We express our best wishes for the complete success of their school.—*Le Laboratoire*, Paris.— C. M. L.

TEETH RECEDING IN VULCANIZATION.—"How is it," asks a dentist, "that the teeth often recede from the caoutchouc, leaving an empty space? I have employed different kinds of rubber and bent the pins, yet experience frequently the same inconvenience."

Answer: Follow closely the instructions explained in every box of the rubber.

Let the temperature of the vulcanizer go up very slowly and vulcanize rather under than above the normal degree. Take more time for the whole process.

Heat your flask in boiling water, and your rubber over steam, taking care that it does not burn. (C. SOULARD, Lyon, *Le Laboratoire*.)—C. M. L.

A NEW PROPERTY OF ALUMINUM.—" A German investigator," says the *Scientific American*, "has discovered an exceedingly valuable and important property of aluminum, which consists in its application as a whetting agent, the effect produced on cutlery set with it being most astonishing. Though a metal, aluminum possesses the structure of a fine stone, has a strong dissolving power, and develops, upon use for honing, an exceedingly fine metal-setting substance of greasy feel, while showing great adhesion to steel. The knives, etc., treated with it quickly obtain such a fine, razor-like edge that even the best whetstone cannot produce a like result. Thus, knives which had been carefully set on a whetstone, when magnified a thousand times, still exhibited irregularities and roughness on the edge, while the edge of a knife sharpened on aluminum, upon exactly the same magnification, appeared as a straight, smooth line."—*British Dental Journal.*

DR. BARTLER recommends a saturated solution of shellac in borax water for the coating of plaster casts. It combines well with the plaster without forming a layer (schicht) upon it. This method facilitates also the separating of the cast from the impression.—(*Asch's Wiener Fachblatt.*)

IF the flask is placed in the vulcanizer so that it stands above the water, a much stronger plate will be the result, as the rubber hardens best in steam. (*Asch's Quarterly Circular.*)—C. M. L.

To prevent the bubbling of the borax during the soldering process, mix a minimum of gum-arabic and water with the borax on a glass slab.

BEFORE closing the flask use a piece of rubber dam coated with soap instead of the muslin. It will give an excellent result. (*Asch's Quarterly.*)

AN "ANTIVOLAT" MEASURE for somnoform, ethyl chloride, or any other liquid anæsthetic, is a double glass graduate with a closed space between the inside and outside to serve as a non-conductor of heat, and provided with a cover. It is extremely difficult to measure accurately very volatile liquids with the ordinary graduate. The heat of the vessel and of the surrounding atmosphere causes a serious loss by rapid evaporation. With this measure, the small portion first poured in, by its rapid evaporation, chills the vessel, reducing its temperature below the boiling-point of the volatile liquid and preventing any further loss. The inner chamber, being insulated, so retards evaporation that if filled a portion will remain after twelve hours' time.

Current News.

OFFER OF PRIZES BY THE NEW YORK INSTITUTE OF STOMATOLOGY.

WITH the desire of stimulating investigation in any field of activity directly relating to dental or oral science, The New York Institute of Stomatology offers two prizes for the best papers submitted to it embodying the results of such original research. The first prize for the best paper will be a gold medal and two hundred and fifty dollars. The second prize for the next best paper, a gold medal and one hundred dollars.

CONDITIONS.

(*a*) The papers offered for competition must be typewritten in English.

(*b*) Must contain not less than fifteen hundred nor more than three thousand five hundred words.

(*c*) Must be signed by a motto or *nom de plume.*

(*d*) Must be accompanied by a sealed envelope marked with the same motto or *nom de plume* on the outside, containing the true names as well as the motto of the contestant within.

(*e*) Must be sent to the chairman of the Executive Committee, Dr. F. Milton Smith, 38 West Thirty-sixth Street, on or before March 1, 1906.

The following gentlemen have consented to act as judges: Dr. C. N. Johnson, of Chicago, Editor of *Dental Review;* Dr. Eugene H. Smith, of Boston, Dean of Harvard University Dental School; Dr. Wilbur F. Litch, of Philadelphia, Editor of the *Dental Brief,* under the following rules:

RULES.

1. The papers will be sent to the judges without the sealed envelopes containing the names of the contestants, which will be retained by the Executive Committee till the decision of the judges is made.

2. In deciding on the merits of papers offered in competition the judges will be requested to take into consideration the value and character of the research work the results of which are presented, more than the literary character of the essays, but to give the latter due credit.

3. The judges are expressly authorized to decide which if any of the papers submitted to them are of sufficient merit to entitle them to the prizes offered, or to withhold the award from all the papers if none are deemed worthy.

4. Authors of the prize papers will be invited to read their essays before a meeting of the Institute, as will the writers of other papers of especial merit, the Institute reserving the right to the first publication of all papers offered in competition.

Papers not used will be promptly returned to the writers. Those read before the Institute will be as fully discussed as possible, and when published will be adequately illustrated.

For further information, address

DR. F. MILTON SMITH.

38 WEST THIRTY-SIXTH STREET, NEW YORK, N. Y.

HARVARD DENTAL ALUMNI ASSOCIATION.

THE Harvard Dental Alumni Association held its thirty-fourth annual meeting in Boston, Mass., June 26, 1905, and elected the following named officers for the ensuing year:

President, Ned A. Stanley, '84, New Bedford, Mass.; Vice-President, Arthur W. Eldred, Worcester, Mass.; Secretary, Waldo

E. Boardman, '86, Boston, Mass.; Treasurer, Harold De W. Cross, '96, Boston, Mass.

Executive Committee.—Waldo E. Boardman, '86, Chairman *ex officio*, Boston, Mass.; Walter A. Davis, '01, Boston, Mass.; Arthur A. Libby, '99, Boston, Mass.

The Council is composed of the officers of the Alumni Association.

WALDO E. BOARDMAN, '86,
Secretary.

COLORADO STATE DENTAL ASSOCIATION.

THE Colorado State Dental Association held its nineteenth annual meeting at the Alta Vista Hotel, Colorado Springs, Col., Tuesday, Wednesday, and Thursday, June 20, 21, 22, 1905. Officers were elected as follows:

President, Wm. Chambers, Denver; Vice-President, J. Allen Smith, Colorado Springs; Secretary, B. Frank Gray, Colorado Springs; Treasurer, Wm. Smedley, Denver.

Fort Collins was chosen as the next meeting place.

H. W. BATES,
Secretary.

MISSOURI STATE DENTAL ASSOCIATION.

AT the fortieth annual meeting of the Missouri State Dental Association, held in St. Louis, May 24 to 26, 1905, the following officers were elected:

President, W. M. Carter, Sedalia; First Vice-President, F. H. Achelpohl, St. Charles; Second Vice-President, F. G. Worthley, Kansas City; Recording Secretary, H. H. Sullivan, Kansas City; Corresponding Secretary, Sam T. Bassett, St. Louis; Treasurer, J. T. Fry, Moberly.

Board of Censors.—J. C. Pasqueth, Mexico; J. L. Bridgeford, Macon; DeCourcey Lindsley, St. Louis.

Committee on Ethics.—J. B. McBride, Springfield; A. J. Prosser, St. Louis; F. M. Fulkerson, Sedalia.

Committee on Publication.—Otto J. Fruth, St. Louis; J. W. Hull, Kansas City.

Committee on Inventions and New Appliances.—Ralph H. Mc-Crum, Springfield.

Committee on History of Missouri State Dental Association.—Burton Lee Thorpe, St. Louis.

Time and place of next meeting, May, 1906, Springfield, Mo.

SAM T. BASSETT,
Corresponding Secretary.

ILLINOIS STATE DENTAL SOCIETY.

AT the annual meeting of the Illinois State Dental Society, held in Moline, Ill., May 9, 10, and 11, 1905, the following officers were elected for the ensuing year:

President, S. Finley Duncan, Joliet; Vice-President, L. W. Skidmore, Moline; Secretary, Elgin MaWhinney, 34 Washington Street, Chicago; Treasurer, Chas. P. Pruyn, Chicago; Librarian, J. T. Cummins, Metropolis City; Programme Committee, J. P. Buckley, Chicago; Clinic Committee, W. F. Whalen, Peoria; Committee on Science and Literature, E. H. Allen, Freeport; Committee on Art and Invention, C. E. Jones, Chicago; Editor of Transactions, Edmund Noyes, Chicago; Members of Executive Council for three years, C. C. Corbett, Edwardsville, M. R. Harned, Rockford, A. D. Black, Chicago; Local Committee of Arrangements, T. P. Donelan, E. F. Hazell, E. A. Kartack, all of Springfield.

The next meeting will be held in Springfield, May 8, 9, 10, and 11, 1906.

ELGIN MAWHINNEY,
Secretary.

THE

International Dental Journal.

VOL. XXVI.   SEPTEMBER, 1905.   No. 9.

Original Communications.[1]

EXTENSION OF PRELIMINARY EDUCATION *VERSUS* EXTENSION OF THE DENTAL COURSE.[2]

BY R. H. HOFHEINZ, D.D.S.,[3] ROCHESTER, N. Y.

A GREAT deal of agitation has recently been exhibited by all men concerned with the education of dental students. Some acrimonious feeling has emanated from the different aspects of the question, and some schools have directly been accused of insisting on returning to a three years' course, because the life and income of the school depended on the brevity of the course. As in all questions of any kind, much has been said and done in the right direction, and much has been said and done that would better have remained unsaid and undone.

It would be carrying water to the ocean should I speak of the gradual developments of the curriculum at our dental schools; they are a matter of history, and form one of the proudest parts of American University development. In this age of keenest competition, there is in every calling and profession a well-founded

---

[1] The editor and publishers are not responsible for the views of authors of papers published in this department, nor for any claim to novelty, or otherwise, that may be made by them. No papers will be received for this department that have appeared in any other journal published in the country.

[2] Read at the banquet given upon the tenth anniversary of the Society, April 25, 1905.

[3] Professor Operative Dentistry, University of Buffalo.

endeavor to raise the professional standard to the highest possible degree. Sense of honor and personal interest of the honest worker, as well as regard for the public welfare, demand it. The inferior work of the poorly educated endangers, always and everywhere, the material and moral welfare of the community. It prevents the public from attaining the best possible products of labor and the highest accomplishments of the pursuit of science; it causes waste of money on work of inferior value and often jeopardizes life and health, by subjecting them to unskilled hands and poorly trained minds. It fosters insincerity and fraud in competing with thoroughly trained and educated workers, by claiming ability to secure results only obtainable by long experience, close study, and application of the well-trained individual.

These facts create an ever-increasing tendency to suppress the quack in every profession, by establishing, whenever possible, a standard of skill and knowledge as a *conditio sine qua non* for admission to practice. Such a standard can only be established by members of the profession concerned, and from the consciousness of this fact arose the tendency to unite for the defence and preservation of common interests. Schools for the proper training of the dental students were established, and thus opportunities were offered for that high degree of special education which has distinguished so many members of our profession.

About fifty years ago the dental colleges had a curriculum consisting of a two years' course, with a term only of four months. Since then the courses have been lengthened to three years, the terms having grown to seven, eight, and even nine months, and a few colleges have a course of four years.

In a paper read by Dr. Truman W. Brophy before Section I. of the International Dental Congress at St. Louis, he said, " The course adopted in St. Louis, in July last, is of three years, each year to consist of thirty weeks, of six days in each week, exclusive of holidays. In thirty weeks of six days each we have one hundred and eighty days. This multiplied by three gives us five hundred and forty teaching days. The advantage in time which the *seven* months' course of four years has over a six months' course of four years is ninety-six teaching days. The advantage of the four years' course of seven months over the three years' course of thirty teaching weeks of six days in each week, is only forty-four teaching days. The advantage of the three years' course of thirty teaching weeks of six days per week over the four years' course of six months each, is forty-two teaching days." This, gentlemen, seems too trifling to make a great difference in learning, with any willing student of diligence and application.

I agree with Dr. Godon when he said, in the discussion of Dr. Brophy's paper, that we should not consider a four years' course of seven months or six months in its comparative value to the one of three years and seven months; but should only consider a four years' course of nine months. This ideal time will come, but not until all States and schools make their preliminary requirements alike.

Education is like freedom,—only a certain amount of it is good for man, and when beyond that limitation, slavery and over-education commence. The conception of education is most varied and elastic. There is a minimum of education which man and beast have in common. Ditte, in his history of education, says, " The sum of all the active services to be rendered by matured individuals to others not yet enabled to self-preservation, in order to secure their existence until they are able to sustain the same by their own powers;" and a maximum being " the sum of intentional and planned influences of developed mankind on the development of others not yet or less developed than their educators." Nature attributes the former to parents assisted in mankind by society. The latter is divided between parents and school,—its centre of gravity lying in the school, the only one of interest to us at present.

The meaning of school education is twofold: (1) the development of humanity to the characteristic of mankind; (2) instruction and training in arts and sciences, necessary for performing a part of the work on which each being depends for its subsistence, its happiness, comfort, and progress. The former begins with our birth and ends with death. Life remains the most permanent teacher, taking all of us to task, either sooner or later, for any carelessness in learning its lessons. The second is the task of the professional school. Proper training must prepare us for both this and the school of life.

The vast difference between the savage and our refined artists, poets, and scientists, lies in the difference of impressions made by the same objects on different minds by means of the very same sensual organs. The school of man must open our eyes for the

evolution of nature and mankind; it must teach us to analyze and
detail our sensual impressions; it must strengthen our power of
observation, concentration, logical conclusions and expression; it
must cultivate a sound mind in a sound body.

All skill and knowledge the school imparts to us must have
this end in view. Our public school must, in the first place, be
an elementary school of preparation for the higher school of life.
enabling us to understand its lessons and profit by them.

The history of education tells us that the neglect of early training of the senses and physical and mental faculties was connected
with a low degree of culture and civilization in knowledge, science.
and art, and also in morals; while the gradual rising of education in this line was accompanied by rapid progress in all.

In Germany, a country of the highest standing in science and
learning in modern time, they had, almost to the sixteenth century, no permanently established schools for the instruction of the
people at large but convent and cathedral schools, considering the
education for priesthood the highest aim for any institute of learning. Virgil was, for them, a magician, and the reader of his works
was in danger of being prosecuted for sorcery by the church authorities. The clergy, educated in such schools, incarcerated Gali-
leo for teaching the motion of the earth around the sun. and for-
bade the study of anatomy and medicine.

Latin grammar, dialectics and rhetoric, music, geometry, arithmetic, and astronomy, or rather astrology, constituted the so-called
higher education. The low standard of the university in the
middle ages is strikingly characterized by the fact that, even in
the sixteenth century, professors of the University of Wittenberg
admonished their students, as Raumer tells us in his " History of
Pedagogy," not to be discouraged in the study of arithmetic by
the difficulty of this discipline, as its first elements were comparatively easy, and although *multiplication* and *division* required application, they might be understood by attentive scholars without
great trouble. What would we think of a university the students
of which must be taught the four elementary principles of addition, subtraction, multiplication, and division by a professor who
considers the two latter of great difficulty, requiring close application?

In this sixteenth century, students entering a university had no previous instruction in geography, history, mathematics, etc. Physics and natural history were unknown to them. They knew nothing but Latin and Greek, which they had not learned in order to study the wisdom of the classics or ancient history, but merely to be able to imitate their style of expression. All preliminary education of those times had no other end in view but the cultivation of the faculty of expression in word and script, training its scholars in Latin, the universal language of the educated classes in the middle ages. All learning was memorizing of words and their connection in phrases,—it gave mere forms without substance. Such questions as, " How old was the angel Gabriel when he brought the message to Mary?" " What language is spoken by the angels?" " How could Christ have accomplished the work of salvation if he had come into the world as a pumpkin?" are a few cited by Raumer in his " History of Pedagogy."

Only a few isolated men obtained a higher standing; they became aware of the truth that all science is based on individual observation of things and facts, which requires training and cultivation in the early stages of life. The educational reformers who have emerged from the darkness of the middle ages, men like Luther, Bacon, Locke, and others, have opened our eyes to the fact that popular intelligence is the source of all human progress, and that it can and must be fostered by proper education in childhood.

Only by a very gradual progress school education was reached. It has become the task of the commonwealth (1) to develop in its children the faculties and endowments proper for the real type of humanity; (2) to equip them by proper training with the knowledge and skill necessary for the entrance in a professional school. Education of the first kind it must make to a large degree obligatory; the latter must be optional. Languages, geography, history, arithmetic, the elements of physiology, natural history, and physics have become the general standard of a common-school education. Modern education has added to these instructions both music and drawing, having become aware of the importance of æsthetics for the development of true humanity which is based on both intellect and feeling.

Manual training has also been added, the educational experiments of Pestalozzi and Froebel having shown the immense educational value of an early training in this line by simply using the child's natural impulses to play and imitate. In a paper read at the National Meeting at Niagara Falls, in 1899, I gathered statistics to show the influence of manual training on general learning. The more complete this elementary department of education fulfils its task, the better will be the work of the later preparatory school, college, or university.

A good deal of the instruction now crowded into the high school might be distributed to the lower grades. The study of history, the elements of natural history, and Latin begin in Germany in the lower gymnasium at the age of eight to nine. Drawing is added in the next year; French, in my own school days; now English; the elements of mathematics in the following grade; Greek, the elements of physics, chemistry, and mineralogy before the pupil has reached his twelfth year. Most of these branches are still exclusively crowded into our high schools, thereby making the work of pupils and teachers burdensome, and not always allowing sufficient time for thoroughness and diversification.

When we consider that there is only a three years' course in most high schools, we shall understand that there can be but little time left for special preparation of any kind, and that its extension to four years is therefore an urgent necessity. Dr. Muensterberg, in his "American Traits," says, "At fifteen I was in the Untersekunda, and there is not the slightest doubt that, at that stage, all my classmates were prepared to pass the entrance examinations for Harvard College."

Dr. G. B. Snow, in an essay on dental education, tells us that the proposal was recently made by the dean of one of the best and most successful dental colleges in the country, that the first year be devoted to a line of subjects which are, or should be, taught in high schools, that the student might have a proper understanding of them before proceeding to his dental course. This would mean a correction of the insufficiencies of our high schools, and really implies that the dental course would be long enough if only the preliminary training were quantitatively and qualitatively sufficient and correct.

With some of the subjects now taught at the high schools referred to the lower grades, and with all States demanding a four years' course of high school training, we would be in a better position to classify the students according to the future study they intend to pursue.

Numerous preliminary studies are less essential to the doctor and the dentist than they are to the engineer. Other preliminary studies are only of value to the future pedagogue and the theologian, and would not deprive the medical or dental student of any necessary acquisition or culture for his vocation. Probably no preliminary studies require more, let me say, specialization, than those applied later on to the surgeon and dentist.

Broad culture can only be obtained by the mastering of manifold studies early in life; but, owing to the enormous extension of all individual sciences, we are apt to be taught far too much, which we cannot assimilate to proper advantage later on. If it is necessary to specialize and sub-specialize every profession, it will become equally necessary to specialize in the preliminary education of the future professional man.

Nothing is more essential than to bring the mind to a properly and correctly trained condition, where it will grasp with ease the scientific and technical teachings of the dental curriculum.

I consider the question of extending the course of dental teaching less important than the improved and extended preliminary teaching. Harvard has answered this question in a very emphatic manner.

Next January the requirements of the State of New York, as to preliminary education for the dental student, are to be raised to four years of high school education, or forty-eight counts. This is a decided step in advance, and the only reason the dental colleges of the State of New York have voted against a four years' course at the present time. If all other States had required similar qualifications for entrance into college, the action of the New York Colleges would have been more open to criticism. The great deficiency of this law remains, the fact that these counts may be obtained by passing examinations in any of some seventy-six branches, many of which are irrelevant to the future dentist.

It is certainly a wonderful progress in comparison to the time when the student was asked what language the angels spoke, but it is also a wonderful progress in comparison to the time when the student came directly from the plough and was told that "Levator labiæ superioris alæque nasi" was one of the many anatomical terms he had to remember for some of the smallest muscles of the body.

The higher the level on which the professional specializing begins, the more effective it is, and I believe also that the earlier we begin, the more effective it becomes. As Professor Muensterberg says, "In the kindergarten I should show my little lawyer two cakes, and explain to him that one is his cake and the other is not,—social information which does not lie in the line of my little naturalist; and I should tell the other little fellow that one cake has plums, and the other has not,—scientific instruction which is without value for the future lawyer."

Many students are destitute of the faculties most needed for the dentist because early training in childhood has been neglected. Manual training, especially, has not begun in the kindergarten and continued throughout the common school in concentric circles. I firmly believe that the principles and aims of general and special preparatory education, and their wants and shortcomings in their present state, form the most important subject for consideration in connection with dental education.

Professor Butler, in an essay on the "Function of the Secondary School," says, "One of the best known academies in the United States requires for admission only some knowledge of common school arithmetic, writing, spelling, and the elements of English grammar, and that the average age of pupils on entering is sixteen and one-half years. At this age the French and German boy is reading Cicero, Virgil, and Horace, Sophocles and Plato, Shakespeare and Tennyson, as well as studying general history, solid geometry, and chemistry. It is very evident that at this point there is a tremendous waste in our educational system. It must be remedied speedily, if our higher education is not to be discredited altogether." When this is happily solved, the proper length of the dental course can easily be ascertained and established.

A great deal of that preliminary education must consist of what I have written in a paper on "Manual and Artistic Training," *Dental Cosmos,* 1899, p. 1099: "Together with the training of the mind must be that of the hand and eyes, if we are not destined to that fatalism in operative dentistry that is beginning to make itself so brutally felt. The intellectual stimulus of constructive art is more vigorous than that of literature; we are continually stimulated by the presence of the object and the operations to be performed. The perceptions become clearer, more positive, more precise. It is a great mental discipline; yes, I go so far as to say it is a great moral discipline. It leads to more exact action; it leads to greater honesty, for honesty is but the moral expression of exactness."

WHAT WILL PROBABLY BE THE DENTAL EDUCATIONAL STANDARD FOR THE COMING DECADE?[1]

BY CHARLES C. CHITTENDEN, D.D.S., MADISON, WIS.

At the last meeting of this Section, at Atlantic City, in 1904, a symposium on dental educational standards was read, which was exhaustive and thorough in its character. In a paper presented at that symposium I had the honor to report chronologically the various facts as they had transpired, during the current year, concerning the attitude of the individual dental schools and the National Association of Dental Faculties toward the newly inaugurated four years' college course.

It had become apparent that a large number of the smaller and financially hampered schools were determined on returning to the three years' course.

This Section, at that time, in its discussions, expressed, in no uncertain terms, its entire disapproval of any such retrograde action.

Immediately following the meeting of this Section came the annual meeting of the National Association of Dental Faculties at Washington, D. C., where the whole subject was gone over and discussed very exhaustively, with the final result that, by a close vote of twenty-four to twenty-one colleges, the four years' course was upheld. This occurred in the early part of June. Almost at once following the adjournment the *ad interim* committee began to receive the resignations from membership in the National Association of Dental Faculties of a number of schools which were opposed to the decision at Washington to continue the four years' course.

---

[1] Read in the Section on Stomatology of the American Medical Association, at the fifty-sixth annual session, July, 1905. From the Journal of the American Medical Association.

These resignations created such a panic in the ranks of the colleges that the *ad interim* committee was finally induced to call a special meeting of the National Association of Dental Faculties to be held at St. Louis, July 18, 1904, whose sole purpose should be a reconsideration of the final decision made at Washington, the month previous, to continue the four years' course.

At this special meeting there were, of the fifty-one colleges in membership, twenty-eight represented. By a vote of 26 to 2 (being by a majority of one of the total membership) the four years' course was revoked and a three years' course of thirty weeks in each year was adopted in its place. The public announcement of this distinctly retrograde step (taken by a bare majority of one of the membership of the college association) came as a distinct shock to the rank and file of the profession. There was no semblance of an off-set in the way of increased standard requirements for admission to the course to, in some measure, soften the baldness of the action. The outside world was simply made suddenly aware that the National Association of Dental Faculties, without waiting to graduate a single class or man under the vaunted higher educational system which that body had spent at least three years in elaborating, and had then declared to the world as absolutely necessary to properly fit the student for the dental degree, had, without explanation, struck its colors and surrendered. The one saving phase of the whole transaction was the fact that practically one-half of our colleges had been opposed to the change and had only acquiesced in it " to save the Faculties Association."

The examiners of the United States had been loyally standing behind and ready to protect the schools in their higher standards in every way. To them this bold retrogressive step called for immediate action. A blow had been struck, for commercial reasons only, at the established standards, and struck, too, by our National Association of Dental Faculties! All the schools of the better class had been obliged to yield to the inevitable and lower their standards— all save one, whose noble independence but makes the situation appear the more pathetic.

The annual meeting of the National Association of Dental Examiners was held late in August, 1904, at St. Louis. It was apparent, from the first news of the " retrogression," that something must be done to retrieve the situation before the world, and the examiners rose at that meeting to the occasion. The following report from the Committee on Colleges, preceded by a careful *résumé* of the entire situation, was unanimously adopted:

> Your committee would therefore recommend that this association establish at once, to go into operation not later than the opening of the school year of 1905–6, the educational requirements, for admission to the dental college course, of graduation from an accredited high school or its full equivalent, all examinations of credentials and equivalents to be placed in the hands of an acceptable appointee of the State Superintendent of Public Instruction where not otherwise provided for by law.
>
> In view of the present disturbed and unsettled conditions existing in dental educational circles, and with a belief in avoiding all unnecessary disturbances of standards at this time, your committee would further recommend that no change be made at this time in the present requirements of this association of not less than twenty-eight calendar months of college attendance for graduation.

By what had occurred the trust of the examiners in the ability of the college association to maintain good faith under certain contingencies was so badly shaken that all standing resolutions which in any way interfered were rescinded, and the Committee on Colleges was instructed to prepare a new list of recommended colleges, based on the acceptance by the individual schools of the standards declared in the above report. The work was to be done independently of the National Association of Dental Faculties.

After having spent many months in correspondence and careful conferences with many of our ablest teachers and scientists, the Committee on Colleges issued the following letter to the deans of this country, February 14, 1905:

> In consideration of the conflicting views as to dental educational standards which have existed for some time, the National Association of Dental Examiners at its annual meeting held at St. Louis, August, 1904, deemed it expedient, and necessary for the upholding of such schools as sought to maintain the standards already published to the world as the minimum that should obtain, to declare what educational standards should be required by the State Boards of Examiners as a criterion of reputability of the schools seeking recognition of their output.
>
> This *ad interim* committee, which is also the committee on colleges, was instructed to inform all schools of the action taken, and directed to prepare a recommended list of colleges on the basis of the standards established at that meeting.
>
> Feeling fully the gravity of the duty imposed, this committee has expended much effort in striving to arrive at a basis of fairness to all

interests concerned, in carrying out its general instructions. The chief requirement established at St. Louis was that of "graduation from an accredited high school or its full equivalent" for admission to the classes of 1905–6.

In several schools and university departments this requirement is already in actual operation, and our committee finds a considerable number of other schools desiring to maintain it. All these, of course, will be placed on the recommended list. There are, however, other schools whose deans assert that to enforce at once this advance requirement would work a serious financial injury to their institutions.

The question of what would constitute a proper length of course for graduation from a dental college has always been left by the examiners to the colleges themselves, except that, after a school has announced to the public a certain course as necessary to properly fit a student for graduation, if it for private or financial reasons deliberately lowers its requirements in any particular, the question of good faith and reputability of that school becomes at once a matter for adjudication by every board in the country.

We, therefore, acting on authority of, and, *ad interim*, representing the National Association of Dental Examiners, which is the advisory body of the various State boards in their official acts, respectfully request that you authorize the Committee on Colleges to place your school on the recommended list of colleges by the acceptance of the following educational requirements for students, viz.:

For matriculation or registration, "graduation from an accredited high school or its full equivalent, all examination of credentials and equivalents to be placed in the hands of an acceptable appointee of the State Superintendent of Public Instruction where not otherwise provided for by law," said requirements to be inaugurated not later than the beginning of the school year of 1906–7; and a college course for graduation optional with you of either four years of seven months each or three years of nine months each, this course requirement to be inaugurated the present year, *1905*.

It is to be expected that schools maintaining these standards will be protected in so doing by the several boards composing the National Association of Dental Examiners.

It is the intention of this committee to prepare and to publish the recommended list of colleges not later than April 1 next, in order to give all schools the earliest opportunity to announce these standards to the public. Therefore information as to your decision is desired as early as possible.

Very respectfully yours,

COMMITTEE ON COLLEGES.

The responses have been quite general and, on the whole, unexpectedly satisfactory. It developed that a large number of schools were only too desirous for the establishment of an educational requirement at once reasonable and at the same time so sufficiently advanced as to not only retrieve the unfortunate back step of 1904, but also to place their schools on a permanent working basis so advanced as not to be liable to material change for several years to come. As one dean expressed it, "This higher standard places us in a position to go ahead with our business, and we will not have to change again unless the Faculties' Association goes one better. It has been this uncertainty as to what was coming or what we were going to do next that had troubled me most. Now I feel as though we had something definite before us."

And thus it has happened that, up to this date, the acceptances have far outnumbered the refusals and the new college list is still growing.

The *rationale* of the matter being that while the National Association of Dental Faculties may and has set minimum bounds of requirement for its members, it can not and never will undertake to prohibit any or all of its membership from placing their individual requirements as much higher as they may see fit. The only chance taken by the individual school in so doing is as to the ability of its product to compete successfully in the market with that of the schools retaining the lower standards.

The question, therefore, resolves itself to this: Will the examiners, with the power of law behind them, keep faith and redeem the pledges made by their authority and in their name by their chosen representatives, *i.e.*, stand by and judicially maintain the advanced educational requirements established by the National Association of Dental Examiners at St. Louis in 1904?

The faith manifested by more than a score of our foremost schools and universities in the integrity and honor of the examiners in this respect would seem to be a harbinger of a new order of things which will be, at least, paramount to commercial success in the conducting of educational institutions.

If the hopes herein foreshadowed shall become realities, a new impetus will be given to dental education, a better class of minds will be attracted to our schools, and for many years to come there will be no further disturbance in preliminary educational requirements for entering our dental colleges.

PORCELAIN INLAYS FROM THE CLINICAL STAND-POINT—CAVITY PREPARATION.[1]

BY JAMES G. PALMER, NEW YORK.

I HAVE prepared a few cavities in some natural teeth which will be passed around for your inspection. These cavities are the most common types of those in which I have inserted por-celain. My work in this direction does not seem to me to have been extensive enough to warrant your committee in their request that I speak upon this subject, and the more intricate cavities, especially restoring contour in the incisors, must be left for those who are better acquainted with such work than I am.

In our ordinary every day work on the labial or buccal sur-faces of the teeth, and in approximal cavities of ordinary char-acter and size—at any rate, cavities not of a complicated character —the first step, of course, is the removal of all decay which is to be accomplished with burs or excavators as the operator pleases.

After the removal of this *débris*, the cavity is shaped with *inverted-cone* burs or square-end fissure burs so that the walls shall be as nearly parallel as possible. Burs of these shapes, with square or flat ends, will form a nearly level floor, within the cavity, of quite a uniform depth, and make the angles at the bottom of the cavity fairly well defined. The edges of the cavity should be shaped in graceful curves rather than irregular out-lines. Many a large contour gold-filling has been made less con-spicuous by proper attention to these curves—to the "line of beauty," if I may use the term—especially on the labial aspect of the tooth, than similar fillings, when attention has not been given to this little detail.

This same principle, I think, applies in some degree to por-celain inlays, and for that reason I say avoid irregular outlines. I have also been impressed with the fact that greater care should be given to preparing the floor of the cavity than has usually been done. If this floor is nearly level and the cavity as nearly as may be of a uniform depth, the inlay will be much more readily retained. In this I find the square or flat end of the

---

[1] Read before The New York Institute of Stomatology, May, 1905.

inverted cone, the fissure bur, and the square-edge wheel bur of great value.

Having thus formed the cavity *in the rough,* as it might be called,—being especially careful, if the cavities are small, that they be deep enough to give sufficient thickness to the inlay so that the "shadow problem" shall be eliminated,—I have used, to finish the edges of the cavities, almost entirely, the fine-cut *plug-finishing* burs.

So much of my work has been in cavities of small size that I have not been able to use Arkansas, Scotch, or other stones to my satisfaction. With a peculiar barrel-shaped plug-finishing bur, having different sizes at hand, I have been able to shape the edges of the cavities quite as I desired. I have also used in connection with these burs a large wheel *plug-finishing* bur with a flat, instead of rounded circumference. When new these burs cut surprisingly well, and with them the walls of the cavity can readily be paralleled. Sometimes it may be desirable to use a stone or sand-paper disk to smooth the tooth itself, so that, with this smoothing or polishing on the outside of the cavity, on the surface of the tooth, and close attention to smoothing the edges of the cavity within, the outlines of the cavity will be almost a knife-edge, so sharply will they be defined. I have always endeavored to avoid sharp or square angles within the cavity or on the line of the circumference, preferring to *round* these corners, if that is understandable.

Where cavities extend underneath the gum, a wisp of cotton tightly rolled and saturated with *adrenalin chloride,* has proved in my hands of great value. This cotton can be tucked well under the gum, even to the point of drawing blood, which the adrenalin promptly checks, and if the mouth and lips have been protected with cotton rolls and napkins, one can frequently complete the entire operation without using the dam.

In some of the larger cavities, by reason of the extent of decay or the shape of the cavity, it may be impossible to adhere to the rule concerning parallel walls. Indeed, I think more stress has often been placed upon paralleling than need be. In some of these large cavities a very long bevel may advantageously be made, with a square floor, something like a cork.

The square end and *long* bevel gives a strong hold when inserted.

In addition to the plug-finishing burs of which I have spoken, the very heavy and *very sharp* chisel is often of great value, especially in the larger cavities.

In very large, but shallow, cavities or restorations on the labial aspect of the six front teeth, where abrasion or erosion has extended a great distance toward the incisal edges, and entirely across the face of the tooth, it is frequently impossible to deepen the cavity on either approximal aspect as much as would seem desirable for purposes of retention. In such cases, however, the wall at the gum line and its opposite toward the incisive portion of the tooth may be made nearly, if not quite, parallel, and will be found quite sufficient to retain such inlays if they fit otherwise.

In large contour work on molars or bicuspids, it has always been my aim to have the floor of the cavity as nearly square or at right angle to the walls as possible, and to cut back the edges sufficiently to make them nearly straight, so that the stress of mastication may be directly through the tooth rather than across it.

I have here one model of a cavity in a devitalized right superior first molar. This cavity is on the anterior aproximal and coronal portion of the tooth, and is presented as a practical case. The inlay was made to-day in my office. You will observe that the floor of the cavity is nearly at right angles to the walls. Of course, such a marked square shape could not be obtained in a live tooth.

BUILDING, BAKING, AND FINISHING AN INLAY.[1]

BY DR. L. A. O'BRIAN, NEW YORK.

GENTLEMEN OF THE NEW YORK INSTITUTE OF STOMATOLOGY.—For many years I have been a member of this society, but visit it to-night for the first time. I wish to thank the society for the honor conferred upon me by the committee in asking me to read a paper on a subject in which I have had many years experience: and although I have had the pleasure of demonstrating before many of you, I feel I shall still be able to offer you something new.

My part of the programme to-night is to tell you of my methods

---

[1] Read before The New York Institute of Stomatology, May, 1905.

of building, baking, and finishing the inlay, and so I will devote myself to these subjects, avoiding digressions as much as possible in the hope that the discussions will give me opportunity to go into details which a ten-minute paper does not permit.

I commence by making a statement, which I hope in the discussion to demonstrate, by telling of my first experiments in producing a so-called low-fusing porcelain thirteen years ago, and also by offering fused samples of some porcelains for your inspection.

My statement is that so-called low-fusing bodies are glass with all its objectionable weaknesses, while the high-fusing bodies are strictly porcelain. I shall confine myself to operations with the latter, and must, in consequence, assume that the matrix is platinum.

This matrix I lay carefully in a platinum tray, in which I have an ample quantity of finely powdered asbestos moistened with alcohol.

After shaking the matrix well into the asbestos, I take a spatula and cover the edges of my matrix to prevent any jar or accident from contorting it; and this tray I now place on the front of the muffle of my Hammond furnace to dry, while I am preparing my body.

I take Close's body for the reason that it has, when fused, the closest approach to the color of the dentine of the human tooth and forms a background such as you will find in the human tooth when denuded of its enamel.

By this time the asbestos is dry, and having moistened the porcelain body with alcohol, on account of its evaporating qualities, I begin to build my porcelain inlay by first dropping into the matrix a drop of alcohol, which acts as a vehicle to float the porcelain body into every crevice of the impression.

Great care is taken to prevent the slightest overflow over the edge, and, as the building proceeds, I bring the moisture to the surface by drawing a file backward on the handle of my melting-pan, absorbing it with small strips of blotting-paper. This is now placed in front of the muffle to dry, care being taken not to hurry it, for nothing kills the success of a porcelain operation more surely than to attempt to hurry any part of it, although the temptation to do so is almost irresistible.

When dry the pan is carefully set into the slightly warmed

muffle and the heat is gradually increased to the highest point of the rheostat. What this temperature is I do not know and do not care, for I never depend upon the pyrometer, but prefer to trust to my more experienced eye. After thoroughly fused, I cut off the current and allow the inlay to remain in the muffle until the glow has disappeared in order not to disturb molecular arrangement by a too sudden change of extreme temperature. On removal I have a foundation no more translucent than dentine itself and resembling that tissue very much. Now we come to the question of color, and here I use the low-fusing bodies which can, when so used, be properly called porcelain enamels.

Ash & Sons make the best as far as material is concerned, but the assortment of colors leaves much to be desired, and here Jenkins enamel helps one out.

The objection to any low-fusing body is, that although you may decide upon a sample which exactly matches the tooth which you propose to restore, if your inlay does not have the same thickness as the sample the color will be different. Put more clearly, I mean to say, that one-half dozen pieces of varying thicknesses made from the same shade and melted together under exactly the same condition, will be of six different shades, all of which will be again changed when the cement is put on.

I am desirous of being very explicit, but some things are easier to demonstrate than to explain, as experience must govern the operation.

I take a shade, or a mixture of shades, much more intense than the shade of the tooth, and cover my inlay with an even coating of it and melt. The body of my inlay is opaque, as is the dentine of a tooth, while the glassy enamel carrying the coloring material is semi-translucent, as is the enamel of a tooth. In no other way can you produce a filling which looks the same from all sides, and you can discard the precarious layer experiments and your cement does not change the appearance of the inlay after setting.

We come now to the last step, the insertion of the inlay. I never use the dam in a porcelain operation, especially if the cavity approaches the gingival margin, but by napkins and cotton rolls I keep the saliva from the tooth and dry it thoroughly with warm air. Ames's cement I use exclusively, and mix it just thick enough to be able to retain it as a globule, which does not drop from the spatula, and this is wiped into the cavity and poked about until every part of the cavity is covered and all air-bubbles have been expelled. The back of the inlay is also carefully covered by my assistant meanwhile, after which I place it in the cavity, pressing it home with a piece of smooth, thin tape, which I remove with a drawing motion which wipes away the overflow of cement. My assistant now hands me a piece of waxed floss silk, about one-quarter yard long, and this I wind in a peculiar manner around tooth and inlay, and this silk, by its elasticity, forces every particle of excessive cement out and holds the inlay securely in place until crystallization has been completed. The more thoroughly to protect the operation, I drop melted paraffine over tooth and inlay, and allow my patient to sit in the waiting-room for from fifteen to twenty minutes, when I remove the silk, and the operation is done. A filling should never be ground because, first, if carefully made by an experienced operator, it will not be necessary, and secondly, if it is ground, one changes the surface angles of refraction by so doing, and in some lights the filling or inlay will look changeable.

My mental picture of this operation has for some reason or other taken the form of a corner to be put upon an incisor tooth, let us say a central, and as the man who first produced a low-fusing porcelain (so-called) and who for thirteen years, in a busy practice, became proficient, if I may be so egotistical, let me say that I never produced, or saw produced, with a gold impression and glass body, any such operations as can be produced in the manner which I have described, and the operator will be spared the shame of failures, especially in such operations as involve incisor corners, which, with low-fusing bodies, show after a few days of use a crevice or depression, caused by chipping of the inlay, on the incisive edge which can be entered by the finger-nail.

Glass, as we all know, is dense and hard, but it is also friable, although it may stand a great strain under slow, crushing force, it will not stand a grinding force, especially on incisive corners, where it must form a perfect right angle with the enamel of the tooth at its incisive edge.

Consequently, I advocate the high-fusing, stronger bodies for such cases.

The ten minutes allowed must by this time have expired, and thanking you for your attention, I shall be pleased to answer

any questions and also to explain the different samples I have
with me should they prove of interest to any of the gentlemen
present. Jenkins's fuses at 1552°, Parker's at 2588°, Close's at
2300°.

THE MATRIX.[1]

BY F. L. FOSSUME, NEW YORK.

MR. CHAIRMAN AND MEMBERS OF THE INSTITUTE OF STOMA-
TOLOGY,—At the request of your Executive Committee it is my
pleasure to-night to describe to you my way of constructing the
inlay matrix. I will do this as briefly as possible and not elaborate upon the various methods which from time to time have been
recommended. Simplicity and practical utility of method must
always be the aim, and although it usually takes but a few minutes to construct a matrix, there are occasionally cavities from
which I find it very difficult to obtain a perfect one. At the
clinic before the International Dental Congress I made eleven
matrices, and, without haste, consumed between five and seven
minutes for each. Dr. Stanton was the patient and the inlay can
be seen in his tooth.

Rolled gold and platinum are the metals used. Gold is superior to platinum by being more pliable and not adhering to the
backed porcelain; it can only be used with a body fusing below
1900°. I prefer No. 60, except in very small cavities, where 30
may be used. Platinum has no peer on account of its power to
resist heat and for holding its shape against the pulling of the
shrinking porcelain body when fusing; one-one-thousandth, one-
twelve-hundredth, and one-two-thousandth of an inch in thickness are used.

When the cavity is prepared, a piece of metal of proper size
is cut, and this is of some importance. For large contours it is
well to have as much of the form of the tooth outlined by the
matrix as possible, so as to guide one when building up the inlay.
In other cavities, especially between teeth, broad laps will prevent
the withdrawal of the matrix and otherwise be in the way.

---

[1] Read before The New York Institute of Stomatology, May, 1905.

For adjusting.the thin metal in place in the cavity I have found spunk the best. A piece more than large enough to fill the whole cavity is placed over the metal and pressed gently against it, driving it in until it is well against the floor, and then considerable pressure is used on the spunk so as to swage the metal in place as well as possible. The spunk is now removed and a band of rubber dam is stretched over the matrix and tooth and the ends held by an assistant or the left hand. The matrix can be seen through the stretched transparent dam, held firmly against the edges everywhere, and it will not rock under the final burnishing. For this purpose I use ivory points; my set is composed of ten instruments, which I will pass around for your inspection. You will notice that some have flat points and sharp edges; this is to fit the form of the cavity, which I always strive to have with reasonably flat floor and straight walls or sides. I wish to call your attention to No. 6, which is for finishing the edges, and No. 8 for pressing the inlay in position when setting with cement and in very large cavities for supporting the matrix with the spunk. Gum camphor is often of great help for swaging the matrix into the cavity, as it can be burnt out of the matrix when removed, or dissolved with alcohol while in the cavity, if it is pressed in so tight as to prevent the removal of the matrix.

When the restoration is to be exceptionally large, and when it is very difficult to support the matrix so as to prevent rocking, I burnish the floor and one wall and then bake some porcelain into this, then reinsert in cavity, and, while the other portions are being burnished, this porcelain serves as a support.

The whole secret in porcelain inlay work is the preparation of the cavity, as this must be prepared in such a manner that the perfect matrix can be obtained from it, and at the same time it must support the inlay with the same strength and accuracy as in mosaic work.

If you with reasonable care have tried to construct a matrix and failed to get a satisfactory result, scrutinize your cavity carefully and you will see that the fault lies there and not with your matrix. If your cavities are correctly prepared, it is practically impossible not to obtain a satisfactory matrix, assuming reasonable skill.

Reviews of Dental Literature.

SOME STUDIES ON THE ANATOMY OF THE TEETH AND THEIR
PRACTICAL APPLICATION.[1] By Dr. W. D. Miller (Berlin).

MR. PRESIDENT AND GENTLEMEN OF THE ODONTOLOGICAL
SOCIETY OF GREAT BRITAIN,—It gives me great pleasure to meet
with you again, and I beg to thank you heartily for your cordial
reception.

Under the risk of trespassing too often upon your valuable
time, I have asked the permission to present a few slides for your
consideration, relating to the hard new formations of the dental
pulp. Every practitioner of dentistry is familiar with the fact
that these formations often very seriously complicate the treatment
of diseased conditions of the teeth. The studies I have the honor
to present to you were undertaken under the supposition that
more exact information regarding the frequency, situation, and
character of these formations, apart from the scientific interest
connected with it, would bring about a more thorough understanding of the difficulties encountered and of the manner of dealing
with them.

[Dr. Miller proceeded to throw upon the screen, by means of
the epidiascope, a series of very beautiful preparations and lantern slides from photomicrographs showing hard new formations
of the pulp in varying positions and extents, a few of which he
described in the following manner.]

The hard new formations of the dental pulp occur almost exclusively as secondary dentine and pulp-nodules (pulp-stones, internal odontomes, odontheles, denticles, etc.). The more or less
diffuse calcifications frequently found in the pulps of senile teeth
and in pulps which have suffered from some nutrient derangement
are brought about by a simple precipitation of lime salts in the
organic matrix of the pulp, and are not entitled to the name of
new formations. Secondary dentine may be found in all cases
where the cusps of the teeth have been worn down sufficiently to
encroach upon the dentine, and usually in cases of chronic caries

---

[1] Read before the Odontological Society of Great Britain, May, 1905.

or other chronic irritations. In the first-named position it does not materially interfere with the process of cleansing the pulp-chamber or root-canals. In the case of chronic caries at the neck of the tooth, however, it may be found in such masses as to obliterate a considerable portion of the pulp-chamber. Where there has been much recession of the gums and a chronic irritation of the root, a formation of secondary dentine may be found at the beginning of the root-canal and very seriously impeding the entrance to the same. The next specimen illustrates a case which I, and no doubt many of you also, have occasionally met with in practice. The patient does not complain of acute pain, but rather of an occasional grumbling, so that he is repeatedly made aware of the fact that the tooth is there, and every time he visits his dentist he again calls his attention to it. The tooth will be found to give no reaction on application of heat or cold, and leaves us to conclude that there must be a dead pulp present. In attempting to treat a tooth of this character some time ago, I bored, as it seemed to me, at least half-way to the apex, and failing to come into contact with the pulp or root-canal, I desisted, and filled up the canal which I had bored with gutta-percha. In such cases we have to do with a more or less complete obliteration of the pulp-chamber and root-canal by a new formation of dentine. In the following specimen there is a still more extensive dentinification of the pulp; in fact, every trace of pulp-tissue to within about two millimetres of the apex of the root had been transformed into a dentine-like tissue.

Those hard new formations, designated as pulp-nodules, are found either embedded in the tissue of the pulp (free) or attached to the pulp-chamber or root-canal (parietal), or in the midst of the dentine itself (interstitial). Regarding the genesis of these pulp-nodules, you are no doubt familiar with the inversion hypothesis of Wedl. Wedl supposed that the layer of odontoblasts, through some cause or other, formed a fold, which dipped or projected into the pulp pretty much as the stratum Malpighii does into the embryonal tissue of the fetal jaw to form the enamel-organ. This fold may become detached from the membrana eboris, and is then in a position to form a free pulp-nodule, or it may remain in connection with it, in which case it forms a parietal nodule, which may subsequently become free by the absorption of the neck attaching it to the wall of the pulp-chamber.

This hypothesis is completely at variance with the experience of all who have made an extended study of pulp-nodules. While it is a most easy matter to find pulp-nodules (according to various estimates, from ten to thirty per cent. of all pulps containing them), no one has ever yet found, among the thousands of pulps that have been microscopically examined, such an inversion of the odontoblast layer as is described by Wedl and his followers. Nor have I, in the hundreds of pulp-nodules of varying sizes that I have examined, ever yet met with a trace of any process allied to resorption.

Personally, I have no doubt at all that all pulp-stones are found free and afterwards become attached to the wall only when it encroaches upon them or they upon it.

Pulp-stones may be limited to the crown portion of the pulp, or they may extend far into the radical portion, and I have occasionally found them quite at the apex. A condition is frequently found in senile teeth in which the gradual growth of a number of pulp-stones has led to their coalescence and union with the wall of the pulp-chamber. In all such cases we experience a special difficulty in devitalizing the pulp, as well as in its subsequent removal. The majority of pulp-stones show a lamellar formation.

I may remark, in passing, that it has been my experience that where severe neuralgic pains have arisen from the formation of pulp-nodules these have been sharply angular in shape. I do not know whether this experience could be borne out by that of other practitioners. We all agree, however, that in the majority of cases pulp-stones do not give rise to any disturbance whatever.

I wish to call your especial attention to the section on the screen, made from a tooth in which a large part of the crown had been destroyed by caries, and the softening of the dentine had quite reached the pulp. We see evidence of extensive suppuration, and note that the pulp, apart from forming a number of pulp-nodules, has thrown up a wall of calcific matter by which it has separated the diseased from the healthy portions; a very remarkable process which shows that the pulp of the human tooth has a considerable power of recuperation, and is a strong argument against the practice advocated by many of devitalizing not only every diseased pulp, but even the healthy pulp accidentally exposed in excavating a cavity. This self-protecting process is very common in the tusks of the elephant, and I have met with it now five times in human teeth; one case has also been recorded by Gysi; and it seems to me that, in view of this evident recuperative power on the part of the dental pulp, we ought to be able in many cases to restore those pulps which have shown evidence of but slight derangements to a healthy condition.

The next specimen is also one which merits our consideration. It shows a condition which, I believe, occurs oftener than is usually supposed. Besides a small free nodule and diffuse formation of secondary dentine along the left margin, we see a large nodule which has become attached to the wall at two points. In attempting to cleanse such a root-canal, we might by good luck succeed now and then in passing a fine broach through the narrow canal at the left of the nodule; more frequently, however, it would catch, and if the tooth had been previously treated by a colleague we would suspect him of having left the point of a broach in the canal. It is in such cases always better to take a more charitable view of the matter, and consider, first, whether we have not to do with a condition similar to that shown by the specimen.

The next slide illustrates a class of cases which, in my estimation, are among the most difficult with which we have to deal. We have here one of the roots of a first permanent molar of a child about eight years of age. The apex is still wide open, and although the tooth is so young a number of pulp-nodules have already formed. One of these nodules has become united to the wall of the root-canal, and every attempt to clean out the pulp-canal below this point would probably only result in pushing its contents farther toward the apex, where, in at least nine cases out of ten, it will sooner or later give rise to serious disturbance. The time may come when radiography will be so simplified and perfected that we may be able to detect such a condition of affairs, and, by boring away the nodule, succeed in removing the contents of the canals below that point. At present, however, we are rather working in the dark when we are treating conditions of this character. Under the most favorable circumstances teeth with open foramina are very difficult to treat successfully. We have here, in my estimation, the only case in which iodoform can be used to advantage.

The next slide shows a condition which is often present, and which may be the cause of our lack of success in treating certain cases. It is a longitudinal section through the root of a lower bicuspid, in which the root is much contracted longitudinally, and

there is an adventitious pulp-canal on one side which is inaccessible
to treatment, and may give rise to disturbance at any time.

[Dr. Miller further showed specimens of interstitial pulp-stones
in human teeth, of pulp-stones in milk-teeth, and diffuse calcification of the pulp, in which he called especial attention to a preparation which had been presented to him by Mr. Mummery.]

The following method was recommended for bringing pulp-
stones very clearly into view: Grind the teeth down from both
sides sufficiently to expose the pulp, then harden them in formalin
or alcohol, impregnate with Canada balsam, after the method of
von Koch and Weil, and after the balsam has become completely
hard grind them down to the desired thickness and subject them to
the action of a one per cent. solution of hydrochloric acid for from
one to two minutes. Then wash them and bring them into the
staining solution, and we shall find that dentine and all the calcifications and pulp-stones, and so forth, which are formed in the
pulp, will be stained bright red, or whatever color we have chosen,
while the pulp-tissue remains unstained. You will see also that
these pulp-stones can be brought to view very easily without the
use of the microscope, and without any photography.

[In conclusion, a number of natural sections of the teeth and
jaws of human beings and of animals, which were particularly
interesting from the point of view of comparative dental anatomy,
were thrown on the screen.] Sections from the teeth of the horse,
warthog, waterhog, etc., can be easily obtained by first dividing
the teeth into sections about three or four millimetres thick by
means of a knife-edged corundum wheel about two and one-half
inches in diameter, and then grinding the sections down to the
desired thickness on a corundum wheel about ten to twelve inches
in diameter, mounted horizontally and driven by a motor of one-
eighth to one-fourth horse-power. For holding the sections while
grinding, a piece of hard cork is far preferable to any means which
have hitherto been devised. After grinding, the sections were
brought for from one to two minutes into a two per cent. solution
of hydrochloric acid, whereupon they were washed with water and
stained in eosin, picrocarmine, or triacid. Very good results may
also be obtained by staining in a thin solution of thionin for twenty-
four hours, then subjecting to a concentrated solution of picric acid
diluted with equal parts of water for about half a minute. Striking
results may often be obtained by a simple staining with eosin. The

enamel remains white, the cement becomes red, while the dentine takes on a bluish tinge.

[Dr. Miller referred to an attempt which he had made in conjunction with, and following out a suggestion of, Mr. Mummery, to find a quick and simple method of preserving the pulp in ground sections.] It is a matter of great difficulty to grind sections of teeth and preserve the hard and soft tissue at the same time. To do that we are obliged to impregnate the tooth with Canada balsam and harden it, which takes six or eight weeks. Mr. Mummery suggested the possibility of freezing the teeth and grinding them, and we carried out experiments which were fairly successful. We placed the teeth in a drop of water on the upper side of a metallic box, froze them by means of chloride of ethyl, and kept chloride of ethyl playing upon it while grinding. You see from the sections on the screen that the results are fairly good, but as we were at an expense of sixteen shillings for chloride of ethyl in making four sections, we left off our experiments for the time being. We hope, however, to take them up again later.

I thank you, Gentlemen, for your kind attention.—*Transactions Odontological Society of Great Britain.*

Reports of Society Meetings.

THE NEW YORK INSTITUTE OF STOMATOLOGY.

A MEETING of the Institute was held at the Chelsea, No. 222 West Twenty-third Street, New York, on Tuesday evening, May 9, 1905, the president, Dr. C. O. Kimball, in the chair.

The minutes of the last meeting were read and approved. The subject for the evening was " Porcelain Inlays from the Clinical Stand-Point."

Dr. J. G. Palmer read a paper entitled " Porcelain Inlays from the Clinical Stand-Point—Cavity Preparation."

(For Dr. Palmer's paper, see page 582.)

Dr. F. L. Fossume read a paper on " The Matrix."

(For Dr. Fossume's paper, see page 588.)

Dr. L. A. O'Brian read a paper on "Building, baking, and finishing the Inlay."

(For Dr. O'Brian's paper, see page 584.)

DISCUSSION.

Dr. H. W. Gillett.—Dr. J. E. Nyman's recent article advocates the combination of high- and low-fusing porcelains. Dr. Nyman's device of a small depression in the floor of small cavities at one end where it would seem to define the position of the inlay, otherwise difficult to place correctly, is of value.

Dr. Ames requests that his cement be allowed to get wet as soon after the setting process begins. This being the case, why use varnishes or keep the patient sitting round with the rubber on.

I use silk or grass line for maintaining pressure on inlays, and think wedges likely to dislodge them from their exact seat. Dr. Head's suggestion of using a separator and then letting the tendency of the teeth to return to place hold the inlays in their proper position, is a valuable point to remember. I am not convinced as to the desirability of porcelain in the posterior teeth except for unusual conditions.

Dr. H. L. Wheeler.—It is especially interesting to hear one who was interested in making the formulæ of the Jenkins body so stoutly assert that the general principles pertaining to high- and low-fusing bodies are, as I have constantly maintained, that the higher the fusing point the better the color and the stronger the material.

The experiment of lining or making the first layers of the inlay of the "Close" body I have not tried, but I believe that this body covered with the Ash & Sons' high-fusing material would make an excellent and strong inlay with great possibilities in shade variations.

Dr. E. A. Bogue.—I showed Dr. Smith an inlay this afternoon that had been in twenty-five years. This inlay was set in the beginning with gum copal, but as that extruded the inlay, it was afterwards caulked on most of its circumference with gold. This porcelain was ground to fit its cavity. One method of holding small round inlays so as to find its proper position in the cavity is to attach it to the end of a stick with wax; it can then be returned to the cavity in the same position it occupied when the waxed stick picked it out.

I do not believe in inlays in crown cavities because they do not wear down evenly with the tooth, hence endanger the teeth later on when perhaps the patient cannot get relief.

I wish to call Dr. O'Brian's attention to the fact that feldspar will melt with all the appearance of glass, if heat enough be applied and the usual amount of potash be present. Hence it was not necessary to show the action of extreme heat on substances not designed to be subjected to such a degree of temperature.

The statement that porcelain fillings are "infinitely more lasting than gold operation hammered in" is also misleading. Time enough has not yet elapsed for us to know how lasting porcelain in approximal fillings may be. I have lately seen five gold fillings forty years old that were not hammered in, and three of those cases were pulpless teeth with the roots filled. These have lasted longer than any porcelain fillings, up to now.

Dr. L. A. Faught.—I am very much interested in this subject and have reached the conclusion that it is not necessary to undercut the inlays in setting. Etching them is sufficient.

One of my early experiences in the construction of porcelain tips was a case involving the six upper teeth. When I did this work I was somewhat of a pioneer, and I found difficulty in inducing the material to fuse so as to build up and out to the shape of the teeth. I think that the little forms which were exhibited here this evening, made by Ash & Sons, would have been a great help.

Adjourned.

FRED. L. BOGUE, M.D., D.D.S.,
Editor The New York Institute of Stomatology.

ACADEMY OF STOMATOLOGY.

AT the regular monthly meeting of the Philadelphia Academy of Stomatology, being the tenth anniversary of the founding of the society, a banquet was given at the University Club, Philadelphia, on the evening of April 25, 1905, at which many prominent members of the profession were guests. The President, Dr. I. N. Broomell, introduced Professor R. H. Hofheinz, of Roch-

ester, N. Y., who read a paper entitled " Extension of Preliminary
Education *versus* Extension of the Dental Course."

(For Professor Hofheinz's paper, see page 569.)

Dr. R. H. Hofheinz.—I rise with a feeling of profound sorrow
for you all. If the Latin adage, " Plenum venter non studet
libenter," which means that a full belly does not like to study, is
true, I think it is also true that a man who enjoys a good dinner
does not like to listen to dry discourses afterwards. It is almost
an infliction, and if any one of you suffer from dyspeptic troubles
to-morrow, I beg you to charge it to Drs. Kirk and Darby. It is
the fault of Dr. Kirk that I came here, and the subject is the
fault of Dr. Darby. I am almost afraid before you get through
you will all feel like the cook who had been employed at the Ox-
ford University. A number of the students complained to the
dean, saying, " We cannot stand John's cooking any longer." The
dean finally went to the cook and said, " John, the students are
complaining about your cooking; they say it is very bad." " Never
mind," replied the cook, " they tell me just the same thing about
your lectures, Mr. Dean."

(The paper was then read.)

DISCUSSION.

Dr. Broomell.—We have listened to this very instructive paper
on dental education and I take pleasure in calling on Dr. E. C.
Kirk, who will open the discussion.

Dr. E. C. Kirk.—I am sure that I voice the general sentiment
of the Academy when I say that we have listened with extreme
interest to this thoughtful and suggestive paper by Professor
Hofheinz. It is extremely instructive, and I feel that there is no
question before the dental profession to-day so great in its possibilities and so pregnant with results to the future as the question of
education. I was called upon at the last moment to open the discussion of this paper, and I have only had opportunity to glance
hastily through it this afternoon, in the midst of distractions, so
that I have hardly had time to digest all that has been brought
before us; yet there are some points which have fastened themselves in my mind, and to them I would like to direct your attention.

I wish to say, in the first place, that I am in general agreement with the argument which the essayist has presented, but I wish to go perhaps a little farther. I want to call your attention to the difference in the attitude of human thought regarding what constitutes education as between our present period and that period to which he referred as the period of the middle ages I doubt, unless you have gone into the subject with some care, whether you have a clear conception of the state of mind or condition of human education at the period to which the essayist has referred in the sixteenth century and even later, and as an illustration which may serve to fasten in your thought the attitude of those who were considered educated at that period, I have brought with me to-night the original record of a controversy which flourished just at the close of the sixteenth century relative to a matter which comes very near to us as dental practitioners. In a book which I have here, which is a German translation of the original publication which appeared in London in 1595, we have the record of an investigation made by a learned professor of medicine and a teacher of his art, with reference to a phenomenon which occurred in Silesia, Bohemia; this phenomenon was the case of a boy of whom it was said he had erupted a golden tooth. To investigate this phenomenon the learned doctor made a pilgrimage to the town where the boy lived and personally investigated the boy's mouth. Having satisfied himself that there did exist in his alveolar border a tooth which was golden in its texture and appearance, and having satisfied himself by various tests that it was *de facto* a golden tooth, he wrote the account and learned treatise which I hold in my hand. In this treatise the author not only stated it to be a fact that the boy did have a golden tooth in his jaw, but he goes farther, and enters into a long and learned philosophical discourse to explain this wonderful natural phenomenon. It is not necessary for me to go over the details of it, but his conclusions were about as follows: The tooth was a supernatural thing in its origin; that it portended the return of the golden age: that because the tooth appeared at a time when certain astronomical conditions indicated or threw corroborative light on the case, it clearly portended that the whole world should be converted to the doctrines of Christianity, the return of the golden age and the ultimate overthrow or downfall of the Turkish Empire. I hold in my hand, again, a learned treatise written by a professor in a Scotch university, twenty years after the publication, in which he tears the whole fabric of the phenomenon to pieces, destroys the arguments of his predecessor, and shows that the father of this boy was nothing more than a mountebank, and that while there was a golden tooth, it was merely a shell crown or shell of gold placed over the tooth, and that there was nothing supernatural about it.

These two books are only two of a series of at least six or eight books that were published by learned men at that time dealing with that particular incident in that way. Think of it for a moment! That was only a little over three hundred years ago. It was a hundred years or more after the discovery of the American Continent by Columbus. In that period it was possible for men justly regarded as the learned men of their time to indulge in such fantastic speculations.

In the intermediate period a great change has come over the mind of humanity with reference to what constitutes education. Professor Hofheinz has clearly shown in his paper that the education of the middle ages was not education at all. It was an education that, I might say, was upon an inflated basis, inflated by ignorance and with little or nothing to give it a basis of truth. They concerned themselves with discovering what language the angels spoke, how old was Gabriel when he made the announcement to the virgin Mary, and other things which have been referred to. Now, we are questioning whether there are such things as angels, and developing an attitude of mind that is not satisfied unless it can be brought face to face with demonstration. That change has largely taken place since Herbert Spencer, fifty years ago, asked his epoch-making question, "What kind of education is of the most worth?" Education simply as an adornment is giving place to the education of usefulness which is derived from the study of observed phenomena.

In the past half-century since Spencer asked that question, we have seen the development of what has been called the scientific attitude of the mind toward the question of human knowledge.

Now, getting closer to the question involved in the title of the paper, and applying to it, as we may well do, Mr. Spencer's question, "What kind of knowledge is of the most worth?" we have to consider, as I understand it, the relative value for dental education of these two propositions, whether it is better to increase the preliminary requirements, or to increase the length of training in technical dentistry of the professional course. It is true, I believe, that improvement is necessary, is needful in the preparation of the mind for dentistry, and I would say that our whole system of preparatory education needs improving. The sentence quoted from President Butler, of Columbia University, of which I have here an abstract from the essayist's address, is as follows: "One of the best-known academies of the United States requires for admission only some knowledge of common school education, arithmetic, writing, spelling, and the elements of English grammar, and the average age of the pupils is sixteen and a half years. At that age the French and Germans have read Cicero and Socrates and Plato. It is very evident that at this point there is a tremendous waste in our educational system which must be remedied." Higher education is not to be discouraged, but we should concern ourselves with the question of this tremendous waste in our system of education and endeavor to stop it. I have, after a careful and thoughtful consideration of the matter, come more and more to believe that the "tremendous waste" is not so much in what children are instructed as it is in the manner of their instruction; it is not so much a question of how much they learn, but of how well they learn what they are taught. It is a question of method rather than of amount, or quality rather than quantity.

We are prone to say that education is the most important thing. I was interested in the reports of the recent yearly meeting of Friends in this city. Some of the questions propounded on this very problem of education they have been treating with that thoughtful consideration for which they are justly so well known, and it was asserted by some of their speakers that we are not sincere in this matter when we say that education is the most important thing. Do we, as a matter of fact, do the best, the utmost that we can do for the education of the young? Is it true that those who are devoting their lives to education are selected with reference to their ability, and are they given sufficient compensation to attract to the profession of teachers those who are qualified to teach, to educate? These are very important things. If we look over the records of the municipal system of education and compare it even with private schools, we find that the amount of compensation for teaching is meagre, and it does not bear favorable comparison with what is paid ordinary clerks. Many teachers who are engaged in teaching the young have less compensation than

23

you pay to the cooks in your kitchen, and with that as the case you cannot attract those most capable of carrying out this work. On the other hand, we have the opportunity to judge of the system of preparatory education by the character of the product that comes to us as the material upon which we are to begin our work as educators for the dental profession. Some careful observation of that matter, some few years of experience in the study of the product which the high schools are turning into the dental colleges has convinced me that the system of education even in our high schools is also imperfect. There are indications there also of a waste of time in the matter of method and quality of instruction. The high school graduate is old enough to reason and to think precisely within the limits of his knowledge, but he comes to us as a confirmed memorizer, not as a disciplined thinker.

Let us bear in mind that education is not what a man knows, but it is the reflex of that knowledge expressed as character and the ability to use the increased power which education brings, which is the real educational result. I know in my own experience that many men who come to us even after high school graduation are wofully deficient in many points, and especially in knowledge of their mother tongue. Not a small proportion of the men who come to us from the high school to-day are ignorant of the elements of the English language. They have not that clear mental conception of the use of words which enables them to use words intelligently or to comprehend the meaning of words when they hear them spoken or read them. Therefore, I believe that the English teaching of our preparatory schools is deficient.

I would call attention, further, to a point which the essayist has brought out very markedly in his paper,—that the question of manual training is one which should be part of the preparatory training not only of the student who goes into dentistry, but should be a part of the education for students of the preparatory school in all departments. We have only begun to conceive the possibilities of manual training and its value; we speak of it sympathetically because we realize that it brings increased skill; but it means much more than that; it is a system of mind training, it is a system of nature study, a system of impressing on the perceptive faculties concrete things and not ideas about things. It is a system of education along the lines of least resistance. Therefore I would emphasize the necessity of manual training, not only for its value in producing finger-skill, but especially as a method of mind training. Dr. Hofheinz spoke approvingly of the advance step, as he calls it, which is to be taken by the regents of the city of New York with reference to increasing the number of academic counts required by law before a man in the State of New York may be permitted to enter a dental college, and that a four years' high school course will be required instead of a three years' course, and yet to my mind he neutralizes almost in the next sentence the value of the step by stating that these forty-eight counts may, in the future, be made up by selection from no less than seventy-six different subjects.

It seems to me the thing to be considered is not the quantity of things that a man may know, but how well he knows a certain number of selected things. I think the utilitarian idea in education is an essential point to be considered, and the training of the prospective students in lines which will subsequently be of use to them in taking up the dental course. I do not wish to be considered as being in a hypercritical attitude toward this question. I am in a critical attitude, but I do not wish to be regarded as an iconoclast,—of tearing down an existing system without offering a suggestion for its betterment. Therefore, in prescribing a course of instruction for a prospective dental student, I would first have him trained in his own language, and that means that he shall not only know English, but he shall also know some other language. I am a believer in the principle which was laid down by Goethe, referring to the study of languages, when he said,—

> " Wer keine fremde Sprache spricht,
> Kennt seine mutter Sprache nicht,"

which means that he who does not know a foreign language does not know his own. He should at least know one foreign language. I would have him know history, that is to say, the general history of the world's development. He must know something of history from its sociological stand-point. He must know mathematics, and why? He must have it for the development of the faculty of precise reasoning and the proper perception of magnitudes. He must learn it to be a fact that two and two make four, and not three and a half or five,—make four and nothing else. He must know science, at least a smattering; he should know enough of it so that he shall be able to comprehend the great fundamental generalizations of science. I plead for a science training so that he may get rid of the last fragment of superstition or mysticism about his work, and because from the training in science he shall be trained to observe phenomena and to assay them at their true value, and not on the inflated basis of ignorance or superstition or mysticism. If he has English, a training in mathematics, a knowledge of history, and a grounding in science, I will trust him to develop well under the dental course.

I have not yet come to the point of the essay. As I comprehend it, the essayist puts before us the problem as to whether it is best, under the circumstances, to lengthen the dental course and hold the preparatory education as at present, or to first increase preparatory education and hold the technical training at its present point. I believe in both of them. I think we need both things. and we need them very badly; but what I have said with reference to the difference between the quality of the preparatory education and its quantity I think will explain my position on that point. I believe it is quite possible, if our preparatory systems of education were so intelligently reorganized as to complete the course of training in three years of high school work, it would be sufficient to fully prepare men for studying dentistry; but to change the existing system of preparatory education is a task to which the cleaning out of the Augean stables would be a mere bagatelle. Possibly we shall have to live another generation before the necessity of changing the present system of preparatory education is realized so that efficiently trained students may be turned out from our schools in a minimum period of time.

I plead for the increased length of the dental course. The argument which has been quoted from the address of Dr. Brophy, that four years of six or seven months is less than a three years' course of nine months, is a specious argument. It was held up by those who advocated the establishment of a four years' course, that if we had four terms of any number of months, we would by that act have fastened the course down to four separate years, and then those institutions which desired to do so would have been able to maintain their four terms of nine months each, and there was nothing to prevent them from doing it. It is true that comparison of four years of six months to three years of nine months is to the disadvantage of the four years' course, but with four annual sessions those who were in favor of the four years' course would have been able to maintain satisfactorily the four annual sessions of nine months each.

I think we need the four years' course of instruction. The total amount of knowledge, the accumulation of data with reference to dentistry, that which constitutes dental knowledge to-day, cannot be put into the head of a dental student so that he can retain and utilize it in less time than four years. We are doing the best we can under the circumstances, but every one of us knows that we could do better with a four years' course of training. I have been told that the late Samuel D. Gross, years ago, when president of the Board of Trustees of the Pennsylvania College of Dental Surgery, was at one time in the institution waiting for a meeting of the trustees to convene, when, incidentally, a plumber's assistant came into the room with a kit of tools. Dr. Gross said to him, "Young man, how long does it take you to become a plumber?" He said, "Four years' apprenticeship." "Why," he said, "come around to the Jefferson Medical College, and we will make a doctor of you in two."

Is it not a wonderful condition of affairs that it takes less time to make a dental practitioner, who, if he is a conscientious man, must know the structure of the human body, its composition and its functions, thoroughly and well, and must erect upon that foundation a special technical training necessary for him to apply the science of dentistry in his profession, to know all that and to make a professional man in less time than it takes a plumber to become proficient. Are we acting sincerely in this matter? I think not. "A stream cannot rise higher than its source" has been said very truly. The source of this question of education is the attitude of the dental profession with regard to it, and just so long as the dental profession at large is willing to stand idly by and see men unfinished in their education turned into the ranks of dentistry, just so long will inferior education be the standard. When they are ready to take that up by enacting a standard that shall be in the form of a statutory law forbidding that these things shall be done, then we shall have a high standard in dentistry.

Dr. Wilbur F. Litch.—I wish first to thank the society for the kind and courteous invitation to be present this evening at this its tenth anniversary, thus giving me an opportunity to enjoy a most pleasurable evening and to listen to the excellent paper of Professor Hofheinz.

My individual society activities have been associated with another society of this city, one which has the distinction of being the oldest dental society in the world, and as a member of that organization I desire to extend to the Academy of Stomatology the felicitations of the old Pennsylvania Dental Association, the mother society, upon this auspicious occasion, and upon the success, prosperity, and usefulness of the Academy of Stomatology.

I have listened with great pleasure to Professor Hofheinz's paper, and the pleasure was the greater because the paper was not a controversial one in any sense, and because it was, as we might well have expected from its source, distinguished by clarity and breadth of vision. Its author has gone into the fundamental principles of education, and has shown us very clearly in what we are lacking in this country. As a teacher for more than a quarter of a century, it has been my fortune to have under me as dental students a large number of gentlemen from the other side of the water, especially from Germany, and I can testify, as can every other instructor, to the general superiority of their educational preparation over that which characterizes the average American student. The magnificent public school system of Germany is at once an honor to that country and somewhat a reproach to our own. It is the crowning glory of Germany that she has a school system so broad in its conception and operation, and so fruitful in results. German students come to us with trained minds, and, notwithstanding the difficulties of listening to technical instruction in a foreign tongue, grapple successfully with the subjects put before them. Not that they are ignorant of our own language by any means, but when they come here they are necessarily without that degree of skill which can only be acquired by considerable training of the ear.

We, in America, have advanced very markedly to-day beyond what was the standard a few years ago, when, as Dr. Kirk has remarked, a plumber's assistant could be taken into a medical school and graduated in two years, but much still remains to be desired. The enforcement of a uniform advanced educational standard for all sections of the country is attended with almost insuperable difficulties. This is a very large country. It contains many classes of people with varying social customs, standards, and possibilities. We have in the southern section of our country States which are just emerging from the devastation and wreckage brought about by civil war, States in which the educational system was very meagre before that conflict, reaching only a small percentage of the white population and, of course, being almost entirely withheld from the negro. These States are to-day doing heroic work in building up their educational system; but it can only be after long years of effort that education can be made as general and as advanced as in the Northern and Western States.

Dr. Hofheinz, in his address, spoke of high schools as having in a majority of instances not more than a three years' course. Not very long ago I obtained from official sources a list of high schools in the State of Pennsylvania having a four years' course, and to my very considerable astonishment the list embraced nearly two hundred schools. I had no idea that Pennsylvania was so rich in high schools. My enthusiasm was dampened, however, when I learned from the same official source that "except in a very few cities, the high schools are very small, with one, two, or three teachers, with courses of study not much, if any, beyond the grammar school course in Philadelphia." The explanation of this anomaly is that the amount of appropriation obtainable from the school fund of the State is dependent on the number of courses given, so the courses are multiplied, although the curriculum is not correspondingly extended. As is well known in Pennsylvania, we are, as compared with many other States of the Union, very backward. It has been officially stated that Pennsylvania stands twenty-third in the list of States as regards high school facilities and money expended for high school instruction.

There is, however, a determination to better this condition of things. As you are aware, the State Legislature has just passed a law by which the public education of the city of Philadelphia is largely taken out of the hands of politicians and placed in the hands of men who will devote their time and attention to education entirely free from political influences. The appropriation for schools has been fixed at a definite sum, and we can hope for a rapid improvement in educational affairs both in the city of Philadelphia and State of Pennsylvania.

These facts, of course, have a very important bearing upon the question of raising the standard of preliminary education as a requirement for admission to the dental schools. Desirable as it would be, I regard it as practically impossible, for the reasons I have stated, to enforce at the present time an entrance requirement, uniform for all the States, much higher than the present standard, a completed two years' high school course. Dental and medical schools are becoming more and more local in their attendance, and cannot successfully keep much in advance of the educational standards and possibilities of their constituency. Nevertheless, I am heartily in sympathy with the view of Professor Hofheinz that the elevation of that standard is the matter of primary importance in dental education. As Dr. Kirk has stated, many of our students holding high school certificates or diplomas come to us sadly deficient in power of analysis and in knowledge of the value of words and the correct use of the mother tongue. The fault is not with the dental college, but with the preparatory school. Colleges must accept students as they come to them and receive educational certificates at their face value. That manual training is not more general is another defect in our common school system. A professor in one of our Philadelphia manual training high schools recently remarked to me that he thought such schools a mistake; that manual training should be a part of every high school course and not restricted to special schools. The training of eye and hand in constructive work he regarded as a valuable educational asset for any boy. He thought, moreover, that the institution of special schools for manual training had cast a sort of stigma upon their students, the students pursuing the academic high school course regarding them as distinctly lower in the scholastic and even the social scale than themselves.

When we come to consider the real objects of education, we can hardly improve upon the analysis of Lord Bacon, that "studies are for delight, for ornament, and for use."

The student who engages in hard study simply for the delight it affords him is, I think, in modern life, very rare. Acquiring culture for culture's sake is not a pursuit which now appeals to the many. There is still a large contingent who take up studies simply as an adornment, to be able to say they know this or that language or that they are graduates of this or that school; but the fundamental thought of modern education is largely the utilitarian one. The high school diploma or degree in art or science is not only becoming a matter of social adornment, but the necessary equipment for a man who would succeed in life; and young men are more and more fully realizing that the great prizes of life even in commercial pursuits are going to the high school or technical school or college men. When this fact is once fully understood, we will have begun to build up upon utilitarian lines an educational system worthy the name. That time is rapidly aproaching, if not already here, and I look forward to the next few years as a period to be marked by the most rapid development in educational interests throughout the country, and have no doubt that as a reflection of that we shall be able in a few years not only to greatly advance the preliminary educational requirements of dental students, but if demanded by advances in dental art and science to still further extend the course of college instruction.

At the present time, I do not see the necessity for giving our students more physiology or chemistry or anatomy or materia medica than they are already receiving. The general consensus of opinion of those who advocate the four years' course is that it is required not so much for advanced theoretical as for further technical instruction, for another year of training in the manipulative process of operative and prosthetic work. If that, under existing conditions, were a practical thing, if it were possible to take the third-year student and pass him on to the fourth year, giving him a little further drilling in theory, but for the greater part of each day keeping him busy in practical work at the chair, then, I would say, by all means, give him the four years' course; it would be money in his pocket, for he would go out better prepared for his life work and more assured of success.

The difficulty in the city of Philadelphia, where we have a number of dental colleges and any number of "dental parlors," is to obtain patients, and it would be practically impossible to keep the fourth-year students busy at the chair each day and still do justice to the second- and third-year men.

We might, by display advertising and other dental parlor methods, make our clinics equal to the further demand, but that would be derogatory to the dignity of the school, a violation of professional ethics, and an injury and injustice to the dental profession of Philadelphia.

Conditions in the future may change, but at the present time that is my great objection to the four years' course.

Dr. Kirk.—Dr. Litch referred to the desirability of the advanced preliminary requirements. Before he relinquish the subject I should like to have him explain what his idea is regarding advanced preliminary requirements, whether the kind of subjects or the quality of training?

Dr. Litch.—My opinion is that they ought to be subjects, if not strictly germane to dentistry, at least in some degree aids to its study and practice as an art and science.

Dr. Inglis.—Dr. Hofheinz has opened the question whether preliminary education should be increased or whether the course should be increased, and in his paper he referred metaphorically to the education of boys. He would offer to two boys two cakes; to the lawyer he would offer one supposed to contain pabulum which would fit him to become a lawyer, and to the other, destined to a commercial life, he would offer a cake containing commercial pabulum. Now, boys in knickerbockers, or even older boys, often have no idea of pursuing the profession of dentistry unless their fathers happen to be dentists, and in the event of a sudden determination to enter upon it they must depend upon their general training.

With reference to early training with a special object in view, I am reminded of a question asked of Dr. Oliver Wendell Holmes as to how early a boy's education should begin. He replied that it should begin about a hundred years before the boy was born. I suppose he meant by that that his forebears, after a thorough education, would transmit a certain quality of mind which would enable him to take in pabulum which would probably fit him for his future work. Now, that a good preliminary education is of great value to a man in whatever walk of life he may take up I think will be granted by any one here. The fairest flowers undoubtedly come from cultivated fields, but the question arises whether the men and women entering the dental profession come with sufficient cultivation for us to take them only from those cultivated fields. We have a certain course for these men; we invite them to come and take the course with us, and we are compelled at present to accept within limitations such material as these persons bring to us. That, of course, brings up the question presented by Dr. Kirk as to the quality of their preliminary education. We are to decide as to whether those presenting have sufficient knowledge to enter the dental college. It is within my own experience at our own school that men have presented themselves who had not quite sufficient preliminary education to enter the college, and it was suggested by Dr. Singer that these men should take the general course, but make up certain subjects which were material; in other words, they entered with conditions.

Some of these men have become exceedingly good students, who turned out to be good mechanics, capable of acquiring the so-called theoretical branches. Now, if the standard of preliminary education had been rigidly enforced, they would have been rejected at the entrance examination. Of course, grossly incapable men should be prevented from entering the profession, but it is a question whether many apparently insufficiently educated have not sufficient intelligence to be received, with great hope of eventual apprehension of their subjects, and I wish to emphasize that point.

I think the New York State requirement of a sufficient number of counts earned upon a variety of subjects is a fair test of intelligence. After all, it is the only important thing, the ability of a man to apply his knowledge, which makes him proficient.

With respect to knowledge of foreign languages, I had occasion not long ago to raise a question in my own mind as to the word " post-extraction." We have had the word " post-mortem" for a long time, and I asked several college-bred men, one of them a Yale graduate, how to best construct the word. I also asked a gentleman who teaches Latin, and I got from him a dictum that " post-extraction" would be a very bad word, that it would be a combination of an English word with a Latin prefix. I asked another, and he had a different idea, and so it went on.

Bearing upon this I recall an incident which happened in my own family. At the time I was in South America acquiring some knowledge of the Portuguese. I sent for my family to come down, and on the way out my wife met a gentleman who was highly educated and who spoke six or seven languages. She told him I had advised her to study as much Portuguese grammar on the way out as she could. He said, " I would not do that; I would study French first. A knowledge of French will help you a great deal in your Portuguese." Now, then, we will suppose the word " star" in French and Portuguese. I question very much if the knowledge of the French word " etoile," or the Latin word " stella," would be of any great help in acquiring the Portuguese word " estrella."

In studying for my examination in Portuguese before the Dental board of Rio de Janeiro, I found that my familiarity with Latin names was of much value, but they were acquired from a study of them at the dental college, and not because I possessed any great memory of my Latin studies at school.

It seems to me that at present the best thing for the prospective dental student to do is to get as much education as he can and then go to college. I firmly believe that while a man should have a fair degree of education, it matters not so much what he has acquired, provided he is able to take up the study of dentistry intelligently, and the course should be so arranged that after he is once in, it will be difficult for him to get out, so that he may be as well educated in dentistry as possible.

As to whether the course should be lengthened depends, I think, on the man. It seems to me a three years' course is quite long enough for some men and not enough for others, and if that course can be arranged so that it will give a student the essentials of dental education, and if he is capable of acquiring these essentials in a course of three years, he should be permitted to go before the State Board, and if he is not prepared for that he should be held back until sufficiently proficient.

It seems to me that there is another important matter to be thought of, and that is the charges of the schools for dental education. I think college fees for education in dentistry are entirely too low when compared with other private school instruction. If the fees were raised to one hundred and fifty or one hundred and seventy-five dollars it would do more toward elevating the standard of education in our dental colleges than any other one thing.

Dr. James Truman.—If I understand the drift of Professor Hofheinz's paper, it is that it is essential to have a higher preliminary education. My experience has been that the higher the preliminary education is, the less satisfactory will be the dentist. Last year, in preparing a paper on this subject for the Dental Congress, I took the trouble, at the University of Pennsylvania, to go through the lists of those who had taken the practical course in the first year of the high school, the second year of the high school, and finally the diploma of the high school, and I found, by taking the average examination in the practical branches, that the men who had only the first year of the high school were as good as the men who went through the four years and received the high school diploma. The higher you go in preliminary training will there be less ability at the end of the fingers to accomplish practical work.

A great deal has been said here regarding the German schools. No one has a higher estimation of the German method of teaching than myself, because I was brought into close contact with it during a residence in Germany, and I am prepared to assert that in my opinion it is the best educational system that the world has ever produced, but the men that come over here from Germany to our schools with this highest education are defective, as a rule, in technical ability, and the reason is that they are too old when they begin to study dentistry. It is not their fault. The preliminary education has not helped them one particle in their practical work.

Allusion has been made by Dr. Hofheinz to the colleges of fifty years ago, and of the course then of four months. We had five months at that time, but all the students, so far as I remember them, had from three to five years with preceptors in dental offices before they matriculated, and then had superadded to that two years of college training, and those men, as a rule, have made a record in their profession quite equal to those with modern training.

I am not in opposition to preliminary education, but, on the other hand, am a strong advocate for the best possible, but I do not want it at the expense of practical ability.

I was surprised when the assertion was made that if we had four years, and the last year entirely devoted to practical work, that it would be absolutely impossible to give a hundred men practical instruction. We are doing that day after day in the University of Pennsylvania, with a hundred chairs filled all the time, and we could carry that on for the next five years if it were necessary to do it. There is something wrong somewhere.

This is a profound subject and I would like to talk on it more than five minutes, but I know very well the hour will not admit of it. We want the four years. The idea has been suggested that it is possible to secure as much from three years of a certain number of months as you can out of four years, but I believe that to be a fallacy. With the mass of study to be digested, it is utterly impossible to accomplish it in three years. The practical must be sacrificed in order to carry the student through the term. The men who brought about this change from four to three years are responsible for lowering dental education in this country.

Dr. Robert H. Nones.—Dr. Kirk's mention of Professor Gross's statement to the plumber that he would graduate him in medicine in a couple of years would have been more applicable had Dr. Gross told that plumber he could be taught dentistry in a couple of years, for the reason that the plumber had practical experience, and that is what counts.

Dr. Truman touched the point which occurred to me,—that is, the immense change which has taken place in the teaching of dentistry, even in my time. But a few years ago men took up the preparatory course with a preceptor, and Dr. Truman spoke of those men becoming better dentists than those of to-day. Why? Because very many of the men who were never fitted in any possible way to continue in dentistry and go to college were dropped before they reached it. Their preceptors very kindly told them to take up something else. To-day the colleges get many men who would not have entered the profession under the earlier method.

Then there is another point that has not been touched upon, and you have probably felt a little hesitancy in doing so, but, to use a very common expression, " colleges are not run to save souls." They are conducted, at least, to meet their expenses and to teach dentistry to the best of their ability. If the dental colleges were so endowed that they could select just what students they wished, what a grand thing it would be for the teachers, the profession, and for the public as well, but unfortunately such is not the case.

If I lived in New York State, I could most heartily agree with Professor Hofheinz in his belief, because the law compels us to do so many things we would not otherwise do. The law of New York says that you must do this, but the law of Pennsylvania and that of other States does not do so. For that reason, possibly, I cannot entirely agree with him. If I were not associated with college work at all, I might also agree with some of the expressions frequently made about colleges.

Dr. Inglis touched on a point relative to " students applying to the different colleges who should not be admitted without the proper preliminary credentials." I would like to ask if we have a right to turn away those who desire to study dentistry because they have not all the requirements? It becomes a serious point and a very vital one. Have we the right to refuse to teach a man dentistry because he has not at that time these preliminary requirements? I think that any one will admit that good environment, as a rule, tends to make better men. I have seen two dental students, one not having these preliminary requirements, —and have been surprised to see how that man has advanced, while the other, who possessed them, proved worthless. Dr. Truman also said that the "best-educated men make the poorest dentists." He does not mean any one to understand that, all other things being equal, the educated man would not turn out as good. I think, under the conditions stated, the man with the better education would certainly turn out the better dentist, but in ninety-nine cases out of a hundred, where he possesses the higher education, he has, in nearly every instance, sacrificed manual dexterity. Does dentistry rest entirely with the brain, or is most of it accomplished with the hands? Which of the two must be sacrificed, if either? These are points we naturally should consider.

I did not for a moment expect to say anything upon the subject, but am somewhat compelled to answer the charge of lowering the four years' course. I do not feel responsible for the three years' course, but we felt that a four years' course was not necessary. In advocating a return to the three years' course we could not have been absolutely in error, inasmuch as institutions which we all respect accepted the shorter course.

We had no intention of lowering the standard of dental education. If there is a school that is endeavoring and has endeavored in the past to advance dental education, to uphold the laws, and make better laws in the State of Pennsylvania, it is the institution with which I am connected. Whenever a four, five, or six years' course seems to be practical, there will be no college more willing to adopt it than ours.

We can make of some applicants dentists in a year, and others cannot be educated in fifty years. Some can be made with a grammar school education, and others not with a collegiate education.

The President called on Dr. Hofheinz to close the discussion.

Dr. Hofheinz.—It is too late to detain you any longer. I agree entirely with Dr. Truman that too much education will make a poorer dentist. I dwelt on over-education in my paper. This really is more or less a continuation of a paper which I read some years ago before the National Society, where I specified what I meant by preliminary education. It is not a question of quantity, but a question of quality, and that is precisely the fault I find with the forty-eight counts. I did not mean seventy-four subjects, but seventy-four branches. English counts for twelve, German three, French three, Latin four, science of all kinds eight, history eleven, other studies twelve, which make seventy-four branches, and not seventy-four subjects. That was a misunderstanding.

What would it avail dentists to know civics or economical history, commerce, home science, and such subjects. It is a satisfaction to have these, of course, as preliminary education, but they are irrelevant to our profession.

Dr. Truman said the reason why the older practitioners were made dentists after two years was not because they had more preliminary education, but they were selected by their preceptors. They were told, You are, or you are not, fitted to become a dentist.

Two or three years ago I had a student, an M.D., and it took him two years to determine the difference between a round and a square hole.

With respect to English, I am reminded of a story. An Hungarian said to an American, " Your English is very difficult. You have such long terms; for instance, you say ' inconvenience,' five long syllables." The American asked him how he would say it, and he answered, " Netlikaplongcheck."

Specific education ought to begin early in life. The child should be taught as early as possible, so that the teacher can train it and lead it to the profession where his natural abilities indicate. If the boy is unable to use his fingers in kindergarten work, he will probably not make a dentist; and if he has manual skill in the kindergarten, he may make an excellent surgeon or an excellent dentist, but may make a very poor preacher.

Dr. Kirk remarked that teachers are compensated too poorly to make ideal teachers. In the secondary schools the teachers are poorly paid, and frequently are of poor quality. The time will come when the American schools will be upon the same level with the European schools, but not until they have been separated from politics will there be an advance in this system of education.

I have been handed a question to answer: If four years are required for dentists, how much time should be given for medicine? That is a question I would not like to answer offhand. Some time ago a gentleman asked me, " If you were a member of a committee in Albany or Philadelphia, and some one offered you two million dollars to do nothing, what would you do?" I said, " I would sleep over it."

In conclusion, permit me to thank you for the invitation to be present and the good time I have had.

On motion, a vote of thanks was tendered by the Society to Dr. Hofheinz and to Dr. Litch for his discussion of the paper.

OTTO E. INGLIS,
Editor Academy of Stomatology.

THIRTY-FIFTH ANNUAL SESSION OF THE NEW JERSEY STATE DENTAL SOCIETY.

THE thirty-fifth annual session of the New Jersey State Dental Society convened at the Auditorium, Asbury Park, Wednesday morning, July 19, 1905.

After the usual preliminaries of opening the session, the President, Dr. W. G. Chase, M.D., D.D.S., of Princeton, read his address. This was brief, and referred to matters of local interest only. The society then, after considering various business matters, adjourned until evening.

At the evening session, Dr. Sinclair Tousey, of New York, read a paper upon " The X-Ray and High Frequency Currents in Dentistry," illustrating by lantern slides the various applications of the X-Ray in dental diagnosis, and a number of instruments to facilitate its use in dental radiography. After reading his paper, the doctor demonstrated his dental fluoroscope, an instrument that is practically a mouth mirror and fluoroscope combined. While it does not reveal to the observer minute detail as does a successful radiograph, it will, in many cases, show all that is required at a glance, and render unnecessary the labor and technical skill involved in developing a photographic film. At present, the required apparatus is somewhat cumbersome; it is expensive, and requires for its proper use a measure of technical skill all dentists do not possess. It is not likely that it will long so remain. We may confidently look for this new aid in accurate diagnosis to become, in the near future, so simplified as to be available to every progressive dentist. Dr. Tousey's dental fluoroscope is a step in that direction.

MORNING SESSION, JULY 20.

Dr. Robert H. M. Dawbarn, of New York, was on the programme to read a paper upon "Adenoids." He had his paper with him, but preferred to lay it aside and make his remarks extempore. Fluently, and in a very interesting manner, he proceeded to give a history of the step by step unravelling of the mystery surrounding and the baneful effects attributed to these growths since they were first recognized some thirty-six years ago. No abstract can do justice to his clear and instructive explanation of their origin, the anatomical peculiarities of the parts near which they are found, and the reasons why their presence as an irritant, as an obstruction, or as an aggravation of diseased or abnormal conditions is so marked and far reaching. He minutely described how they are diagnosed, and laid especial stress upon the more noticeable signs which indicate their presence. Inability of a very young infant to continuously nurse usually indicates the presence of adenoids; the nasal passages being partly closed, the infant is compelled, after a few efforts, to stop to breathe. Later in life may be noticed mouth-breathing, a peculiar facial expression, and changes their presence brings about in the maxilla, the relation of the maxilla to the mandible, and in the arrangement of the teeth. A change in the voice, and more serious and far-reaching disturbances, mental and physical, due to their interference with respiration, are noted later.

He spoke at length of the general prevalence of adenoids in cities on the coast-line, suggesting that this was due to climatic conditions, to frequent and sudden marked changes in humidity and temperature. Some children seem to be afflicted with them almost from birth; he had removed them from infants of but a few months. He advised their prompt removal as soon as discovered, under a general anæsthetic, preferring for this purpose "ether." In the case of very young children, he inquired of the mother when the child took the usual mid-day nap, and selected that time for the operation, operating at the child's home. On arriving, he cautiously, and noiselessly, approached the sleeping infant, and, with care not to disturb it, administered a minute dose of chloroform. This acts quickly, the little patient passing quietly from normal sleep to partial anæsthesia without being aroused, —inhaling a few drops is frequently sufficient. This is followed by ether until the full anæsthetic stage is reached. The operation is then performed, and after it is over the infant is returned to its couch to find its nap. On awakening, it scarcely knows that anything unusual has taken place. Careful attention to diet for a few days, and the little one's trouble is over. By this procedure the child is saved the fright from which it otherwise would have suffered before the operation, and the reaction following this excitement. For this the mother is duly thankful.

He was not favorably impressed with the use of cocaine in this operation, preferring a general anæsthetic. He directed attention to the profuse hemorrhage frequently attending the removal of adenoids, and to the care necessary to prevent this becoming a serious complication. This he controlled by the application of very hot water. He dipped a napkin in boiling water, and after lightly wringing out the excess of water immediately applied it to the parts. The patient, being under an anæsthetic, felt no pain; it acted promptly, and he had not in any case seen any but beneficial results follow its use. It had been suggested that the application of water so hot would be followed by sloughing; this he had never seen.

He urged the importance of prompt action in all cases of adenoids; they never get better of themselves, and it is very important that they should be removed before they have caused structural changes that will be permanent, or have set up a diseased condition difficult to control, or it may be incurable.

He next referred to the tonsils, which frequently are involved, or are a complication in cases of adenoids. They may be the seat of operative procedure as the result of adenoids, in connection with them from causes not due to their presence, or on account of abnormal or diseased conditions peculiar to the tonsils themselves, and in cases where adenoids are not found. He described minutely the anatomy of the tonsils and their surroundings, pointing out the special features which make these glands so liable to give trouble, and which so greatly favor microbe invasion. He made the broad distinction between operations for the removal of adenoids and operations upon the tonsils. While the first rarely, if ever, results fatally, the latter is much more serious, and has repeatedly compromised life. This he urged as another reason for the prompt and thorough removal of adenoids, lest its neglect should make necessary the more serious and more dangerous operation. He objected to the use of cocaine when the tonsils are to be extirpated on account of its causing contraction of the tissues, which may lead to some portion of the organ being overlooked, and necessitate a second operation. If a local anæsthetic is used he preferred beta-cocaine, which, while equally efficient as an anæsthetic, is not open to this objection. Hemorrhage, in operation upon the tonsils, is frequently dangerously profuse. The danger is not alone from blood flowing into the air-passages, etc. The abstraction of blood, especially if the patient be anæmic, he considered more dangerous to life than the so-called surgical shock, especially when it comes from, and lessens the normal blood-pressure in vessels concerned in the proper nourishment of the brain. This hemorrhage can be controlled, and in many cases may be absolutely prevented by first ligating the gland in a manner he described and illustrated, but which cannot be explained without a diagram.

The subject presented he considered proper for discussion by a dental society. It is one of much importance to the dentist, and to the stomatologist, not solely because it concerns territory adjacent to that especially under dental care, but rather because the dentist far more frequently and more carefully examines this field than does the medical practitioner. His opportunity and his special training enables him to quickly detect abnormal conditions in and about the oral cavity, and whether or not he undertakes their treatment, he should be able to appreciate their character and importance. By announcing the presence of such as require prompt surgical interference, he not only renders his patient an excellent service, but advanced his own reputation with the community, and the standing and importance of the profession he honors.

The discussion added but little of importance; it, however, enabled the doctor to elucidate some points upon which further information was desired, and to know that his remarks were fully appreciated.

THURSDAY EVENING, JULY 20.

Dr. A. W. Harlan, of New York, read a paper entitled " Food in its Relation to Teeth—Their Sockets and Adjacent Structures."

The paper was somewhat lengthy. It brought up to date matters which have been in the past frequently discussed. The essayist made free and discriminating use of information derived from experiments recently made at Washington, to determine by actual tests under exacting scientific control the value of various foods, the effects of food preservatives upon the human economy, and the relation of diet to nutrition.

To counteract the probable effect of reading a somewhat prosy paper, the doctor ingeniously followed it by a few humorous lantern slides of subjects presumed to be related to that of his paper. It was well done. The slides and his witty remarks were well appreciated.

The discussion was along lines that developed nothing especially new. The paper, indeed, was not one that could be profitably discussed by those who had not made of the subject a careful and continued study. It will read well, and will be instructive.

This was followed by the reading of a paper upon "Sensitive Dentine," prepared by Dr. C. S. Stockton, who, on account of recent illness, was unable to be present. It detailed a method the doctor has recently been using with satisfaction for obtunding sensitive dentine, in which dryness and warm air seemed to play an important part.

These four papers completed this portion of the programme.

Of the fifty-three clinics on the programme, the writer saw but few. Probably the most novel, and the most instructive, was a collection of anatomical sections of the head and face from the museum of the Dental Department of the University of Pennsylvania, presided over by Dr. F. A. Faught, of Philadelphia. These were made by Dr. Cryer during his study of the anatomy of the head and face with special reference to the various cavities which so frequently become the field of surgical operations. The human head has been "sliced" into parallel sections showing, graphically, the exact relation, at all points, of its various parts as could be done in no other way. This instructive exhibit was made much more so by the lucid explanations Dr. Faught was able to give of its purpose, and of the various points of dental interest invisible in an undivided skull, many of which are but imperfectly shown in anatomical plates. Indeed, until Dr. Cryer devised this method of investigation they were but imperfectly known.

The manufacturers' exhibits were not equal to the best of

former years. This was due, no doubt, to the extra effort to display their goods made so recently at the meeting of the Pennsylvania State Dental Society, in Philadelphia. They were, however, numerous and instructive, and proved a convenience to those living at a distance from the large cities.

The Ransom & Randolph Company, of Toledo, Ohio, had a new anæsthetic apparatus by which it is said prolonged anæsthesia can be maintained without loss of consciousness. This is said to have been in use, experimentally, for several years, and to be safe and satisfactory. 'It is known as "Weisell's Airoform and Airoform Appliance." The Airoform is a proprietary preparation consisting of chloroform, cologne spirit, amyl nitrite, and oleum unonæ. The apparatus is so constructed that the exact proportion of the anæsthetic and atmospheric air passing through it can be determined; this is so regulated that sufficient only of the anæsthetic is used to produce the desired effect,—insensibility to pain without loss of consciousness.

Dr. Brinkman, Chairman of the Clinic Committee, has overcome the difficulty so frequently encountered, of providing chairs for operative clinics. An ordinary steamer chair is fitted with a head-rest. A box to contain it when folded for packing, is furnished on one side with cleats to hold the chair in position, and serves as a platform on which the chair stands when in use. This box will hold not only the chair, but also a folding-table, a basin, a water-pitcher, and a cuspidor—a complete outfit. When in use, the chair, table, cuspidor, basin, and water-pitcher provide each operator with a very serviceable and convenient suit of furniture that, with a white paper table-cover, looks neat and inviting. The outfit is quite inexpensive, and packs not only into a small compass, but into a form that is readily and safely stored with the least possible loss of room, and when needed is quickly unpacked, and easily handled. The society has provided a number of these, and has thus happily solved the chair question. They were used for the first time at this session, and well filled the bill.

WILLIAM H. TRUEMAN.

Editorial.

THE CONVENTIONS AT BUFFALO.

THE conventions held at this season of the year are, in one sense, a professional thermometer, indicating, through the rise and fall of the spirit manifested, the temperature of the national body. It may not always be truly indicative of the character of the impulses governing the entire number of the 25,000 practitioners in this country, but, while possibly defective in this respect, it is the only standard of judgment we can use as the years go by.

The present period seems to mark an advance as far as the National Dental Association is concerned, for, notwithstanding there were many criticisms regarding its value, these, it seemed to the writer, were not altogether just. The papers presented were, upon the whole, of better quality than we are generally called upon to hear on similar occasions. Yet, while this is true, there should be a greater cultivation of the critical spirit in those having charge of this matter and eliminate all essays that have not, at least, a flavor of originality.

It was given out that the experiment of holding but one section daily would be tried. Why this was not done is not known, but it was unfortunate that the opportunity was not grasped. The experience of running several sections at the same time had been tried previously at the Columbian Congress and at St. Louis, and had in each instance proved a dismal failure. The holding of one section daily promised good results, as it would have brought all together at the same time and place, and virtually would have become a general meeting. The officers controlling this matter should seriously consider this problem, and either abandon the sections absolutely or else arrange these, as stated, and confine the essays to the number necessary to fulfil the daily needs of the association.

The number in attendance was larger than expected. The counter attraction on the Pacific Coast, and the State conventions at this season, necessarily kept many away, yet the interest was sustained from the first day to the last. The climatic conditions were all that could be desired. The cool weather was particularly grateful to the parboiled denizens of the Atlantic Coast, and this contributed not a little to the energy and life of the meeting.

It was unfortunate, in some respects, that the clinics were forced so far away from the general meeting-place. The Buffalo Dental College was, however, well adapted for the purpose, and the crowds in attendance attested to the interest. This contributed, in a large degree, to reduce attendance at the sections and general meetings. Unstinted praise must be given to Dr. Wedelstaedt for his untiring labor in producing one of the best managed clinical exhibits it has been the pleasure of the writer to see. From the lower floor to the upper the rooms were filled with workers. It is rare to find so many fine gold operators brought together as upon this occasion. This was especially satisfactory in view of the fact that the porcelain craze has, for some time past, thrown the old reliable methods somewhat in the shadow. We cannot afford to lose any of the good things that have been proved of value in the past.

Valuable as these clinics are from a practical view, they must become a serious problem for the future in connection with dental conventions. With the divided interest between clinics, trade exhibits, and sectional meetings, something must suffer loss. The interest, with the average operator, lies naturally with the practical. and the meetings are more and more taking a second place, and the scientific side of dentistry is a sufferer thereby. The solution of this serious matter is not, at present, attainable. The Section on Stomatology, American Medical Association, has settled this question for itself, but in eliminating all practical matters it has developed a one-sided dentistry, excellent in itself, but impossible as a means of perfecting dental practitioners.

The National will meet next year at Atlanta, Ga. It was necessary under the rules that it should go south next year, and this city seemed the most available place. Meeting in the early September is, in the view of the writer, a grave error. Very few members from the North will be able to attend at that period. The vacation time is practically over, and few will care to extend it beyond September 1.

The most important matter decided upon by this national body was the decision to publish a journal as the organ of the association. This matter has been under consideration for the past two years, it having been placed in the charge of a committee at the meeting held at Asheville, N. C., in 1903. This committee was unable to report in 1904, as the National Association passed its regular meeting in deference to the Fourth International Dental Congress.

The report was very fully considered in council, and was finally sent to the general meeting, and it was there unanimously decided in favor of establishing a journal independent in character and representing the interests of the dental profession in this country. A committee of five was appointed to arrange for the early publication of this journal upon a permanent financial basis. It is probable that this committee will mature its plans during this early fall, so that the journal can be launched on its career of hoped-for usefulness at the beginning of the year.

The National Association of Dental Examiners held its annual meeting at Buffalo, but, as these meetings are held with closed doors, it is always difficult to learn the result of its deliberations. As far as the writer was informed, the conclusions were about as Dr. Chittenden has outlined in his paper published in this number. The association, it is understood, made it very clear to the dental colleges that they must come up to a certain standard and, failing in this, would not be regarded as acceptable institutions. Up to the close of the meeting some twenty-two colleges had accepted the conditions. If there be no further additions to this list, it will leave twenty-nine colleges in a peculiar position.

The Association of Faculties met in annual meeting, with forty-five members present.

It is difficult to determine the position that this body occupies at the present time. It was very evident that the members felt they had lost strength through the irregular action at St. Louis and were incapable of holding the membership to the rules, as had been the case for the past twenty-one years. The writer introduced a resolution at the opening meeting, with the object of repudiating the action of the meeting held at St. Louis. This was, as anticipated, laid on the table, but one member voting in the negative. This settled the question whether the Faculties intended to abide by its own constitution, violated at the aforesaid meeting. As they decided to confirm that action, they practically destroyed all the rules passed since 1884 for the government of the colleges under its jurisdiction. In doing this they eliminated all power once possessed over the educational institutions in membership.

That this was the feeling was very evident, for the several sessions lacked force. No business of any importance was transacted. The matter of fees claimed attention, and a motion was finally passed to raise the yearly fee to $150, beginning with the session 1906. It will probably be carried out by a few, but concert of action upon this minor matter is not to be expected.

A matter which would have been of vital importance to dental colleges under former conditions was a report from the Committee on Schools, Dr. A. O. Hunt, of Omaha, chairman. This was a very elaborate paper and closed with the following suggestions, "To secure a standard and have it properly administered, so that it will command the support of all interested.

"To select from this body ten persons, whose tenure of office shall be ten years (or, what is better still, for life), to be known as Dental Regents, with absolute authority to create and administer a standard for entering upon dental courses and requirements for graduation.

"That all schools of this association shall be bound by their action," etc.

Under the peculiar ruling of the acting president, a motion to adopt was permitted and carried, with the understanding that it be held over for next year for final action. As each session of the Faculties is a new body, it will puzzle the astute parliamentarians, at that time, to find a way to reconsider a question already decided at a previous annual meeting. It is not, however, probable that this very crude suggestion will pass then, or, if it should, that it can ever be enforced. There is not a dental school of any standing that would submit to any such interference with educational methods.

It is impossible to feel otherwise than discouraged at the future outlook for this body. It has performed a great work for the regeneration of dental education in this country during less than a quarter of a century of existence. The four men who called it into being in 1884 had no conception of the extended influence that this body would exert in the future upon dental education in the United States, moulding it into form and giving it an ethical character previously unknown. The life of all organizations is necessarily limited. The conflict of opinion at no very remote period weakens and causes disruption, and it is, therefore, not to have been expected that this body would have been an exception to the universal rule. It is, nevertheless, a cause of profound regret that it should thus early have entered a period of senile decay. Its power has passed into other hands, and, while it may linger for a time as a moribund body, its moral force in dental educational circles has departed, and those who have the training of young men must seek a broader ethical life for their standard of work.

The hospitality of the dental profession of Buffalo was not the least of the pleasant things that goodly city offered to visitors. Everything was done to make the sojourners feel at home, with the result that there was a unanimous feeling that Buffalo was an ideal convention city, and the dentists within its gates were worthy representatives of the true professional spirit.

THE OATH OF HIPPOCRATES.

WHILE our readers are doubtless familiar with this oath, as usually published in condensed form, the translation in full, furnished by a valued correspondent, and published elsewhere in this number, may be of special interest.

Hippocrates, born on the Island of Cos, about 400 B.C., and dying in Larissa, Thessaly, about 377 B.C., is recognized as the Father of Medicine, probably as much from the high ethical character of this oath as from his writings, voluminous as these were.

The republication of this oath at this time seems appropriate at this season of conventions, for if it have no other object, it will, at least, remind dentists that they are a part of the great healing art, and that the ethical laws, as laid down by the Master, are as forceful in their line of work as in that of general medicine.

There never has been a period when the true professional idea requires inculcation into the dental mind more than to-day. The dental profession is apparently drifting away from the ethical tenets of Hippocrates and absorbing the commercial spirit of the age. The true professional spirit is gradually being lost in the financial sophistries of the hour, practically taught by example in dental colleges, and practised by graduates and practitioners. It is well, therefore, to recall the foundation principles upon which the healing art is founded, and which are as true to-day as they were twenty-four hundred years ago.

Domestic Correspondence.

THE OATH OF HIPPOCRATES.

BOSTON, May 12, 1905.

To THE EDITOR:

Sir,—Appended please find the Oath of Hippocrates. This, as you know, is the basis for professional ethics to-day. This is the line in which the dental profession is lacking, I think.

HORACE L. HOWE.

" I swear by Apollo the physician, and Æsculapius, and Health, and All-heal, and all the gods and goddesses, that, according to my ability and judgment, I will keep this Oath and this stipulation—to reckon him who taught me this Art equally dear to me as my parents, to share my substance with him, and relieve his necessities if required; to look upon his offspring in the same footing as my own brothers, and to teach them this art, if they shall wish to learn it, without fee or stipulation; and that by precept, lecture, and every other mode of instruction, I will impart a knowledge of the Art to my own sons, and those of my teachers, and to disciples bound by a stipulation and oath according to the law of medicine, but to none others. I will follow that system of regimen which, according to my ability and judgment, I consider for the benefit of my patients, and abstain from whatever is deleterious and mischievous. I will give no deadly medicine to any one if asked, nor suggest any such counsel; and in like manner I will not give to woman a pessary to produce abortion. With purity and with holiness I will pass my life and practise my Art. I will not cut persons laboring under the stone, but will leave this to be done by men who are practitioners of this work. Into whatever houses I enter, I will go into them for the benefit of the sick, and will abstain from every voluntary act of mischief and corruption; and further, from the seduction of females or males, of freemen and slaves. Whatever, in connection with my professional practice or not in connection with it, I see or hear, in the life of men, which ought not to be spoken of abroad, I will not divulge, as reckoning that all such should be kept secret. While I continue to keep this

Oath unviolated, may it be granted to me to enjoy life and· the practice of the Art respected by all men, in all times! But should I trespass and violate this Oath, may the reverse be my lot."—*From " The Genuine Works of Hippocrates," translated by Francis Adams, LL.D.*

TEETH RECEDING IN VULCANIZATION.

BUFFALO, N. Y., August 3, 1905.

To THE EDITOR:

SIR,—On page 563 of the INTERNATIONAL DENTAL JOURNAL for August, there is a paragraph headed " Teeth receding in Vulcanization." As the advice given does not fit the case, may I venture to add something to it?

The phenomenon alluded to is a consequence of the shrinkage of rubber in vulcanizing. It often occurs when it is not suspected, and is the reason why, if it becomes necessary to remove a gum section from a vulcanite plate which has been worn, there will be found under it an exceedingly malodorous and nasty magma of particles of decaying food and mucus. To demonstrate this shrinkage, let a small cube of rubber be vulcanized in a plaster mould. say half an inch in size, carrying the temperature not above 280° or 300°. The time must, of course, be lengthened accordingly. It will be found impossible to. do this, and preserve flat sides to the cube. One or more of them will be concaved, unless the temperature has been high enough to render the rubber spongy. By a specific gravity test, the vulcanite will be found to have from three per cent., for pink, to six per cent., for black rubber, more density than the rubber compound before vulcanization.

To overcome the difficulty, if the plate does not call for a very thick layer of vulcanite, use a flask which is closed by spring pressure, and cut a gateway which encircles the plate. with no leaders passing to the cavity of the mould in which the plate is to be formed. Cut away all the surface of the plaster. except a narrow margin, not over an eighth of an inch wide, around the mould. Then the rubber in the mould is imprisoned when the mould is closed, and it becomes very difficult to entirely close the flask. It is not necessary to close it. The spring pressure on the flask will close it as the rubber shrinks in vulcanizing, with the effect of hold-ing the rubber up against the teeth, and preventing the formation of cavities under them.

For very heavy sets, where a greater thickness of vulcanite is necessary, the flask should be propped open at first by inserting thin pieces of sheet metal, from 22- to 30-gauge, and partially vul-canizing the plate. After about half the time for vulcanizing has elapsed, the vulcanizer should be cooled sufficiently to allow of the removal of the flask, the props removed, the flask immediately re-placed in the vulcanizer, and the operation finished by continuing the heat, after it has reached the vulcanizing point, for the re-mainder of the time.

Vulcanizing in steam is preferable to vulcanizing under water, if for no other reason because the plaster does not soften so much.

Geo. B. Snow.

Miscellany.

Caution: Death from Blood-Poisoning, following Local Anæsthesia for Tooth Extraction.—A case is recorded in the *British Journal of Dental Science* for July 15, 1905, page 664. that deserves more than a passing notice. A woman called upon " an artificial tooth-maker" (this is a new vocation, having its origin in the peculiar provision of the British Dental Act, which forbids those not legally qualified assuming the name of " dentist" without forbidding them to practise the art. To evade this act, the unqualified call themselves " tooth-makers" and " tooth-extract-ors") for the purpose of having several teeth extracted. On the first visit six were removed, and three on a subsequent visit a week later. On both occasions " White's" anæsthetic was injected with a hypodermic syringe. About a week after the second visit, suffer-ing pain in her head and being unable to open her mouth, she called upon a physician for relief. She was then suffering from lockjaw, which continued to the end. Five or six days later a large abscess developed upon the jaw. This was promptly opened and freely drained; notwithstanding this, she developed an acute attack of blood-poisoning, from which she died. At the inquest the operator testified that at the second visit there was a little matter (*i.e.*, pus) around the seat of the previous extractions; that while the wound was not entirely healed, it did not seem to be in a serious condition. He testified that he kept his needles in alcohol to keep them from rusting, and boiled them fifteen minutes before using them again. The testimony seemed to show that the untoward result was due to pus present on the gums near the site of the first extractions being injected into the gums with the anæsthetic used preparatory to the second operation.

Notwithstanding that it was shown that the operator had commenced practice after only six months' instruction, the woman's death was not charged to his incompetency. This was doubtless just, from the fact that the importance of sterilizing the field of operation immediately before making a hypodermic injection is not generally appreciated, nor yet is it generally practised by dentists.

The jury returned a verdict of "Death from blood-poisoning," adding that there was nothing to show how the poison had been absorbed.

It is remarkable that so few cases like this have been recorded, since hypodermic injections for tooth extraction has become so general, and the precautions adopted to avoid this danger are usually limited to sterilizing the needle. Would not a like result be liable to occur were one of a series of teeth or tooth-roots subjected to this treatment preparatory to extraction abscessed?—W. H. T.

For cleansing bridges and regulation apparatuses a saturated solution of caustic soda will prove very efficient. It will render them aseptic. (*Le Laboratoire.*)—C. M. L.

Current News.

FIRST ANNUAL CLINIC OF THE FRATERNAL DENTAL SOCIETY OF ST. LOUIS.

THE first annual clinic will be held November 20 and 21, 1905, at the Barnes Dental College. Special features of the meetings will be a series of lectures on "Cavity Preparation," "Methods and Principles of packing Gold," and "Methods and Principles of finishing Fillings," by Dr. E. K. Wedelstaedt, of St. Paul; Drs. A. C. Searl, of Owatonna, Minn., J. F. Wallace, of Canton, Mo., and numerous other members of the Black and Wedelstaedt Clubs, and other prominent men in Operative and Prosthetic Dentistry will give clinics. Complete programme will be announced later.

All ethical practitioners are invited to be present and clinic. Please send your name and subject of clinic to the secretary. Exhibit space to be obtained by application to the secretary.

A cordial invitation is extended to the profession to be present and make this meeting limited in scope but limitless in importance, the best ever held in this section.

BURTON LEE THORPE, President.
S. H. VOYLES, Secretary,
3201 Washington Avenue.

THE

International Dental Journal.

Vol. XXVI.   October, 1905.   No. 10.

Original Communications.[1]

SOME EFFECTS OF INEBRIETY ON THE TEETH AND JAWS.[2]

BY T. D. CROTHERS, M.D.[3]

SOME years ago, through the courtesy of Dr. Talbot, my attention was called to the degenerations of the teeth and jaws in persons who had used spirits and drugs to excess. General marks of degeneration seen in the head and face and other parts of the body have been commonly noted in inebriates, but we owe to Dr. Talbot the credit of showing that certain of these defects were traceable to spirit- and drug-taking both as an active and predisposing cause.

My work for nearly thirty years has been almost exclusively confined to the study of inebriates from spirit- and drug-taking. This has given me an opportunity to note many facts along these lines and confirm and verify the statements of others. In an analysis of the histories of a large number of inebriates, at least seventy per cent. will be found to inherit from their ancestors neurotic defects and faults of vitality and nutrition. The remain-

---

[1] The editor and publishers are not responsible for the views of authors of papers published in this department, nor for any claim to novelty, or otherwise, that may be made by them. No papers will be received for this department that have appeared in any other journal published in the country.

[2] Written for the Section on Stomatology of the American Medical Association.

[3] Superintendent of Walnut Lodge Hospital, Hartford, Conn.

ing thirty per cent. are traceable to injuries, diseases, bad nutrition, and environment. The first class show marks of this neurotic heredity in defects of the body and deficient vitality. The second class are more prominent in general symptoms of anæmia, starvation, and poisoning.

The brain, nervous system, and functional activities reflect these conditions in many ways. Thus in the inherited class the head, face, teeth, and maxillaries all show degrees of symmetry which point to irregular and retarded growths and faults of nutrition. In the acquired class the faults of nutrition with irregular control and feeble brain function and vigor are prominent.

The direct action of spirits on the mouth and teeth is due in some degree to the rapid water-absorbing qualities of alcohol. Alcohol on the surface absorbs the moisture so rapidly that it becomes an irritant, corrugating the tissue. In the mouth, it has the same effect, which is neutralized in a measure by the excessive salivary discharge.

It has been noted that spirit- and beer-drinkers who take small quantities of spirits, sipping them over long periods of time, have defective teeth and gums, while others who drink spirits with large quantities of water, swallowing them rapidly, do not suffer so much. Persons who use beer and spirits to gratify the sense of taste and enjoy the flavors always suffer from degenerations of the mucous membrane, gums, and teeth. Often such defects are unnoticed until the spirits are withdrawn and the anæsthetic condition which has existed passes away; then the exposed nerves and crumbling teeth call for help.

The use of alcohol produces vasomotor paralysis, by which the circulation of the blood is retarded and deranged. The nutrition of tissue and cell is lowered and impoverished. Added to this there is an increase of toxins with leukocytes and deficient power of elimination; hence both starvation and poisoning follow. The terminal arterioles are deranged and the cell and dentrites suffer from defective nutrition and the irritation from the toxins. I think that the same process takes place in the terminal nerves of the teeth and gums that is noted in the nerves of the extremities in neuritis. There is, without doubt, a very close association between neuritis and dental degeneration, and in my experience they frequently follow each other.

Spirit- and drug-takers who complain of so-called rheumatism.

particularly pain, stiffness of the joints, and defective locomotion, have neuritis and toxæmic states affecting the cell and dentrites at the extremities. The crumbling teeth and shrunken gums is another symptom of what appears to be the same pathological process of acute nerve poisoning.

The toxin of syphilis shows itself often in the faulty growth and condition of the teeth and gums. Lead and other poisons are manifest in the same way. The profession is not aware that alcohol is a toxæmic in its effects on nutrition, and it is only recently that we are confronted with the evidence that alcohol is cumulative in its effects.

The steady use of spirits, even in small doses, such as wine at meals taken with the utmost regularity for a long time, is a source of degeneration that is as clearly traceable as that of syphilis. In physics the continual tapping by a hammer on the hardest steel will after a time break up its tenacity and cohesiveness, causing it to crumble like chalk. In like manner the continued use of small doses of spirits acting on the vasomotor centres, deranging circulation and nutriton, increasing the toxins, and diminishing the power of elimination, produces permanent erosions and degenerations of cell and tissues. Fibrinous deposits and sclerosis of the nerve and tissue are always present in such cases. Metabolism and vitality are slowly and surely destroyed, and this condition is transmitted to the next generation, appearing in convulsive degenerations, recurrent insanities, and morbid impulses for spirits and drugs.

So-called moderate drinkers, who imagine that their temperate use of spirits is a virtue, with increased enjoyment of life, in reality cripple and destroy the next generation by transmitting to them defects that are continuous evidence of the degeneration from the use of spirits.

Dentists as well as physicians are constantly confronted with these evidences of the failure of parents to transmit to the next generation normal vigor and vitality. If associated with the use of spirits, either in excess or moderation, there is hypernutrition, the person using foods in excess, the toxæmic conditions are very greatly increased, and this is seen in the teeth and mouth.

Formerly unthinking physicians prescribed alcohol and drugs as remedies which covered up this condition. Often persons who have local inflammation of the dental nerves find that spirits and drugs give temporary relief, and very soon continue their use and become habitués. The defects of the teeth become intensified, and finally they are removed as a remedy.

Many persons believe that the local inflammation of the gums and teeth was the active cause of the drug addiction. Cocaine-taking is frequently contracted by the use of this drug for the effects on the gums. Other drug addictions may spring from the same cause, but it is evident that the localized effect on the teeth and gums point to some grave condition affecting the entire body, and the spirit- and drug-taking are only culminations of degenerations beginning long before.

Morphia-takers have defective teeth and a general marasmic condition of the mouth. The continued anæsthesia of the sensory centres not only increases the degeneration, but covers up all evidences of it. In some of the opium addictions there is great hyperæsthesia of the gums and teeth; in others marked anæsthesia appears. In most of the persons I see who use this drug to excess the active degeneration goes on in the mouth without any recognition of it, but the moment the drug is removed the condition becomes intensified and very prominent. Occasionally teeth that are sound become the centre of extreme pain. The entire dental nerve and its branches seem to be in a condition of acute inflammation, and even after the teeth have been removed obstinate neuralgias continue. A sudden acute localized inflammation of the dental nerves should be regarded as neuritis with distinct causes, prominent of which are alcohol and narcotics, also lead and mercury. I have met a few persons whose morphinism developed an acute hyperæsthesia of the maxillary nerves. Every effort to remove the drug was followed by a return of the pain and suffering, until finally the case became chronic and all treatment was abandoned. I have seen two such cases who are comfortable while using morphia, but the removal brought on the most aggravating suffering. In one instance reported to me, where the morphia had been removed, a surgical operation was resorted to and the nerve severed, but the pain continued. The removal of the teeth does not always check the pain. The nerve becomes permanently disorganized.

It is an interesting question in the study of the causes to know how far alcohol or other narcotics have had primary or secondary effects on the teeth and gums. Where dental defects existed before drug-taking some constitutional condition existed, usually manifest in that way. Some very unusual cases have come under my observation where profound shocks and derangements of nutrition have resulted in inflammation and erosion of the teeth. The following is an example:

A business man, aged forty-five years, temperate, with no heredity, was made unconscious by a lightning stroke in his immediate vicinity. Invalidism without any distinct symptoms lasted for two months; then suddenly he began to use spirits to great excess, and came under my care. In a short time the craze disappeared entirely, and acute maxillary inflammation began, extending to every tooth of the mouth. There was no evidence of decay, only extreme hyperæsthesia of the gums and tenderness of the teeth. All local and general treatment failed, and he went under the care of a nerve specialist. A year later he returned as a morphia-taker. His teeth had all been removed, but the pain along the maxillary continued except when under the narcotism of morphia.

A second example was a similar temperate business man, in good health up to the death of his wife from an accident. A few weeks later acute inflammation of the teeth and gums, with great sensitiveness to heat and cold in the mouth, came on. Active treatment by a dentist, with the removal of the teeth, was followed by improvement. He then became an alcoholic inebriate. Under my care he was treated with electricity, and recovered both from degeneration of the mouth and the use of spirits.

There was probably in these cases some profound toxæmic condition associated with the psychical shocks in both cases which localized in the maxillaries. I have the histories of several persons who before all use of spirits and drugs had a prolonged period of dental troubles in which nearly every tooth was filled, and later they all broke down. The history of specific taints with salivation from mercury and loss of teeth, than spirit- and drug-taking, are very common. In some persons forms of neurotic exhaustion precede the breaking down of the teeth; then comes spirit- and drug-taking as a local and general remedy.

A very interesting question is frequently asked concerning the effects of tobacco on the teeth and jaws. Evidently cigarette smoking is the most marked form of tobacco that appears to have its specific effect in the mouth, and persons who urge the antiseptic action of tobacco find it very difficult to substantiate their claims from any data known at present. Another interesting fact probably has some influence in this direction, although it cannot be very clearly made out. Thus the perversion and diminution or obliteration of the sense of taste follows the use of spirits. Such persons show abnormal impulses and crave for acids, sugars, salts, and irritant condiments, which influence the nerve terminals of the teeth and the mucous membrane of the mouth and its nutrition. The obliteration of the sense of smell is another factor encouraging localization of acute degeneration of the teeth and gums, or in the liver and kidneys.

I think that it can be clearly established that alcohol taken to great excess, either continuously or at intervals, has a profound influence on the teeth and gums. In paroxysms followed by a distinct free interval in which the anæsthetic effects pass away and a degree of restoration follows, the effects are less prominent. In the continuous use, as before mentioned, the nutrition and vigor of the teeth are always seriously impaired. Of course, there are certain distinct pathologic conditions which may concentrate and produce more serious effects in some particular organ of the body, and the teeth and gums may be one of these locations. The mucous membrane of the nose and throat is another. The liver and heart are also among the organs that register these special effects. Occasionally drug- and spirit-takers exhibit great fragility of the osseous system associated with degenerate teeth. This is probably owing to some faults in the diet, with absence of proper mineral matter and nutrition.

An observation made by the late Dr. Wright, some years ago, has been amply confirmed by my studies,—namely, that when syphilis and alcoholism are combined, degeneration of the teeth and maxillaries is a very common result. Both of these diseases are toxic and the teeth and jaws should be examined for evidence of their influence.

Another observation has been confirmed in many ways, and is this: In certain families, notably those who began with alcohol degeneracy, a marked persistence of diseases of the teeth and jaws is noted, extending through two or more generations and appearing in every member of the family. I have seen two incidents of this in which a great-grandfather, who was an inebriate, was followed by a numerous family, all of whom had defective and diseased teeth in early and middle life. This degeneration continued into the next generation, and was most marked. There were only three inebriates in a family of twenty-six, but every one had degenerate teeth.

I have been told that this form of degeneration is sometimes seen in syphilitic inheritance, and no doubt this is true.

I conclude these observations with a general summary: (1) Spirit- and drug-taking is a very potent cause of defective teeth and gums. It may be stated that a large percentage of degenerations of the mouth come directly or indirectly from this source. (2) Conditions of degeneration which localize in the teeth and gums may be the exciting causes of spirit- and drug-taking. The increasing prevalence and demand for narcotic drugs indicates low vitality of which the vigor of the teeth is a prominent part. (3) A study and correction of the injuries or beginnings of diseases in the mouth may be the removal and prevention of serious drug neurosis which may follow.

ERRORS, MISTAKES, AND FAILURES, OLD AND NEW.[1]

BY DR. C. W. STRANG, BRIDGEPORT, CONN.

MR. PRESIDENT, AND GENTLEMEN OF THE INSTITUTE OF STOMATOLOGY,—In casting about in my own mind for a subject for this occasion, of some that suggested themselves were "Successes and Achievements," and "Errors, Mistakes, and Failures." I have selected the latter, believing it will prove more interesting to my audience, inasmuch as it is the successes and achievements that we hear of or are most frequently recorded in our dental publications.

I congratulate myself that the subject is a broad one; the material is genuine, for it has been personally made, and whatever may be said, I shall hardly be wandering from the text.

While it may be true that too much brooding over one's failures is depressing to mind and body and productive of harm, yet most of us have learned from experience and observation that failures many times have been blessings in disguise and the stepping-stones to success and renown.

---

[1] Read before The New York Institute of Stomatology, June 6, 1905.

The words error, blunder, mistake, and failure, while sometimes used interchangeably, are not synonymous, but in the order named stand somewhat in the relation of sequence, the one leading up to the other.

Recalling my advent as a dental practitioner, without any training along the lines of practical business, the unsuitable light for operative purposes had in the first two offices occupied, the scanty equipment, both at the chair and in the laboratory, my heart goes out in sympathy to any struggling young man who is similarly situated; and the wonder is that failures are not more numerous and success less frequent.

In our early days it was strenuously advocated by some eminent in the profession that if teeth are worth filling at all, they are worth filling with gold.

I absorbed enough of that sentiment to warrant me in now declaring that the experience gained in the manipulation of gold was purchased at a high rate, in so far as the interests of our patients were concerned.

Cohesive gold fillings inserted in the anterior teeth of children twelve or fifteen years of age, no rubber dam, no obtunder, a wooden wedge crowded or driven between the teeth against the gum—the thought of the anguish then inflicted makes us shudder now.

It was a mistake, for in a year or two I had the great mortification of seeing much of that work failing at the cervical border. and had it not been for the operations made in the masticating surfaces of the molars and which generally did fairly well, I would have been left without a reputation, or possibly with a bad one.

Prior to the introduction of the rubber dam the large percentage of failures arising from the impracticability of properly treating and filling the root-canals of posterior teeth, particularly the inferior molars. stimulated experiment along the line of conservative pulp-treatment. Of all the agents employed for capping exposed pulps. oxychloride of zinc received the greatest boom.

We can recall as though it were but yesterday hearing Dr. Atkinson tell how the operation should be made. It ran something like this: Remove the decay from the cavity, prepare cavity as indicated for filling to be inserted, thoroughly dry out the cavity, sop the exposed pulp with creosote,—the creosote unites with the albumin and forms an insoluble compound. That insoluble compound, what hopes we built upon it! Mix the oxychloride to the consistency of cream, place into the cavity, and gently coax it over the pulp. After it has had time to harden put in the filling. Kiss your patient good-bye and all will be well. I took up pulp-capping and tried faithfully to follow Dr. Atkinson's directions, cutting out the kissing part. Josh Billings said, when he heard them sing, " Come where my love lies dreaming," he never went because he did not think it would be right.

What were the results? Just what we would now expect where little or no thought is given to pathological conditions. A few thus treated remained comfortable and retained vitality for longer or shorter periods; but many became so painful that relief was sought in extraction or other treatment. In some instances, where actual exposure had been repaired by a deposit of secondary dentine and conditions promised well, congestion set in, and it became necessary to devitalize the pulp and treat accordingly.

It was the failures of long years ago to treat successfully or give much relief in those cases, where pyorrhœa alveolaris was getting in its work, that gave a stimulus to be thorough in the care of the mouths of our patients, systematically and regularly removing the foreign deposit, believing that under those conditions the dreaded disease would not be as likely to develop.

I have been abundantly rewarded for the time and labor expended in this particular kind of work, though it has not been as fascinating as making gold operations, and not as remunerative.

Personal experience with an exposed pulp in each of the inferior sixth-year molars in my early teens afforded an opportunity to obtain knowledge concerning that malcondition that certainly could not have been procured in any other way, and I also retain pronounced recollections of agonies endured from an occasional accidental impacting of some foreign substance upon a congested pulp.

An alveolar abscess at the root of each of these molars for ten or twelve years afforded an opportunity for the acquisition of more valuable information.

The possibilities lurking in pulpless teeth made such a profound impression upon me that I was stimulated in after years in our examinations to be scrupulously careful not to overlook or fail to locate cavities in obscure places, avoiding as much as possible the necessity of devitalizing pulps.

With the introduction of the dental engine and its equipment, many of the instruments employed in cavity preparation prior to that time have gradually become obsolete, and presumably there are few dental operators who have come into the profession during the last score of years whose instrument cabinet contains a good assortment of excavators, chisels, hand cavity burs, and plug finishing burs; and this we regard as a mistake, and as a result of the mistake more pain is inflicted, frail walls are unwittingly left to be broken down at a later time, necessitating a repetition of the operation of filling.

A few well-directed strokes of the enamel chisel in the hand of the skilled operator will, in a moment or two, effectually remove that which should be sacrificed, and with the infliction of less pain and discomfort to the patient than that produced by abrasive wheels and burs revolved rapidly in the hand-piece of the dental engine.

Again, with the advent of the dental engine the final polishing of the teeth with stick and pumice-stone was very generally abandoned by most operators, and the rubber cups and points substituted for that purpose, and this, in the light of present developments, we believe has been a mistake, and my convictions are deepened and strengthened by almost daily experience and observation.

A recent case in practice, which with your permission I will cite, has a bearing upon this point; and although medicaments were also employed in the treatment of this case, the chief factor in bringing about a normal and healthy condition of the mouth was absolute cleanliness of the teeth obtained by the frequent and thorough use of the orange-wood points carried in the porte-polishers and loaded with pumice-stone.

The case is as follows: In the afternoon of the last Sunday of October a gentleman, by direction of his family physician, called upon me and requested me to treat his wife, who was suffering with a badly inflamed mouth. The case, he stated, had been treated from time to time by a dentist for about three months; but, as it grew worse rather than better, had been transferred to an oral surgeon, who, after a few days' treatment by spraying the mouth, advised the patient to consult a physician, that she might also receive systemic treatment. Under these circumstances the patient decided to return to her home for treatment.

An examination revealed the following condition: The lips and a space extending for a half-inch from the border of the mouth was a solid mass of ulcers resembling very much the fever sores that are commonly seen about the mouths of children. Around all the molars, both inferior and superior, the gums were spongy and puffed and rolled over upon the masticating surfaces of some of them, and hemorrhage was induced by slight interference. The tongue, roof of the mouth, and, indeed, the mucous membrane of the mouth everywhere was thickly studded with ulcer patches. Articulation was so interfered with by the excessive inflammation that it was almost impossible to understand the patient in conversation. The treatment consisted, first, of an application of rose water and glycerin to the lips and surrounding parts, to render them as pliable as possible, then the removal of whatever of hard deposit that was attached to the teeth, and this was not abundant; then about two hours was spent in polishing the teeth with the orange-wood points loaded with pumice-stone moistened with phenol sodique. As each tooth was polished the gum tissue about it was syringed with tepid water.

The patient was directed to rinse the mouth every hour with Phillips's milk of magnesia, every other day alternating with precipitated chalk, 2 parts, carbonate of magnesia, 1 part, mixed to the consistency of cream, a tablespoonful to a glass of water. At the end of five days the case was again seen. No perceptible improvement was observed. The polishing and cleansing was repeated, and the antacid treatment continued. At the end of another period of five days the case was again seen, and the improvement was remarkable.

The treatment as described was continued for one month, at intervals of five or six days, when the patient was dismissed with the mouth in a perfectly normal condition.

In conclusion, I desire at this time to tender to Dr. D. D. Smith, of Philadelphia, acknowledgments for courtesies extended to me nearly two years ago at his office. Also to say that through his teachings came a preparation that has enabled me to treat so successfully not only the case just referred to, but others of a serious, if not similar nature.

About seven years ago a lady, who had been a patient of mine for twenty-five years, consulted me with regard to a pain that she had in the left side of the lower jaw, beginning at about the median line and extending back to the ramus of the jaw. This disturbance had gone on for five or six weeks before she came to see me. There was over the ramus of the jaw a little swelling. The second bicuspid and the first molar had been removed a number of years before, and the lady was wearing a partial plate. The second molar had been badly worn away. I diagnosed the case as probably a dead pulp in this molar. Upon entering the tooth, I found the pulp dead in the anterior but alive in the posterior root. I devitalized the pulp in the posterior root, but to my surprise I could not find any opening into the anterior root; it seemed to have closed. After treating the tooth for a while I filled it temporarily. The pain continued. There was no change, especially in so far as the prominence on the face was concerned. I opened into the soft tissues, but found no pus, only a slight discharge of serum. I said to my clerk, "We have a malignant case here." I wrote up the history of the case and advised the patient to consult a specialist in this city. She consulted with him, with the result that he advised certain treatment, stating that he found nothing of malignancy in the case. She went under the care of her family physician, and I saw nothing of her for a week, when the physician came to me saying that there was pus somewhere in that region, and that if I would open into the pus cavity he would stand back of me. I did not care to go on with the case without having something more definite, so I telegraphed the specialist the opinion of the family physician. He advised a free incision. I met the physician at the home of the patient and made the incision. We found no pus there. The physician said there would be pus in three or four days. The wound was packed with iodoform gauze. On the following day the patient's face was badly swollen, but no pus had made its appearance. I insisted upon getting the advice of another specialist in this city, who also said that he saw nothing of malignancy. He believed it was a case of necrosis, and advised immediate operation. The patient came to this city and was operated upon. The molar tooth was removed. That tooth which was very firm at first, too firm I might say, at the time of the operation had no bone about it. It was removed without using any force whatever. Considerable disorganized bone was removed at that time. The patient remained in New York under treatment. In about six weeks I received a letter from the surgeon stating that he would again operate, and invited me to be present. I could not leave. A specimen was prepared at this time for microscopical examination, and the case was found to be malignant. The patient returned to her home about the holidays and lived until the following April. Somebody made a mistake in this case.

In June last a young man called upon me at the request of his physician. There was a growth under his tongue extending back as far as the second bicuspid on either side. It had been increasing for about a year, and had been, very annoying for the last few months. I think if that case had come to me three years before, about the first thing I would have done would have been to put a knife into it. I know now that if I had done this I would have made a mistake. There was much deposit on the lower teeth. The teeth were thoroughly cleansed. In two weeks there was a marked improvement in the case. In about a month the mouth had returned to a normal condition.

SOME PARTIAL IMPRESSIONS.[1]

BY DR. S. E. DAVENPORT, NEW YORK.

THE advantages possessed by modelling composition over plaster, in some cases, are well understood and appreciated by most practitioners, and, in spite of a rather general feeling to the contrary, the successful handling of composition requires quite as much skill as does plaster.

Among the disadvantages of plaster as an impression material, mention may be made of its lack of firmness and consequent failure to press the soft parts into the position they would naturally occupy under a plate.

The greater one's experience with modelling composition, the more positive is the opinion, I think, that the best results are to be obtained when the least thickness possible of the softened material is used.

This means one of two things, either the cup must conform very closely to the mouth or a preliminary impression of composition must be taken and, after being chilled out of the mouth, cut away slightly over the whole surface for the addition of a thin layer of soft composition for the final accurate impression, the

---

[1] Read before The New York Institute of Stomatology, June 6, 1905.

hard composition underneath serving merely as an addition to the cup to force the soft composition into all inequalities.

While plaster is a more reliable material for impressions of hard upper jaws, when the plate decided upon is to depend for its retention upon atmospheric pressure, the very soft upper gums occasionally met with may be more accurately duplicated by skilful use of modelling composition, and the resultant "suction" will therefore be greater.

It has been my custom for a number of years to use composition almost entirely for the taking of difficult impressions for lower partial plates, the method being the same whether the plate was to be of gold, rubber, or other material.

A composition impression is first taken in a cup which conforms as closely to the desired parts as will any ready-made cup. This composition impression is then poured with plaster as usual, and the resultant model is used for the making of a special cup which will quite accurately fit the parts to be duplicated.

These special impression cups may be made in several ways, two of which I have found most useful.

Exhibit No. 1 represents a swaged cup. A die and counter-die having been made from the plaster model of the preliminary impression, copper plate No. 28 is swaged, then thickened and stiffened by the addition of pure tin flowed over the reverse side with a soldering iron. A wire handle is soldered on, as represented in the one exhibited.

Exhibit No. 2 shows a cast impression cup of pure tin. Upon the plaster model from the preliminary impression a wax form is made of the size and thickness desired, the wire handle being bent and placed in its proper position in the wax. This form, being removed from the plaster model, is then invested with plaster and sand in an ordinary vulcanizing flask in two parts, the wax form in the lower part, the wire handle in the upper.

The flask then being separated and the wax removed, two holes are made through the plaster and sand in the upper half of the flask, connecting from the top of the plaster and sand, the metal cover of the flask being left off, with each extremity of the cavity previously occupied by the wax form.

The melted tin then being poured into one of the holes until it oozes from the other, the cup is made, needing only some trimming and smoothing.

Before taking the final impression, the new impression cup, which already fits the first model, should be carefully adjusted to the mouth so that it will easily go to place by the use of a certain practical movement, and if the design is carried out, the cup will fit the gum and necks of the teeth so accurately that but a thin layer of composition will be necessary.

In taking the impression the cup and composition should be carried to place with considerable force, which should be as evenly distributed over the whole surface as is possible.

No effort should be made at this time to secure an accurate impression of the crowns of the teeth, it being unnecessary to have them represented at this stage of the process, whether the plate is to be of gold or rubber.

If gold is to be used, the plaster teeth would be cut from the model before it is moulded in the sand; and if the plate is to be of rubber, the better way in these difficult cases is to vulcanize the plate upon the model first, using it then for taking the bite, as we would a wax form or a gold plate.

I am reminded of a recent case in which I was asked to make a complicated lower partial plate to take the place of a poorly fitting rubber plate, which the patient had vainly attempted for two or three years to get good use from.

As I was about to take the preliminary impression to have the special cup made the thought came to me that I might use the old plate for the cup. Then adding a thin layer of composition to its under surface, I carried it to the proper position, and the plate made upon that model fit like the proverbial " duck's foot in the mud."

Emphasis should again be given to what in my use of composition has been an established fact: the greatest accuracy of result is obtained with the thinnest possible quantity of the softened material carried to its place in a positive and forceful manner.

A PRACTICAL WAY TO IMPROVE DENTAL COLLEGE INSTRUCTION.

BY DR. WILLIAM H. TRUEMAN, PHILADELPHIA.

"At the Princeton Commencement President Wilson announced the new departure in instruction which he has been planning for some time past to introduce. A committee of the alumni has assured the University of additional income exceeding one hundred thousand dollars a year. This money is to be spent in adding to the Princeton faculty fifty preceptors, who are to do, apparently, what tutors do in the older English universities,—that is, they will keep in constant touch with the students, ' as guides, advisors, and testers of their learning.' Less reliance than formerly is to be placed at Princeton on recitations and examinations, and more on conferences of individuals and small groups of men with their instructors. Not only the new preceptors, but the older members of the faculty, are to take part in these conferences." (*Harper's Weekly*, July 1, 1905, page 931.)

This new departure is in line with the change that has been slowly going on in educational institutions. The instructor is being brought closer to the pupil. "Telling how," is giving way to the much more practical "showing how;" the gulf between the desk and the benches is slowly being bridged, and the printed text-book will soon be supplanted by well-trained, properly qualified demonstrators, who will interpret to individual students the instruction formally imparted from the lecture-table. This will call for a large increase in the teaching staff, a higher intelligence, and a marked aptness for teaching that will demand and merit a more liberal recompense. It will also make needful more room and more appliances. All these things are costly. The fees received from students do not, in the higher educational institutions, provide the facilities required.

While this fact has made an impress upon the community that has borne fruit. it does not seem to be appreciated by members of the dental profession. Judging from remarks now and again recorded as having been made at dental gatherings, the impression prevails that dental colleges are mines of wealth, and a dental professorship is a short cut to fortune. This is far, very far from being the case. While the cost of instructing has very much increased, the college fees have not been materially advanced, so that, notwithstanding the larger classes, that portion of the income charged to profit, from which the teaching staff is paid, is far below a just recompense for service rendered. The dental graduate seems impressed with the idea that his diploma is a *quid pro quo* for the fees he has paid; with its reception the transaction is ended; he has no further use for the college, and its future welfare is no concern of his.

It is very fortunate that this feeling does not extend to other vocations, otherwise educational facilities would be very meagre in this country. The medical fraternity contributes very largely to maintain the varied educational facilities of the medical profession. Its members give freely of their time, talent, and earnings, to found, maintain, and improve their colleges, hospitals, and libraries; and their example has prompted the laity to liberally assist. Their unselfishness is appreciated by the community, and in return the profession is freely accorded a social distinction and a place of honor as public benefactors.

The dental profession does not receive, and has done nothing to merit, any further consideration from the public than that accorded other artisans. The dentist does his work and gets his fees as a *quid pro quo*. While it is generally recognized by the profession that dental college training could readily be made more effective, any suggestion of providing the means is coldly received. A far less sum than that provided by the alumni of Princeton would enable any one of the dental colleges to vastly improve its teaching facilities, would attract to its teaching staff men of talent and ability who under present conditions forsake the schools for private practice, and the mere fact that if it had been done would raise the profession in public esteem. The excuse that the profession is poor is false. It is not dollars and cents, it is *esprit de corps* that is wanting. It is high time the dental profession fell in line, and in a practical way contributed to improve its own educational facilities. Let the faculties be assured that they will be financially supported in advancing the educational standard, and they will as readily respond as have other educational institutions. Loudly proclaiming that we are not commercialists, but professional men is idle talk so long as there is nothing publicly seen to show the existence of the dental profession but its business signs. We do nothing for the community but that which we are paid for, and for this we are constantly scheming for higher fees. The example of the Princeton alumni is an excellent one to follow, and the method of instruction liberally provided is just what is wanted to make the dental college course what it should be.

STUDY OF THE PITHECANTHROPUS ERECTUS, OR APE-MAN.[1]

BY EUGENE S. TALBOT, M.S., D.D.S., M.D., LL.D.

HAECKEL suggested many years ago that in a hypothetic continent called Sumeria, of which Java, Borneo, etc., were the remains, as having a continual fauna, man originated. From time to time pithecoid types of skull, like the Neanderthal and Spy type, were discovered in Europe, albeit comparatively late in geologic history in the pleistocene rather than the tertiary (eocene, miocene, and phocene). The face type was pithecoid, but the skull, while low in cranial capacity, was far above the highest anthropoid ape. Evidences of man in the shape of cut whalebones had been found in the pleocene to the Neanderthal and Spy type of man, despite the fact that his ape-like face and femur was not the oldest type.

In 1892 there was much excitement in the biologic world over the discovery by Dr. Dubois, in Java, of a few bones and teeth at a distance of thirty-two feet six inches below the surface of the ground upon a river bank. Great stress was laid upon the antiquity of these fossils, because of the distance below ground, the character of soil, etc., but Dubois believed them to be pleistocene. " The first sight of the fossils was a surprise, as they were evidently much older than appeared from Dubois's description. All the physical characters impressed Marsh with the idea that the remains were pliocene and not pleistocene. The discoveries consisted of a tooth found first in the bank of the river thirty-nine inches below the water-level during the dry season. A month later the skull was found a short distance from the tooth; two months later another tooth was found ten feet from where the skull was located; still later a femur was discovered. These bones were

---

[1] Read before the Chicago Academy of Medicine, June 27, 1904.

carefully studied by Dubois, who believed them to belong to a new family which he named the pithecanthropidæ, distinguished mainly by the following characteristics.

The brain cavity is absolutely larger and, in proportion to the size of the body, much more capacious than in the Simiadæ, yet less so than in the Hominidæ. Cranial capacity about two-thirds the human average. Inclination of the nuchal surface of the occiput considerably greater than in the Simiadæ. Dentition, although retrogressive, still the human type. Femur equal in its dimensions to that of man, and like that adapted for walking in an upright position, unlike the Spy femur here, which was more pithecoid.

Of this skull the upper portion alone is preserved, the line of fracture extending from the glabella backward irregularly to the occiput, which it divides somewhat below the upper nuchal line. The cranium seen from above is an elongated oval in outline, dolichocephalic, and is distinguished from that of other anthropoid apes by its large size and its higher arching in the coronal region. The greatest length from the glabella to the posterior projection of the occiput is 185 millimetres; the greatest breadth is 130 millimetres; and the smallest behind the orbit is 90 millimetres. The cranium in its original condition must have been of somewhat larger dimensions. The upper surface of the skull is without ridges, and the sutures all appear to be obliterated.

This dolichocephalic skull, with an index of seventy degrees, is readily distinguished from the brachycephalic orang-outang skull. The absence of the characteristic cranial crests separate it from the dolichocephalic skull of the adult gorilla. In its smooth upper surface and general form it resembles somewhat the chimpanzee skull, and still more that of the gibbon (Hylobates).

In this hurried communication I had no means of obtaining a more complete study of the cast. There are, however, two or three points of interest which seem to indicate that this skull belongs to a type neither man nor ape. The first is the peculiar length and shape of the orbital ridges. If the animal had walked upon all fours, such prominent ridges would have been unnecessary for the protection of the eyes from the sun and violence of all kinds. They are much more prominent and thinner than those of the Neanderthal, Engis, or Spy skulls. If he had walked continually upon all fours, the occipital protuberance and the superior curved line for the attachment of strong muscles would have been excessively developed. In the place of occipital protuberance appears a depression.

The tooth, of which I have only a picture, is the last upper molar of the right side in good preservation. It indicates an adult. The crown is subtriangular in form, with the corners rounded and the narrowest portion behind. The antero-posterior diameter of the crown in 11.3 millimetres and the transverse 15.3 millimetres. The grinding surface of the crown is concave and less rugose than in existing anthropoid apes. The diverging roots are a pithecoid feature.

How Dubois decided that the tooth was a right superior third molar, or even a third molar at all, is a mystery to me. The picture (a drawing) shows a very small crown as compared with the roots. The roots are short and strong. The third molars in human beings usually have their roots close together, crowns small, with long, thin enamel, flat grinding surface. The short crown, heavy enamel, concave grinding surface, a few rugose, short, thick, heavy, diverging roots all indicate a lower type than those of man.

SOLBRIG'S PORCELAIN JACKET CROWN.[1]

BY JOHN H. SPAULDING, D.D.S., PARIS, FRANCE.

MR. PRESIDENT AND GENTLEMEN,—Before entering upon a description of the technique used in the operations which are the subject of this paper, I wish to call attention to a few facts which show to whom the profession is indebted for the original idea of such a crown, as well as for the procedure which has resulted in improving and perfecting it, and placing it before the profession as a practical and artistic reality.

In the early Summer of 1903, one of my patients who had very unsightly teeth, owing to extensive erosion, followed by dark brown discoloration, asked me if there was not some way of re-enamelling them. I told her that I did not know of any. Just at this time, I read the article in the *Dental Cosmos*, June, 1903, written by

---

[1] Read before the American Dental Society of Europe, at Geneva. Switzerland, April 21, 1905.

Dr. C. H. Land, of Detroit, in which he speaks of "enamelled caps or jacket crowns." This article interested me so much that I called the attention of my assistant to it. I left in July for America, and promised myself a visit to Dr. Land to inspect his method personally, but was prevented from seeing him.

Upon my return home in September, 1903, my assistant placed in my hands three of the most beautiful, all porcelain jacket crowns which it is possible to imagine,—the result of his experiments during the summer. I was simply delighted with the beauty and natural appearance of these crowns, and we immediately put to a practical use this most artistic invention. I wish to give credit to Dr. C. H. Land for the original suggestion, of which it is the evolution and perfectionment. Judging from the facts related in an article by Dr. Henry W. Gillett, D.M.D., of New York, in the INTERNATIONAL DENTAL JOURNAL for May, 1904, under the title "Spalding's Porcelain Jacket Crown," we have here an undoubted case of coincident and simultaneous invention on the part of Dr. Edward B. Spalding, of Detroit, and Dr. Oscar Solbrig, of Paris, and I believe it to be the most artistic, as well as practical, of anything which has ever been given to our profession, excepting, perhaps, porcelain enamel inlays.

I believe, further, that they will ultimately almost entirely take the place of pivot crowns in any of the six anterior teeth, because the bulk of the natural tooth just where the strain is greatest—at the gum line—does not have to be cut away, the entire strength of the tooth being thus retained, and this is augmented by the porcelain crown.

We have twelve of these crowns doing solid service for many months, some as long as one year and seven months, and we have the greatest confidence in their long durability.

Dr. Solbrig's procedure originated entirely with himself, having for its point of departure nothing but the somewhat vague suggestions contained in the article by Dr. Land, above referred to, and, while arriving at the same practical result as Dr. Edward B. Spalding's, is quite different, and would appear to give a more absolutely exact and certain result with the least trouble to both patient and operator.

Dr. Solbrig makes no shoulder at or under the gum margin, but first removes all existing natural enamel and gives the tooth a conical shape and shortens it as much as possible if living, as much as prudent if dead.   (See Fig. 1, *a*, showing tooth with enamel; *a*, *b*, and *c* showing side and front views of prepared stump.)

Fig. 1.

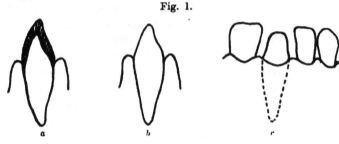

a   *b*   *c*

An ordinary plate tooth (we use English teeth which permit of shaping and polishing at will) is then ground out concave on the under side, making a fine, almost feather-edge, where it slips under the gum margin and is exactly fitted to the stump at this point.   This we will call the porcelain facing or veneer.[1] A strip of rolled cohesive gold-foil No. 40, the width of which corresponds to the length of the stump, is then placed around the latter and slipped as high as possible under the gum and held in position laterally by pieces of spunk wedged against the adjoining teeth. (See Fig. 2.)   This band is then folded with pliers both on the

Fig. 2.

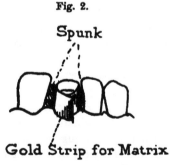

Spunk

Gold Strip for Matrix

palatal and labial sides (see Fig. 3, *a*), drawing the gold as tightly as possible to the contour of the stump.   This is now lifted off the stump and annealed, and the excess of gold where folded is then cut away with scissors, which welds the gold at these points (front

---

[1] Porcelain veneers are now produced by the manufacturers of porcelain teeth in America, and I hope Ash & Sons will also do so very soon.

and back), leaving a conical cap, or matrix, of gold (Fig. 3, *b*). This cap is now replaced on the stump and reburnished over its entire surface. A little beeswax is then placed on the labial surface of this gold matrix, as well as in the concave of the porcelain

Fig. 3.

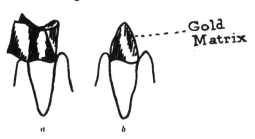

facing; also a small softened piece against the lingual side of the matrix; the facing is then placed in position and pressed home, if necessary, with a warm spatula. (See Fig. 4, *a*, *b*, and *c*.) When cool, the whole is removed from the stump and invested in

Fig. 4.

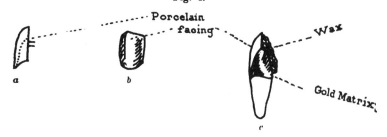

powdered asbestos paste. It will be noticed that the relative positions of porcelain facing and gold matrix, as well as the adjustment on the stump are absolutely exact and the investment in powdered asbestos maintains these conditions, *and also enters the matrix, taking the place of the stump itself.* After drying, the wax is removed by warming and, finally, burning out, and its place between the facing and the matrix is filled with porcelain, which is then fused, thus uniting the facing and matrix.

Additions of porcelain and repeated fusings are made until this space is entirely filled. The investment is then entirely removed, *except that part which enters the matrix,* and which represents the stump of the tooth. It is very essential to retain this part of the investment until the crown is entirely finished, as it prevents any possible change in the shape of the matrix or gold cap during manipulation. Subsequent additions of porcelain and fusings are then made until the lateral and lingual aspects of the crown are covered and the crown is complete. There is no necessity to have the patient return for reburnishing of the gold matrix.

When the bakings are finished, the gold matrix is stripped out, leaving a porcelain cap exactly the same shape and form as would be the natural enamel were it possible to lift it off from the dentine, but it is much thicker and stronger, except at the margins where it is made exactly to represent and replace the natural enamel. There is no shoulder to fit, therefore no joint, and in the case of recession of the gum the tooth would not be more unsightly than a natural tooth under the same condition.

I wish to call your especial attention to the great value this method has, apart from its artistic appearance, over the ordinary pivot tooth of any system in the matter of strength. When a canine or incisor is cut off even with the gum, and the strongest pivot tooth that is possible to make has been adjusted and cemented in, you have still the weakest point just where the greatest strength is required,—viz., at the gum margin, and the frequent bending or breaking of the pivot at this point is a witness to its weakness and to the stress which it is called upon to support. A porcelain jacket crown made and set as herein described not only makes it unnecessary to weaken the natural tooth in the slightest degree, but it gives it added strength and solidity. In the case of dead teeth, the remaining dentine may be reinforced by cementing a thick, strong, metal pivot into the tooth. Before setting, the interior of the jacket crown should be roughened or etched with hydrofluoric acid, thus giving a surface much better adapted for the attachment of the cement which insures the maximum of strength between the porcelain and the stump. For setting, we give the preference to Harvard cement, as it is very tenacious and becomes exceedingly hard with time.

We use Dr. Jenkins's new porcelain enamel, or prosthetic porcelain which fuses just under the fusing point of pure gold, and is exceedingly strong and fine grained. It unites perfectly with the English teeth and can be ground and repolished as circumstances and convenience require. We consider it the *ne plus ultra* of strength, reliability, and convenience of manipulation.

Reviews of Dental Literature.

-- --- --

THE ANTIMICROBIC ACTION OF IODINE.[1] By Guy C. Kinnaman, M.D., Assistant Instructor in Skin and Venereal Diseases, Chicago Policlinic, Chicago.

PREFACE.

The uniform satisfaction given by the iodine catgut prepared after the method of Claudius,[1] which has been used by Dr. Nicholas Senn in his clinical work, led him to employ a solution of iodine for irrigation in infected wounds and also for hand sterilization. The results obtained demonstrated, clinically, the marked potency of iodine in solution as an antiseptic. Its continued use for several years has shown it to be far superior to any antiseptic previously employed.

In order to determine the absolute value of this solution, a series of experiments have been carried out on a number of different micro-organisms *in vitro*. A sufficient number of different organisms and a great number of tubes have been used. Therefore one is justified in assuming that the conclusions arrived at from a careful study of the series of experiments represent as nearly as possible the position of iodine in the family of antiseptics. When we try to make an accurate comparison between the members of this numerous family, however, we find we cannot do so because of the widely different methods of procedure employed by the different investigators. In addition, the majority of the methods show one or more points of possible error. Not for the purpose of comparison, but with the idea in view of presenting the experimental findings of various men on the more important antiseptic substances, there has been incorporated in this research a short bibliography of antiseptics in general.

Bichloride Mercury.—Kyle[2] found that it took $^1/_{1000}$ solution bichloride ten hours to insure no growth of tetanus bacillus. Koch[3] determined that a $^1/_{2000}$ solution killed anthrax spores in ten minutes. Klein,[4] how-

---

[1] Work done as Fellow in Surgery at the Senn Laboratory, Rush Medical College. An abstract prepared from the original article in the Journal of the American Medical Association, with consent of the publisher.

ever, found that anthrax spores were not influenced by a $^1/_{10000}$ solution acting for one hour. Evans,[5] from experiments on *Bacillus anthracis* in liquid media, reported that a $^1/_{15000}$ for one mniute and a $^1/_{20000}$ for thirty minutes were effective. In regard to the spores he found that a $^1/_{100}$ for fifteen minutes and $^1/_{1000}$ for one hour were effective. Likewise, a $^1/_{1000}$ for five minutes gave growth. On *Staphylococcus pyogenes aureus*, the same author states that a $^1/_{200}$ solution for fifteen minutes killed, while a $^1/_{200}$ solution for one hour impaired vitality. Tarnier and Vignal,[6] using thread method of Koch, found that a $^1/_{1000}$ solution for two minutes killed both *Streptococcus* and *Staphylococcus pyogenes aureus*. Harrington,[7] employing the same method, states that where the threads are moist an exposure of over fifteen minutes to a $^1/_{1000}$ solution is necessary to kill the *Bacillus pyocyaneus*, while if threads are dry five seconds are sufficient. On *Staphylococcus aureus*, either on moist or dry threads, from five to ten minutes kills. On *Bacillus anthracis*, either dry or moist threads, an exposure to a $^1/_{1000}$ solution for thirty minutes has no bactericidal effect. Hence, he states that bichloride of mercury is a greatly overrated disinfectant. Burgess,[8] who also used the thread method in his experiments on *Bacillus coli communis*, found that a $^1/_{100}$ solution for one minute was effective, as were a $^1/_{2000}$ solution for five minutes and a $^1/_{1000}$ for ten minutes. Sternberg,[9] from experiments on gonococcus, states that 0.005 per cent. bichloride solution for two hours kills. He concludes that in bichloride we have a germicidal agent of the highest value.

Carbolic Acid.—Kyle[3] found that the tetanus bacillus had to be exposed to a five per cent. carbolic acid solution for six hours in order to assure no growth. Cabbot,[10] on adding five per cent. carbolic acid to a putrefactive solution and then transferring several drops of mixture to an aseptic medium, discovered that after five seconds' exposure no putrefaction occurred in fresh tubes. Evans[5] found that on anthrax bacillus a $^1/_{100}$ solution for five minutes, a $^1/_{150}$ solution for fifteen minutes, and a $^1/_{175}$ solution for thirty minutes, were effective. On the spores, he got a growth after four hours' exposure to a five per cent. solution. A twenty-four hours' exposure, however, was sufficient to insure no growth. A $^1/_{40}$ solution on *Staphylococcus aureus* for fifteen minutes gave no growth. Burgess,[8] in his work on *Bacillus coli communis*, states that a ten per cent. solution kills in one minute, a 2.5 per cent. in five minutes, a one per cent. in thirty minutes, and a 0.75 per cent. in one hour. Blyth[11] found that a ten per cent. solution for four hours had no effect on anthrax spores. A twenty-four-hour exposure, however, proved efficient. He used the glass-rod method. On the gonococcus and micrococcus of abscess pus, Sternberg[9] found that the action of an 0.8 per cent. solution for two hours killed the organisms.

Alcohol.—From experiments on the germicidal effect of alcohol, Harrington[12] concludes: " Alcohol of any strength has absolutely no effect on anthrax bacillus; sixty to seventy per cent. alcohol is the most efficient strength against non-spore-forming bacteria, i.e., *Staphylococcus pyogenes aureus* and *albus*, typhoid bacillus, bacillus of diphtheria, being usually effective in five minutes."

Salzwedel and Elsner,[12] using thread method, state that fifty-five per cent. (by weight alcohol) was most destructive to staphylococcus pus, requiring in fresh pus from five to six minutes to be effective. They state that this solution is not quite equal to a $1/1000$ solution of bichloride, but is as efficient as a three per cent. carbolic solution. Sternberg[9] found that with a two-hour exposure, a ninety-five per cent. alcohol was fatal to gonococci, while a forty per cent. solution did the work on the micrococcus of abscess pus.

Hydrogen Peroxide.—In his work on the tetanus bacillus, Kyle[2] states that after a forty-eight-hour exposure to hydrogen peroxide the bacillus still grew. On the other hand, Gibier[14] finds, from experiments he has made with a 3.2 per cent. hydrogen peroxide solution in water on *Bacillus anthracis, Bacillus typhosus, Streptococcus pyogenes*, etc., that after some minutes of contact (exact time not stated) the bacteria could not be cultivated from bouillon, hence were destroyed.

Formaldehyde.—Shaw[15] determines that a $1/200$ solution of formaldehyde broth prevented the growth of *Bacillus pyocyaneus*. Pottevin[16] finds that five centigrams of formaldehyde to a litre of bouillon stops growth of *Bacillus diphtheriæ, pyocyaneus, typhosus* and the *Staphylococcus pyogenes aureus*. Burgess[8] concludes that on *Bacillus coli communis*, a $1/20$ solution is destructive in one minute, a $1/40$ solution in five minutes, and a $1/100$ solution in thirty minutes.

Lysol.—Burgess,[8] who included lysol in his experiments on *Bacillus coli*, found that a $1/10$ aqueous solution killed it in one minute, a $1/40$ solution in five minutes, a $1/200$ solution in thirty minutes, and a $1/300$ solution in one hour.

Boric Acid.—Burgess[8] also found that a saturated solution of boric acid was entirely wanting in antiseptic powers, no matter how long the exposure. Sternberg[9] came to a like conclusion from his work on gonococcus and micrococcus of abscess pus.

Phenic Acid.—On streptococci and staphylococci Tarnier and Vignal[6] state that a three per cent. aqueous solution of phenic acid is efficient in seventeen minutes, a two per cent. solution in eighteen minutes. Chamberland,[17] from his experiments, finds that anthrax bacilli are killed by a forty-eight-hour exposure to a $1/400$ solution of phenic acid.

Salicylic Acid.—A $1/240$ solution of salicylic acid for three minutes kills putrefactive organisms, according to Cabbot.[10]

Methyl Violet.—Stillings,[18] as his findings from experiments, states that methyl violet is three times as strong as bichloride in its action on anthrax bacillus and quite as effective as it is on *Staphylococcus pyogenes aureus*.

Nicotine.—Herbert,[19] reviewing the work of Pécholier (1883) on the action of nicotine in alcoholic solution on bacteria; that of Vincent Tassinari de Pise (fumes of tobacco, in 1888); and that of Vissalli (fumes of tobacco, in 1888); and from added experiments of his own (nicotine in alcohol solution), says in conclusion that "nicotine does not appear gifted with very powerful antiseptic properties, for one-third of a drop (sufficient to kill a pigeon in a few seconds) does not prevent the development of certain bacteria in three cubic centimetres of bouillon." But he concludes from experiments of Tissinari on tubercle bacillus and spirillum of Asiatic cholera, and from his own on bacillus diphtheria that it attenuates the virulence of microbes. Junor[20] reports a case of tetanus cured by local application of infusion of tobacco.

Mercuric Cyanide.—Harrington,[21] using the thread method, found that a ¹⁄₁₀₀₀ solution of mercuric cyanide had to act in thirty minutes to kill *Staphylococcus pyogenes albus*, while a three-hour exposure on *S. aureus* showed no antiseptic effect. Hence it is impractical.

Radium.—It was found by Van Buren,[22] from his experiments on *Bacillus typhosus*, *Bacillus pyocyaneus* and *Staphylococcus pyogenes aureus*, that radium, acting from eight to thirteen hours, was negative in antiseptic action. Pfeiffer[23] also shows its negative action on *Bacillus typhosus* and the cholera spirillum.

Collargol.—Fortesque-Brickdale[24] states " in solution of 0.5 per cent. and under, collargol has no bactericidal effect on *Streptococcus pyogenes* or *Staphylococcus pyogenes aureus* after a twenty-four-hour exposure to a one-day-old culture. (Plate Method.)" A one per cent. solution gave no growth. ,

Turpentine.—Marx[25] found that it required ¹⁄₁₀₀ turpentine acting for an hour to hinder the growth of anthrax. Forty minutes was required for *Staphylococcus pyogenes aureus*.

Glycerin.—Copeman.[26] from numerous experiments, fully covered by controls, on *Staphylococcus pyogenes aureus* and *albus*, *Streptococcus pyogenes*, *Bacillus anthracis*, *subtilis*, *coli communis*, *pyocyaneus*, *diphtheriæ*, and *tuberculosis* determines: " (1) No visible development of organisms employed takes place in presence of more than thirty per cent. glycerin in beef peptone broth; (2) all organisms, except coli and subtilis, are killed in less than one minute in the presence of thirty per cent. to forty per cent. glycerin in the cold."

Potassium Permanganate.—According to Cabbot,[16] a ¹⁄₆₀₀ aqueous solution of permanganate potassium requires over six minutes to stop putrefaction in a putrefactive solution. Sternberg[9] found that 0.12 per cent. permanganate acting on gonococcus and micrococcus of abscess pus destroyed them.

BIBLIOGRAPHY OF ANTISEPTICS CONTAINING IODINE IN CHEMICAL COMBINATION.

Biniodide of Mercury.—On the *Staphylococcus aureus* and the *Streptococcus,* Tarnier and Vignal[6] have shown that a 1/1000 solution of biniodide of mercury is destructive in nine minutes; a 1/2000 solution in twenty-two minutes. On *Bacillus coli communis*, Burgess[8] states that " biniodide of mercury is by far the strongest and best antiseptic (of the ones he tried), and it is not affected by albumin." In his table he places 1/1000 solution effective in one minute; 1/5000 in five minutes; 1/20000 in ten minutes; 1/80000 in thirty minutes; 1/200000 in one hour.

Lithio-Mercuric Iodide.—Rosenberger,[27] working with lithiomercuric iodide (thirty-four per cent. mercury, sixty-five per cent. iodine, one per cent. lithium) and using thread method, found that on *Staphylococcus pyogenes aureus,* when threads were moist, 1/1000 solution for thirty seconds killed; 1/5000 for one minute did the same. When threads were dry, 1/1000 for one minute killed; likewise 1/5000 for three minutes. On *Streptococcus pyogenes* (dry threads) 1/1000 for thirty seconds killed; 1/5000 for thirty seconds killed; threads moist, 1/1000 for thirty seconds was effective; 1/5000 required two minutes. On anthrax bacillus 1/1000 solution was necessary for fifteen minutes when threads were dry, and for thirty minutes when moist threads were used. He concludes that this is a much more powerful germicide than the usual mercuric salts.

Iodoform.—The experimental results differ greatly from the clinical. A great deal of experimental work has been done on iodoform. Its action has been tested on various organisms by numerous investigators, and their findings seem to indicate that it possesses no bactericidal properties of any moment. The men who have so determined are Heyn and Rovsing,[28] Riedlin,[29] Baumgarten,[30] Kronacher,[31] Buchner,[32] Kunz,[33] Schnirer,[34] Lubbert,[35] and Tilanus.[36] On the other hand, the work of Mikulicz,[37] who, on adding iodoform to putrefying liquids, saw putrefaction sometimes stopped and sometimes to continue; that of Maylard,[38] who states that it retards but does not stop the development of anthrax bacillus; and that of Stohegoleff,[39] who found that tubercle bacilli inoculated on five per cent. iodoform bouillon were dead in forty-eight hours, seems to indicate that under certain conditions (*i.e.,* where free iodine is eliminated) it has a slight antiseptic value.

Clinically, when the iodoform comes in contact with tissues, more free iodine is eliminated, hence the results are much better than experiments would indicate. Its use in tubercular joint injections needs no comment. Vinke[40] reports favorably in two cases of anthrax dressed with iodoform. Sormani[41] found by wounding rabbits and guinea-pigs and injecting them with tetanus bacilli and then treating them with different antiseptics that iodoform was the most active of all, and if applied at once tetanus did not appear. Pryor[42] reports thirty-seven cases of puerperal sepsis with but four deaths treated by packing uterus and widely opened cul-de-sac with iodoform gauze, free iodine being liberated and shown to be present in the urine.

Iodine.—The antiseptic action of iodine was discovered by Davaine [43] in 1873. He found that a 1/12000 solution caused the virulence of anthrax to disappear in thirty minutes. Tarnier and Vignal,[6] in their work on *Staphylococcus pyogenes aureus* and *Streptococcus pyogenes*, found that a 1/1000 solution of potassium iodide required over an hour to kill, a 1/500 solution required fifteen minutes, and a 1/300 solution required eight minutes. White [44] states that he has made a number of tests and observed that " in strength of 1/1000 iodine solution in bouillon no growth of streptococcus occurs. *Staphylococcus aureus* will not grow in strength of 1/5000." Davaine [45] determines that a 1/170000 solution of iodine in contact with anthrax blood for fifty to sixty minutes renders it harmless to inject into guinea-pigs. Sternberg [9] states that a 0.2 per cent. solution destroys gonococcus acting for two hours. Claudius,[1] in his article describing his method of sterilizing catgut by immersing in a solution of one part iodine, one part potassium iodide, and water one hundred parts, for eight days and then transferring to three per cent. carbolic acid to rinse off excess of liquid iodine, remarks that from his experiments he has found that a one per cent. solution kills *Staphylococcus aureus* in three minutes and anthrax in twenty hours. He states further that such a long contact is unnecessary (1/5000 solution kills anthrax spores in a short time).

Clinically, iodine solutions have been used with excellent results in treating anthrax. Sereins [46] reported two cases of anthrax cured by injecting a 1/100 solution around and into pustule. Brochin [47] has also reported two cases successfully treated by the same method. Human actinomycosis has been cured by the daily injection of two cubic centimetres of a ten per cent. iodine solution, as shown by Gaucher.[48]

In concluding the bibliography, it is only necessary to call attention to the great number of different substances employed as antiseptics to show that, as yet, the ideal germicide is a negative quantity.

TECHNIC OF EXPERIMENTAL RESEARCH.

Solution Employed.—A solution of iodine in sodium iodide and water was prepared after the following formula:

Iodine .... 2.5 gms.
Sodium iodide .... 5.5 gms.
Aqua (sterilized) ....250.0 cc.

This gave a 1/100 solution. From this solution, by aqueous dilution, strengths of 1/200, 1/300, 1/500, and 1/1000 were made. In preparing the mother solution, accuracy was observed in weighing the iodine and sodium iodide. The same care was followed in making dilutions. The glass containers were sterilized.

Asepticity of Solutions.—The varying strengths of solutions were now tested to see whether or not they were, of themselves, sterile. For this purpose the plate method was employed. Three drops of solution were used to inoculate a melted agar tube from which a plate was made. From each strength solution three plates were made. After incubating six days every plate was free from colonies, hence sterile. To confirm results inoculations from the different strengths were made on six per cent. glycerin potato and incubated six days. The result was again negative in character.

METHOD OF CONDUCTING EXPERIMENTS.

In conducting the several series of experiments, an effort was made to employ a method which would offer the minimum possibility of error, and, at the same time, approach, as nearly as possible, to the exact relation of bacteria to the body in disease. In other words, the media employed were solid in every case, and the growths on them were allowed to become marked, both in extent and thickness, before beginning experiment. Thus, by the thickness of the growth, the penetrating power of the liquid could be ascertained.

The micro-organisms on which the action of the iodine solutions was tried were various enough to permit of definite deductions being made from the results on the antimicrobic action of iodine. These micro-organisms were: (1) *Bacillus prodigiosus;* (2) *Bacillus anthracis* and spores; (3) *Bacillus tuberculosis;* (4) *Staphylococcus pyogenes aureus;* (5) *Streptococcus pyogenes;* (6) *Blastomyces dermatitis;* (7) *Actinomyces bovis.* On these various growths in the test-tubes, the iodine solutions were deposited by means of a sterilized pipette until the surface of the growth was completely covered. After varying periods of time, which are designated in the tables, small loops of growth, thus acted on, were

transferred to tubes of sterile media and well inoculated, and then
put in incubator and watched for growth. No effort was made
to wash the inherent iodine solution from the loops because of
the danger of washing away the bacteria. For each time of exposure, four tubes were used, each one being covered by a control
tube. It is well to note that the bacterial growths transferred were
macroscopic and not microscopic in size.

SUMMARY OF EVIDENCE ON ANTHRAX.

Considering first the strength of solution and time of exposure
to same necessary to produce the death of *Bacillus anthracis* plus
spores, the evidence shows that a 1/200 solution for one hour or
a 1/100 solution for ten minutes procures death. An exposure to
a 1/100 solution for less than ten minutes gives a growth. The
second consideration or the inhibitory effect, depending as it does
on the two factors,—*i.e.*, time of exposure and strength of solution,—first shows itself after an exposure of the organism to a
1/1000 solution for sixty minutes. The inhibitory effect is marked.
The effect is also shown by an exposure of fifteen minutes to a
1/500 solution, but to a lesser degree. As the time of exposure
is increased, the inhibitory effect becomes more and more marked.
Likewise, as the strength of solution employed is increased, the
inhibitory action becomes progressively more powerful. If, after
the death point is reached, we decrease the time of exposure, we
again come into the sphere of diminishing inhibition.

SUMMARY OF EVIDENCE ON PRODIGIOSUS.

In making a summary of the evidence, there are two factors
to be considered: (1) The strength of solution and time of exposure to same necessary to produce the death of the micro-organism; (2) the inhibitory action of solutions. Considering (1).
therefore, we find that a solution less than one per cent., acting
for an hour, does not destroy *Bacillus prodigiosus*. To cause the
death of this organism it is necessary for a 1/100 solution of iodine
to act for ten minutes. A shorter period of exposure,—*i.e.*, nine.
eight, and five minutes,—gives a growth. On considering (2) it is
readily seen that two items have to do with the inhibitory effect.
These are, strength of solution and period of exposure. Thus. a
solution acting for a certain period of time shows no inhibitory
effect, but if the time of exposure is increased, such an effect ap-

pears. Conversely, as the strength of the solution is increased, the time of exposure necessary to produce an inhibitory effect becomes less. Bearing these two facts in mind, we find that in this series a slight inhibitory effect is first shown by a 1/1000 solution after an hour's exposure. A 1/500 solution begins to show this effect after thirty minutes' exposure; a 1/300 solution after fifteen minutes. Thus, progressively, as the time of exposure to each strength of solution is lengthened, and the strength of the solution itself is increased, the inhibitory action becomes more marked until the death point of the germ is reached. And, if we try to decrease the time of exposure necessary to produce death, we reach the inhibitory stage again.

SUMMARY OF EVIDENCE ON TUBERCULOSIS.

The evidence shows that to produce the death of the *Bacillus tuberculosis* an exposure to a 1/200 iodine solution for one hour or to a 1/100 solution for seven minutes is necessary. An exposure of less than seven minutes results in a growth. When we come to the consideration of the inhibitory effect we find that a 1/1000 solution for one hour is without effect. Inhibition begins to be shown slightly by a 1/500 solution for fifteen minutes. From this point on, as the period of exposure is increased and as the solution employed becomes of greater strength, the inhibitory effect becomes progressively more and more marked until the death point is reached. Then, if we try to lessen the time of exposure to the necessary strength, we come into the sphere of inhibition which decreases as the exposure decreases.

BIBLIOGRAPHY.

1. Claudius: Deutsche Zeitschrift für Chirurgie, 1902, vol. lxiv. pp. 489–494.
2. Kyle: Therapeutic Gazette, 1892, vol. viii. p. 163.
3. Koch: Mittheilungen aus dem k. Gesundheitsamte, vol. i. 1881.
4. Klein: Local Gov. Bd. Rep., London, 1885–86.
5. Evans: Guy's Hospital Report, London, 1890, 3 s., vol. xxxii. pp. 195–252.
6. Tarnier and Vignal: Arch. de méd. expér. et d'anat. path., Paris, 1890, vol. ii. p. 477.
7. Harrington: Boston Medical and Surgical Journal, 1903, vol. cxlviii. pp. 445–439.
8. Burgess: Lancet, London, 1900, vol. i. p. 1798.
9. Sternberg: American Journal of Medical Science, 1883, vol. lxxxv. pp. 321–343.

10. Cabbot: Boston Medical and Surgical Journal, 1870, vol. ci. p. 75.

11. Blyth: Proc. Royal Society, Edinburgh, 1884, vol. xii. p. 638.

12. Harrington: Boston Medical and Surgical Journal, 1903, vol. cxlviii. p. 551.

13. Salzwedel and Elsner: Berliner klin. Wochenschr., 1900, vol. xxxvii. pp. 496–500.

14. Gibier: Verhandl. d. X, International Medical Congress, 1890, Berlin, 1891, v. 15 Abth., pp. 124, 125.

15. Shaw: Journal Hygiene, London, 1903, vol. iii. p. 162.

16. Pottevin: Annales de l'Institut Pasteur, 1894, p. 804.

17. Chamberland: Acad. de Science, Paris, 1883, vol. xcvi. p. 1088.

18. Stillings: Lancet, London, 1891, i. p. 872.

19. Herbert: L'art méd., Paris, 1896, vol. lxxxiii. pp. 176-193.

20. Junor: Edinburgh Medical Journal, 1866-67, vol. xii. p. 684.

21. Harrington: Boston Medical and Surgical Journal, 1904, vol. cl. p. 43.

22. Van Buren: American Medicine, 1903, vol. vi. p. 1021.

23. Pfeiffer: Berliner klinische Wochenschrift, 1903, vol. xl. p. 641.

24. Fortescue-Brickdale: Bristol Medico-Chirurgical Journal, 1903. vol. xxi. p. 343.

25. Marx: Centralbl. f. Bakteriol., Jena, 1902, vol. xxxiii. p. 75.

26. Copeman: Rep. Brit. Assn. Adv. Sc., London. 1896, p. 987.

27. Rosenberger: American Medicine, 1904, vol. vii. p. 1021.

28. Heyn and Rovsing: Fortschritte der Medicin, 1887, Bd. V. pp. 33-47.

29. Riedlin: Arch. f. Hyg. München U. Leip., 1887, vol. vii. p. 310.

30. Baumgarten: Berliner klinische Wochenschrift, 1887, vol. xxiv. p. 354.

31. Kronacher: Münchener med. Wochenschrift, 1887, vol. xxxiv. p. 545.

32. Buchner: Münchener med. Wochenschrift, 1887, vol. xxxiv. p. 465.

33. Kunz: Arbeiten a. d. Pathologische Institut zu Königsberg. 1887.

34. Schnirer: Wiener medicin. Presse, 1887, Nos. 36-38.

35. Lubbert: Fortschritte d. Medicin, Bd. V, 1887, pp. 330-345.

36. Tilanus: Münchener medicinische Wochenschrift, vol. xxxiv. p. 309.

37. Mikulicz: Langenbeck's Archiv, vol. xxvii. pp. 196-239.

38. Maylard: Annals of Surgery, 1890, vol. xi. pp. 17-33.

39. Stohegoleff: Arch. de méd. expér. et. d'Anat. Path., 1894, vol. vi. pp. 813-837.

40. Vinke: St. Louis Courier of Medicine, vol. xiii. p. 125.

41. Sormani: Riforma Medica, 1890, January, pp. 11-13.

42. Pryor: New York Medical Journal, 1903, vol. lxxviii. p. 356.

43. Davaine: Dictionaire Encyclopédique des Sciences méd., p. 335.

44. White: Amer. Jour. of Obstetrics, 1904, vol. xlix. p. 605.

45. Davaine: Bull. Acad. de méd., 1880, 2 S., vol. ix. p. 763.

46. Sereins: Union méd., Paris, 1887, 3 S., vol. xliv. p. 470.

47. Brochin: Gaz. d. hôp., Paris, 1880, vol. liii. p. 1010.

48. Gaucher: Ann. de Derm. et Syph., 1903, 4 S., vol. iv. p. 837.

AN INTERESTING CASE IN PRACTICE.[1] By J. H. Carter, L.D.S.I., D.D.S. (Phil.).

The following case, which first came under my notice in 1899, has been treated off and on by myself and partner up to the present time, puzzling and worrying us both very much.

Mr. ——, a gentleman about fifty years of age, residing near Leeds, of fair complexion and healthy appearance, called, desiring me to scale and polish his teeth; also to remove any sharp edges I could find in connection with them. This I promptly did. I should explain that his mouth appeared normal and his natural dentures better than the average. In a little time he came again, complaining of roughness behind the lower incisors. These were carefully re-examined and some further scaling done to remove any possible fraction of tartar that might have been overlooked on the previous occasion; also I thoroughly polished the lingual surfaces again. To my surprise, in a week or two he again called, with the same complaint as before, especially in connection with the two central incisors. I did not quite know what to do, being so satisfied this roughness did not exist, but as he was so persistent, I repeated the polishing process and polished as I have never polished before, particularly their approximal surfaces. Each time on going away he expressed satisfaction and said they were better.

In a month or so, on my way to the station one day, a gentleman driving a carriage stopped me; well, it was my patient, who said he was no better, and would I see him again. When he called, he remarked that he was more convinced than ever that there was a roughness; that this bothered him extremely, his attention being perpetually drawn to it by the annoyance it caused. He compared it to the feeling as if the tip of his tongue was rubbing against sand-paper; indeed, he had been to his doctor, who could find nothing wrong, and who referred him back again to me, as it was quite a dental case. My patient suggested the advisability of having the two centre teeth extracted; to this, of course, I demurred. Wondering if there was anything wrong with his tongue, I examined this organ, but it appeared quite healthy and normal. Thinking the trouble might be partly mental or imaginary,

---

[1] Read before the Leeds and District Section of the North Midland Branch, March 14, 1905.

and feeling that doing something was the best way of getting the thing off his mind, I did still further polishing. Time went on, and again he hailed me from his carriage, stating that he was no better and what was to be done? In my despair I suggested his calling again, an appointment was made, but, not being able to find anything wrong when he came, I told him to divert his mind from his teeth; that his tongue must be morbidly sensitive, and that he had got into a way of fidgeting about it. In order to thoroughly polish the sides of these teeth, as they were set very closely together, I got my patient to wear some tape between them for the purpose of separating, so that I could use a polishing disk or other means. At the next visit he cheerfully informed me that the presence of the tape had nearly cured him. This gave me the idea that if only all the interstices were filled up I should succeed, so, putting on rubber dam, I packed each space with gutta-percha and made all very smooth. To my great annoyance in a little time he called, saying this material had become loose and come away. I saw there was no good in renewing it, for the little movement in each tooth had destroyed the adhesion, and I was sure nothing would hold. Feeling that my patient might be losing confidence in me and perhaps go elsewhere, and thinking a change of dentists might be of advantage, also being heartily weary of the matter, I suggested that my partner should take him in hand. He, knowing the history of the case, adopted very heroic treatment, passing files and disks between the incisors, rounding off everything in all directions, and polishing to such an extent that even the cutting edges were made round like knobs. As all this treatment failed as before, my partner recommended the wearing of a gold shield or plate, covering the lingual surfaces of all the six front teeth and affixing by clasps to the bicuspids; this arrangement afforded some relief, and it was worn for a considerable period.

About this time I was again accosted in the street by my patient, who complained that he was not comfortable and did not like wearing the plate; also he did not know why I had transferred him to some one else, and desired me to take him in hand again. Feeling that this plate was likely to cause damage, a happy inspiration came to me. I suggested discarding it and crowning, or rather encasing, the two offending teeth with gold. This I did, and I am glad to say matters were improved a good deal; yet the case is not altogether satisfactory. I should explain that one of the lateral incisors, not being crowned, is sensitive where the enamel has been polished away; this tooth is now much shorter than its neighbors, and appears to be getting much abraded. I saw the patient quite recently, and was much discouraged on being told that his thoughts were still constantly recurring to his teeth. Almost from the beginning my diagnosis was that either something was wrong with the tongue or the evil was imaginary; if the former, then it must be due to exaggerated or enlarged papillæ, or abnormal sensitiveness. This troublesome case got at last on my nerves, and I was in dread, when on my way to the station, lest I should again have my friend stopping me to say that he was no better, and what was to be done?

I have recently been in correspondence with his doctor regarding him, and he writes: " I am of the opinion that, for the last two or three years he has suffered from neurasthenia, connected with or due to business anxieties. During this time he has had the great responsibility of a failing business, in which not only his own fortune, but those of his brother and sisters, have been involved. Two or three years ago he complained much of right brachial neuralgia, after this had troubled him for some months, he suffered from left intercostal neuralgia and wandering pains about the neck and sternum, making himself and his doctor anxious as to the possibility of angina; finally, a spasmodic condition of the tongue muscles, with complaint of the sharp edges of his teeth, revealed the neurasthenic neurosis. I must say that I for a long time attributed all these things to irregular gout, as there was often an accompanying lithæmia." One authority says of neurasthenia, it is " a peculiar condition of the nervous system, a deviation more or less from the normal state and characterized by a loss of resistance, the latter in its turn producing an increased irritability and debility." Another says it is " a morbid irritability, an irritable weakness, an exaggerated sensibility. All kinds of unpleasant sensations and even vivid pains are of usual occurrence in neurasthenic individuals. The development of neurasthenia is specially favored by overwork, more particularly of a mental kind, by late hours, disappointment, grief, and care. It is of a subjective nature, and even in the most painstaking examination no objective foundation can be found, so that it is generally regarded as imagination or exaggeration; it causes the patient, however, enough trouble and discomfort to make him lose his happiness for a considerable period of his life."

In conclusion, this case may serve to suggest that we occasionally have mysterious and inexplicable symptoms presenting themselves, without sufficient or assignable cause; cases which we are unable to diagnose satisfactorily, and which perhaps belong more to the domain of the medical man than the dental surgeon.— *British Dental Surgeon.*

Reports of Society Meetings.

THE NEW YORK INSTITUTE OF STOMATOLOGY.

A MEETING of the Institute was held at the Chelsea, 222 West Twenty-third Street, New York, on Tuesday evening, June 6, 1905. the President, Dr. C. O. Kimball, in the chair.

The minutes of the last meeting were read and approved.

COMMUNICATIONS ON THEORY AND PRACTICE.

Dr. H. W. Gillett.—I wish to call attention to the little paper points put up by Johnson & Johnson for drying out pulp-canals. At my request they have made some a little shorter and thicker than their regular stock. I find these a very great convenience. It may be a convenience to members to know that they can get these special points by ordering a quantity.

Dr. F. Milton Smith.—I wish to offer a suggestion in regard to a method of evacuating pus from a cavity. The case where I had occasion to use the method was a right lower bicuspid tooth. I mentioned it to Dr. Bogue, and he said that he had never heard of it before. It is sometimes difficult, after the opening is made through the root of a lower tooth, to get the pus to come up through it. To facilitate this I took a little Dunn syringe and placed the point into the canal. After squeezing the bulb together and holding it there, I packed the space around the point with gutta-percha. Then releasing the bulb, I found the suction sufficient to bring up the pus.

Dr. Sinclair Tousey presented a little appliance to be used in connection with X-ray work in making skiagraphs of the jaw. It consisted of a film-holder to which was attached an indicator so arranged that it would facilitate the adjusting of the apparatus for any particular field in and about the mouth. Negatives made in this way were more quickly done, but were not quite so sharp. Dr. Tousey exhibited the apparatus together with some of the negatives.

Dr. Leo Green mentioned a case of fracture of the inferior maxilla which was readily reduced by means of an aluminum cap splint. This did away with the necessity of feeding through a tube. He thought with a little more attention to details the interdental splint might be discarded.

Dr. S. E. Davenport read a paper entitled " Some Partial Impressions."

(For Dr. Davenport's paper, see page 645.)

DISCUSSION.

Dr. Strang.—I can indorse Dr. Davenport's method of taking a preliminary impression and making therefrom a cup. I frequently have had occasion to take my first impression without regard to the teeth, simply vulcanizing on that model the base on which the teeth are to be articulated, and with that in the mouth getting the correct articulation. I remember about ten years ago I had a very perplexing case. The difficulties of getting a good impression of that mouth seemed insurmountable. I made the plate upon which the teeth were finally mounted in two sections. I took the impression of one side of the mouth first and vulcanized this half, and then got my correct impression of the other side and vulcanized that. Placing them together, I had a correct plate on which to articulate the teeth. The result was very satisfactory.

Dr. F. L. Fossume.—In difficult cases where undercuts exist, I use smooth, nickel-plated impression cups. which are oiled, and after the plaster is hardened in the mouth the impression cup is slipped off and the plaster is split with a knife and removed in sections, and these are again placed back in the cup.

Where a metal plate is to be struck up on such models. the teeth forming the undercut should be sawed half through and then broken off, and after the metal die is obtained and the plate swaged the teeth are carefully placed back on the model and waxed in position with hard wax. In this way the whole denture with clasps and lugs can be completed on one model, which is of great importance, as it avoids taking another impression.

Dr. C. W. Strang, of Bridgeport, Conn., read a paper entitled " Errors, Mistakes, and Failures, Old and New."

(For Dr. Strang's paper, see 639.)

DISCUSSION.

The President.—I had the other day a personal illustration bearing out some of the points in Dr. Strang's paper. My second son, an interne in one of the New York hospitals, while fooling with one of his associates, acquired a twisted fracture of one of the metacarpal bones. He came down with his wrist all done up in the proper manner. He told me that he had learned more in twenty-four hours regarding such fractures than he had learned during his entire medical course. He proceeded to enumerate the things he had found out from this personal experience that he could not have gotten from his teachers.

I am sure that any of us who, in the course of our experience, have required the manipulation in our own mouths of some other practitioners, have learned more than we had learned in long years of ordinary practice. It has been said that no one ought to practise dentistry who did not have a tooth to be filled at least three or four times a year, so that he might know something about the way in which he is treating his friends.

Dr. E. A. Bogue.—It has seemed to me that Dr. Strang's experience is the experience of us all. He has stated that at first he tried to follow the teachings of Dr. Atkinson, but after abandoning them he did better. I remember at one time having consulted thirty-two of my fellow-practitioners in regard to a certain point, finding eventually that every one of them was in the wrong. That is why I have my thousand models now for reference.

I saw to-day a case that seemed to me to be one of extreme error. It was one of ten or more inlays. They were of metal and on the grinding surfaces of the anterior teeth above and below. All of them had pins set into the pulp-chambers of the various teeth. The articulation was such that none of the upper incisors met the lower. These heavily armored teeth did not touch each other at all. Why these teeth should have been shod to that extent I do not know.

Regarding the case mentioned by Dr. Strang, I could not help wondering why he did not have a microscopical examination made.

Dr. Strang.—That was seven years ago, and the facilities for such an examination were not as available as now.

Dr. F. Milton Smith.—I am thankful, gentlemen, that I have not a monopoly on this subject. I am delighted to hear of Dr. Strang's mistakes. One or two of my own mistakes are still in my memory.

I have not in years gone by regulated sets of teeth as I should have done, and I am beginning to have patients come in to me who have been my patients for fifteen, twenty, twenty-five, or twenty-eight years, and I am beginning to realize my former neglect. This is one of the mistakes that I have made.

Another very serious mistake that I have made is that in order to make room in certain cases I have sacrificed an upper bicuspid and a lateral incisor, lower. I wish some of you gentlemen could see that mouth.

Dr. Bogue.—Another mistake. Last Friday a young lady was in my chair, and she wanted to know why her teeth were decaying between the molars, as she was very careful in cleansing them. I explained to her that the reason was that when she was a child I did not know enough to regulate her teeth properly. " If I were doing it to-day I should see to it that all the thirty-two teeth articulated as nature had intended them. If I had done this you would not have the trouble you are now having."

It is not more than three years since our president said to me, at a meeting of the Reform Club, " Why, the first thing we know, this fellow will be claiming that the articulation of the teeth has something to do with the deposition of tartar." Dr. Davenport, who was with us at the time, immediately spoke up, " Well, it does." And he was right.

The wisdom-teeth, situated as they are at the angle of the jaw, are the key of the other teeth. They are the braces against which the other teeth rest. They are the bumpers set up at the station house against which the trains are to hit. Remove the braces, and what happens? The other teeth begin to separate a little bit, food crowds in between, and then deposits of tartar will begin to be found, and you may be pretty sure decay will go on there sooner or later.

Dr. Gillett.—I often feel thankful that two cases of first molar extraction are out of my reach and that I see them no more. One of them I never saw after the extraction was done. A case that I do see is one in which I insisted on having the deciduous molars extracted because they remained some time after their normal time. I did this with the assurance that the bicuspids would soon be making their appearance. I see that patient occasionally, but those bicuspids have never appeared, and it is a pretty sorry set of teeth. Of course, we do not do those things since we have had the X-ray, and the younger men may avoid such mistakes.

Dr. Strang.—Referring to Dr. Bogue's contention that the wisdom-teeth should always be saved, suppose, for example, in a patient eighteen or nineteen years of age the wisdom-teeth erupt and almost immediately begin to break down, and this in a mouth where all the other twenty-eight teeth are in good condition. It has seemed to me that in these cases, where it seems hopeless to save the wisdom-teeth, it would be better to take them out and preserve the remaining teeth in a fairly sound condition. The wisdom-teeth are not always good bumpers, because sometimes they point the other way.

Dr. Bogue.—The normal articulation of the teeth at about eighteen years of age involves twenty-eight teeth. Later on it may require thirty-two, but when the articulation is normal these teeth are almost self-cleansing. They do not need a brush, and they do not need a dentist very often, and when they wear down they leave cusps.

Dr. L. C. LeRoy.—I have in mind a case where the upper wisdom-teeth seemed to be not merely unnecessary, but positively an injury to the mouth. Before the third molars erupted the arch was practically perfect, with the exception that the lateral incisors were apparently too wide for the size of the upper centrals. This disarranged the anterior arrangement a little. The point I wish to make is that the cuspids, bicuspids, and molars occluded perfectly. When the upper wisdom-teeth erupted they caused considerable crowding and overlapping of the lateral incisors and disarrangement of the occlusion until the eruption of the lower third molars.

Regarding the surfaces of molars that are so prone to decay, I have treated such surfaces with nitrate of silver previous to filling with phosphate. The advent of copper marks the advent of a new era in the treatment of these cases and many so-called "soft" teeth of children.

Dr. Gillett.—Dr. Strang speaks of the nearly perfect mouths in which there have appeared these very imperfect wisdom-teeth, the extraction of which he advocates. It would be very interesting if he would go over these mouths again as they come to him and ascertain if possible if any of the things spoken of by Dr. Bogue have occurred, and show us casts to demonstrate whether the extraction of the wisdom-teeth in these cases has resulted in harm. Those of us who have been in practice know that it often takes more than ten years to develop results in the mouth. We so often misunderstand each other because the same words do not always mean the same thing to speaker and hearer. Casts showing results would be of great value in discussing this point.

Dr. Strang.—I might say that this suggestion of Dr. Gillett's has been followed, and that I have as yet seen no ill effects from these extractions.

It was moved and carried unanimously that a vote of thanks be extended to Dr. Strang for his very helpful paper.

Adjourned.

FRED. L. BOGUE, M.D., D.D.S.,
Editor The New York Institute of Stomatology.

ACADEMY OF STOMATOLOGY.

A SPECIAL meeting was held Tuesday, June 20, 1905, at eight P.M., the President, Dr. D. N. McQuillen, in the chair.

INCIDENTS OF PRACTICE.

Dr. Dudley Guilford.—I have some bur-holders that I procured in Paris that may be of interest. They are gotten up by Raymenfrayer. The holder consists of a nickel-plated brass frame, into which are put the glass tubes with the head of the bur sticking up. It is a neat arrangement, and at the bottom there is a sterilizing apparatus. I have here a drawer with the same arrangement, except that the tubes are placed in a little frame in the drawer.

Another arrangement which I have not seen before is that of keeping the Swiss broaches wrapped in cotton in a Petrie plate, by which means they can be sterilized dry.

Another useful device is a cotton-holder, which I also procured in France, though it may be an American invention.

Dr. Otto E. Inglis.—The remarks of Dr. Guilford suggest a little point which I make use of. It is sometimes necessary to sterilize the broach quickly, and this is rather better accomplished by placing the broach in water and then dipping it into dry sodium. This gives a more reasonable assurance that the cotton is sterile.

Dr. Boenning.—I think the suggestion of Dr. Inglis is a good one. I believe that one reason why we have unsatisfactory results is that we have not been sufficiently careful to sterilize instruments and materials. Thorough sterilization is almost as necessary as in abdominal surgery.

I would like to speak of a case of a child who at four years of age, and though in perfect health, has lost her lower centrals. She is now four and a half years of age, and is losing the four molars. There is no history of any injury, and the child is well nourished. I have assured the mother that there is no doubt about the second teeth coming in. I have seen probably one or two cases in which the deciduous teeth were lost at five years, but not in a child of four years. The upper teeth are loosening, and will probably be lost within the next six months. The roots of the teeth lost were absorbed. Dr. Pearce, whom I consulted, has seen two or three cases, and he assures me that the permanent teeth came through normally.

Dr. Otto E. Inglis.—Dr. Boenning's case recalls one of a child six years of age with a very deformed mouth and no occlusion at all. There is some hypertrophy of the alveolar process, and the teeth are in such bad condition that I have decided to have chloroform administered and extract all of the deciduous teeth. I had another case of a lady who had a reasonable number of teeth, which looked fairly well, but there was no occlusion whatever. The occlusion was between the ramus of the lower jaw and the tuberosity of the superior maxilla. I have been unable to secure an impression of her mouth.

Dr. Boenning.—I have received a letter asking for my experience with the apparatus for drawing pus from the tooth socket. The writer of the letter had used it on a patient and had drawn what appeared to be pus. He was much elated, but the next day the patient returned, saying that he had suffered greatly through the night. Dr. Gaylord, I understand, has been making some experiments with the apparatus, and I would like to inquire of his success.

Dr. Gaylord.—I purchased one of the appliances made by the Keystone Electric Company similar to the one shown by Dr. McPherson, and used it in a most pronounced case in which the pus had burrowed through the bone. The mucous membrane in certain lights had a yellowish cast, which would prove to any one that pus was present. With the electrode applied over this area there was gathered an accumulation of material which resembled pus. It was about of the consistency of pus, was of a greenish-yellow color, and I think anybody would have called it pus. A specimen was submitted to a bacteriologist and pathologist whose opinion no one would question. He made a careful examination, and said that no pus was present. The only abnormality was its richness in albumin; otherwise it would have been called saliva. There was nothing to indicate that it was pus. The fact bears out my argument, the night the subject was presented, that things are not always what they appear and that it is better to go at things carefully and with scientific investigation prove them rather than to guess at the results. I have the apparatus, and would be willing to sell it at a greatly reduced price.

Dr. Otto E. Inglis.—I have seen and used the apparatus once, and do not desire to purchase Dr. Gaylord's. The gentleman on whom I used the apparatus had the tooth opened in the usual way, but without relief. Suction was made and an effort made to get through the apical foramen. For twenty minutes I applied this battery which had been left at my office by the Keystone Company. No relief was secured, and the tooth was subsequently removed. I could see nothing having the appearance of pus. What I did see was a little frothing about the gum. Personally, I cannot see why the electricity would not follow the easiest channel, going through the soft parts and creating electrolysis.

The President.—Personally I have had no experience. Dr. Head tells me that he is very well satisfied with his results in its use.

Dr. Gaylord.—I think the instrument is of value as a counter-irritant.

The President.—One patient told me that the pain from its use was worse than the pain he was bearing.

Dr. Inglis.—My patient complained of a great deal of burning from the use of the apparatus.

OTTO E. INGLIS,
Editor Academy of Stomatology.

NINTH ANNUAL MEETING OF THE NATIONAL DENTAL ASSOCIATION.

THE ninth annual meeting of the National Dental Association, held at Buffalo, N. Y., convened in the auditorium of the Central Y. M. C. A. building at ten o'clock, Tuesday morning, July 25. 1905, the President, Dr. Waldo E. Boardman, of Boston, Mass., in the chair.

Dr. Charles S. Butler, of Buffalo, delivered the address of welcome on behalf of the mayor of Buffalo, who was unable to be present.

The session was then opened by the President reading his address, which, after a short discussion, was referred to a committee.

The first business transacted was on a motion by Dr. H. J. Burkhardt, of Batavia, N. Y., to amend the constitution and by-laws, changing the basis of representation so as to admit to membership in the National Association delegates from State and Territorial societies only, thus restoring a basis which proved so unsatisfactory, after trial, early in the career of the organization, that it was promptly changed.

Notice of this was given last year, and it was brought up at this meeting as unfinished business. It provoked an angry discussion, took up much valuable time, and was finally passed by a small majority, and was made to take effect immediately, notwithstanding that the announcement for this session distinctly states that " Members of the profession are cordially invited to this meeting. and may join the association by presenting delegates' certificates from their State or local societies." In the face of this, making the amendment immediately effective was an outrageous proceeding. and placed a number who had come to the meeting with certificates from local societies in an embarrassing position. The writer suggests that in all future announcements the clause defining conditions of membership be immediately followed by the words, *"subject to change without notice,"* in conspicuous display type. This action is the more indefensible from the fact that it was not prompted by any desire to benefit the society, but for the purpose of keeping out a single individual who, having been expelled from the leading dental society in his locality, had gathered around him a sufficient number of associates to organize a new society, and came as their delegate. Rather than assume the responsibility of declaring this new society or its delegate unworthy, the majority of those present preferred that the association should place itself on record as inviting members of the profession to unite with it on terms distinctly stated, and then, after these had been complied with, and the candidates were present, without cause refusing them admission. The injustice of this was so evident that the Council advised that it be recalled. It is a dangerous thing for associations like this to take part in local quarrels, and unwise to change its general rules to meet special cases.

This was followed by a long report from the Committee on Army and Navy Legislation. Such long reports should always be printed and distributed, so that members may read them at their leisure. However interesting or important, or however well read, they are tiring to the audience, and very few indeed can follow their reading sufficiently well to fully understand their import.

This was followed by adjournment.

The afternoons and evenings were allotted, according to programme, to meetings of sections, and accommodations were prepared at Hotel Iroquois, head-quarters of the Association, for the three sections to meet in separate rooms, at the same time, for reading of papers and discussions. For an association so few in numbers as is the National, this is a very unsatisfactory arrangement. While the list of papers was long, very few in attendance heard many read. There was, in the first place, no certainty when any particular paper would be presented, so no one could select any one section without risk of disappointment; and the effort of some to overcome this caused a to-and-fro movement from one section to another that was distracting. Of the thirty-two papers on the programme, the greater number were, judging by their titles, not such as should be brought before a National Association. Some were, practically, second-hand; others, while good, were upon subjects far more suitable for local society discussion; others, again, were on subjects quite threadbare, and would find their proper place in an undergraduate student's society. Were these eliminated, and the time of the association properly utilized, all that remained could have been properly cared for in general sessions.

Very much time was wasted by not beginning the meetings of sections at the time appointed. By means of placards the various events were fairly satisfactorily announced, but (the evening meetings especially) they were not promptly called. Frequent changes were made, and the meetings of general sessions, of committees, and of sections, were very confusing. Not only was this time-wasting, but the delay and the uncertainty discouraged that keen interest in the proceedings so essential to a successful meeting. Members, after standing around half an hour or more waiting for a session to open, strolled off, to straggle in later, when the session was half over.

The preparation and proper presentation of scientific matter for information and discussion is admittedly a vexed question. The present scoop-net method is faulty. Selection by invitation, as the profession is now organized, would probably prove equally unsatisfactory. Any censorship, unless tactfully exercised, invites trouble. Should the Association succeed in launching a journal of its own, this might prove an acceptable outlet for papers prepared for the association meetings that in either subject or treatment were not deemed the best to bring before it. They need not be rejected: they could be read by title and accepted for the journal by a complimentary vote of thanks to the writers. Papers on subjects of general professional interests, education, legislation, etc., original research, matters pertaining to practice that are entirely new, seem to be much more appropriate for presentation to a National Association than variations of old methods or matters which have been frequently discussed.

Meetings conducted as was this, while a social success, fall far below what they might be in helpfulness to professional growth. There is nothing in them attractive to the new-comer, one who is not yet initiated into the inner circle. This is serious, for the new-comer is very important to a society's progress, indeed to its very existence. Without a constant influx of new life, of new ideas, and new ideals, the period of decadence is soon reached, and " race suicide" invited. Only those born later can keep in close touch with men and affairs of later days.

The multiplicity of fraternities, and of associations meeting at the same time and place as the National Association, and under its shadow and wing, is a growing evil. However worthy and useful in themselves, they are intruders and parasites when permitted to interfere with the more important body, as they undoubtedly did at Buffalo.

There was far too much disorder on the platform. During the opening session, at one time, all on the platform, except the member speaking, were engaged in an animated discussion among themselves. This is distracting alike to the speaker and to the audience. At the general sessions and the section meetings a constant running to the platform of this one and that kept up a commotion that was annoying to the speaker, and divided the attention of the audience. Such thoughtless actions detract very much from the dignity of the proceedings, and should be by all means avoided.

Enthusiasm is necessary to a thoroughly successful meeting of a body like this. That is best promoted by a series of properly conducted consecutive sessions, well attended. Vacant chairs are not inspiring.

No one individual could hear enough of either the papers or the discussions at Buffalo to pass judgment upon their merit, or to give an idea of their value, scope, or character. In that respect the meeting was unsatisfactory. The profession must wait for this perhaps a year or more, and accept it in driblets. It will come to them in time, like the "left-overs" of a forgotten feast—much of it insipid and useless. The same is true, in a manner, of the business transacted.

The manufacturers' exhibits lost much of their impressiveness by being displayed in a number of small rooms. This, however, to the writer seemed an advantage. It gave the attendants a much better opportunity to present their wares, and the dentist a much better opportunity to examine and select, than when jostled by a crowd. The exhibits were excellent, varied, and instructive. They were unobtrusive without being in the least degree suppressed. Of late, the tendency has been to permit commercial interests to occupy so prominent a place that professional interests have become a mere annex. It was not so at Buffalo.

The clinics, held the mornings of Wednesday and Thursday,

July 26 and 27, in the Dental Department building of the University of Buffalo, were the most satisfactory part of the meeting. The various rooms, and their furnishings afforded excellent accommodations. The clinics had been well advertised, and the supply of patients was abundant. Every thing was well ordered, and promptly and without confusion each day's work was commenced. Every opportunity was afforded onlookers at the operative clinics to inspect each critical stage of the operation as it was reached at the various chairs. This was an excellent feature. Having opportunity to examine the field of operation before anything was done, knowing what the operator proposed to do, again examining the cavity when ready to receive the filling, and having the special points of interest in its preparation pointed out, and later, under like favorable circumstances, being able to note the progressive steps by which the filling was constructed, and finally, at leisure, to critically inspect the finished work, made the operation interesting and instructive. This was done in all cases that admitted of it. It was more helpful, indeed, to the observer than to watch an operation from start to finish in that more than one operator's work was seen. It was helpful also to the operator; it relieved him of a distracting crowd when the work in hand most needed his undivided attention, and the intervals when his work was inspected gave him needed rest. As many like operations were going on at the same time, the onlookers were kept busy going from chair to chair in response to the announcement that so and so had reached an interesting stage of his work. To enter into a description of the operations performed is beyond the scope of this brief sketch. Suffice it to say that interest centred in the work of members of the G. V. Black Dental Club of St. Paul, exponents of the much talked of "extension for prevention" ideas, etc., of later days. There were other operators, but these attracted the most attention in the room in which the gold-workers were located.

The writer was impressed by the great change which has taken place in later days. A few years ago nearly all the gold operations here performed would have been done with an electric mallet. Not one was seen in the clinic. All the work was done with a hand mallet in the hands of a trained lady assistant. The businesslike ways, the non-obtrusiveness, the precision of movement, the patient attentiveness of these lady assistants in anticipating and supplying the operators' needs was quite marked.

Nearly all the gold-workers were *sans* coat and vest, in "shirt sleeves," an attire out of place at a dental chair, even at a clinic. It is true that the room was warm; a light coat adds but little to one's discomfort, however, and looks far more professional than a day-laborer's garb. The "slouchy" positions some assumed while working were justly criticised; such positions are as unnecessary as they are unhealthy and ungraceful. Operators at a dental clinic should remember that they themselves are part of the exhibits, quite as much so as is their work, and conduct themselves accordingly.

Porcelain work held second place; it was not, however, neglected. A number of skilled operators, located in another room, by constructing and inserting practical work, demonstrated their methods and, at the same time, the distinctive features of several different electric furnaces used.

The new anæsthetics, narcotile and somnoforme, were used, practically, for tooth extraction; and in addition they were administered to any dentist who desired to personally experience their effects.

Several surgical clinics were on the programme, but as these were held at the Buffalo General Hospital, and at the same time as these clinics were going on, they were missed by the writer.

The table clinics were an interesting feature. Among those which especially attracted the writer's attention was a press exhibited by Dr. J. A. Brown, of Morrisville, Vt., especially designed for swaging aluminum plates. He claimed for this method not only ease of working and accuracy of adaptation, but a better plate, inasmuch as the hard surface given to sheet aluminum by rolling was not impaired. It may not be generally known that when aluminum is rolled into plate the surface immediately in contact with the rollers is condensed and thereby becomes more resistant to wear and to corrosion. Swaging between dies usually roughens this surface so that in the smoothing and polishing processes it is entirely removed. Dr. Brown claims that by the method he demonstrated this was avoided.

Dr. L. L. Bosworth, Toledo, Ohio, exhibited an electric furnace for gold soldering. This was not a muffle furnace. It was shaped somewhat like a round asbestos soldering-block; the depression, however, was deeper, and sufficiently large to hold a full denture invested and ready for soldering. This cavity, its bottom and sides fitted with thin platinum wire, as is the muffle of porcelain electric furnaces, becomes evenly heated when the current is turned on. In simple cases the blow-pipe may not be needed; in others it is used while the case is still in the furnace to direct the flow of the solder. It is claimed for this furnace, greater convenience, safety to the porcelain teeth, and less risk of the plate warping.

Dr. A. L. Haas, of Des Moines, Iowa, demonstrated an appliance for swaging gold or platinum caps to the end of tooth-roots prepared for crowning. All the work is done upon the root itself, in the mouth. The gold or platinum plate is roughly shaped to the root, and the dowel passed through. A punch, provided with a series of removable faces to suit different sizes of tooth-roots, with a hole loosely fitting the dowel, is then adjusted over it, with a piece of unvulcanized rubber between the plate and the face of the punch. A sharp blow with a mallet on the end of the punch drives the plate into close contact with the root, and marks its outline. It is now removed, and the dowel soldered to the plate. The edges of the plate are now bent so as to fit over the root, and so form a seamless cap fitting over the face of the root and extending rootward as far as desired. This is fitted to the root and the punch applied as before, to correct any change made by soldering and bending. It seemed to be a practical idea.

Dr. W. B. Dunning, of New York City, demonstrated a method of packing non-cohesive gold that to the writer was quite new. He formed the gold into small, soft, almost square pellets, and packed them into position, using an instrument with a sharp edge, very like a large hatchet excavator. This edge was kept quite sharp and smooth by frequent application to an Arkansas stone. The doctor especially recommended the method for small, irregular cavities. The method was not rapid; it made, however, a solid, very hard filling, that finished as nicely as though of molten gold.

Dr. L. C. Taylor, of Hartford, Conn., showed how to combine gold and cement. The cavity need not be prepared so carefully for retention as is usual when gold alone is used. The cement, he mixed to about the same consistency as it would be to retain an inlay, and with it partially filled the cavity. He then took a pellet of crystal gold large enough to nearly fill the cavity, heated this quite hot, and immediately pressed it into the cement. By heating the gold the air in its interstices is expanded, as this contracts when it is forced into the cement, the cement is drawn up into it.

making a more reliable union between the two than would otherwise take place. The heat also hastens the hardening of the cement.
The gold is held firmly in position until the cement hardens. It
is then packed, more added if needed, and finally well burnished
and finished. Dr. Taylor has made free use of this method in filling children's teeth, fissure cavities where he did not desire to
extensively excavate, and in cases where an easily introduced filling
is called for. He found fillings so inserted satisfactory and durable.
He laid particular stress upon having the gold quite hot when it is
pressed into the cement.

An interesting exhibit, occupying a small room, was made by
the Dental Department of Harvard. In the collection the writer
observed a series of lantern slides, such as are used in class instruction; instruments used by the students in making dental alloys,
and for testing the expansion and contraction of amalgam; and
several microscopes with slides showing specimens of crystals
brought to professional notice by recent researches regarding saliva.
Crystals from saliva and crystals of corresponding salts artificially
produced were shown side by side. The collection was well selected,
to show methods and means of instruction employed in the Dental
Department. It would be a good idea if the colleges generally
embraced the opportunity afforded by these large professional gatherings to show advanced methods for imparting instruction now in
use. So few dentists ever enter a college after they graduate that
it is not generally known how much change has been made of late
years in their methods and means.

Eighty-five clinics were on the programme for each day. One
hesitates to criticise, especially after seeing an exhibit, that seemed
too trifling for notice, surrounded hour after hour by an interested
crowd; yet, looking over the list, an impression remains that a
judicious pruning would have done no harm; not that there was
anything objectionable, but rather a lack of novelty and importance
in many of the table clinics, and in some of the chair clinics. It
seems a useless waste of time to demonstrate matters that have
been accepted facts for many years.

The number in attendance was said to be very satisfactory; it
was less, however, than the writer recalls at meetings of the American Association of more than a score of years ago. The conditions
of membership have not been changed, while the number of practising dentists, the contributing societies, and the membership

therein have very materially increased. This is not encouraging. This would have no meaning if the National Association was a strictly representative body. This is not the case. It is very largely composed of permanent members who owe no allegiance to the body through which they came to the Association. To a local society it is a matter of no moment whether all of its members or none are connected with the National Association, and makes no difference whether its appointed delegates attend or not. From one year's end to another it is very seldom, indeed, that anything occurs to remind the members of a local society that there is in the United States a National Dental Association, and equally rare that the local societies are referred to, helpfully, in the National Association proceedings. The National Association does not concern itself in making known its doings to the profession at large, and is practically unknown. At Buffalo, the section best attended was one not on the programme, the social section, almost continuously in session in the hotel lobby. To its own members accustomed to meet year after year, and to those well known to its members, it was very interesting, enjoyable, and will be longest remembered. To the "young fry," however, while it may have proved interesting and instructive,—far more so than attractive,—it is not likely that it tended to an increase of membership. They were left out in the cold. There seems to be a need for reorganization on lines better suited to geographical conditions, a reorganization which shall definitely define the position, the work, and the relations to each other of local, State, and national bodies; a reorganization from which the permanent membership idea is entirely eliminated in all but the local societies. They can then work together, and form an harmonious, compact body commanding the respect and support of the profession at large.

WILLIAM H. TRUEMAN.

Editorial.

PAST, PRESENT, AND FUTURE OF MECHANICAL DENTISTRY.

THE question of serious import in dentistry at the present time is, What shall constitute the fundamentals in teaching and practice? The dental world is apparently fast drifting into three classes. One regards mechanical dentistry, in its broadest sense, including operative, as the foundation of all our work and the one thing most necessary in the equipment of every practitioner. Another holds that this is altogether a minor qualification,—in fact, may be entirely set aside as unworthy and left exclusively to the one with mechanical tastes and experience. This man regards the medical school and all that is therein implied as the foundation of dentistry, and that nothing more is needed. The third holds that dentistry is a complex profession based on mechanics, nurtured through many years upon the idea that teeth to be saved must be defended from the inroads of destructive environments through the mechanical substitution of lost parts, and, failing in this, after an indefinite period, through the same mechanical skill substituting for the lost teeth artificial dentures.

That medical science, in its various branches, is of vast importance in the building up of dentistry needs no argument with the advanced thinker of the present period, but that it covers all that is necessary in the training of the dentist cannot be conceded.

The dental practitioners of a half-century in the past had no difficulty with these several divisions in thought and practice. That this has been materially changed is unfortunate, as it has created an antipathy detrimental to the best progress of the art. At this period there was but one dentistry, and its bounds were well defined and thoroughly understood. In time there came into it men from the medical schools too late in life, as a rule, to become proficient in the mechanical and operative side of the profession. These, very naturally, sought to separate the purely medical and surgical from the mechanical and relegate the latter to the secondary position it properly occupied, in their estimation. This was strength-

ened by the views held in Continental Europe and also by the
prejudice that has always existed against it by the medical profession universally and an unwillingness to recognize it as a part
of the great healing art.   It was assumed by this class that all
connection with mechanical dentistry must be severed before it
could be classed as a learned profession.   While at present it has
not gone so far as to include operations upon the natural organs, the
evident tendency is eventually to place that in the same category
with the worker upon the laboratory bench.

It seems to the writer that the time has arrived for a clear and
positive affirmation, on the part of the constituted professional
bodies, what should or should not be classified as dentistry.   If the
men who repudiate all mechanical knowledge are worthy to fill the
honored place of practitioners of the dental art, it will be to the
interest of the world to know it; but if, on the other hand, the
said world cares very little for the scientific attainments of the
individual, but does care very much for his ability in his mechanical
operations, it will be of vast importance that this should be most
thoroughly cultivated, that humanity may reap the benefit.

The writer occupies the position that there need be no real lines
of demarcation between the purely mechanical, operative, scientific,
and medical branches.   They should be so completely dovetailed,
each to the other, that the lines of separation should be indistin-
guishable.   This is, beyond all question, the true stand to take.
Neither of the four divisions can be lopped off without serious loss:
indeed, each is indispensable to the perfection of the whole.   It
seems, therefore, that those who are working to effect a separation
are straining to produce something based on false ideals, and these
latter never can result satisfactorily.

Mechanical dentistry, in its broadest acceptation, has been one
of the most important factors in the hygienic improvement of
human life.   Until mechanical dentistry began to assume proportions of value to the masses, their condition was of the most serious
character.   From the dawn of civilization the world had had no
means of preserving, much less to have inserted a substitute for, lost
organs.   It is within the memory of many still living that there
was a period when there existed a strong prejudice against any
attempt to thwart the destructive action of what were called the
natural processes of destruction, and that the word *false*, in connection with the human body, was regarded as antagonizing the

will of the Creator, and he or she who attempted to subvert this will by any substitute came under suspicion and reproach. The early practitioners had, therefore, a difficult task, and one not appreciated at the present period of more intelligent enlightenment. The advantages of a substitute for lost dentures were but slowly comprehended. This was due, in a measure, to imperfect skill on the part of dental mechanicians, for ability in this direction was of slow growth. As this was developed through years of experimentation, there came a different feeling, prejudices slowly vanished, and the skill of the mechanical dentist was more and more brought into requisition.

Upon the advent of the rubber base for dentures there came an increased, but in some respects an inferior, mechanical ability. The skill of the jeweller, the pride of the earlier dentist, was lost and has never yet been wholly regained; in fact, it is mainly due to this that the demand has been made for a separation from mechanics. While it is true much has been lost through the advent of rubber for dental purposes, much has been gained. That which has been lost to dentistry has been to the increase of health and happiness of large numbers of the human family. Dental workers have been multiplied by the thousands, enabling other thousands to have artificial substitutes at very moderate cost, not possible fifty years ago.

The result of all this work is beginning to make itself manifest in a remarkable manner. The individual who has passed the years of the Psalmist can well recall the appearance of the grandfathers and grandmothers of his youth. Bowed with the infirmities of age at sixty, toothless and with elongated mandibles, these caricatures of humanity were doomed to give their comparatively short lives as an evidence of the fact that nature is far from perfect, and that man, in numerous instances, is required to step in and remedy destructive effects. It was everywhere in evidence that the old men and women, through lack of proper digestive ability, failed rapidly physically and mentally. The so-called period of dotage was expected as a matter of course. The individual of middle life looked forward to this time with a feeling of horror. To the woman it was the period of the mob-cap and the witch's face. This the mechanical dentist has changed to a large degree, and eventually must be a condition obliterated. All that he has done has not been artistic,—far from it,—but he has given the larger number the means of masticating food properly. He has enabled the wearer of an artificial denture to be assured that, however imperfect it might be, it will aid, better than any other means, in keeping the stomach in reasonably good order, and with this in proper condition. mental force may be indefinitely continued. It is recognized that there are other factors that enter into and produce a loss of mental vigor, but it is nevertheless beyond question that, given a good digestion, mental activity will be prolonged to an age not possible, as a rule, a hundred years in the past.

It is then of vital importance that mechanical dentistry should not only be fostered to the fullest extent, but it should be held to be worthy the best efforts of the most cultivated. It is the art of all arts that appeals most to humanity, or should appeal, for it places the vestibule of the entire organism in a fit condition for the reception and comminution of the food necessary for the mainte-nance of the body in health. The same may be said equally of the operative branch; in fact, these two constitute a dentistry worthy the most extended efforts for their perfection.

Dentistry, as a whole, must be regarded as a failure if its mission is confined to the salvation of the natural teeth. While prophylaxis has, undoubtedly, a great future, and will be eventually a specialty in itself, it will fail, as all efforts have failed, to keep the natural organs to an advanced old age. Dentists, many of them at least, have yet to learn that the destructive processes are sure, in the future life of the individual, to end the life of the teeth. The exceptions to this are too few to be considered. Some operators still persist in regarding the destruction manifest after sixty as pyorrhœa alveolaris, but this is only in part true. The pulps die: the tubulated structure has long since ceased to fulfil its function. being closed and obliterated by secondary deposits; the teeth are no longer nourished by the peridental membrane; osteomalacia sets in, and the teeth become foreign bodies, are acted upon by the environments, and go down to destruction. The labor of the dentist has been of immense value in prolonging the usefulness of the teeth, but in the end it is written, failure.

The work of the mechanical dentist, then, is to fill this gap and make the skill of the dentist continuous. It commenced with the cradle, and it should follow humanity, through the added decades of life, to the grave.

With this view of prosthetic dentistry, and its twin brother operative dentistry, it seems almost a crime against humanity that there should be any effort to belittle this work. It should be welcomed as the handmaiden of our profession. And while dentistry, as a whole, may change, it seems reasonable to expect that the future of mechanical dentistry may be regarded as being co-existent with the life of the race on this planet. Therefore, while leaving nothing in the realm of scientific medicine untouched and unexplored, let us still cling to the foundation of that dentistry that has divested life of one of its many terrors and made the old man and the old woman more worthy of our respect and veneration, for the reason that our profession has made youth perennial.

Miscellany.

An Automatic Anæsthetic Capsule-Holder and Breaker (designed by Mr. Vernon Knowles).—There is little doubt but that the capsule form of the more volatile anæsthetics, such as ethyl chloride, somnoform, etc., has "come to stay," since the advantages obtained are many and obvious.

In the first place, they can be kept any length of time, in any climate, without the slightest risk of deterioration, or diminution of their contents. Then, again, exact and known quantities can be relied upon, a very important factor, as the risk of overdosage, with its distressing and sometimes fatal symptoms, is entirely eliminated. They are open to one great objection,—viz., the difficulty of their manipulation.

Some makers advise cutting off the tips with a pair of scissors; others, that the necks should be nicked with a file. Neither are satisfactory. Not only is there danger of the operator being wounded by glass splinters, but ofttimes their contents are lost through fracture of the capsule, or by being forcibly expelled.

To overcome this, various inhalers have been introduced containing contrivances whereby the capsules can be fractured inside the same. This is an objectionable, if not a dangerous method, in that particles of glass are scattered in all directions. This device overcomes these difficulties in a simple and practical manner.

It is small and compact, and, being of metal throughout, is

unbreakable; owing to its simplicity of construction, it is little liable to get out of order.

It consists of four parts, which when put together form a metal case completely enclosing the capsule,—the body which holds the capsule, a sheath which keeps it in position, a ball-and-socket nozzle, and a nozzle cap. These are held together by bayonet catches.

When the capsule is inserted and the parts are put together, the neck of the capsule projects into the ball-and-socket nozzle; it therefore follows that when the latter is deflected in any direction the neck is fractured, and the contents projected on to or into any medium that may be selected for presenting the anæsthetic. a properly placed fine gauze screen effectively holding back any glass particles. The device is manufactured by the Dental Manufacturing Company, of London.—(*Dental Record*, vol. xxv., July, 1905, p. 342.)

THE INFLUENCE OF THE FIRST AND SECOND DENTITION PERIODS IN THE ETIOLOGY OF EPILEPSY.—In the course of an article bearing this title in the *Medical News* of December 10, 1904, Spratling gives us the following views which bear on treatment. He thinks it is always a mistake to regard the convulsions of dentition, or the convulsions due to any other cause in early life. in any other than a serious light. They are never positively benign—at least, we have no right to regard them so. That infants who have convulsions escape serious consequences in the future is always a matter for congratulation, but the physician should never assume that this is the outcome to be expected. When disease tendencies are so strongly marked as these morbid manifestations so plainly indicate, the most constant care and treatment should be undertaken at once in every case with a view to preventing epilepsy, or idiocy, or insanity, or other states of degeneracy destined to destroy the mental life of the individual in question.

In conclusion, the author's views in the matter may be briefly summarized as follows:

1. Difficult dentition—*i.e.*, the piercing of the gums by the tooth

—may, in suitable subjects, constitute a sufficient irritant to cause convulsions.

2. In suitable subjects these convulsions may ultimately lead to epilepsy.

3. By suitable subjects is meant infants who inherit a neuropathic tendency to disease; whose parents have epilepsy, or insanity, or who are alcoholic, or suffer from some other general vice that could be transmitted to the offspring in some form capable of vitiating its powers of resistance to disease.

4. The author does not believe that difficult dentition alone in a child who inherited no ancestral taints, and who at its birth is free from a tendency to nervous disease, can cause epilepsy.

5. Great caution must always be exerted to lay the true cause in cases of this kind where it belongs; for the reason that gastro-intestinal disorders, the sequelæ of the eruptive fevers, and other factors common at this age, may produce similar results.

A NOVEL HEAD-REST, ESPECIALLY USEFUL IN TOOTH-EXTRACTION.—An article in the June number, 1905, of C. Ash & Sons' Quarterly Circular, page 189, credited to Mr. W. Orr Gray, L.D.S. (Eng.), D.D.S., describes and illustrates a novel head-rest, invented by Dr. Frank Nyulasy, of Melbourne, Australia, especially useful in tooth-extraction under a general anæsthetic. This head-rest is shaped very much like a bowl, and is intended to be fixed, by means of adjustable arms, to an ordinary surgical operating-table, or to a common deal table, to support the patient's head while he is recumbent upon the table. The bowl-like rest is fixed a few inches below the level of the table, and supports the head comfortably and firmly in a position not only favorable to operations within the mouth, but in a position especially favorable to easy respiration. It was originally designed to facilitate operations for post-nasal growths, for operations upon the roof of the mouth and upper jaw, for excision of the larynx, and for endoscopic examinations of the œsophagus. Its chief advantages to the dentist are: (1) The absolute prevention of all danger from ingress of teeth, roots, etc., to the respiratory passages. (2) Complete and unhampered use of the respiratory mechanism, in contradistinction to the strained position of the anterior muscles of the neck when the patient is in a dental chair. (3) The facility with which lower back roots or impacted wisdom-teeth can be removed, as well as all the other teeth. (4) The almost total prevention of the passage of blood to the stomach during anæsthesia.

The recumbent position is especially favorable to safety in administration of general anæsthetics, and to rapid recovery from their effects.

The article closes with the remark that " for further information as to the head-rest, the *British Medical Journal* of April 20, 1904, may be consulted."

W. H. T.

Current News.

MISSISSIPPI DENTAL ASSOCIATION.

THE twelfth annual meeting of the Mississippi Dental Association, held in Jackson, April 19 to 21, 1905, elected the following officers:

President. Dr. A. B. Kelly, Yazoo City; First Vice-President. Dr. L. B. McLaren. Natchez; Second Vice-President, Dr. J. F. Scott. Summit; Secretary, Dr. E. Douglas Hood, Tupelo; Corresponding Secretary, Dr. W. H. Reaben. McComb City; Treasurer. Dr. C. C. Crowder, Kosciusko.

Executive Committee.—Dr. W. O. Talbot, Biloxi; Dr. C. F. Boger, Natchez; Dr. E. Douglas Hood. Tupelo. Chairman. *ex officio.*

The next meeting promises to be the best ever held, and preparations are now being made for a good series of papers and some interesting clinics.

The thirteenth annual meeting will be held in Gulfport. between the 1st and 15th of June. 1906. Exact date to be fixed by the Executive Committee.

E. DOUGLAS HOOD,
Secretary.

OFFICERS OF THE NATIONAL ASSOCIATION OF DENTAL EXAMINERS.

PRESIDENT, H. W. Campbell, D.D.S., Suffolk, Va.; Vice-President from the West, F. O. Hetrick, D.D.S., Ottawa, Kan.; Vice-President from the South, F. A. Shotwell, D.D.S., Rogersville, Tenn.; Vice-President from the East, George E. Mitchell, D.D.S., Haverhill, Mass.; Secretary and Treasurer, Charles A. Meeker, D.D.S., Newark, N. J.

Committee on Colleges.—J. G. Reid, D.D.S., *Chairman*, Chicago, Ill.; George E. Mitchell, D.D.S., Haverhill, Mass.; J. J. Wright, D.D.S., Milwaukee, Wis.

Committee on Conference.—J. F. Dowsley, D.D.S., *Chairman*, Boston, Mass.; F. O. Hetrick, D.D.S., Ottawa, Kan.; R. H. Walker, D.D.S., Norfolk, Va.

Membership Committee.—M. F. Finley, D.D.S., *Chairman*, Washington, D. C.; Thomas Cole, D.D.S., Newman, Ga.; C. R. Taylor, D.D.S., Streator, Ill.

State Advisory Committee.—Henry Barnes, M.D., Cleveland, Ohio; George E. Mitchell, D.D.S., Haverhill, Mass.; E. P. Dameron, D.D.S., St. Louis, Mo.; C. H. Oakman, D.D.S., Detroit, Mich.; W. G. Mason, D.D.S., Tampa, Fla.

Committee for Promoting Relations with Foreign Examiners.— T. J. Barrett, D.D.S., *Chairman*, Worcester, Mass.; F. A. Shotwell, D.D.S., Rogersville, Tenn.; F. C. James, D.D.S., Winona, Minn.; C. Stanley Smith, D.D.S., Cincinnati, Ohio.

Committee on Resolutions.—H. C. Brown, D.D.S., Columbus, Ohio; C. S. Stockton, D.D.S., Newark, N. J.; F. F. Drew, D.D.S., Baltimore, Md.

Committee on Contracts.—Charles A. Meeker, D.D.S., Newark, N. J.

Committee on Tabulation of Examiners' Reports of Examinations.—Alphonso Irwin, D.D.S., Camden, N. J.

MISSISSIPPI VALLEY MEDICAL ASSOCIATION.

AT the next meeting of the Mississippi Valley Medical Association, to be held at Indianapolis, Ind., October 10, 11, 12, 1905, the annual addresses will be delivered by Dr. Arthur R. Edwards, of Chicago, and Dr. W. D. Haggard, of Nashville, Tenn.

Dr. Edwards has chosen for the subject of his address, "Certain Phases of Uræmia: Their Diagnosis and Treatment," and Dr. Haggard will discuss, in his address, "The Present Status of Surgery of the Stomach." In addition to these addresses there will be the annual address of the President, Dr. Bransford Lewis, of St. Louis.

A cordial invitation is extended to every physician in the valley to attend this meeting, for which a large number of interesting and valuable papers have been promised.

HENRY E. TULEY, M.D.,

Secretary.

NATIONAL ASSOCIATION OF DENTAL FACULTIES.

THE twenty-second annual meeting of the National Association of Dental Faculties, held at Buffalo, N. Y., July 27 and 28, 1905. resulted in the election of the following officers and committees:

President, J. H. Kennerly, 2645 Locust Street, St. Louis, Mo.: Vice-President, J. I. Hart, New York; Secretary, George Edwin Hunt, 131 East Ohio Street, Indianapolis; Treasurer, H. R. Jewett, Atlanta, Ga.

Executive Committee.—D. J. McMillan, Kansas City; L. P. Bethel, Columbus, Ohio; J. B. Wilmot, Toronto; R. M. Sanger. East Orange, N. J.; H. B. Tileston, Louisville.

Ad Interim Committee.—S. H. Guilford, Philadelphia; M. C. Marshall, St. Louis; J. P. Gray, Nashville.

Foreign Relations Committee.—G. V. Black, Chicago; W. F. Litch, Philadelphia; D. R. Stubblefield, Nashville; William Carr. New York; J. D. Patterson, Kansas City.

Forty-three of the fifty colleges holding membership were represented by delegates, and a most harmonious meeting was held. United States Consul J. H. Worman, Munich, Germany, was present at one session, and told what was being done to rehabilitate the American degree in that country. Announcement was also made that the United States government had recognized the National Association of Dental Faculties in its act regulating the practice of dentistry in the Philippine Islands.

GEORGE E. HUNT.

Secretary.

THE

International Dental Journal.

VOL. XXVI. NOVEMBER, 1905. No. 11.

Original Communications.[1]

SURGICAL ASPECTS OF DISTURBED DENTITION OF THE THIRD MOLARS.[2]

BY M. L. RHEIN, M.D., D.D.S., NEW YORK CITY.

THE third molars generally make their appearance between the ages of sixteen and twenty. The final development of the length of the maxillæ posterior to the mental foramen in the lower jaw and the maxillary sinus in the upper, takes place during this period, and in this manner sufficient space is provided for the proper alignment of the third molar when it breaks through the gum tissue. Where this development proceeds without any disturbing constitutional causes, no difficulties attend the eruption of these teeth. As, however, all inflammatory actions that arise during this period, either from local pathological causes or by virtue of constitutional disturbances, have a marked effect on the osseous development of these parts, we find the normal type of development to be the exception. These departures from a purely normal type vary greatly according to the amount of disturbance that has taken place,

---

[1] The editor and publishers are not responsible for the views of authors of papers published in this department, nor for any claim to novelty, or otherwise, that may be made by them. No papers will be received for this department that have appeared in any other journal published in the country.

[2] Read at Portland, Ore., July 12, 1905, before the Section on Stomatology of the American Medical Association. Published with consent of the Journal of the American Medical Association.

and in a large number of cases interfere with the normal eruption of the third molars. This interference with the eruption of these teeth is confined more particularly to the lower jaw. The reason for the lower third molar being exceptionally liable to serious disturbances is due to the difference in the anatomy of the two jaws. On account of the limitations of time, and small percentage of troubles encountered with erupting upper molars, these remarks will be confined strictly to the inferior teeth.

The necessity for sufficient room at the angle of the body and the ramus is shown in Fig. 1 (Cryer). Fig. 1 shows the mandible of one of the Fan tribe of West Africa, and there is abundance of room for the third molar. Fig. 2 (Cryer) is a picture of a Caucasian lower jaw of normal type where there is just barely sufficient room for the third molar. The lessening of this amount of space is one of the most prolific sources of disturbed dentition in this locality. Too frequently there is no room left between the second molar and the ramus, and as a result the third molar finally erupts in some unusual position. During this effort at unnatural eruption, grave disturbances are very liable to occur. The close proximity of the cribriform tube (Fig. 3, Cryer) to the roots of the third molar is another anatomical feature which has a marked bearing on the etiology of disturbances in this region. In many anatomical specimens the incompleted roots can be seen penetrating the canal itself. The cribriform tube or inferior dental canal (Fig. 4, Cryer) furnishes a pathway of slight resistance to infection, and once involved leads to serious septic conditions. Another marked pathological condition, that results from the close proximity to the inferior dental nerve, is that the irritation of this nerve is very likely to produce a stimulation in nutritional supply at this point. so that the normal cancellated bone (Fig. 5, Cryer), through which the erupting tooth can readily force its way, is replaced by the hardest of osseous structure which attempts to force the tooth aside and seek some easy but unnatural mode of eruption. This excitation of bony development sometimes proceeds to such extremes as to encapsulate the tooth in a dense bony cyst (Fig. 6, Cryer), in which it becomes impacted. The study of this condition will not be considered at this time, but it is merely mentioned as a possible result where this undue eruption proceeds to its extreme limit.

The unnatural increase in osteoblasts with all its attending inflammatory conditions, produces a marked effect on all the sur-

Fig. 1.

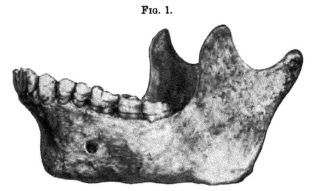

Mandible of a member of the Fan tribe, West Africa, showing abundance of room for third molar. (Cryer.)

Fig. 2.

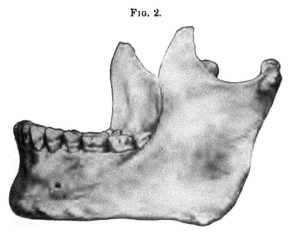

Caucasian lower jaw of modern type, with barely sufficient room for third molar. (Cryer.)

FIG. 3.

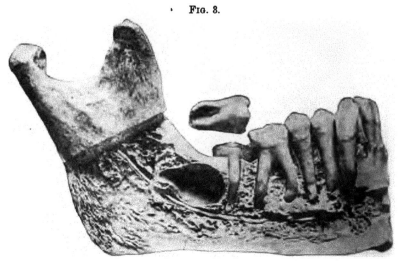

Close proximity of cribriform tube to root of third molar. (Cryer.)

FIG. 4.

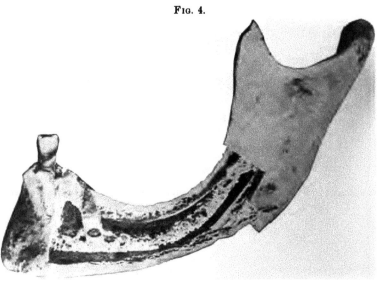

Showing cribriform tube. (Cryer.)

FIG. 5.

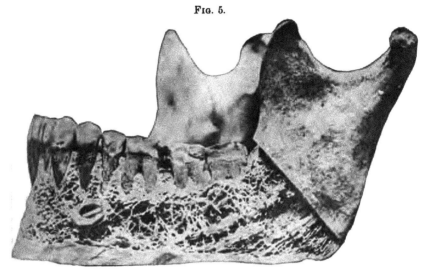

Normal cancellated bone. (Cryer.)

FIG. 6.

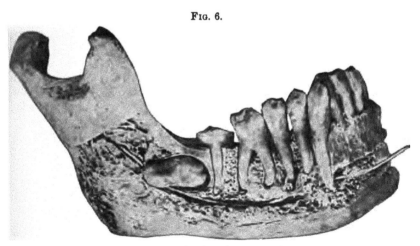

Tooth encapsulated in dense bony cyst. (Cryer.)

rounding tissue. Their tone of resistance is depressed in proportion to the degree of irritation, and this is also further influenced by any disturbances of the general system. When this decreased resistance has reached a certain stage, the parts become an easy prey to infection. In this way we find the eruption of the third molar, which should be a natural physiological action, complicated by more or less severe pathological disturbances.

Another etiological factor, that sometimes plays an important rôle in depressing the local vitality, is found in mouths where on occlusion the two jaws come so close together that traumata of the gums over the erupting tooth are constantly taking place, caused by the upper teeth constantly biting the gum tissue over the erupting tooth, and infection frequently ensues.

Another marked point of irritation is found in such mouths where, on account of lack of space between the second molar and the ramus, the third molar is pushed forward and its eruption is impeded by coming in contact with the distal side of the second molar. Frequently only the slightest impingement on the territory of the second molar will start up an inflammatory action, and the parts become rapidly infected.

Since 1828, when Toirac gave the first accurate description of this disturbance, French and German authorities have written extensively on this subject. In 1878 Heydenreich reviewed the list of writers on this subject up to that date. According to Magitot and David, complications ensue in the eruption of seventy-five per cent. of third lower molars. Some very unique etiological theories are advanced by some of these authorities. Moty, in 1901, tries to show an analogy between suppurating dermoid cysts and infections of erupting third molars. He finds the cause at the end of the root, and speaks of it as an "epithelial inclusion," and it will be instructive to quote from him. He says, "In our opinion these phlegmons are due entirely to a collection of epithelial cells enclosed at the bottom of the alveolus. This enclosed epithelium is found as a fungous mass which has gradually infiltrated the wall of the alveolus without enlarging the latter. In some cases this neoplastic tissue becomes encysted. In nearly all cases these epithelial inclusions cause abscesses at the time of eruption of the wisdom-teeth, or later on. Early extraction may be necessary on account of the pain, even before suppuration has set in, but the latter invariably occurs in cases left to themselves. The cause of this non-bacterial suppuration is due entirely to these cells acting as a foreign body.

"Epithelial inclusions may be found with other teeth, but only rarely. It is very probable that the enamel body may leave an epithelial focus in the gums which may develop into a tooth (giving rise to a third dentition). These cases themselves are very rare, but grouped with other anomalies (single cusps, an additional cusp or round root added to a molar, a large tooth, an extra tooth not growing from the gums, etc.) make a large class. Abscesses associated with healthy wisdom-teeth and commencing in the depth of the alveolus are generally sterile. The pus has no bad odor unless a secondary infection has supervened. An odor generally indicates a carious tooth."

If views such as these are correct, it upsets all our ideas of the pathogenic conditions at work in these cases. It is wise, however, to have our attention directed to the different views that are held on this subject, and I have quoted the latter one because it is so remarkably well expressed.

Careful observation of clinical data impress us with the view that there are many predisposing factors to be considered in the etiological study of different cases.

For the sake of convenience the subject can be considered in two divisions. First, disturbances which antedate the appearance of the tooth. Second, those which take place after the partial eruption of the tooth. Symptoms in the early stages are not much more marked than in ordinary physiological dentition. There is the usual amount of pain accompanied by congestion of the gums overlying the erupting tooth. The œdema becomes more marked, rapidly progressing in every direction, involving the pillars of the fauces and the various glands in the mouth. Neuralgic pains radiate to the ear and eye, and as the submaxillary glands become involved, they extend to the neck, shoulders, and even to the arms. The patient finds it more and more difficult to open the mouth. As infection progresses, the pulse becomes more rapid, and temperature may even rise to 103° F. A careful digital examination over the gums will readily detect the presence of the tooth underneath. In some cases the gum becomes attenuated and pale, as in ordinary dentition, but, as a rule, this is not the case, but the opposite condition results, which is that of excessive congestion.

Prompt excision of the entire hood of gum tissue is at once

called for. The resection of the gum should be so thorough as to completely expose the four sides of the tooth. Many authorities recommend the cautery for this purpose, but the knife is a more valuable adjunct, as the blood-letting itself is very beneficial. Every possible means should now be used to aid in the rapid eruption of the tooth and the prevention of reinfection of the parts. Foreign writers all unite in a plea for extraction as the only radical cure in these cases. Whenever it becomes evident that the third molar, by reason of its irregular position and a lack of space in the jaw for its proper berth, can never become a useful organ, the earliest extraction of the tooth is called for.

On the other hand, in a large percentage of cases, the tooth can be brought into proper alignment and occlusion, and under such circumstances there is no valid excuse for its extraction. A strip of gauze should be packed between the gum and tooth around its entire circumference. In case of the second molar acting as an obstruction, this gauze will act to some extent as a wedge in making a proper place for the third molar. The gauze packing should be frequently changed. If possible, the mouth should be sprayed at intervals with a hot borinated wash, which, at any rate, should be used by the patient frequently as a mouth lotion. The focus of infection in most cases under sufficiently energetic treatment will soon find an outlet, either into the mouth or the fauces, and the symptoms will rapidly abate.

The trismus, paralysis, and œdema symptoms in these cases involve so much surrounding territory that they are frequently mistaken by the medical attendant for adenitis, stomatitis, pyorrhœa, parotitis, and diseases due to other teeth. An error in diagnosis in these cases generally means an error in treatment, and usually results in an unnecessary disfigurement of the face. The frequency of errors in diagnosis of these cases is one of the strongest pleas that can be made for the education of medical men in the principles of dentistry.

The following notes taken from a typical case will illustrate this fact:

Miss A., between the ages of sixteen and seventeen, had been convalescing for two weeks from an attack of measles, when she commenced to have paroxysms of pain in the posterior portion of the mouth. This was accompanied by œdema and a steadily rising temperature. The physician who had attended her with the measles

was sent for, and he made a diagnosis of adenitis of the submaxillary glands. The temperature twenty-four hours later had
risen to 102.5° F., and her pulse was 120. Under his direction,
Credé's ointment was liberally spread over the neck at the angle
of the jaw, and this was covered by rubber tissue. The expectation of the attending physician was that the absorption of the
silver salt would arrest the infective infiltration. The result, however, was that it acted as a poultice, and drew the inflammation
and infection within the mouth to the outer tissues.

Forty-eight hours after this treatment had been commenced
I was called to see the patient, because the mother had a suspicion
that the teeth might be involved, the patient having continuously
complained of pain at the angle of the body and the ramus of the
mandible.

Examination.—I found the patient suffering severely from neuralgic pains, with a great amount of œdema, extending through the
entire cervical region, and involving most of the hyoid muscles.
A very careful external examination failed to discover any sign
of any glandular enlargement, but simply an œdema penetrating
through all the tissues. On this account it was difficult for the
patient to open her mouth, yet a careful digital examination over
the mandible, between the second molar and the ramus, readily
distinguished the outlines of an erupting third molar. The attending physician had reached the point where he expected to call
in a surgeon and make an external incision into the infected area.

Treatment.—The case being turned over to me, I at once dis-
sected away the entire hood of gum tissue which was covering the
erupting tooth, and found that the mesial approximal surface of
the third molar was impinging slightly on the distal approximal
contour of the second molar. Iodoform gauze was packed around
the entire circumference of the tooth, special attention being paid
to the space between the second and third molars.

Result.—The temperature of the patient dropped immediately
to 100.5°, and the pulse to 100. Naturally, the ointment and rubber tissue were at once removed from the neck, and hot borinated
mouth lavations were ordered every fifteen minutes, with the hope
of bringing the inflammatory action back again into the oral cavity.
A blood-count showed twenty thousand leukocytes.

There were many unpleasant instances connected with this
case on acount of the ill-feeling engendered in the mind of the

physician, because of the necessity of my making so radical a change in the treatment of the patient.

The patient was constantly under the care of a trained nurse, and for the following five days the temperature varied between 99.8° and 101°. At this time results of the treatment prevailed, and a purulent effusion made its escape from the tonsils. The packing of the gauze between the two molars was persisted in for about ten days, when sufficient space between the two molars was obtained, and the third molar was finally erupted into a position of correct occlusion and alignment.

The most serious type of cases are those where disturbances do not abate after partial eruption of the tooth has taken place. Writers frequently speak of the purulent troubles of third molars that exist even after eruption of the tooth has been completed, but a careful anatomical examination will generally show that the eruption of the tooth has not been entirely completed, some obstacle being present which prevents the tooth coming out as far as it naturally would. This is the class of cases that Moty, quoted above, speaks of, in which he classifies the cause as an " epithelial inclusion."

The undue osteoblastic stimulation that would result from the inflammatory action present in these cases is sufficient to account for this condition, which he so graphically describes as " epithelial inclusion," but which is nothing more than an overstimulation of peridental membrane, which, if persisted in, frequently leads to a complete ossification of the parts and produces an impacted tooth.

In all these cases every effort should be made in the line of proper orthodontia, so that, if possible, the tooth can be properly erupted and preserved. The value of the retention of the third molar in a mandible large enough to contain it should never be overlooked. If, however, it is found impossible to bring the tooth to its proper height and alignment, extraction should be resorted to at the very earliest moment. In such cases it makes no difference how difficult it is to extract the tooth; if necessary deep narcosis must be resorted to, and a portion of the mandible cut away, so as to remove every portion of the tooth. The longer there is any delay in such cases, the greater is the danger of severe neuralgic complications and infiltrative osteomyelitis through the passageway of the inferior dental canal. For this same reason, if extraction of such a tooth has taken place, the greatest care should be taken to keep the wound packed with sterile gauze, in order to avoid reinfection which may lead, by means of the cribriform tube, to an extensive osteomyelitis. The same rule obtains in cases of abscessed or necrotic conditions where there is any danger of reinfection, and especially where the field of operation is in close proximity to any of the osseous sinuses. This does not necessarily include healthy alveolar sockets in other parts of the jaws.

The following clinical case will illustrate the danger resulting from neglecting to attend to the sterilization of such a socket:

Mr. S., bachelor, aged about thirty years, had a third molar extracted which had never completely erupted, but had been a constant source of irritation for many years. The extraction was performed by a specialist in this line, and was said to have been a very difficult one. The later surgical operation demonstrated definitely that the roots of the third molar penetrated the cribriform tube, as shown in Fig. 3 (Cryer). Inadequate attention to keeping the wound sterile (no packing having been used) was followed by an infection in the alveolar sockets. This spread without any difficulty to the inferior dental canal, and when I saw the patient for the first time in the hospital on July 3, 1900, in consultation with Dr. Howard Lilienthal, he was not far from a moribund state. There was a very rapid and weak pulse, with a temperature of 105.5°. Our diagnosis was an infiltrative osteomyelitis progressing through the passageway of the cribriform tube. The patient was immediately anæsthetized, and an external incision made at the angle of the body and the ramus. The bone was chiselled away at this point until the interior of the tube was exposed, where there was an effusion of a large mass of purulent matter, grayish in color, and most foul in odor.

The condition of the patient at this time was so serious that the operation was made as short and rapid as possible, great fear being entertained that he would not survive the ordinary surgical shock. Drainage was established through the external opening thus obtained, and the recovery was very slow. It soon became evident that an entire infected zone of bone had not been removed, and on October 27 a subperiosteal resection was performed, extending from the symphysis of the body to a considerable portion of the ascending ramus. After this the case went on to complete recovery.

Figs. 4 and 5, taken from Cryer, will illustrate most beautifully the parts operated upon. The prognosis in such cases is remarkably good, as long as correct surgical principles are used in the operative procedure.

Summarizing, it would appear that the medical profession are remiss in their failure to call on stomatologists for consultation in obscure cases of infection in the oral regions. Frequent errors of diagnosis made by medical men have been the cause of numerous cases of unnecessary facial disfigurement.

On the other hand, the stomatologists themselves should realize the value of retaining all of the molars, if possible. When extraction has to be resorted to, too much and too harsh criticism cannot be used against those members of this specialty who are negligent in taking proper precautions against infection of wounds in this locality.

BIBLIOGRAPHY.

1. Jourdain: Revue Médicale, 1829, p. 396.
2. Thirly: Geneva, 1857.
3. Robertson: Dental Cosmos, vol. v., 1863, p. 243.
4. Heydenreich: 1878.
5. Magitot: 1879.
6. Trudeau: Medical Examiner, vol. i., 1838–58.
7. Cobleigh: Cin. Med. News, 1880, vol. ix. p. 433.
8. Magitot: Contribution à l'étude des accidents de l'éruption de la dent de sagesse inférieure, Gaz. hebd. de méd., vol. xvi. p. 3.
9. Delacour: Accidents de l'éruption de la dent de sagesse, Bull. Soc. Anat. Clin., 1892, vol. vii. p. 169.
10. Gutman: Verhandlung d. deutsch. odont. Gesellschaft, 1892, vol. iii. p. 292.
11. Dunogier: Contribution à l'étude des accidents lies à l'évolution de dents de sagesse, Mém. et Bull. Soc. Méd. et Chirurg., 1893–94, p. 11.
12. Davezac: Gaz. des hôp. de Toulouse, 1894, p. 25.
13. Demons: Gaz. des hôp. de Toulouse, 1894.
14. Redier: Des accidents de l'éruption de la dent de sagesse, Journ. de Soc. Médicale de Lille, 1895.
15. Bourgogne: Un cas de lymphangite, Odontologie, 1897, v. p. 254.
16. Heydenreich: Rev. Méd. de l'est, Nancy, 1898, vol. xxx. p. 285.
17. CauMartin: Accidents provoqués par l'éruption de la dent de sagesse, L'Écho Méd. du Nord, Lille, 1901, v. p. 15.
18. Moty: Accidents de la dent de sagesse, Rev. de Chirurg., vol. xxiii., 1901, p. 617.
19. Beltrami: Sur quelques dus à l'évolution de la dent de sagesse, Marseilles, Méd., 1902, vol. xxxix. p. 429.

20. Nogue: Arch. de Stomatol., 1902, vol. iii. p. 590.
21. Witzel: D. Monatschrift f. Zahnheilkunde, 1902, vol. xx. p. 590.
22. Guittermin, L.: Schweizerische Vierteljahrschrift für Zahnheilkunde, January, 1903.
23. Williger: D. Monatschrift f. Zahnheilkunde, 1903, vol. xxi. p. 57.
24. Kollbrunner: Schweizerische Vierteljahrschrift für Zahnheilkunde.
25. Turnbul: Dental Record, 1903, vol. xxi. p. 36.
26. Frey: L'Odontologie, October 30, 1904.
27. Dunogier: Gaz. des hôpitaux de Toulouse, 1894, vol. vii. p. 17.
28. Cornudet: De la dent de sagesse, Lille, 1887.
29. Chevassu: De quelques accidents causés par l'éruption et les déviations de la dent de sagesse, Paris, 1873.
30. dit Orme: De quelques accidents causés par l'éruption de la dent de sagesse, Montpelier, 1880.
31. Gallas: Quelques considerations sur les accidents dus à l'éruption de la dent sagesse inférieure, Bordeaux, 1889.

INAUGURAL ADDRESS.[1]

BY WILLOUGHBY D. MILLER, A.M., D.D.S., M.D., SC.D.[2]

THE provost of your university has done me the honor of inviting me to address a few remarks to you at the opening exercises of the new term of work and study which now lies before you. As I have the distinction of being an alumnus of the Dental Department, I felt that it might appear ungrateful for me to decline the invitation, and so I am here before you, notwithstanding many misgivings as to my fitness for the function which I have undertaken.

These initial exercises in which you are annually invited to participate appear to me to be of very vital importance. As you are all aware, every inert body set in motion has a tendency to go on moving forever in a straight line and in the direction originally imparted to it. And, in like manner, every receptive mind, such as that of the young student, has a decided inclination to follow along certain lines of thought or activity which have been imparted to it by those with whom it has come into contact. Hence

---

[1] Delivered at the opening exercises, October 2, 1905, of the twenty-eighth annual session of the Department of Dentistry, University of Pennsylvania.

[2] Professor University of Berlin, Germany.

we see how important it is that the young man, in setting out upon a career of whatever nature, receive his first impulses in the right direction, and how great a responsibility rests upon the one whose duty it is to impart these impulses.

Preliminary instruction or advice as to the general lines which a student should follow in acquiring his education, whether scientific, political, or ethical, might perhaps be better dispensed with here at the University of Pennsylvania than at many other institutions.

In foreign, especially German, universities, the student enjoys absolute freedom. He may attend the lectures or not, at his own discretion, and is obliged to pass no examination until he comes up for his degree. As a result, he may be, and sometimes is, matriculated at the university for months and even years without coming into contact with the teachers under whom he is supposed to be studying. This condition of affairs is exemplified by the anecdote of the man who, being asked the way to the university by a student, replied, "I don't know. I am a student myself." Here, the student is not only required to economize his time and to acquire habits of industry from the very beginning, but he is brought into closer relation with his teachers, and the opportunity of seeking and receiving advice from time to time is always present, and forms a safeguard of inestimable value if the student will but avail himself of it.

You, gentlemen, are particularly fortunate in having for your teachers and advisers a corps of men who are esteemed the world over as dentists, as scientists, and as men, and I have no better advice for you than that you put yourselves implicitly in their hands and follow their directions and their examples in every particular.

I have naturally no means of knowing what the motives were which determined each of you to take up dentistry as his life work. But of whatever nature they may have been, one thing is certain, that in acting upon them you have taken the most important step of your lives, a step, in fact, which fixes at once the whole configuration of your future lives, your occupation, your success, and to a great extent your happiness, and every one should be continuously awake to the fact that it is a very serious matter to take such a step, and, having taken it, he should bend all his energies toward successfully and honorably carrying it out.

A quarter of a century ago one of Germany's most famous surgeons, Professor von Mussbaum, characterized dentistry as a great and beautiful science. If this was true twenty-five years ago, it is doubly so to-day, for we may say, without fear of being accused of exaggeration, that, with the exception of bacteriology, no specialty of medicine has advanced more rapidly than, and very few as rapidly as, dentistry. Few accomplish as positive results, none repair injured or restore lost organs with the same degree of success, or with the same perfect imitation of nature, as is accomplished by the dentist. Moreover, in the same degree as a knowledge of the intimate and causal relations of the diseases of the teeth and mouth to the most diverse local and general disorders becomes more wide-spread, so, too, a more thorough appreciation of the importance of the science of dentistry is rapidly making its appearance everywhere, and especially in the ranks of the medical profession. It is, or soon will be, familiar to all of you that diseased conditions of the teeth are the cause of the most various local and general disorders of the human body. To say nothing of the inflammation of the dental pulp, of alveolar abscesses, periostitis, necrosis of the jaw, suppuration of the antrum and frontal sinuses, we know that neuroses, neuralgias, serious disorders of the digestive organs and of the air-passages and lungs, troubles of the ear, eye, and nose, as well as meningitis, septicæmia, chronic pyæmia, etc. very frequently have their origin in diseased teeth. More recently, moreover, Professor Bunge has shown that lactation is very markedly influenced by the condition of the teeth. The statistics of Röse and others reveal a striking percentage of recruits rejected because of bad teeth, and, what is of particular interest, various observers have found that the capacity of school children for giving attention to their lessons and for learning bears a direct relation to the condition of the teeth, and that good grades are indicative of good teeth. I need not dwell upon this point, for it is now universally known and acknowledged that the physical well-being of a nation, its progress and development, are in no small degree dependent upon its teeth; and we need not hesitate for a moment in placing the specialty which you have chosen, in respect to its capacity for relieving human suffering, for healing disease, and improving the general health and comfort, for intensifying capacity for work, physical or mental, on a perfect level with the other specialties of medicine.

A knowledge of all these facts has been for years, and still is, rapidly spreading among all classes of people, with the result that a demand for well-educated and skilful practitioners is rapidly increasing, so that the outlook for those who are now entering upon or already engaged in the study of dentistry is very encouraging. And with the opportunities which are afforded you here, it lies with great certainty in your power to attain success in your life work, with all the pleasures and comforts and power for doing good which accompany it. But you must not imagine for a moment that success comes of itself. It has been said that some men are born great, some achieve greatness, and some have greatness thrust upon them. But this does not apply to the dentist. The only way in which he can become great is by achieving his own greatness; and that he can do only by most diligent application and by taking advantage of every opportunity that is afforded him for perfecting himself in every branch of dental science and dental practice.

And you must not forget, gentlemen, that dentistry is a science so broad and comprehensive that to master it every moment of time at your disposal must be called into requisition, and anything short of that will not guarantee your success. It may entail your failure. For, while there is always room, and always will be room, for eminent workers in every profession and trade, there is but little place for the mediocre, and none at all for the inefficient or lazy.

It is said that the young are inclined to be optimistic, but this idea does not tally with the fact that our most pessimistic systems of philosophy of life, which are so well adapted to wreck the happiness of millions of otherwise contented beings, were brought out by men scarcely out of their twenties, while many of our most ardent exponents of a more hopeful and faithful view of life, have been men well advanced in years. I should say, therefore, that it is not optimism, but rather criminal thoughtlessness, when a student goes through his college days with no thought of the future, and doing only just the amount of work necessary to secure his degree. In fact, the student often makes the mistake of supposing that he is studying only for a degree, and that, the degree once obtained, everything else will come of itself. This is a great mistake, and the sooner it is remedied the better. The degree is simply an outward decoration, a guarantee that the holder has gone through with a certain amount of study and work; it adds nothing whatever to his capabilities.

Never forget that your chief object here is not to secure a degree, but to prepare yourselves for a great life work, and that your future happiness, success and position will depend upon the more or less perfect manner in which you carry out this object. Work always with this aim in view, and the degree will come of itself.

If you will permit me, I will give you in as few words as possible my conception of the ideal dentist of to-day.

In the first place, he must have a broad, liberal education to begin with, since it is folly to attempt to erect a beautiful superstructure upon a weak or rotten foundation. The dentist will be seriously handicapped in the pursuit of his professional studies if his liberal education and training have been deficient. A man, moreover, whose calling is at the same time scientific and humane, and brings him into contact with all classes of people, must be an educated man in order to uphold his own dignity and that of his profession. He must also be prepared to think and act intelligently in all social, political, and educational problems of the day.

The dentist must be thoroughly posted in all branches of general medicine which have a direct bearing upon dental science or practice. As a matter of fact, the question may be asked with perfect propriety, " Is there any reason why the dentist should not take exactly the same preparatory studies as the other specialists?" Certainly the relations of the teeth to the neighboring parts, and through the nerve-vascular and lymphatic systems to remoter parts, are quite as manifold and complex as those of the eye or ear; and why should the dentist be expected to know less of anatomy than the aurist or ophthalmologist? The same question may also be asked in respect to physiology, hygiene, general pathology, bacteriology, etc. I personally would say, in answer to this question, that the science of medicine in all its branches is growing so rapidly, and has already become so extensive, that no one, even though he may have five, ten, or even twenty years for study, will ever be able to master all parts of it equally well, and that it will be expedient if not necessary in the future that every specialist restrict himself more or less to those branches of study which have a direct bearing upon his own specialty. There is no more reason for the aurist than for the dentist to devote months to acquiring a thorough knowledge of obstetrics or gynæcology, or even of the anatomy of the extremities, physiology of the spleen, etc. On one ground only we may be possibly justified in limiting the general medical studies of the dentist somewhat more than those of other specialists, and that is because he requires more time than they to master his own special studies and operations. We must, however, carefully avoid going too far in this direction, since, as already indicated, to use a geographical expression, dentistry is absolutely bounded on all sides by the science of medicine, and must stand on the same or at least on as firm a foundation as the other branches of medical science.

The dentist must naturally be particularly proficient in all special subjects relating to the science and practice of dentistry. He must also possess a high degree of manual dexterity, in view of the exceeding delicacy required for the carrying out of many operations which he is called upon to perform. The want of this dexterity has been the cause of the failure of many dental practitioners, and the student who is not endowed with it by nature should make every effort under the direction of his instructors to acquire it. He must not forget that dental operations are to many patients exceedingly painful, and he should take every precaution to reduce their discomforts to a minimum. The idea that the excavation of a tooth, to be perfectly done, must of necessity be painful always seemed to me to be a bit barbarous, and sometimes made use of as a mantle to cover lack of care or the use of improper instruments.

The dentist must be a most strict observer of the fundamental principle of modern surgery,—*i.e.*, of the rules of asepsis. In no department of medicine is a demand for asepsis—*i.e.*, cleanliness—greater than in the practice of dentistry, both on account of the danger of transmitting diseases and because the dentist is brought into more intimate contact with his patients than the general practitioner. The student of dentistry should, accordingly, from the very beginning, cultivate habits of the strictest cleanliness, not only in respect to his person, especially the hands, but also to his napkins, his instruments, materials, and everything which comes into contact, directly or indirectly, with the mouth of the patient. An experience of twenty-one years of teaching has taught me that one cannot insist too strongly or too often upon this point. He must studiously avoid getting into the habit of degrading his profession to the level of a trade, or of putting to himself the question, "How many dollars and cents are there in this mouth for me?" instead of "How can I best save these teeth and make them comfortable and useful to the patient?"

No dentist can conduct a practice on such a principle without dishonoring himself and his profession. Certainly it is right and honorable that he receive a fair remuneration for his work. It is right that he should accumulate enough of wealth during the long years of a responsible and trying practice to enable him to meet old age free from care. But to make everything else subordinate to the one thought of getting money, and possibly to sacrifice the best interests of those who intrust themselves to his care, for this aim, is to do violence to the ethical principles by which every member of the humane professions is inexcusably bound, and the dentist who conducts his practice on this plan is little better than a parasite.

I may also say in this connection that an institution which exists ostensibly for the purpose of preparing men for the practice of dentistry, but which sacrifices what is acknowledged to be the best interests of its students in favor of a greater balance in the cash account, deserves no better consideration, and the sooner it goes out of existence, the better for all concerned.

The dentist should not be over hasty to criticise the work of a colleague, as he cannot know the exact conditions under which it was done, nor can he by any means always trust the statements of the patient in regard to it. Above all things he should never, by a shrug of the shoulders or by silent acquiescence in erroneous statements of the patient, sanction an unjust accusation against a colleague. No dentist who has a proper feeling of self-respect would do a thing so mean, to say nothing of the fact that the patient usually sees through the object of it. On the contrary, it is the simple duty of every dentist to strongly and unequivocally defend the character of a brother dentist when he sees that it has been unjustly attacked.

There is still another matter to which I wish to call attention. The patient-material upon which the student operates in the dental college is recruited largely from the poorer classes,—servants, day-laborers, etc.,—and the student easily acquires the habit of thinking that it is not necessary for him to have the same respect of person, or to carry out the treatment with quite the same care or consideration, that he would observe in his private practice. This is a grave mistake, for habits acquired during your college practice are difficult to change later on, to say nothing of the fact that the poor man has the same sensibilities, and, as patient, is entitled to just the same respect as the rich man. You should, accordingly, in your college practice, observe in every particular the same degree of care as will be demanded of you in your private practice later on.

I have been in the habit of pointing out to my students a certain criterion by which they, in a way, are enabled to foretell their success or lack of success in their future practice.

If the patients are satisfied with the treatment which they have received, and if, on returning later on, they ask to be treated by the same student, and bring their friends with them for treatment, so that the student in a way accumulates a practice about him in the dental college, I do not hesitate to say that his future success is assured.

If, on the other hand, patients complain of his treatment and apply to the demonstrator to be put into the hands of some other student, then it is time for him to seriously inquire whether he is not in some vital respect at fault, and to give himself the greatest pains to remedy the fault; for if he is not able to give satisfaction in his college practice, he will do it much less later on.

Do not forget that you have duties to perform in the interest of your profession. A member of a family, a society, community, or profession cannot isolate himself from his surroundings, or honorably escape from the performance of his duties toward the organization of which he is a part. The dentist owes all he has to his profession, and if he does not seek to make some return, he is either very selfish or, at best, very thoughtless. It is his duty to support the societies which are the nerve-centres of the profession. He should do all in his power to advance dental science. He should extend his aid and encouragement to the less fortunate brothers, and help to elevate the standard of his profession by living a righteous and just life and by seeking the advancement of his profession as well as his own. Above all things, he should not make use of any influential position which he may have acquired in any dental organization for carrying out his own devices.

A young man beginning the practice of dentistry should be

prepared to undertake the treatment of all diseases of the teeth and contiguous parts which present themselves; excepting, of course, surgical cases requiring a more special training than he has been able to acquire, which he should refer to some colleague who has made a specialty of such operations. It does not follow from this, however, that it may not be advantageous for him, as well as for his patient, to restrict his practice to some particular branch of dental surgery; in fact, the practice of dentistry has become so extensive and is growing so rapidly that the time will soon come—if not already here—when it will not be advisable for the dentist to attempt to do all operations which come within the scope of his profession. And if you find that you have a special aptitude for any particular work, whether it be for the preservative treatment of the teeth, for dental surgery, for prosthetic dentistry, for crown- and bridge-work, or porcelain, give your particular attention to such work, if circumstances permit, and eventually you may be able to restrict yourself to that alone, with the result that you will work with much more satisfaction and less strain to yourself, and serve your clients better.

Great opportunities are offered to the young man now entering upon the practice of dentistry. Our profession is as yet only in its infancy, and the work so far accomplished, great as it is, is small in comparison with that which is still to be done. At present the great aim of medical science is to prevent disease by restricting its courses, by assisting the body in the use of those powers of resistance with which it is naturally endowed, and by inciting such powers where they are wanting, and we, as dentists, following out the same line of thought, have our problem of immunity to caries, as observed in individual persons to deal with, and the practically still more important problem growing out of that of conferring immunity upon persons naturally disposed,—*i.e.*, the problem of the prevention of the decay of the teeth,—and the man who succeeds in solving this problem will confer a greater boon upon humanity than resulted from the discovery of the X-Ray, or of the diphtheria heil-serum.

Another great problem with which you will have to grapple is that of making the blessings of dentistry accessible to the great masses of the people. Dental operations as now carried out are disagreeable, if not absolutely painful, to the patient, as well as trying to the operator, and, in particular, they require an expendi-

ture of time which appears to be out of proportion to the operation itself. We consume more time in filling a simple cavity in
a tooth than the surgeon in amputating a leg or performing a
laparotomy, and when we have to do with a pulpless and diseased
molar, the amount of time spent may be five to ten times as great
as is necessary for a difficult surgical operation upon which the
life of the patient is depending. The result is that the care of
the thirty-two permanent teeth becomes a very expensive matter,
and many a father of a family pays more to the family dentist
than to the family physician,—*i.e.*, more for the care of the teeth
than for that of all the rest of the body together. We are also forced
to admit that for the same reason the blessings of preservative
dentistry are a luxury far' beyond the reach of the great masses
of the people. Taking it the world over, not one person in five
hundred could afford the expense of having his dead molars properly cared for. In European countries the percentage will be
about one to twenty-five or thirty. In America, where there is
much more money in circulation among the middle and labor
classes, it may possibly be as high as one to five. Nor does it
appear to me that the development of dentistry in the last few
years has been such as to make it more accessible to that class of
people which in the daily struggle for existence suffers much more
from the lack of sound teeth than the opulent classes who stand
above the struggle and are better able to compensate for the lack
of sound teeth by other means. At present dentistry is developing
most rapidly in the artistic direction, and there is a great cry
for artistic operations. Everything must be made of porcelain,—
porcelain bridges, porcelain crowns, porcelain fillings,—and everything carried out with such a highly developed sense of the artistic
that the artificial nature of the work shall be absolutely unde-
tectable to the unskilled eye.

And we must admit that there is a great future for the dentist
in this class of operations, and great credit is due to all who have
done anything to perfect this particular line of work, and it is to
be hoped that the time is not far distant when the gold crown
on an incisor root will be a thing of the past. But, nevertheless,
this class of work tends to render dental aid still less accessible to
the poorer classes, and its particular culture cannot be regarded
as an unmixed good unless at the same time an equal development
takes place along other lines.

We need materials and methods which will render it possible to shorten and cheapen dental operations so as to bring them within the reach of every one. We need, accordingly, a filling-material of the nature of a cement which can be quickly and easily inserted and will preserve the teeth permanently. We need some way of shortening and simplifying our present long and complicated methods of treating root-canals, and the one who discovers and introduces such material and methods will confer a greater boon upon humanity than those who have contributed to the development of the art of employing porcelain in the preservative treatment of the teeth, for we must always bear in mind that it is the object and evident duty of our as of every other humane profession to do the greatest possible good to the greatest possible number of people.

Professors of a great and beautiful science with a constantly widening sphere of activity, with manifold great and complex problems, both scientific and practical, to be solved, a great future lies before you, and if you are willing, I doubt not that you will also show yourselves capable of meeting all the requirements that your profession justly exacts of you. Liberally educated, well posted in all collateral branches of medical science, master in the science and practice of dentistry, unerring in the performance of his duties, ethical and Christian to his patients, his colleagues, his profession, and his country,—this is my conception of what the dentist ought to be, and of what I trust each of you will be, never forgetting that, however great a thing it may be to be a good dentist, it is far greater to be a good man.

THE DENTISTRY OF TO-MORROW.[1]

BY HARRY P. CARLTON, D.D.S., SAN FRANCISCO, CAL.

SEVERAL years ago I had the opportunity to read before the Odontographic Society of Chicago a paper on " University Train-

---

[1] Read in the Section on Stomatology of the American Medical Association, at the fifty-sixth annual session, July, 1905, and republished by consent of the Journal of the American Medical Association.

ing and Dental Education," in which I took the ground that dentistry would only be a full profession and recognized as such when the character of the men who comprised it brought its recognition up to what it should be; that as this increase in dignity and professional status must come from within the body of the profession itself, a high grade of young men must be added to its ranks. I outlined the demands of the day and the way to meet those demands, making a plea for better educated material with which to begin our dental training, claiming that with these superior men we could shut the doors of our profession against the trifler and the tinker, and reserve the training of our schools for those who brought to the work the instincts, traditions, and outlook of the scholar; the result, real doctors of dental surgery.

I look on this occasion and this paper as but another chance to express my thoughts, to take another step forward, and to prophesy what seems to me the inevitable outcome. If dentistry is to continue to advance, along what lines must it go? It is pretty well conceded that mechanically we are close to the top notch, and only moderate advance can be looked for in that direction. The advance must then be along scientific lines, higher education, and the encouragement of research and investigation.

Dentistry is a specialty of medicine, but the only specialty not universally requiring the degree of doctor of medicine. Indeed, dentistry should be one of the most important branches or specialties of medicine, for in the mouth begin all those processes of nutrition and metabolism which of recent years have attracted so much attention. Thus far neither the physician nor the dentist has given enough scientific study to this special area of the human anatomy, and neither knows what the other has been doing or learning or is doing and learning.

Medicine and dentistry, though cognate sciences, have always been separately studied. This dissociation is now seen to be a great error, due not alone to the fact that the relation of the mouth and teeth to the rest of the anatomy was not understood, but also because only the mechanical aspect probably appealed to those who first considered the matter; no doubt dentistry had its beginning in the pulling of a tooth. This conception of dentistry as an entity and not as an integral part of medicine has made it an art, possibly a trade, rather than a science. A correct appreciation of physiology, pathology, and bacteriology—physiology representing the normal relation between the mouth and the rest of the alimentary canal; pathology showing the relation between the deranged functions of the mouth and abnormal conditions of other portions of the alimentary system; and bacteriology as an outgrowth of the study of pathology, showing the causes of the pathologic conditions of the mouth—necessitates an entirely different attitude, and is rapidly bringing the child, dentistry, back to its real parent, medicine. It has been said that " Dental science has brought the diseases of the mouth, jaws, and teeth so obviously under the domain of general pathology, that somatic problems elsewhere presented in the body are best and easiest studied in the mouth."

The opportunities of modern dentistry are so new and vast that not only is more manipulative skill demanded, but ampler education, more insight, more sagacity, faculties to whose development nature and elaborate training must both contribute. And this training must be given under the guidance of scientific teachers, non-practitioners, men of productive scholarship, men who devote their lives to the special work of teaching the various subjects which are embodied in a medical education, instead of by those who give instruction during the intervals of a busy practice.

There are new duties calling for a high degree of disciplined intelligence; to quote a recent article, " The knowledge of life and disease represented by the average D.D.S. degree is certainly deplorably deficient." How are we to remedy this? Give our young men a thorough medical training. Dentists are specialists only in their own handiwork, but the groundwork is uniform, and the demand for individualized education emphasizes the whole difference in our chosen tasks and ignores the great similarities. The technic of our branch of the profession, then, appears only as a small variation of the work in which we all share. The higher the level on which professional specialization begins, the more effective it is. And, again, " the higher the profession, the more nearly is the whole man working in every act, and the more, therefore, is a broad general education necessary."

How well I remember Professor Joseph Le Conte's likening of the modern system of education to the great sequoia, in which the primary and secondary schools were the rootlets and roots, the college culture courses the great bole, and the coming out from it at various altitudes as specializing branches, were the group of professional schools that make up the university. The trunk thus dividing grew higher and smaller, but persisted as the principal member all the way, until the topmost reach of pure culture was highest of all. Specializing without culture he likened to the low-branching bush, with no hope of reaching any fair height, and that the great branch of this tree of knowledge that deals with the study and care of the human body should spring from the main trunk after a considerable height of culture, at least that of the college curriculum, which Dr. Le Conte likened to the unbranching trunk, was the contention made in the former paper already mentioned. Without this no standing among the learned professions can be had at all. The half-light of the forest depth cannot be grown out of at any less altitude.

It is equally clear, also, that the great branch, the study of the human frame I have spoken of, must go out from the culture trunk of the university tree as a whole. The least consideration of its logical relations to the general culture and to other branches of knowledge will show the justness of this statement. And, having thus gone out from the main trunk, there is plenty of room for a considerable outward and upward reach of this great branch before it begins to subdivide into the various specialties, as the care of the various portions of the human body. So viewed, the mouth has as much relation to medical science, as a whole, as has the care of the eye, the ear, or, indeed, any other organ or group of organs.

He would be a superficial reasoner who could deny the great culture value of the medical course. Dr. Le Conte himself found it a firm foundation in its hold on physics and chemistry and a whole group of other sciences, and yet more in its cultivation of the habits of scientific observation of facts and logical reasoning from them for the stately structure of his own scientific attainments. The man who has taken it is a doctor, with none of the weakening qualifications of D.D.S., connoting a lesser scientific rank.

Most dental schools of the present time are at the mercy of the demands of the day and age, and their students are the product of the surroundings, not the choice of the school. An ideal professional school would be one that exists for its work alone, for scientific investigation and practical instruction not given by busy wage earners.

The dentist of to-morrow cannot be the same sort of man as the dentist of the past, whose own little sphere has been bounded

by thirty-two teeth. He must be the carefully educated student
in the medical branches, plus the dental specialties, and you can
only make him so by following the same educational plan as in
preparing the doctor of medicine. Without the requisite medical
education, the ordinary mechanically expert dentist is not competent to practise his profession—he can only exercise a mechanical
dexterity, but with the proper education he not only exercises the
same dexterity, but he has professional ability.

The mouth is a fairly good barometer of the whole system,
but your merely mechanical man, as contrasted with the dental
specialist in medicine, is not competent to read it, and he does not.
Why? How can any man untrained in medical science understand
the problems presented to him in the condition of the mouth? We
all know how exceedingly often some affection of the mouth or
teeth is but an indication of a general systemic disturbance of
metabolism; and, on the contrary, how frequently we see a faulty
dental anatomy causing nutritive derangements which are puzzling
to the physician who is ignorant of the large part played by the
mouth in general alimentation. These things cannot be comprehended by the merely mechanically trained dentist, as distinguished
from the dental specialist, any more than they are intelligible to
the physician whose training has omitted all reference to the mouth
as a vital part of the alimentary canal. He who would in the
future confine his professional work to conditions involving the
mouth and teeth—the dental specialist—must be a broad diagnostician; he must know the relation of the mouth to the general
system, and he must interpret what he sees in the mouth in the
light of his general medical education.

To bring about this condition—a condition which must surely
come with the passage of time—the same preliminary training in
the academic sciences will be required, whether the student intends
to practise general medicine or surgery, or to specialize along the
lines of ophthalmology, dermatology, orthopædic surgery, or dentistry.

The same general medical education must also be required, no
matter to what special region of the anatomy nor to what special
line of work the student intends to confine himself eventually.

What will be the results of this medical education? When this
is accomplished what is going to become of your dentist? Practical life demands a division of labor; therefore, the specializing

of the individual. There will be a division of the product just as in general medicine, and the natural ability of the individual will show itself. Some are going on plugging teeth, but better able, not less equipped for that work, for this higher education is not a question alone of preparing great men for great things; it must also prepare little men for greater things than would otherwise have been possible. Another lot are going to take up broad scientific work and research—not merely the mouth, but the mouth as merely a part, and the world will be spared from lots of trouble. But he who takes up the mechanical side of dental medicine has a broad and an inviting field of work before him. Thus far the orthopædic surgeon and the ophthalmologist who confines himself to refraction are most highly skilled mechanical specialists in medicine, but the medical dentist of the future will stand with them.

Consider the remarkably high degree of mechanical skill developed in the proper adjustment of a plaster jacket! Think of the tremendously complex Wullstein apparatus, devised for this purpose, and consider a man with no mechanical skill, in spite of any amount of medical education, attempting to apply such a jacket!

Dentistry, as well as orthopædic surgery, requires this highest kind of mechanical ability—take the apparatus used in orthodontia, for example; its construction and application call for the best mechanical skill, but they need back of that the academic training, or they do not reach the elevation. The real professional man should possess the resources of a highly developed, reasoning faculty, which comes only after years of systematic pursuit of what might be called higher or university study. It is this broad mental training that makes better dentists and better men. We are not only professional wage-earners—we live for our friends and our nation; we are in contact with nature and science, with art and literature; we shape our town and our time. Let us, then, provide the kind of men who know how to think.

Imagine a profession of mere operators; professional men! Not so; mechanical artisans. The hope of the profession lies not in fitting a system of instruction to the capacity of unpromising students, not in "substituting intellectual milk for intellectual meat,—aye, even in giving this milk in small quantity because of the puniness of the babes; but in choosing students equal to the requirements of an advanced method of instruction and substituting capable men for the class that now fill our colleges."

Turning out men with broad, well-balanced minds, with the faculty of judgment, strengthened by the mastery of principles rather than the acquisition of information. So much of the groundwork of medicine and dentistry is held in common that it is a wasteful folly to teach it in separate schools rather than in one well-equipped and well-manned institution. The cutting out of this unnecessary duplication of work is the spirit of the age and the method of much that we call our modern advance.

To summarize this point: The things that are purely groundwork, physics, inorganic chemistry, and all the branches that make for the building up of the man able to see clearly, to imagine vividly, and to reason correctly, as Dr. Henry Van Dyke puts it— these should be given in college. Then, all the studies necessary to the understanding of the human anatomy, physiology, and hygiene should be taken in a medical course; then, and then alone, is it time to specialize on oral surgery to make a dentist. It used to be said of Cuvier that, given a single bone, he could construct a whole animal, but he never arrived at that point by the study of one kind of bones only. Rather it is the method of to-day to study the whole skeleton, yes, and all the other parts of an animal as well, in order to understand one bone.

" Great truths approach slowly and dwell a long time with small minorities." Progress is the law of this American race, which stands for all that is best; truly it is a race which knows no rest. Was it not Macaulay who said, " A standing point which was yesterday invisible is the goal to-day and will be the starting post of to-morrow"?

DISCUSSION.

Dr. F. L. Platt, San Francisco, said that a degree from a university is certainly commendable and necessary, but he thinks that it is hardly all that is required. A large part of dentistry is mechanical and must necessarily continue to be so. He believes that in addition to a university degree, if a young man is going to study dentistry, he should also attend a school of manual training. Dr. Platt has noticed that the students who have had some manual training do superior work. There must be a combination of these two kinds of training before one can become a good dentist. After a man has gained a knowledge of chemistry, physics, bacteriology, and therapeutics, his training should be largely clinical. The greater part of dentistry can be taught by clinics, and Dr. Platt believes that each member of a class should be required to demonstrate his ability in the presence of others, and should not wait to learn to do this after he has acquired a degree. Experience in teaching operative technic has convinced Dr. Platt that so far as operative work is concerned, clinical instruction is far ahead of the lecture. He does not believe that dental colleges should be private corporations. Schools of law, medicine, theology, and dentistry should be integral parts of State universities, with funds provided by the State and faculties paid by the State. At the end of the first six months, if a student does not display aptitude for the work, he should be advised to take up something else. Dr. Platt agreed with Dr. Carlton that a high school education is not sufficient. Dr. Platt attended a pedagogic meeting a year ago, and heard many people speak who were in favor of a four years' course in dentistry, but did not hear a single sound argument in its favor. He thinks that the course should be at least nine months a year and four years if necessary, but to make the course four years at the expense of cutting down the length of each year, is not advancing. Students who have five months' vacation will not graduate from college as well equipped as students who have only three months' vacation. Some argue that the students get so tired they need five months' vacation. Others argue that students ought to have five months to work to earn money to finish their course. Neither of these arguments is worth considering. If the course is to be lengthened, let it be made four years of nine months each. A plan could be adopted requiring a degree in arts and letters for admission, as well as a manual school training, and then three years of good, earnest work would turn out good dentists.

Dr. M. L. Rhein, New York, said that possibly the colleges that have a six months' course are in the South, and they would have a six months' course whether it was three years or six. It has always seemed difficult to get Southern colleges to give any lengthy term. The tendency in the Northeast has been to increase the teaching term whatever the number of years. Dr. Rhein thinks the basis for dental education should be absolutely as high as that of medical education, and until that standard is reached dentists are below their true standard, and that is the only thing that keeps dentistry from being recognized as it should. It is the one thing that keeps students of the proper caliber from taking up this specialty. They do not care to place themselves on a lower plane than any of the other branches of medicine. This section should strive to make the requirements of dental education as high as that required for medicine, and to keep them up to that standard. Dr. Rhein thinks it impossible for a man to practise this branch of medicine without being thoroughly grounded in general medicine. The groundwork of medicine is recognized as being not only of value, but of necessity, and while dentistry is a technical work, and while a technical school is of the utmost importance, without the scientific knowledge of medicine the dentist is at a loss to properly apply his technical knowledge.

Dr. A. H. Levings, Milwaukee, said that there are many subjects in the medical curriculum which would be of no use to the dentist, though a dentist must have some knowledge of the fundamental branches, such as chemistry, pathology, bacteriology, histology, and therapeutics. He must have some knowledge of surgery and perhaps a smattering of medicine, but Dr. Levings thinks that the study of neurology, gynæcology, obstetrics, dermatology, otology, and allied subjects would be of no benefit to the dentist commensurate with the time spent in study. If the coming dentist were required to take a full course in medicine, he would have to spend an extra year in mechanical work, because the medical student's time is fully occupied. He cannot complete the course of to-day in less than four years of eight or nine months each. Dr. Levings said that he has heard many say that the requirements should be put so high that but few dental students could meet them. The only consideration should be what is best for these prospective dental students. Dr. Levings appreciates as much as any one that the more culture, refinement, education, and mental training an individual has, the higher he can rise in his profession, and the more easily he can maintain himself, but it is not within the possibility of every prospective dental student or every prospective medical student to secure the standard. Such a course as is given now in dental colleges will train any man who has a high school education so that he can master all the problems pertaining to either dentistry or medicine. Those who have the time and money may take a medical and a dental degree, and before this an A.B. degree, and polish themselves as much as possible.

Dr. M. I. Schamberg, Philadelphia, said that it may take some time before dentists will reach a higher standard than that existing at the present time. To his way of thinking, there are two things of prominent importance in taking up this subject: one is the raising of the standard of the profession, and the second, which he considers even more important, is the placing of such men in the dental world as are able to render the best possible service to humanity. The financial status of the dental college should be absolutely ignored. It may be that the work of the stomatologist and the dentist will ultimately become separated before arriving at the desired goal. If that be the case, it will probably be best for humanity at large. Dr. Schamberg would prefer to see the various dental institutions under the control of State universities, so that the financial side of the question would not enter into it so much as the educational.

Dr. G. V. I. Brown, Milwaukee, said that in this question of dental education a distinct advance of some kind is wanted. The purpose of Dr. Chittenden's paper is to fulfil the crowning act of a long life that has been given freely to the upraising of the standard, that before he dies something definite may be accomplished in the establishment of a higher standard of dental education. Dr. Brown said that he drew the resolution in the faculty association regarding the four-year term, and he has made more or less of a battle at different times for the four-year course. It is useless to discuss at this time the value of such a course, because for the time at least it has been decided to be inadvisable. He believes that the additional year could be secured with less hardship to the schools and with more likelihood of its being practical than any other advance. He believes every argument that has been made about the mechanical side of dentistry, and that since there cannot be a four-year course there ought to be higher entrance requirements, and that the course should be at least nine months, or as near that length as possible. Dr. Brown is connected with schools in the South and in the West. He sees both sides of the question, but at the present time no plan has been suggested which is practicable for meeting the situation. When some one presents a plan which will carry with it a distinct advance, so long as it is an advance which will enable the colleges of the South, West, and elsewhere to continue and to prosper, that plan will meet with approval, and when that time comes he has no doubt the examiners' and faculty associations will again be on an harmonious basis. Dr.

Brown believes in the value of having dental colleges under State control, but even under this condition it is not all smooth sailing by any means. At this time it seems nothing beneficial can be accomplished by discussion alone.

Dr. H. P. Carlton said that he has never yet written a paper of this character nor spoken his thoughts along this line, that the discussion did not at once turn to the question of courses and years. He wants to establish foundation courses and to leave the length of courses and curricula out of the question. He hopes to live to see it proved that the dentist of the future is going to be a medical man. The more a man gets in brain development the better dentist he will be. A man cannot be too broad and too scientifically trained to be a dentist.

THREE CASES IN ORAL SURGERY.[1]

BY THOMAS FILLEBROWN, M.D., D.M.D., BOSTON, MASS.

I HAVE had in my practice the three cases which I have contemplated for some time bringing to the attention of the Academy. The first one I mention particularly to illustrate what the X-rays might have done. Some years ago, before Dr. Clapp had his X-ray machine, and before the value of X-ray examinations was realized, a young woman about twenty-eight years old came to me, showing a trouble in the region of the left inferior third molar, evidently caused by a tooth. She had had an attempt made once or twice to get the tooth out, but the operators had been unable to reach it. It was then discharging continually. I probed the matter through the fistula, and it was plain that there was some part of a tooth there, but it was so low down that a considerably serious operation was demanded to reach it. I took her to a hospital, where she could remain, and with a trephine in the dental engine I cut down the lingual wall of the alveolus of the jaw to, as I thought, about the level of the apex of the root of the second molar. I carried my trephine down, thinking that

---

[1] Read before the American Academy of Dental Science, Boston, February 1, 1905.

I might bore out the substance of the tooth that was remaining. The jaw-bone was so dense that I could not in that case determine, as I usually can, the line of demarcation between the root and the bone. There is usually to my touch a difference in feeling sufficient for me to recognize bone from tooth. I got down until I thought I had all of it out.

The lady had to go away before it had healed. Her duties called her to Europe, and the jaw set seemingly well. She later went South, I think to Washington, and as it then gave her some trouble, a surgeon operated on it, and attempted to remove the same. Some three or four years after I had first operated she drifted back to Boston, and came into my hands again. I probed around it, and plainly felt the outline of a root of a tooth. After all that time, and the many operations, the parts had greatly softened up and the tooth had risen a little, and I found a point that seemed to be favorable to getting hold of it. I took an elevator and, using it carefully, drew out the remains of a wisdom-tooth. Of course, the patient got well in a short time after that. The point I make in reporting this case is, that had we known of the X-ray and realized its value, and had I used it on this lady, I should have found an embedded wisdom-tooth and known how deeply it was buried. I think it was more deeply embedded than the famous case Dr. Cryer has figured in his work. There is another point to consider. Had it been diagnosed at the time, would it have been wiser to remove it at the time, or wait and temporize with it, as was done? The patient would have been saved much annoyance had it been done at once, though it would have required quite an extensive and severe operation.

The second case is quite peculiar. In February, 1903, a lady, aged about forty, married, came to my office, with partial ankylosis of the jaw. She could open her teeth but very little. Gradually the mobility had been lessened until at that time it was with difficulty that she could get food enough between her teeth to sustain life. There were two lower inferior molars, one on each side, so that from the bicuspids to the first molars there were no teeth. She had had trouble with them before. Both had been devitalized and were filled. I did not think it best at first to interfere with this. At that time, as now, I was using suggestion considerably, and I concluded to try its merits. Between then and April I saw her quite a number of times, and she got great relief, so that she regained half of the mobility which she had lost, and was able to feed herself fairly well. But there was considerable pain. I could not detect that there was anything abnormal about the articulation of the jaw, although she suffered much pain in that region, as it did not get well. In April I concluded that I would prove the quality of the operations. I removed the fillings and examined the pulp-chambers, and found in one of them very sensitive pulp in the root. I treated this awhile, removed the sensitiveness, and refilled the teeth. There was still more improvement, but not great. She did not get entirely well, and in May we finally concluded that she had better have the molars out. The desire to save them was for the purpose of using them later as abutments for bridge-work. Although improvement followed, she did not fully recover. Near the last of my treatment I learned that her husband was suffering from a trouble from the effects of which he died in June. The great mental strain the patient was under, and she being so reduced physically, retarded the cure. Of course, being relieved of all that care, responsibility, and worry, she improved in health, and as she improved in health the gain that she made in the mobility of the jaw was maintained and increased and the pains disappeared, and when I saw her last she was in very good condition. It was trying to me to take out two strong, firm teeth, but I could see no other way. There is some excementosis on the roots, but not enough to account for so much trouble.

Speaking of excementosis recalls a case I had thirty or more years ago, where an upper molar in a gentleman's mouth was causing him to suffer extreme pain. I removed the pulp, and tried all sorts of treatment, which failed to give any relief. By exclusion, I diagnosed excementosis. I extracted the tooth and found a large deposit. The patient was entirely relieved from pain. Within a year or two he had another tooth that acted just the same way, and, guided by my former experience, I extracted it, and found it in the same condition.

Dr. Wilson.—Did these two teeth you extracted have any cavities in them?

Dr. Fillebrown.—I do not remember that there were any cavities in them. The memory of the case is called up suddenly. I am not positive.

My third case is of a man about thirty, who called on me in

1902. Some four years before that he had had the right inferior first molar tooth extracted, a root being left. His face continued to give him much trouble, with some swelling for about two years. He had called once or twice on the dentist who had extracted the teeth, and did not get much satisfaction, and finally called on another and had the root out. Trouble continued. He consulted several other dentists, and got no relief. Finally, a lawsuit for damages was the result, and he lost his case. He had consulted so many dentists that the responsibility, if any, was too much divided. He came to me after the matter was quite far advanced, and I operated on it, hoping to stir up the matter so as to get some activity in the parts, but I did not succeed, although I tried three times. Finally, the trouble seemed to locate in the anterior portion of the diseased part, and a great deal of pus was continually welling up from the vicinity of the root of the second bicuspid. I examined his bicuspids carefully many times, and there was no visible sign of trouble with them, and it was impossible for me to believe that they were the source of any constantly discharging abscess. I made up my mind to sacrifice the bicuspids, and I extracted the teeth. I broke open the second bicuspid and found that the pulp was completely calcified, white in color. There is the root, and the pulp standing up intact, seemingly of perfectly natural shape. It was a surprise to me. I saw him later, and the abscess caused by the tooth was cured, but there was well-developed necrosis in the region of the first molar, the exfoliating process being extremely slow, it will be some time before he gets entire relief. I did not feel warranted in cutting to any great extent at that time.

DISCUSSION.

Dr. Hopkins.—I should like to ask Dr. Fillebrown, in regard to the first case, the wisdom-tooth, whether it would have been possible to have done anything by extraction of the second molar?

Dr. Fillebrown.—Possibly, if we had known what was there. It seemed hardly reasonable to do so at that time.

Dr. Hopkins.—I had such a case in the Massachusetts General Hospital last summer. I went down there on call by one of the surgeons. I had the assistance of the hospital. By getting out the second molar I was able to get out a wisdom-root that was difficult of access where there was partial ankylosis of the jaw.

Dr. Fillebrown.—That certainly was a good thing to do.

Dr. Potter.—I would like to report a case that came to me two or three years ago, a case of a young lady about eighteen or twenty years of age, who had a fistula through the face, about opposite the superior first molar. She had been in the hands of a well-known surgeon of this city for treatment. He was washing out the fistula and trying to heal it up. I could never find out just what his diagnosis of the trouble was. On examination of the left superior maxilla, I found a suspicious second bicuspid. The bicuspid had the history of being a tooth in which the pulp had died. The patient said that she had been treated. The root-canal in this tooth had been treated, so that one would naturally expect that the second bicuspid was the source of this trouble. That was the natural supposition. I percussed the first and second bicuspid, and the first molar. The only indication of trouble was in this second bicuspid. I naturally opened into the root of the second bicuspid, to see if there was any action between that and the fistula. After opening it and undertaking to force a stream of water through, I found there was no free opening. There was a large filling in the proximal surface of the first molar, and although this molar gave no indication of trouble, I thought I would open into it, which I did, and found a dead pulp, and it was not long before I had forced a stream of water through the first molar and out through the cheek. The case is singular, in that the first molar had never given the slightest symptom of trouble. The patient could remember nothing unfavorable from that first molar, and yet there had been sufficient trouble there, sufficient force and energy in the pathological process, to force the fistulous opening through the cheek. The case healed quickly with the renovation of the first molar, and the scar was extremely slight.

Dr. Fillebrown.—In a condition where a fistula appears in the region of a bicuspid on the cheek, is it not evident that the trouble is with the molars and not with the bicuspid?

Dr. Andrews.—I had a case brought to me by one of the physicians of Cambridge, a case of a fistula under the chin. Several dentists pronounced the teeth all right. It was curetted, but it did not heal. I examined the lower incisors carefully. There was no sensation on percussion. I thought I would use my electric light. I found one of the centrals much darker than the other. I drilled in and found a dead pulp. I brought that on in three weeks' time, and it commenced to heal, and healed up in good shape. So that we cannot always tell by the appearance of the teeth where there is a dead pulp.

Dr. Potter.—I would like to ask Dr. Fillebrown if he would not expect soreness and trouble from all teeth that had produced a fistula?

Dr. Fillebrown.—Yes; but there are exceptions enough to that to put one continually on his guard.

Dr. Wilson.—I think I can answer that question. I remember a good many years ago a young patient came to me with her mother, a young girl, I should think fifteen or sixteen years old, and I noticed a little bunch under her chin. I asked what that was, and she said, " I think it is a tumor, and Dr. —— is going to take it out, as it does not heal." The gentleman named was one of our most prominent surgeons in Boston. I did not say anything at the time, but I suspected it was a tooth. I made a very careful examination, and found it was the sixth-year molar tooth. I told the mother so at the time, and said, " I am quite sure that I can cure this, and there will be no need of an operation." She was quite sceptical at the time, because the man who was to perform the operation was one of the most skilful surgeons in Boston. To make a long story short, I probed the tooth, the fistula healed up, and she has never had any trouble since. There was no pain or soreness. The tumor dried up. It was a little cauliflower excrescence.

Dr. Lett.—I want to relate a peculiar case. A lady was sent to me when in her eighth month of pregnancy with a small tumor, the size of a large pea, right under the second bicuspid tooth. The bicuspids were perfect, without any fillings. The second and first molar had been extracted. On account of the closeness of the period of delivery, her physician advised that nothing be done then. Two months later I saw her, and the tumor had grown to the size of a pigeon's egg, and went down through to a thin layer of bone, in which there was an enormous pus socket, which looked like this Golden Flake sealing-wax. The bicuspid teeth were sensitive at the cervical margin, so I did not disturb them. This woman had fallen out of a third-story window when about two years old. It was a very interesting case for the surgeons of Boston, who did not see how she could live. She had a third molar tooth that had two small gold fillings and a vital nerve. The cervical margin was quite sensitive. I could get a probe as far as the mesial root of the second molar. I thought of extracting that tooth, but was very much in doubt about it, when the lady's relatives partially decided for me by demanding the extraction of the tooth. I did not see its use, so I decided to take it out, and found quite a severe necrotic condition. The apex of the two roots had been eaten away by this necrotic process. Immediately after this it started to heal, and accomplished this beautifully and entirely. I do not know why I took the tooth out; it was under the impulse of the moment. I do not see why that necrotic condition existed there and caused the condition so far anterior to it.

Dr. Fillebrown.—Dr. Lett's remark leads me to express a conviction that I have had for a good while, that where we have these serious troubles with the jaws, that cannot be controlled, it is advisable, and is demanded of the operator, that he make examinations, and seek for a cause which is oftentimes remote from the effect. I believe it to be our duty not to be too conservative in the matter of removing teeth, because health is worth more than any one tooth.

Many of you perhaps remember the article by Dr. Seton, of New York, who said that there was too much saving of teeth, speaking particularly in regard to troubles of the ear and the eye, and also making the statement that dentists were saving too many dead teeth. I remember that Dr. Abbott took umbrage at it, and wrote several severe articles in reply. I believe Dr. Seton was right. There is something besides teeth in the human system, and when teeth are less useful than the parts to which they are doing damage they ought to be removed.

Dr. Potter.—As an incident of office practice, I want to report the use of a very satisfactory instrument that one of our members has been working over for several years. You have heard Dr. Merriam speak with some feeling of the fact that he had introduced something here in the Society long ago, and no notice was ever taken of it. I think that when our members do anything in the way of processes or instruments, we ought to take some notice of it.

I have been using Dr. Wilson's plugger for only a short time, but it seems to me rather a valuable thing. If any of you have not been using it, I think you ought to try it. It seems to me that it manages the gold better than a spring mallet. It requires less muscular energy to work it. It is refreshing to get hold of a plugger that works so easily.

Dr. Bradley.—Speaking of Dr. Merriam's introduction of gutta-percha, I do not know that there is any formal record of his work in gutta-percha, but almost every one knows that he was one of the pioneers in the use of it. I remember twenty years ago when he demonstrated the use of gutta-percha and the oil of cajuput and taking impressions in the root-canals, and I know that he has visited Rhode Island and demonstrated the use of gutta-percha and talked about it there. He not only spoke about it and demonstrated its use, but left a box for every member that was present. I was looking over my things recently, and found some of his gutta-percha. I feel sure, Mr. President, that we want to give Dr. Merriam a great deal, if not all, of the credit for unfolding to us a more complete knowledge of the possibilities that are in gutta-percha.

Dr. Fillebrown.—I wanted earlier to say a word on that very point. I think Dr. Merriam is acknowledged as being the pioneer in the use of gutta-percha. I think it is on record sufficiently. He wrote a paper, and read it here and in other places. It has been in general use ever since that. I am sure that if you speak to the Harvard alumni, you will find very few of them ignorant of his use of gutta-percha. Dr. Hamilton did not claim to originate the use of gutta-percha. He was only using what others were using.

H. S. PARSONS,
Editor.

THE SUCCESSES AND FAILURES IN OUR DAILY WORK.[1]

BY DR. HARRY F. HAMILTON, BOSTON, MASS.

MR. PRESIDENT, AND GENTLEMEN OF THE ACADEMY,—Instead of presenting a paper for your consideration this evening, I have

[1] Read before the American Academy of Dental Science, Boston, February 1, 1905.

thought it might be of more interest to take a few subjects, in which I had been working, and briefly present them for your consideration. While there is nothing perhaps distinctly novel, yet the successes and failures, the methods and results, of our daily work is always of interest and advantage to others.

NAPKINS.

I wish to show first the napkins I use. We cannot control the laundry, and do not know what other articles are in the tub besides napkins, so that, while they look clean, I do not feel that they are so, and prefer not to use them a second time. After some search I found a heavy bleached cotton, rather stiff with dressing, which answers admirably, and after use is thrown away. It is the Anchor brand; one yard of it costs twelve and one-half cents and makes sixteen napkins; so you see the daily cost is small. Before being used I put them in the formalin sterilizer, so there is no possibility of odor. A pile of these new clean napkins in the drawer is a daily satisfaction, which I hope you will all try.

RIBBON.

I next submit something, not as necessary, but which in many cases is useful. It is a very thin ribbon, without any extra thickness at the selvage, called lute string or taffeta ribbon, and which I use in cleaning teeth; and sometimes I can get patients to use it themselves, a few times a week with tooth-powder. It is not very strong, and in many places tears, but where it does go in will do its work quickly and well.

I pass around enough silk and napkins, so each gentleman may take one as a sample if he desires.

NITRATE OF SILVER.

About twelve years ago I began using nitrate of silver, at first carefully, as I had some fear of its deep staining, but later I used it freely, and for ten years I have made it a rule to see that all the teeth back of the cuspids were given a good treatment of the saturated solution as soon as possible after eruption. I simply dry off the surfaces and put on the solution with a small swab, letting it stay a minute, during which time I push it with an explorer down into the sulci. I merely wish to give this as an invariable rule, carried out with great success for this length of time. The staining is only surface, and decay is generally prevented, and in cases where it does occur is greatly delayed. Teeth given this treatment need as careful watching as if untreated, for in a few cases it seemed that the nitrate did not go to the bottom, and decay went on, deep down, without showing on the surface. Our big operations give a certain satisfaction, but it is not to be compared to that of feeling that we have actually kept the teeth from decay.

CROWNS.

I have done much crown-work, my experience even going back to resetting a few old hickory pivots. I have followed all the fortunes, good and bad, of Bonwill and Richmond, and all their modifications, and I have arrived at the conclusion that there is only one crown, possessing all the qualifications of beauty, strength, and durability, and that is a porcelain crown on a banded platinum base,—the Richmond crown with platinum band and solid porcelain top.

There is one point I wish to bring out first, which I do not remember having seen in print, and that is the tolerance of the gums to platinum bands and bridges. The gums do not recede, but, on the contrary, embrace the band, and are perfect in color and cleanness. Gradually I have worked out a method which is simple and easy, and the result is quite perfect; but yet it takes much time, and I hope I shall be able to shorten it. I dare say you have all made similar crowns, but my method may be of interest.

I trim the root, as for a Richmond crown, only smaller, fit a copper band to the root, and, with that as a model, have a seamless platinum cap struck up, which I fit to the root. I then decide whether the pin is to be a part of the root or of the tooth. Generally I prefer to set a screw pin in the root. In this case, I put a hole in the cap, and solder a very thin platinum tube to it, through which the pin projects when set. The tooth is carved and baked on this base, and generally set with gutta-percha. It is equally valuable for bridge-work piers; and so easy to do that wonderfully good work can be done in the back of the mouth.

In the other case the pin is soldered to the cap, which it goes through, and is left projecting above it, to aid the porcelain's hold.

While these crowns may take a little more time to make, yet it is a straight operation; that is, each piece fits as it goes along, so when the crown is ready it goes perfectly into place, and there is no splitting, no decay of the root, but a crown absolutely strong, beautiful, and permanent as anything the dentist is called on to do.

INLAYS.

Two years ago I read a paper that Dr. Wassell, of Chicago, had delivered in Stockholm, the previous summer, telling his method of making inlays by the impression method. It seemed feasible, and later I chanced to see some of his work, which was superb. On my way to California I stayed over in Chicago, and saw much more of it; and it was a revelation. I saw mouths where careful examination was necessary to discover the inlays, and yet they comprised fillings in all sorts of places, and including large portions of the teeth. After seeing that beautiful exhibition of skill, I could not be satisfied with the inlay work which I had been doing, and which I had, indeed, been rather proud of, but I took steps to learn his methods, which are well described in the directions coming with Brewster's porcelains, and which, I presume, are familiar to you all.

The impression of the cavity is taken in cement, and the counter-die from it also in cement; the platinum matrix is swaged, and the inlay built to shape by trying in a plaster case of the teeth. With this method it is possible to build up corners even, and whole crowns, and have all the contours accurately reproduced, as in the original tooth. My first step on beginning was to install a young man in the laboratory to work up a knowledge of the methods. We have worked long and hard, and with many trials and discouragements, lightened by seemingly wonderful successes, until now it is comparatively easy for both, and we are looking toward the rewards.

You may recall, at an Academy meeting, a few years since, my showing the Jenkins apparatus, the first which we had seen. Before that I made some few inlays, with platinum matrix and Downie body, which, by the way, are excellent now; but when the elaborate Jenkins porcelains and furnace came, Dr. Hadley and I used it with much success, because we never ventured beyond the limitations of a low-fusing body. The inlays were quickly made, and little trouble arose from shrinkage. With the desire to build up the missing portions of the back teeth, new problems in shrinkage and repeated fittings arose, which could not be done in the mouth, and which in the laboratory need the greatest care to solve.

To better show the difficulties, I ought to say that although the man who has taken this in charge has shown much cleverness in his work, yet the result is that he can turn out only about fifteen satisfactory inlays a week; but as he now knows porcelain better, and has a helper for making the matrices, he will be able to furnish all we need.

This brings me to the point I wish to make, and which I have not seen made in inlay discussions, and that is, that the large inlays, involving more than one surface, can not be successfully made at the chair by a dentist with a large practice. We do not do our own artificial work; we do not make our own instruments; and yet this is infinitely more delicate, and, from my experience, I do not believe that any dentist, in the course of his daily work, can fit matrices, carefully dry his porcelain, and accurately bake it, with the pressure of coming patients hurrying him on. I have no doubt but that in the future some methods may be found to shorten and simplify this, which will modify this statement, but I believe the inlays, such as I show, should be made in a public or private laboratory.

I will pass around a few specimens, duplicates of actual cases that I have set. In these cases the maker of the inlays has not seen the tooth. I took the cement impression, and also one in impression material, gave them to him with the color, and he sent back the inlay.

As to inlays coming out, I regard that as a bugbear, and where they fail it is from the improper shape, or, more often from not keeping them absolutely dry for the hour needed while the cement is hardening. We never pay much attention to the shape of a cavity for a cement filling, and as inlays are at present made, they are nothing but cement fillings with nearly the whole of the cement replaced by porcelain.

At one time it looked as if inlays were to be permanently discredited, by the failures caused by dentists putting them in mouths before they had mastered the methods; but the successes have more than offset the failures, and little is heard now from the patients, to their discredit.

Before a discussion of these subjects, I would suggest that if any member would like to ask further information, I would be pleased to answer now.

QUESTIONS AND DISCUSSION.

Dr. Piper.—I would like to ask Dr. Hamilton about the platinum cap for the crown. Does he swage that in the office?

Dr. Hamilton.—No; I send it to the Paine Crown Company, who are expert in making them.

Dr. Piper.—I am glad to know that; I make the same thing on a Richmond crown. I would like to ask why you make your measurement in copper rather than in wire measurement?

Dr. Hamilton.—It gives the gum contour better.

Dr. Clapp.—Do you ever have any trouble with this thin edge of body running down over this band and cracking off after it has been in the mouth for some time?

Dr. Hamilton.—Very little. In one case it was on the inside, and I didn't mind it at all. If at any time it cracks off, I can heat it, take it off, roughen the platinum, and put more body on, with very little trouble.

Dr. Baker.—Give the method of setting with gutta-percha?

Dr. Hamilton.—I have used gutta-percha for some time by having it made in a big lump, and then with a rubber file having it filed down into a powder, and with oil of cajuput, a small amount, I would put it on a slab and warm it, and that would soften it up. About burning, I made a rule that if I could hold it in my fingers, the patient should be able to bear it on the gum.

Dr. Cook.—What form of gutta-percha do you use?

Dr. Hamilton.—Red base plate.

Dr. Cook.—Do you put anything with it?

Dr. Hamilton.—No, just as it comes.

Dr. Merriam.—I am somewhat in doubt whether I ought to speak on this matter of gutta-percha again or not, but this whole matter in relation to the setting of crowns over gutta-percha, the use of the essential oils for softening gutta-percha, and the setting of crowns by methods of impression, was brought before this Academy by a member long years ago, and, like many suggestions of the kind, it has never received recognition until brought back again from some other city. I will say that this matter of setting crowns in gutta-percha was presented also in New York at one of the meetings of the society there, and I presume it was recorded, although I am not sure.

Dr. Werner.—Many seeming innovations are only rehashed and reapplied methods. Take, for instance, our turbine engine, reinvented about thirteen years ago by a Swedish engineer. Hieron, in Alexandria, about the beginning of the Christian era, had it and used it.

Speaking of gutta-percha and the oil of cajuput and other essential oils, I remember Dr. Merriam speaking about it in the Odontological Society when he was a member there. He taught us that.

When I set a crown in gutta-percha I do not dance around in the way Dr. Hamilton speaks of, but let my patient do it. I simply have two or three finger cloths on my hands, and have an instrument carved out of wood on which I put my crown and warm it, and try that on my own hand, to see how well the patient can stand it. If I can stand it on my own hand, the patient can stand it very much better on a partially cocainized gum.

I have often thought that the crowns do crack if baked over this platinum. I also find difficulty with my platinum bands. They do not take very kindly to the gum. The gums that I have treated did not take kindly to bands of any kind. Seemingly they did take very kindly for three or four months, and sometimes for a year or two, but later those crowns look very bad.

I am not talking against inlays at all, for, however limited their usefulness, they have come to stay, but all of you have equipped yourselves with furnaces and complicated machineries, and the dental depot men will have much less interest in your buying teeth. There has been a great overdoing in inlays. In their proper place they are very good things, and should be studied by all of us.

Dr. Allen.—I want to ask Dr. Hamilton if he has ever used an iridio-platinum plate for bands. I find in my experience that the platinum bands made in this way cause trouble by binding and breaking off porcelain, and I use No. 30, as Dr. Hamilton has indicated, but I find that I can use No. 35 or 36 iridio-platinum, having it much thinner and safer, and with less danger of breaking.

Dr. Hamilton.—I have made some bands, but never a cap of iridio-platinum for crowns. I do not think it would be a good plan, as it. has a way of cracking when stretched, and might develop an incipient crack which would open later.

Dr. Allen.—I have used them as I would make a Richmond

cap, soldering platinum over the band instead of iridio-platinum. For the cap, on the edge of the band, I would use pure platinum.

Dr. Merriam.—I think that the soldering on platinum or iridio-platinum is apt to be treacherous. I find, in making the band for bicuspid crowns, we can make crowns entirely of iridio-platinum, and it appears to be strong, but after a time it peels off.

Dr. Baker.—I would like to ask Dr. Hamilton how he shapes his root?

Dr. Hamilton.—I have no particular way of shaping the root. Just with the disks and some good strong scalers.

Dr. Werner.—I would like to ask Dr. Hamilton how long he has used the swaging process in the laboratory?

Dr. Hamilton.—Since a year ago last October.

Dr. Porter.—Will you tell us in a few words just what you do in making an inlay?

Dr. Hamilton.—I open up the cavity with the rapid chisels, and do nearly all the excavating with the new Gem cavity wheels. These, if used under water, are not very painful. Then adjust a copper matrix, dry the cavity thoroughly, and polish well with common talcum powder (not the perfumed kind). Then fill with Fellowship cement, well over the edges. After it hardens, remove matrix and start impression by putting a piece of wood against a strong edge and striking the other end of the wood with a small hammer. This impression is set in plaster, face uppermost, and the die obtained by putting Ames's cement into it, after it has been well rubbed with talcum. This gives the working model, which is set in plaster, in the steel cup of the Brewster outfit.

The platinum matrix, one-thousandth of an inch thick, is adapted to the die by swaging and burnishing. I do not know that this gives a more perfect fit than if adapted in the cavity, but it is done in the laboratory, and does not take my time, which is the special plea for it that I am advocating this evening.

Reviews of Dental Literature.

CONTRIBUTION TO THE PATHOLOGY AND TREATMENT OF TIC
DOULOUREUX OF THE FACE.[1] By J. Besson (de Grenoble).

I report five observations of tic douloureux of the face which
I have made during two years. Fortunately the patients have
been willing to submit to a surgical treatment not often resorted
to in cases of chronic neuralgia.

This treatment, however, is not new. In 1894 Dr. Jarre spoke
in the *Revue de Stomatologie* of the pathology and treatment of
tic douloureux, based on the latest works of stomatologists.

According to him it is not logical to attribute tic douloureux
always to a central nervous origin. The frequent infection of the
mouth, the composition and structure of the teeth, easily penetrated by the products of fermentation, the sensitiveness of these
same teeth, the frequent lesions of the gums, of the alveolus, and
the adjacent osseous tissues, appeared to explain sufficiently the
nervous lesions of the adjacent tissues. It was here that we had
to look for a pathology and the logical treatment of tic douloureux,
which was probably caused by peripheral nerve-filaments of the
trigeminus. In order to support his hypothesis, Dr. Jarre reports
a series of tics cured through the extraction of all the teeth on the
affected side, and especially the removal of the diseased alveolar
walls.

The communication of Cruet at the International Congress of
Medicine, 1903, and the theses of Gaumerais and Gillet confirmed
this theory.

In December, 1902, Dr. Hermite de Grenoble sent a patient to
me who suffered for thirteen years of an intermittent tic douloureux. The attacks recur, from month to month, lasting several
days, sometimes weeks. When I saw him he was suffering from
a severe paroxysm of pain. The right side of the face was affected
by spasms, especially at the level of the eyelid and the lips. The
lips were paralyzed, the saliva was constantly running from the

---

[1] Translated for this journal from the February Number, 1905, of the
Revue de Stomatologie, by Clara M. Lötschert, D.D.S.

mouth. The equally paralyzed tongue articulated with difficulty some vague sounds. The skin presented an unusual hyperæsthesia. The slightest contact of the right side of the face with a foreign body increased the pain. Here was, indeed, a typical case of tic douloureux of the face.

As predisposing cause, hereditary and personal, the history revealed only articular rheumatism.

I examined the mouth. It showed the characteristics of gouty condition,—congested and spongy gums inclosing some loose elongated teeth covered with tartar. Four teeth only remained in the superior maxilla, which was the seat of the neuralgia. I decided upon extraction, which was followed by the free use of hydrogen peroxide.

The conditions, however, remained unchanged; other remedies had to be resorted to. The idea that the bone was involved had presented itself from the very first. In order to generalize, we decided to direct our operation only to the superior maxilla, which seemed to be the seat of the trouble, especially the canine region. The slightest touch on the skin in this portion of the face brought on a severe attack of pain.

We applied the chisel and the bone forceps to the whole bony area situated between the sinus, the nasal fossa, and the supraorbital canal. The operation was then completed with the removal of the alveolar walls behind the canine region.

One incident during the operation caused some annoyance,— the accidental opening of the sinus.

The result was immediate. In waking, the patient declared himself entirely relieved; the spasms and the pain had disappeared. Our operative interference had occurred during one of the paroxysmal crises.

The cure continues until this very moment. But an infection of the sinus through the buccal opening necessitated frequent antiseptic injections. Dr. Hermite was called to close the opening by a suture; a cutaneous entrance was established for our preventive measures, the protection of the mouth from bacterial influence.

The patient, the janitor of the faculty, sleeps and eats normally. During the past two years he has hardly felt a vague shooting sensation in the supra-orbital region. His awaking in the morning is now a pleasant sensation after the horrible nightmare of thirteen years.

This clinical observation called our attention to two points: first, the fixed point of the pain located on a level with the canine fossa; second, a peculiar circumstance revealing itself during the operation,—the compact, ivory-like appearance, the excessive hardness of the osseous tissue in the canine region. Both are of special value when we consider the result obtained through the operation. New cases were studied more methodically.

Two months later, in January, 1903, M. C., sent by Dr. Perriol de Grenoble, presented himself.

The same symptoms—paroxysms of pain dating back fifteen years with rare intervals; the whole organism considerably weakened by intolerable suffering.

The mouth was intact in spite of the advanced age of sixty-five. Not one tooth was missing, but it showed the characteristics of a long-standing pyorrhœa alveolaris.

Three to four teeth were suspected and extracted without modification of the pain. Definitive interference followed a few days later,—the extraction of all the teeth on the affected side and the "resection" of the osseous part of the canine region with the help of Dr. Perriol.

The result was marvellous. Previous to this operation the inferior maxillary nerve had already been removed by Professor Jaboulay de Lyon without marked effect. Two years later Dr. Perriol removed the supra-orbital nerve. After each of these operations the patient, in waking from the anæsthesia, experienced the sensation that the intensity of the pain was the same as before. After our surgical interference, however, he awoke with the conviction that he was cured, for all pain had disappeared.

Unfortunately, the weakened constitution of the patient could not stand the violent shocks of the treatment. He died a month later from phlebitis of the lower limbs.

Here again had been the symptoms of the tic douloureux,—spasms, pain located in the canine region. All had yielded to the surgical operation performed during a period of the paroxysms. The maxilla showed at the mentioned area an excessive compactness. The mouth had been long since the seat of pyorrhœa alveolaris.

In May of the same year, with the assistance of the doctoress Bruyant and that of my brother, I performed the same operation on a woman of the suburbs, fifty-five years of age, suffering for two years from facial neuralgia of light spasmodic character. Extracted eleven teeth on the affected side. Then a month later, the pain having continued meanwhile, removed the osseous part of the canine region. Immediate cessation of the pain without recurrence. The same observation as before regarding the location of the pain and the compactness of the bone.

In August, operation on a woman sixty years old. Mouth very much affected by chronic pyorrhœa; neuralgia dating two years.

Three or four remaining teeth were extracted; a few days later, resection of canine area. The result was even more complete. We have seen our patient again. She does no longer suffer.

The last operation on record took place August, 1903. At the distance of one month we performed two partial resections of the superior maxilla on a woman fifty years of age, suffering for ten years from tic douloureux. The first surgical interference brought no relief. At the second we approached the supra-orbital nerve. She felt a slight decrease of pain for a period of three months. But the pain has recurred since then. Grateful for the relief, she came back desiring that we should go farther. Here again we had to do with a mouth of arthritic character undermined by pyorrhœa alveolaris. Once more the paroxysms appeared to take their origin on a level with the canine fossa, and the superior maxilla was at that period very compact. It remains to state that in three cases of those operated upon the teeth showed signs of old arthritis with calcified pulps.

From all these operations I have only marked out the most striking points. I will repeat them in a few words.

1. The neuralgia or chronic facial " névritis" is an affection of advanced age. It seems to manifest itself more in gouty persons whose tissues undergo senile or sclerotic changes.

2. The seat of the pain seems to be more that portion of the trigeminus which expands on a level with the canine fossa, that is to say the anterior dental branch.

3. The "névritis" of these nerve extremities is accompanied by a marked compactness of the bone tissues.

4. In five cases operated upon the canine fossa, the results have obviously been far superior to those obtained by extirpation of the nerves.

5. We conclude with Dr. Jarre that the chronic facial névritis appears to be the consequence of oral infection in gouty persons

and of the osseous transformations which take place in the length of time. It is a neuralgia through infection and pressure of bone, comparable to the dental pulpitis.

6. We agree, with Jarre, Cruet, Gaumerais, Gillet, when they regard tic douloureux in the majority of cases as a peripheral "névritis." We consider a surgical operation upon the peripheral region logical; one, limited to the alveolar region, insufficient.

7. We add that it must be made on the superior maxilla in general; in particular, on the canine fossa. Our clinical observations prevent this, while the following anatomical facts reinforce our opinion.

If we consider the character of the superior and inferior dental plexus, we find that throughout the nerve-endings detach themselves from the trunk in order to disappear almost immediately in the dental canal, except on one point. The anterior and the middle dental branches, branches of the superior maxillary nerve take their origin before the entrance of the maxillary nerve in the superior orbital sinus. From this they take their course through two special bony canals enclosed in the thickness of the wall of the sinus. Thus we have here two long osseous canals, each embracing a nerve branch, being at the same time in direct connection with the alveoli of the incisors and canines, also with the sinus.

When one knows the frequency of chronic alveolar infections in arthritic patients, when one thinks of the frequent existence of obscure (ignored) sinuses, then it is permitted to think that the osseous tissue transforms itself under these influences; that it slowly compresses (smothers) the nerve branches of which the pulp extremities are often already dead.

At any rate, this hypothesis presents itself after having seen the dense, compact, ivory-like aspect of these tissues, the calcification of the pulp, and, above all, the cessation of the pain after the operation.

For us tic douloureux of the face is a peripheral nervous affection; it is curable through a surgical operation upon the canine region.

WHY USE LOW-CARAT SOLDER ON NEW DENTAL WORK? By William H. Trueman, D.D.S., Philadelphia.

The time was, and not so very long ago, when gold solder kept for sale at the dental depots was so brittle and so broken that it might be handled with a scoop. This is now changed. Firms catering to the wants of dental mechanics have brought skill and science to bear upon their metallurgical departments, and as a result the needed precious metals are obtainable in better form and in greater variety. The tendency, however, to debase the solders, while no doubt in response to a demand for solder of easy flowing qualities, is not to be commended. The fault, however, is not with them, but is due to faulty teaching in our schools and text-books. The time was when solders of a standard carat were for sale; now they are advertised and branded, not as of a certain carat, but as *solder for a certain carat plate*, special stress being laid upon their easy flowing qualities and good color, rather than upon their fineness. The reduced price plainly indicates that they are debased.

In an excellent text-book upon prosthetic dentistry, now before me, I find the following formula for a gold solder, which, it states, " may be used in connection with eighteen or twenty carat plate:"

> 6 dwts. pure gold.
> 2 dwts. rosette copper.
> 1 dwt. fine silver.

That such a formula should be published in a dental text-book of so recent a date (1897) is a disgrace, and yet it is a fair sample of those set before dental students by their class teachers and their text-books in this year of grace, 1905, copied without change from ancient text-books.

In the first place, it is not explicit, nor yet in accord with usage in scientific works. Why should the reader be compelled to work out a mathematical problem in order to obtain information that should be conveyed by the formula itself?

Let it read:

> 16 parts (or dwts. or grains, it is immaterial which) pure gold;
> 5½ parts rosette copper;
> 2⅔ parts fine silver;

and the reader knows at once that the resulting solder is sixteen carats fine. It may be used, of course, upon eighteen- or twenty-carat plate; but why should such low-carat solder ever be used in connection with eighteen- or twenty-carat plate? This is followed by two others, one a fraction over fifteen carats fine, and another eighteen, both naming gold coin and brass as components. Now let me ask, What is "rosette copper"? What is "gold coin"? What is "brass"? When this formula was first written, some seventy or more years ago, "rosette copper" might possibly have been some special brand of that metal; it has no meaning now. Brass, fine brass, brass pins, etc., are of as uncertain composition as is a low grade of boarding-house hash. Regarding "gold coin," nothing is certain beyond its containing a definite amount of pure gold. No doubt, when the mouth blow-pipe was in general use, with the well-remembered alcohol lamp, that now and again blew up, or more frequently "went out," like those of the unwise virgins, and from the same cause, before the soldering operation was completed, or in prolonged operations blinded one by its irritating fumes, a solder fusing at a few degrees less heat was appreciated. All that is now of the past, and it is high time that expedients made necessary by meagre facilities were erased from dental college teaching and dental text-books.

All the needed metals—gold, silver, copper, and zinc—are now readily attainable, as nearly absolutely pure as chemical processes carefully conducted can make them; and they only should be used. The difference in cost between pure gold and pure silver, and coin gold and coin silver, is trifling. Pure gold costs, at the refiners, one dollar and ten cents per dwt. for any amount less than an ounce, and twenty-one dollars an ounce. This never changes. Pure silver fluctuates; its present price is about seventy-five cents an ounce; pure copper is about twenty cents an ounce; pure zinc about fifteen cents an ounce. The base metals may be obtained from dealers in fine chemicals, who provide these metals for use in delicate chemical processes. There is no excuse for using, and no excuse for advising the use of commercial metals or alloys in making either plate or solder for dental use. They all contain harmful impurities.

Now, it is not every dentist who has facilities for making his own plate or solder, and when it can be purchased from reliable parties it is better to do so. It is well, however, to understand that eighteen-carat gold solder and solder for eighteen-carat gold plate are not the same. The latter is usually about two points lower carat.

If in the formulas for plate and solder given in the text-books the number of grains of the precious metal in each pennyweight is first given, the formula itself announces the carat. It is rather more scientific to state the parts in thousands; either, however. is explicit. The use of alloys should be discarded. There is no advantage in their use; they are confusing and unreliable.

The following formulas I use in my own laboratory. They are all I need for new work, and I find them quite satisfactory. They flow freely, have good color, and are as tough and pliable as plate. Between their fusing point and that of the metals for which they are intended there is ample margin. The eighteen-carat will flow freely upon silver plate, and the twenty-two-carat upon eighteen-carat plate without in either case the plate being overheated. This is my test of their fusibility.

Twenty-two-carat gold solder:

> 22 parts pure gold;
> 1 part pure copper;
> 1½ parts pure zinc.

Eighteen-carat gold solder:

> 18 parts pure gold;
> 3 parts pure silver;
> 2 parts pure copper;
> 1½ parts pure zinc.

Silver solder:

> 19 parts pure silver;
> 1 part pure copper;
> 4 parts pure zinc.

There is a slight loss of zinc, especially in making gold solder, not from oxidation, as the books generally state, but from volatilization, which is quite a different thing.

A fraction of a grain is added to allow for this. If pure metals are used, there is so little oxidation that as a rule the crucible from which the solder is poured is left perfectly clean; so clean, indeed, that they are promptly broken to avoid the temptation of using them again; a dangerous experiment, as the borax usually penetrates the bottom and causes them to leak when used a second time.

Either in safety to the porcelain teeth or to the plate, the slight difference in the fusing point between the high and low grade

solder is of no practical advantage, and for new work a solder of
a lower carat than the plate is inexcusable. The lower-grade solders are occasionally required in making repairs, and should be
used for that purpose only.

Silver, being more fusible, requires a solder a little less fine,
but there is no excuse for using a silver solder composed of equal
parts of silver plate and brass.

While zinc is a base metal, and is credited with causing brittleness when alloyed with the precious metals, the character it has
acquired as a component of precious metal alloys is not deserved.
It is due to the impurities found associated with it rather than to
the metal itself.

Notwithstanding that the solder sold as solder for eighteen-
carat plate is but little if any finer than sixteen-carat, I am told
by dealers that many dentists when purchasing eighteen-carat gold
purchase sixteen-carat solder to use with it, so that as a matter
of fact they are using on new work fourteen-carat solder. I wonder why! It cannot be economy; the difference in cost is too
insignificant. I take it to be ignorance, or it may be that they
do not possess proper heating arrangements, or lack effective blow-
pipes.

With the advent of crown- and bridge-work, a handy form of
blow-pipe has come into general use. For small, delicate operations they are very convenient, especially when the work is done
in the office on an office work-bench. None that I have tested
have proved satisfactory for serious work. The old-fashioned large
gas flame and the old-fashioned blow-pipe, operated with a foot-
pump or bellows, may make things hot on a warm day; may
occasionally singe the hair or burn the fingers; but when their
use is once mastered, soldering with honest, high-grade solder is a
pleasure.

As gold solders are now graded, a solder two carats higher than
the plate should always be used. It would be better, however, if
the dealers would cease to equivocate, and sell their gold solders
for what they really are.

Another reform. Our text-book writers should discard all the
old out-of-date formulas. There is no necessity for a multiplicity
of formulas, one for each grade is amply sufficient; and they
should teach that the plate and solder should be of the same fineness.

As before remarked, the difference in the fusing point of solder differing slightly in carat is no help to the workman constructing a new denture, but it makes a great deal of trouble at times, when that piece of work requires repairs or alterations, and these are attempted with "honest" solder.—*Dental Office and Laboratory.*

Editorial.

THE POSITION OF DENTISTRY IN RELATION TO MEDICINE.

WE are beginning to receive from various sources the results of the dental meetings in the East and the West, from national, State, and local organizations, and the two volumes of the Transactions of the Fourth International Dental Congress. While the proceedings of the less pretentious associations are not all in the hands of readers, and probably will not be until the summer solstice is again upon us, there is sufficient to form an opinion that the papers, as a whole, will average about as usual; some scientifically valuable, but the majority seemingly hurriedly put together to fill a gap in the programme. It is not necessary to criticise this, for it always has been and probably always will be, yet these papers, notwithstanding an ephemeral existence, have a certain value.

The subject of dental education has, as usual, been quite thoroughly threshed out, and it is very evident that no new thought can be forthcoming from that quarter.

We have become accustomed to long and labored articles from the pens of medical graduates on the position of dentistry in its relation to medicine, in which these earnestly endeavor to convince the dental mind that there is but one course to reach perfection in dental practice, and that is through the medical school. These articles would be more convincing if the graduates with the M.D. degree would universally show a superior ability in the work of the modern dentist. The writer has failed to discover this superiority, although he has numerous professional friends in possession of medical diplomas. If a careful examination of results be made, it will be evident that it is rare to find that these are any better qualified to treat pathological conditions, met with in the oral cavity, than those educated in the higher dental schools of the present time. It seems a waste of time to argue this question upon theoretical grounds when the results are all around us.

While we have had much from the medical side, and mainly partisan in character, it is not often found that a D.D.S. will present the question so decidedly one-sided as does Dr. Carlton on another page. His argument contains nothing specially new, for, as before stated, there is nothing new to be written upon this well-worn theme; yet, while this is true, his paper is of special note, as it is the product of one of the most cultivated members of our profession on the Pacific coast. It is, however, with some feelings of regret that he has been willing to lend his mental force in what seems to be in the direction of lowering the professional standing of dentistry. The trend of the article is evidently to make the D.D.S. degree a synonym of partial culture, but it is practically no culture at all, for he says, " Medicine and dentistry, though cognate sciences, have always been separately studied. This dissociation is now seen to be a great error, due not alone to the fact that the relation of the mouth and teeth to the rest of the anatomy was not understood, but also because only the mechanical aspect probably appealed to those who first considered the matter. . . . This conception of dentistry as an entity and not as an integral part of medicine has made it an art, possibly a trade, rather than a science." And further, he quotes from another that " The knowledge of life and disease represented by the average D.D.S. degree is certainly deplorably deficient." We are accustomed to this kind of talk from the self-appointed critics of the medical school, and may have the privilege of estimating it at its real worth, but it is not pleasant to have this kind of thought spread upon the pages of a medical journal, and that from the pen of a D.D.S. If it were absolutely true, it would be proper to let all the world know of it, but as it stands it creates the idea that the better class of dentists are ashamed of their calling, because it is not an " integral part of medicine." Its tendency must, therefore, be to give strength to the prejudice existing in the mind of the average medical practitioner against dentistry and dental schools.

Those who have entered dentistry in recent years have but a limited conception of the struggles made to overcome this unjust depreciation of it by medical men. It began openly when Harris failed to convince the medical thought of his day that dentistry was worthy of acceptance as a distinct part of the healing art. He was rejected then, although an M.D., and the D.D.S. has been rejected ever since.

When the amount of superior culture obtainable in that day by the student of medicine is considered, the claim to superiority becomes farcical. It is a matter of medical history, in comparatively recent years, that medical science embraced certain foundation studies, with certain others deemed of vital importance to-day omitted, because practically unknown. The man of less than forty years in the past took his degree in two years of six months, and was not aware that histology was vitally important to the study of general anatomy, or that bacteriology had any close relation to pathological conditions. The question of preliminary education was not considered an important factor, and it is doubtful whether it was regarded as essential, although the advanced social position accorded the medical practitioner drew a larger proportion of educated men to the medical schools.

The higher dental schools of the present time are not only better equipped for the teaching of all the foundation branches of medicine, but the subjects, with the exception of anatomy, are far more thoroughly taught than they were in the medical schools of 1870. This statement cannot be successfully controverted. Not only are these more thoroughly acquired through individual teaching, but instead of two years and sessions of six months, the dentist of the present must take a course of three years of eight to nine months' sessions each. It is true that there are dental schools of a high order and schools that may be termed mediocre, but the same may be said of medical colleges which are turning out yearly imperfectly trained medical practitioners.

The question of what is the best course to pursue in dental schools has not as yet been satisfactorily answered. The practical man has long since recognized that the study of medicine, following the scholastic period, carries the youth beyond the time to begin mechanical training; that the head at this period is being cultivated at the expense of the hands. The other side deems this of no importance, and assumes that the mechanical, including operative, can be performed by specialists, who deserve, from their trade affiliations, no claim to professional consideration. The true dentist of the future is, in their estimation, one who knows nothing of these, but much of so-called medical science, and he will be the oral pathologist of the future. This may possibly come true in the generations yet to be, but what kind of dentistry will that be that knows nothing of that mechanical skill that preserves the natural organs, or substitutes when these are destroyed by age or disease. In a word, the great benefit that has accrued to humanity through dental mechanics would have been lost. Fortunately this is an impossible supposition.

What may be the developments in the future, or the place which dentistry will occupy, may not be possible to foresee, for the problem is one incapable of solution, but dental educators are trying to lay a sure foundation that it is hoped will lead to a system of practice that will measurably be free from criticism.

It must be evident to the careful observer that advanced training has its drawbacks so far as dentistry is concerned. It is unnecessary to dwell upon these, but the man who has graduated in medicine subsequent to his dental college training seems to lack something that the D.D.S. alone possesses. He may have all the skill requisite, and certainly he possesses superior knowledge, for he has spent some six years in obtaining it, but he appears to have come to occupy the position of being neither a good medical man on the one hand, or a happy member of the dental fraternity on the other.

This difficult question will probably be settled in the future by the dental colleges being brought in closer affiliation with the university system of the United States, and then, as now, the dentist will be trained in medicine and dentistry during the undergraduate course of five years' duration. He may carry then the M.D. as a badge of higher professional culture, but the world will know him as a dentist, and not as a stomatologist or as a practitioner of the healing art. It is not believed by the writer that his standing then will be regarded as being equal to the mother from which he sprang. It is a safe rule to always calculate that the man who works with his hands will always occupy a lower level than the individual who labors with his brains, and the dentist of the future must rest content with the conviction that his work, properly conducted, has a value far superior to the average medical practitioner, for the certainty in results of the one and the uncertainty of the latter will in time come to be understood better than it is to-day, and then the practitioner of the healing art will be judged more directly by results obtained.

Obituary.

RESOLUTIONS OF RESPECT TO DR. GEORGE E. NETTLETON.

New Haven, Conn., September 20, 1905.

Whereas, By the death of our friend and co-worker, Dr. George E. Nettleton, this Association records the loss of one through whose efforts, to a very great degree, we are indebted for our existence as an organized body, and while of an extremely retiring disposition, he was always on the alert in consideration of the Association's welfare; and

Whereas, Our profession loses a representative member, an earnest worker, who for more than thirty years had been honored and trusted by a large clientele. His positive yet affable nature won for him more than usual the respect and confidence of his patients. He was also a warm friend and helper to many young men entering our profession. During many years' association we never heard him speak a harsh or unkind word. His memory will always be cherished by this Association, never ceasing to mourn his loss; therefore, be it

Resolved, That we extend to the family of our departed brother our sincere sympathy in this hour of their bereavement; and be it further

Resolved, That these resolutions be spread upon the records of this Association, and a copy sent to his family.

E. S. Gaylord,
C. W. Strang,
H. A. Spang,
Committee.

Hartford, Conn., September 11, 1905.

Whereas, We, members of the Hartford Dental Society, have learned with profound sorrow of the death of Dr. George E. Nettleton, of New Haven; therefore be it

Resolved, That we deeply sympathize with his family and present our condolence to the New Haven Dental Association in the loss they have sustained. Honored and respected, he was for years regarded as one of the leading practitioners of dentistry in our State. We shall ever revere his memory and deplore his departure; and be it further

Resolved, That a copy of these resolutions be sent to his family, likewise to the New Haven Dental Association, and also that they be entered upon the records of this Society.

ALBERT E. CARY,
Secretary.

Current News.

XV CONGRÈS INTERNATIONAL DE MÉDECINE, LISBONNE, 19-26 AVRIL, 1906.

REGLEMENT.

ARTICLE 1.—Le XV Congrès International de Médecine s'ouvrira à Lisbonne le 19 avril 1906 et sera clos le 26 du même mois. Son but est exclusivement scientifique.

ART. 2.—Seront membres du Congrès:

1.°—Les Médecins qui en feront la demande.

2.°—Les savants qui seront présentés par le comité exécutif portugais ou par les comités nationaux étrangers.

ART. 3.—Tout membre du Congrès recevra sa carte d'identité, après avoir fait parvenir sa cotisation au Trésorier général du Congrès. Cette carte sera nécessaire pour pouvoir profiter des avantages faits aux Congressistes. Le versement à faire est de 25 *Francs* ou 20 *Marks* ou 1 *Livre Sterling* pour les Membres étrangers; de 5$ 500 *réis* pour les membres nationaux.

Les comités étrangers peuvent recevoir les adhésions de leurs nationaux. Ils en transmettront les cotisations au Secrétariat général portugais, qui leur enverra immédiatement un nombre de cartes égal à celui des cotisations transmises.

ART. 4.—En faisant parvenir leur cotisation au trésorier, les membres du Congrès devront indiquer lisiblement leurs nom, qualités et adresse, la section où ils veulent s'inscrire, et joindre leur carte de visite.

ART. 5.—En dehors des autres avantages, chaque membre du Congrès aura droit au volume de la partie générale du Congrès et aux travaux imprimés de la section dont il fait partie.

ART. 6.—Les sections du Congrès sont les suivantes :

(1) Anatomie (anatomie descriptive et comparée, anthropologie, embryologie, histologie).

(2) Physiologie.

(3) Pathologie générale, bactériologie et anatomie pathologique.

(4) Thérapeutique et pharmacologie.

(5) Médecine.

(6) Pédiatrie.

(7) Neurologie, psychiatrie et anthropologie criminelle.

(8) Dermatologie et syphiligraphie.

(9) Chirurgie.

(10) Médecine et chirurgie des voies urinaires.

(11) Ophthalmologie.

(12) Laryngologie, rhinologie, otologie et stomatologie.

(13) Obstétrique et gynécologie.

(14) Hygiène et épidémiologie.

(15) Médecine militaire.

(16) Médecine légale.

(17) Médecine coloniale et navale.

ART. 7.—Un Comité exécutif et une Commission générale d'organisation sont chargés de la préparation et du fonctionnement du Congrès.

ART. 8.—Le Congrès tiendra séance chaque jour, soit en assemblées générales, soit en réunions de sections.

ART. 9.—Deux assemblées générales auront lieu, l'une le jour de l'ouverture, l'autre le dernier jour du Congrès.

Il y aura en outre les assemblées extraordinaires que l'on jugera nécessaires pour la discussion de sujets généraux ou pour la présentation de conférences scientifiques ; leur programme sera fixé par le Comité exécutif.

Les conférences ne peuvent pas être suivies de discussion.

ART. 10.—Il sera procédé le jour de la première assemblée générale à la proclamation des présidents d'honneur du Congrès.

ART. 11.—Les assemblées générales d'ouverture et de clôture seront consacrées aux discours d'usage et aux vœux à émettre. Ne pourront prononcer de discours dans ces assemblées générales que les membres qui auront été désignés et invités par le Comité exécutif du Congrès.

ART. 12.—Toutes les propositions relatives aux travaux du

Congrès devront être notifiées au Comité exécutif avant le 1.er janvier 1906. Le Comité décidera sur la suite à donner à ces propositions.

ART. 13.—Les communications se référant aux travaux du Congrès doivent parvenir au Secrétariat général avant le 1.er janvier 1906; celui-ci se chargera de leur transmission à la section respective.[1]

Les titres des communications devront être accompagnés d'un court résumé (en forme de conclusions, si possible); cet extrait sera imprimé par les soins du Comité exécutif du Congrès et distribué aux membres de la section correspondante.

ART. 14.—On pourra présenter des communications après le 1.er janvier 1906 et même pendant le Congrès, mais elles ne pourront être mises à l'ordre du jour qu'après discussion de celles présentées dans le délai prescrit.

ART. 15.—Chaque Comité de section organisera son programme de travail (audition des rapports et discussion des sujets proposés, communications diverses).

ART. 16.—Deux ou plusieurs sections peuvent se réunir en une seule assemblée pour des travaux en commun.

ART. 17.—Les membres du Congrès peuvent prendre part aux travaux des sections où ils ne se sont pas fait inscrire.

ART. 18.—Les discours prononcés en assemblée générale et les rapports faits dans les sections seront publiés dans les comptes rendus des travaux Congrès; pour les communications diverses et discussions, le Comité exécutif se réserve tout droit d'examen. Le temps assigné à chaque communication ne pourra pas dépasser quinze minutes, et les orateurs qui prendront part à la discussion ne pourront parler plus de cinq minutes chacun.

Les auteurs des rapports et communications auront dix minutes pour leur réponse générale.

ART. 19.—Le texte écrit des rapports, communications et discussions, devra être remis le jour même au Secrétaire de la section respective. De même pour les discours en assemblée générale à remettre au Secrétaire général.

---

[1] Les *communications libres* ne doivent par être confondues avec les *rapports officiels*. Pour ceux-ci, le Comité exécutif a fixé le 30 septembre 1905 pour la présentation au Secrétariat général, a fin qu'ils puissent être imprimés avant l'ouverture du Congrès (*Note du Secrétaire général*).

ART. 20.—La langue française est la langue officielle du Congrès pour les relations internationales. Dans les assemblées générales ainsi que dans les sections, les langues allemande, anglaise et française pourront être employées.

Dans les sections on pourra faire usage d'une autre langue, pourvu qu'un des membres présents en fasse la traduction immédiate dans une des langues permises.

ART. 21.—Toutes les questions ayant trait aux travaux scientifiques des sections doivent être soumises et adressées au Président du Comité de la section intéressée. Pour tout ce qui concerne l'organisation et le fonctionnement du Congrès, on devra s'adresser au Secrétaire général.

ART. 22.—Dans sa dernière assemblée générale, le Congrès désignera le siège de sa prochaine réunion et en elira le bureau.

ART. 23.—Les dames des congressistes auront leur entrée au Congrès dans des conditions qu'on réglera, moyennant le versement d'une demie cotisation.

Comité exécutif.—Président, Cons. Costa Alemao; Secrétaire général, Prof. Miguel Bombarda (Hôpital de Rilhafolles, Lisbonne); Trésorier, Alfredo Luiz Lopes; Secrétaires, Antonio de Azevedo, Mello Breyner, Azevedo Neves, Mattos Chaves (Fernando); Membres, Annibal Bettencourt, Prof. Clemente Pinto. Prof. Daniel de Mattos, Prof. Ricardo Jorge, Silva Carvalho, Zeferino Falcao.

SECTIONS.

1.re—Président, José Antonio Serrano, Lisbonne; Secrétaire resp., Marck Athias, Rua de Santa Martha, 144, Lisbonne.

2.me—Président, Philomeno da Camara, Coimbra; Secrétaire resp., Arthur Cardoso Pereira, Rua Conselheiro Pedro Franco, 42, Lisbonne.

3.me—Président, Pedro Bettencourt Raposo, Lisbonne; Secrétaire resp., Annibal Bettencourt, Real Instituto Bacteriologico, Lisbonne.

4.me—Président, Raymundo Motta, Coimbra; Secrétaire resp., Brito Camacho, Hôpital de Rhilhafolles, Lisbonne.

5.me—Président, Bettencourt Pitta, Lisbonne; Secrétaire resp., Benjamin Arrobas, Campo dos Martyres da Patria, 28, Lisbonne.

6.me—Président, Dias d'Almeida, Porto; Secrétaire resp., Jayme Salazar De Sousa, Avenida Fontes Pereira de Mello, D. Lisbonne.

7.me—Président, Caetano Beirao, Lisbonne; Secrétaire resp., Virgilio Machado, Avenida da Liberdade, 200, Lisbonne.

8.me—Président, Zeferino Falcao, Lisbonne; Secrétaire resp., Mello Breyner, Rua da Junqueira, 59, Lisbonne.

9.me—Président, Oliveira Feijao, Lisbonne; Secrétaire resp., Augusto de Vasconcellos, Rua Nova do Almada, 80, Lisbonne.

10.me—Président, Moraes Caldas, Porto; Secrétaire resp., Arthur Furtado, Rua de S. Roque, 100, Lisbonne.

11.me—Président, Sousa Refoios, Coimbra; Secrétaire resp., —— ——.

12.me—Président, Gregorio Fernandes, Lisbonne; Secrétaire resp., Avelino Monteiro, Avenida da Liberdade, 91, Lisbonne.

13.me—Président, Candido de Pinho, Foz, Porto; Secrétaire resp., Daniel de Mattos, Hôpital de Rilhafolles, Lisbonne.

14.me—Président, Ricardo Jorge, Lisbonne; Secrétaire· resp., Guilherme Ennes, Rua do Livramento, 50, Lisbonne.

15.me—Président, Cunha Bellem, Lisbonne; Secrétaire resp., Manoel Giao, Avenida da Liberdade, 115, Lisbonne.

16.me—Président, Silva Amado, Lisbonne; Secrétaire resp., Lima Duque, Calçada da Estrella, 131, Lisbonne.

17.me—Président, Cons. Ramada Curto, Lisbonne; Secrétaire resp., Silva Telles, Rua Saraiva de Carvalho, 14, Lisbonne.

FIRST ANNUAL CLINIC OF THE FRATERNAL DENTAL SOCIETY OF ST. LOUIS.

SPECIAL features of the meeting to be held November 20 and 21, at the Barnes Dental College, will be a series of lectures on "Cavity Preparation," "Methods and Principles of packing Gold," and "Methods and Principles of finishing Fillings," by Dr. E. K. Wedelstaedt of St. Paul.

The following well-known members of the Black and Wedelstaedt Clubs will be present and clinically demonstrate "extension for prevention" to its fullest extent: Drs. A. C. Searle, Owatonna, Minn., J. F. Wallace, Canton, Mo., C. W. Booth, Cedar Rapids, Iowa, J. J. Booth, Marion, Iowa, William Finn, Cedar Rapids, Iowa, J. B. Pherrin, Central City, Iowa, Ed. S. Brown, Edina,

Mo., W. T. Rutledge, Monroe City, Iowa, and S. E. Wallace, La Belle, Mo.

Porcelain work will be fully demonstrated by Drs. F. E. Roach, Chicago, W. L. Ellerbeck, Salt Lake City, Geo. T. Banzett, Chicago, W. H. Cudworth, Milwaukee, and Craig W. Work, Ottumwa, Iowa.

Other clinics, on various subjects, will be given by Drs. W. L. Reed, Mexico, Mo., J. B. Howell, Paducah, Ky., C. L. Rose, Fargo, N. D., F. B. Lawrence, Eldorado, Kan., Geo. D. Sitherwood, Bloomington, Ill., A. Gaiser, Davenport, Iowa, Fred. Westerfield, St. Charles, Mo., Otto J. Fruth, St. Louis, Richard Summa, St. Louis, and others.

The following dealers have signified their intention to be present and display their exhibits: S. S. White Dental Mfg. Co., Dr. Jenkins Porcelain, Klewe & Co., A. C. Clark & Co., St. Louis Dental Mfg. Co., John Nolde Dental Mfg. Co., Risey Dental Mfg. Co., Denthol Chemical Co., Lambert Pharmacal Co., Lee S. Smith & Sons, Century Dental Laboratory Co., W. M. Berry Dental Laboratory Co., Sanitol Chemical Co., R. C. Brophy & Co., Keeton Williams Gold Co., Horlicks Food Co., Kress & Owens, Oakland Chemical Co., McKesson & Robbins, and others.

The Western Passenger Association and South Western Excursion Bureau have granted a rate of one and one-third fare, plus twenty-five cents validation fee, certificate plan, for this meeting for the States of Missouri, Iowa, Minnesota, Kansas, Nebraska, and Illinois, on and west of the line of the Chicago and East Illinois Railroad.

Headquarters will be at the Jefferson Hotel, Twelfth and Locust Streets. Rooms for one, without bath, $1.50 and up; rooms with bath, $2.50 and up. Rooms for two, without bath, $2.00 and up; rooms with bath, $3.00 and up.

Exhibit space may be obtained by application to the Secretary. If you have a clinic to give, send your name at once to the Supervisor of Clinics.

A cordial invitation is extended to the profession to be present and assist in making this meeting, limited in scope but limitless in importance, the best ever held in this section.

D. O. M. LeCron, *Supervisor of Clinics.*

S. H. Voyles, *Secretary.*

Burton Lee Thorpe, *President.*

THE

International Dental Journal.

VOL. XXVI.   DECEMBER, 1905.   NO. 12.

Original Communications.

THE INFLUENCE, ON DEVELOPMENT, OF ARRANGING IRREGULARLY PLACED TEETH INTO NORMAL POSITIONS.[1]

BY E. A. BOGUE, M.D., D.D.S., NEW YORK CITY.

BEFORE starting to consider the question that I am about to bring before you, let me say that I have not been unmindful of the influence of adenoid vegetations in producing the irregularly placed teeth which are so generally, if not uniformly, found in connection with mouth breathing, high arches and nasal stenosis, but all that has been purposely left out, that our attention may be drawn to certain features that have been less discussed, if indeed discussed at all.

I am clearly of the opinion that neglect is at the bottom of the worst cases we have to treat, that early treatment of the conditions now to be considered will result in the prevention of much of the evils of those conditions, and that preventive medicine is the highest level of that art.

---

[1] Read at the annual meeting of the British Medical Association at Leicester, July 28, 1905.
Republished from the Journal of the British Medical Association, with added illustrations.

Mr. President and Gentlemen: I was invited by your committee to furnish something of dento-surgical interest to be read at this meeting, for instance, " The Influence of Development on the Arrangement of the Teeth." This invitation furnishes me with the title of my subject, which will be " The Influence, on Development, of Arranging Irregularly Placed Teeth into Normal Positions."

Many of the evils that we as orthodontists are called upon to treat, and many of the diseases which confront the rhinologist,

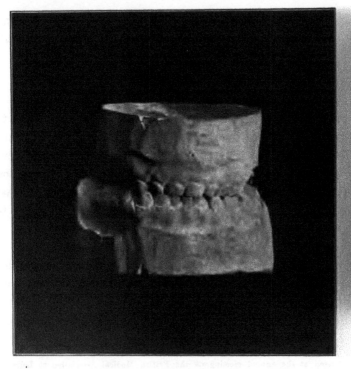

Fig. 1 shows the upper temporary molars inside the arch of the lower molars.

arise from a deficiency in the vital force of the child—an inability to overcome some mechanical obstruction.

Every developmental process is an expression of vitality. Every defect in formation or function is an indication of a deficiency in a motor centre of power sufficient to overcome obstructions. The expression of deficiency is various.

One of the most common expressions, and one that every dental surgeon and rhinologist should recognize, is irregularity in the arrangement of the teeth of the child. Sometimes this irregularity shows itself in the temporary, teeth, sometimes it shows first in the malarticulation of the first permanent or principal molars.

The lower principal molars of man have upon their outer or buccal side three cusps or tuberosities; upon the inner or lingual side they have two.

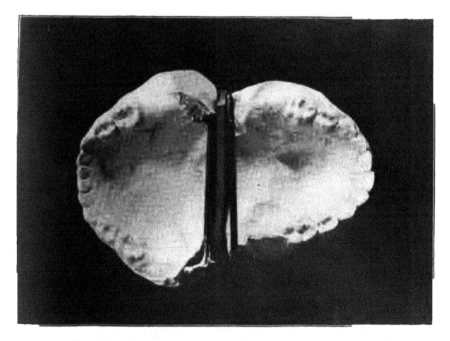

FIG. 2 is the same mouth open, showing the smaller upper arch of temporary teeth and therefore indicating contracted arches of permanent teeth not yet erupted, and contraction or non-development of contiguous bones.

The upper molars have two on either side. In the normal position of these teeth when closed the anterior buccal cusp of the upper molar and the anterior lingual cusp sit astride of the outer ridge of the lower first molar, just posterior to, and nicely fitting in with, the anterior buccal cusp of the lower molar.

This arrangement is made necessary by the greater width of the upper incisor teeth over the lower incisors.

The same general arrangement exists in the case of the tempo-rary teeth, so that the careful observer may detect irregularities in

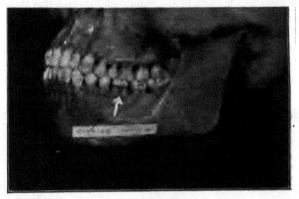

Fig. 3 shows a normal articulation of the permanent teeth.
· I am indebted for this slide to Dr. Summa of St. Louis.

the positions of the temporary teeth that are sure indications of malpositions among the permanent teeth *that are not yet erupted.*

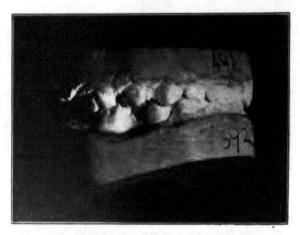

Fig. 4 shows an excessive overbite that would indicate irregularity in the lower arch.

Whenever there has been loss of temporary teeth, or even exces-sive decay, and a loss of considerable portions of the temporary teeth, the principal molars, which are either in the process of development or are just erupting, are pressed forward by the eruptive processes and seek to occupy the places of tissue lost by decay or of the missing temporary teeth.

For example, a temporary tooth becomes decayed, the pulp is exposed and dies. The process of absorption of the roots, so far as

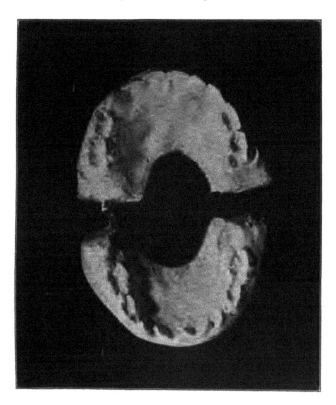

F₁ɢ. 5 shows the irregularity, being the models of the same mouth opened

such absorption is dependent upon the pulp, ceases, solution from whatever cause is slower, hence this pulpless tooth is an obstacle to the regular development of the tooth beneath, and if this tooth succeeds in emerging from beneath the temporary tooth it is deflected from its proper place in the arch.

If the cavity of decay be upon the posterior approximal side of the temporary tooth, toward the erupting first molar, this first molar sometimes leans forward into such a cavity enough to lose its proper position and its antagonism with the lower molar.

If, as in the illustration, the last temporary molar is lost, and the first molar is also decayed on its posterior approximal surface.

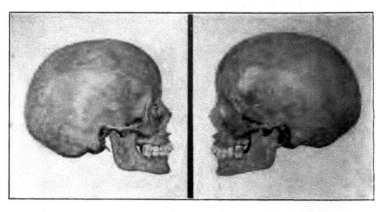

Fɪɢ. 6 is a case of mal-articula-tion on the right side of the mouth, temporary teeth.

Fɪɢ. 7 shows correct articulation on the left side, temporary teeth. Same mouth.

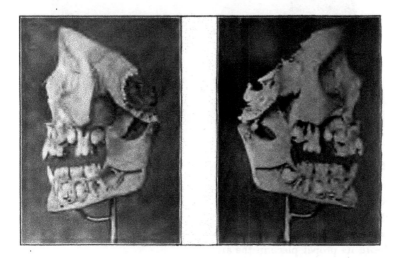

Fɪɢs. 8 and 9 show the loss of a temporary molar at such a stage of development that the permanent molars adjoining will inevitably tip forward to occupy the spaces left by the lost temporary molars, and so will destroy the normal articulation with the lower molars.

the tendency of the incoming first permanent molar is to occupy both vacancies and to come forward the full width of a tooth or more.

Not only will it come forward, but in coming forward it advances on the lines of the arch of the jaw, and the further forward it comes the narrower becomes the space between it and its opposite molar on the same jaw.

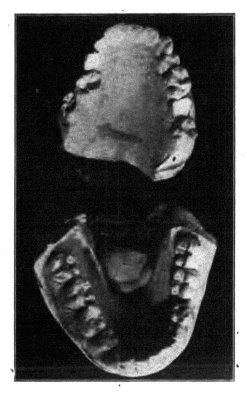

Fig. 10.—This illustration shows on the right side, above a second permanent molar that has come forward until it touches the cuspid.

It is plain to see that extraction has not "made room" here, but has greatly diminished the arch.

These principal molars occupy in the adult normal jaw the middle of the arch from before backward between the cuspid and the wisdom tooth.

As they are in a sense the keystones of these antero-posterior arches they become, upon their eruption, the keys to the situation, for if these four keystones or pillars to the dental arches are *normally* arranged at the period of their development they support the jaws during the shedding of the temporary teeth and their replacement by the permanent ones, and we are almost certain that all the other molars posterior to these will be correctly arranged. It is also almost certain that the teeth anterior to these keystones

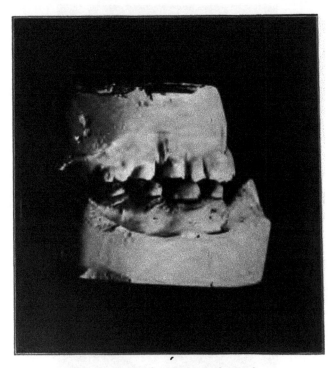

Fig. 11 shows the same mouth closed.

with whose development and proper placing in their alveoli we have to deal may be easily inducted into their places, should they erupt irregularly, practically without pain, and therefore without detriment to the well being of the child, whose growth is not thereby inhibited, and whose usual avocations are but slightly interfered with.

These permanent molars, then (let us suppose a case of upper teeth), which have been deflected from their normal positions, occupy a certain amount of room (space) anterior to what they should, and consequently they crowd out of place the other permanent teeth anterior to the molars, either by a narrowing of the arch and a protrusion of the incisors, or a bunching of the bicuspids or both.

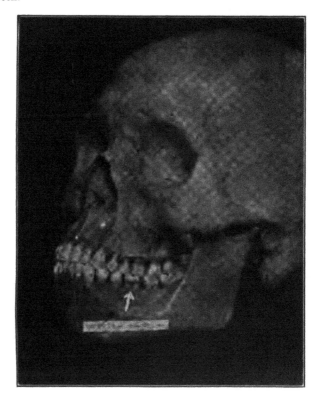

Fig. 12 shows a skull belonging to Dr. Summa of St. Louis, that exhibits, see arrow head, the first molar occupying the centre of the arch from the cuspid to wisdom tooth.

For it must be remembered that the teeth of any given individual are adapted to the size of that individual's jaws and alveolus. (There is no such thing as large teeth in small jaws and alveoli, for the alveolus is formed upon the jaws after the crowns of the teeth are complete, and it forms around the roots of those teeth that are themselves in process of formation.)

But there is still further mischief caused by the decay of these temporary teeth.

The development or displacement of even one permanent molar further forward on the arch than it should be, therefore narrowing the arch, confines and cramps to a considerable extent all those contiguous bones that are in process of development at just this period, and obstructs their growth; so that unless aid is rendered and the

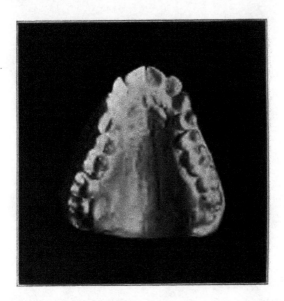

Fig. 18 shows the narrowing ot the arch and a slight protrusion of the incisors. By courtesy of Dr. Ainsworth, Boston.

mechanical obstruction is removed, the face never gets its full development, the vault of the palate is more or less deformed, there is not room for the tongue, still less for the free use of it, nor for vocal resonance, which fails unless there is ample room and a broad and well-formed palatine arch; nor for full and free inspiration, owing to a diminished nasal meatus, so that often we find mouth breathing supervening upon the loss of certain of the baby teeth and the development of the permanent molars too far forward in the arch.

It will be perceived, therefore, that if at a very early age we can positively diagnose for impending irregularities of the permanent teeth, it will also be possible in most instances to correct those irregularities, *and without extraction,* during the eruption of the permanent teeth, beginning the operations while the temporary teeth are still among the instruments to be acted upon, broadening the arches and correcting the articulations of the principal molars. If this is done at this early age not only will the growth of the

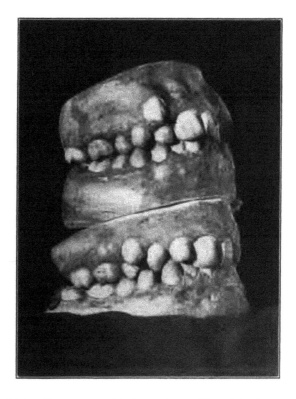

Fig. 13 A.—The upper model shows the cuspids and the lower model the bicuspids crowded out of place by the molar being too far forward.

superior maxillæ and the alveoli be promoted, but the growth of the adjacent bones of the nose, palate, head and face will also be promoted. Instead of narrow or saddle-shaped jaws with deficient nasal passages, obstructed oftentimes by undue and excessive convolution of the turbinated bones and by recurring lymphoid growths, which growths are promoted by the contracted regions in which they lie, we shall have a resumption of growth in the maxillæ, palate bones and nasal bones, and probably as well in the ethmoid and sphenoid bones. The nasal septum will be straightened considerably by broadening the arch of the upper jaw and so lowering it, and as this broadening relieves the pressure and tends to straighten the septum so proper nutrition is encouraged and Nature is allowed to exert her influence toward a development of all the sinuses, which become freer and more nearly normal.

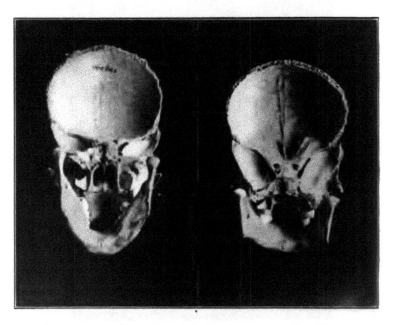

FIG. 14 shows the relation of the nasal meatuses to the adjacent bones, and how the enlargement of the superior dental arch must inevitably have an influence upon them, and tend to promote their growth.

As this gives better respiration, the lungs themselves become enlarged, the strength of the patient increased, and the dignity of expression, which comes with distinct speech, good articulation and resonance of voice follows as a matter of course.

I will try to exhibit a few specimens of these results as I close.

I am aware of the objections raised to these views, especially on the part of those who say that having been brought up to extract teeth, both for children and adults for the correction of certain irregularities, they cannot see why patients should be allowed to seem " all teeth" when the extraction of a few of the seemingly superabundant ones would so easily correct the difficulty. It is evident that those who make this claim cannot have considered with sufficient care the processes of growth and the results of a little easily obtained expansion in the regions under discussion.

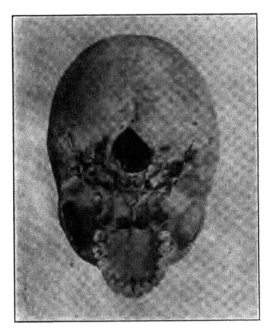

FIG. 14A is a photograph of a skull in the museum of the Harvard Medical College at Boston, showing the entire right side of the skull, including the dental arch, the nasal meatus, and even the foramen magnum out of proportion to, and smaller than the left side, yet to a casual observer the nasal meatuses and the dental arch seem normal.

At birth the ethmoid bone is small, very incomplete, and imperfectly ossified. The hard palate at the height of the arch is above the eustachian tube. In the adult the hard palate is below this tube, consequently, as Dr. Swain, Professor of Otology and

Laryngology, Yale University, has correctly observed in one of his papers, "the palate has grown away from the base of the skull. What has accomplished this? It has been the downward growth of the superior maxillary bone, the septum and the pterygoid processes of the sphenoid, so that in a certain sense of the word the palate of a young child is supposed to grow down instead of up. It is safe to assume, therefore, that this downward growth is an extremely important process in our present consideration, and it may be looked upon as a part of the normal growth of the superior maxillary bone."

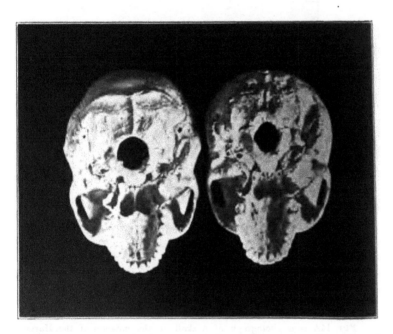

Fig. 14B are Dr. Hawley's two skulls, showing two apparently good arches having good contact, yet, the nasal meatuses of the narrower arch are as much too small, as the arch is too narrow, while with the wider normal arch the meatuses are ample.

Now it happens that the sutures of most of the bones of the head and face do not solidify until adult life, some of them not until middle life; they are, therefore, during all this time subject to change, and if expansion of irregular dental arches is accomplished previous to solidification, it is almost always the case that, stimulated by the removal of undue repression of the parts seeking development, renewal of growth will take place, and one or two

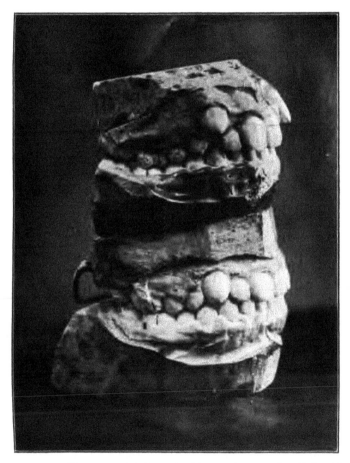

Fig. 15.—The top model shown in Fig. 15 is that of a little girl ot 12 years.
The lower model is the same mouth 18 months later.

years is quite sufficient time for the changes of such growth to produce a nobler countenance out of a most unpromising one.

These changes can be best noticed by photographs taken before and after the operations, by models of the teeth made at the same time as the photographs, and if the operator so wills by plaster casts of the face, which are easily made, and are unimpeachable witnesses as to what occurs.

I have been working along these lines for about five years, aiming to correct irregularities in the positions of the teeth as early as I could get control of them, and that is often from the fifth to the seventh year, the very climacteric in the child's life, when growth begins to manifest itself most strenuously. The results not only in my own hands, but in those of my son, and one of

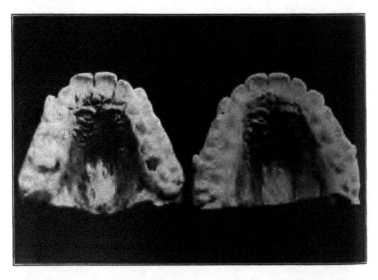

Figs. 16 and 17.—Shows the upper half of the same models, from the occlusal sides.

my former pupils, Dr. Kelsey, of Baltimore, and in a few cases in the hands of other practitioners, have gone far to convince me of the soundness of my position not only, but of the soundness of the hypothesis upon which I have worked.

I find by an examination of many hundreds of aboriginal skulls in the development of which Nature has been free to work her will without the assistance of man, and where the so-called accidents

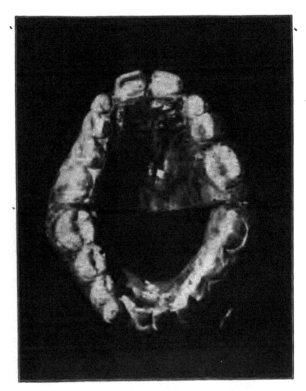

Fig 18.—John M., 8 years old, open. April 19, 1900.

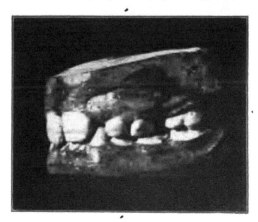

Fig. 19.—John M., Same model closed.

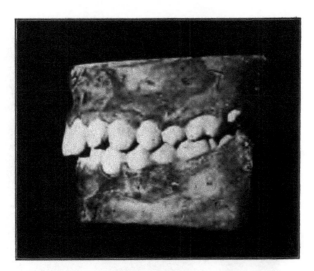

Fig. 20.—Same model John M., May 1902.

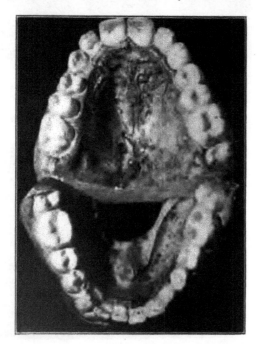

Fig. 21.—Same model open. John M., May 1902.

of development occurred as they do with us civilized races, though probably not with the same frequency, that in all those cases where irregularities in the development and positions of the upper teeth exist there are also irregularities, more or less strongly marked in the development of the maxillæ and the palate bones, and seemingly in the vomer, the sphenoid and ethmoid as well, and that the nasal septum particularly is sure to be crooked and the turbinated bones

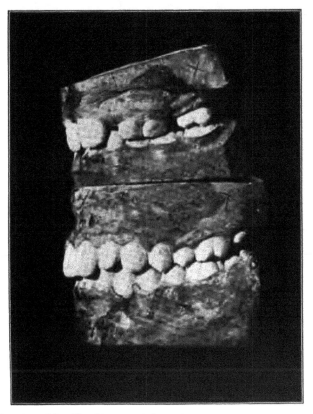

Fig. 22.—John M., Upper model, April 1900.
Lower model, May 1902.

so excessively curved as to materially interfere with the proper openings of the nasal meatus. And when I say irregularities of the upper teeth, I am not forgetting that the upper jaw with its teeth is dependent upon the lower for correctness of position.

Per contra, by just so much as the permanent teeth are

regular in their development, and are regularly placed in their arches, all the sinuses of the maxillæ and facial bones are better developed, the nasal septum becomes straighter, the turbinated bones less obstructive, the sphenoid and ethmoid larger proportion-

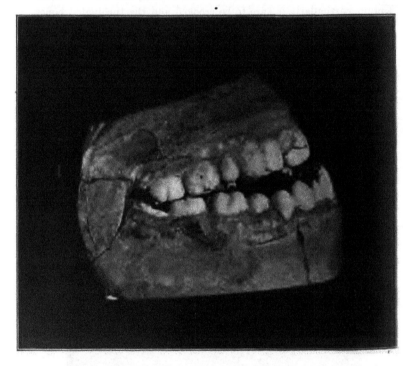

FIG. 23.

ately to the size of the skull, and the facial bones occupy positions that add the dignity of strength to the individual.

Illustration: John M., 8 years old; began May 6, 1900. Last illustration made May, 1902. Fixtures remained on for two years from the time they were placed. Actual time occupied in moving the various irregularly placed teeth into their present positions, sixty days interspersed in different periods during those two years. Absolutely no pain.

Adenoids have been removed in this case prior to the enlargement of the arch. No recurrence of that tissue. Face and nose both show the enlargement and the teeth retain their normal positions, breathing normal, general development rapid.

Applications of apparatus for regulating have been irregular,—on and off almost at the will of the patient,—but the last illustra-

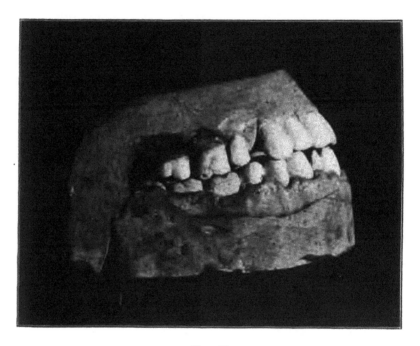

Fig. 24.

tion shows the stage which the boy had reached when 14 years of age, at which time he had nearly lost his stooping shoulders, entirely quit mouth breathing, strengthened and developed in a remarkable degree, and, I am told, is now willing to wear an apparatus continually. No thought of improving his breathing or his general health was entertained when the enlargement of the arch was undertaken.

Do not understand that the single phase that I have to-day presented is any more than one phase in conditions that have taxed

the intelligence and the patience of both rhinologists and dentists
to the last degree, but if my confreres may be helped over some few
of their perplexities by a recognition of their causes and a prompt
and early application of the simple mechanical apparatus necessary
to correct these deformities, I shall be very glad to have been the
instrument through which such a presentation has been made.

Four days after mailing this essay to your committee, I noticed
in the *Dental Cosmos* for May, 1905, a paper by Hofzahnartz W.
Pfaff, of Dresden, Germany, entitled "Stenosis of the Nasal Cavity,
Caused by the Contraction of the Palate and Abnormal Position of

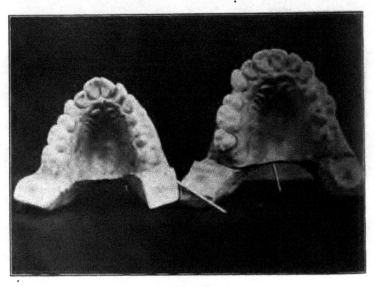

FIG. 25.

FIG. 23. Models taken from young man, 25 years of age.   Patient of Dr.
Kelsey, Baltimore.   Fixtures placed May, 1904.

FIG. 24. Same mouth May, 1905.

FIG. 25. Same mouth before treatment and after.   The two upper arches
side by side for comparison.

Upon asking the patient whether he could breathe any better than before
the operation, his reply was: "Breathe! I never could breathe before; but
now I breathe with perfect ease."

the Teeth; Treatment by Expansion of the Maxilla," that had been
read at the St. Louis Congress while I was ill in the hospital, and
is along almost precisely the same lines as my paper.

I take pleasure in calling your attention to this paper as strongly confirming the views just presented for your consideration.

As the two papers were the results of two persons, the one in Germany, the other in America, working unknown to each other on the same subject, the results are worthy of note.

And while both papers are far from being exhaustive, they at least indicate a subject for further investigation.

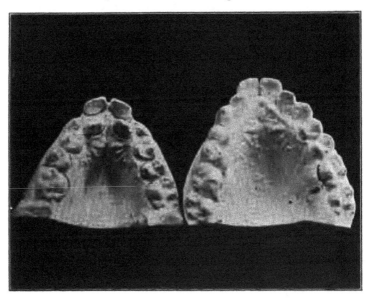

FIGS. 26 and 27.

FIG. 26 and 27. Patient of Dr. J. G. Palmer, New York. Boy 10 years of age—a stooping, round shouldered, mouth breathing, delicate boy, whose very walk betokens his feebleness.

A CONSIDERATION OF THE OCCLUSAL BALANCE.[1]

BY LAWRENCE W. BAKER, BOSTON, MASS.

ORTHODONTIA is a science broad and interesting. The illustrations which I wish to show you have been selected and arranged to prove the truth of this statement. The subject is so broad that I can only bring out a few fundamental principles on which the science is based; but by exhibiting the results which I have obtained by working on these principles I hope to hold your attention this evening.

In dealing with the subject I shall depend largely upon the stereopticon; in fact the paper will consist principally in the description of slides which have been selected, grouped, and arranged to bring out a few fundamental principles underlying this work.

The first group of illustrations deals with the application of force and Fig. 1 shows the old well-known expansion arch appliance in its simplest form adjusted to a typical case for treatment.

The true progress of orthodontia,—and this is one of the very few unqualified statements I shall make this evening.—depends upon this appliance and its modifications. The single fact that it is the only appliance in which the necessary forces are reduced to their lowest terms is sufficient proof of the truth of the statement.

The appliance as we see it represents the results of centuries of work in simplifying. Even as far back as Fauchard's time these same principles were well-known and practiced. Each true step in advance from that time to this was a more direct and simple method in the application of force, until the appliance now has reached perfection. The appliance is perfect because, as I say, the forces are reduced to their lowest terms; that is, to three distinct and positive forces: the spring of the arch-wire, the ligature force, and the screw force. All these act and react in harmony upon the arch through the anchorage and arch-wire. These three primary forces can be applied in many combinations; in fact, they are capable of as wonderful and innumerable combinations as those of the ever-changing kaleidoscope.

---

[1] Read before the New York Institute of Stomatology, Nov. 4, 1905.

FIG. 1.

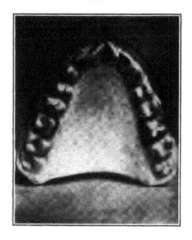

FIG. 2.

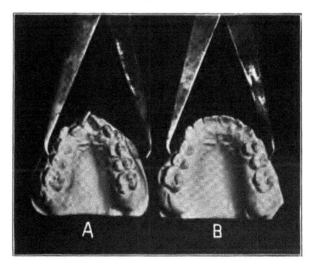

FIG. 3.

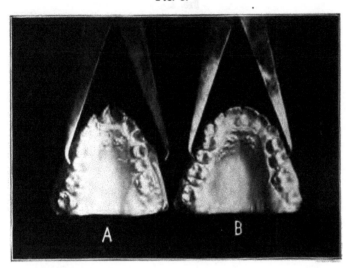

FIG. 4.

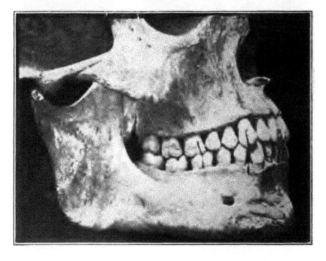

FIG. 5.

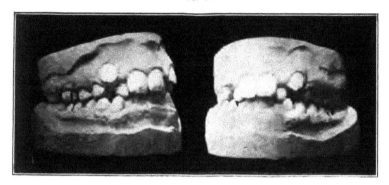

FIG. 6.

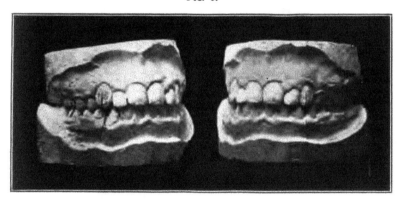

FIG 7.

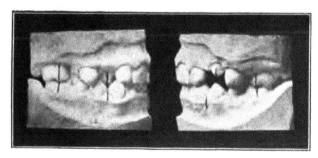

FIG. 8.

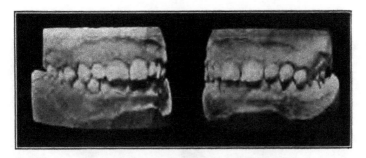

FIG. 9.

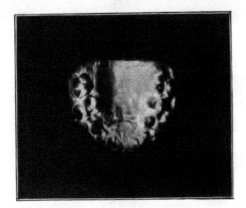

FIG. 10.

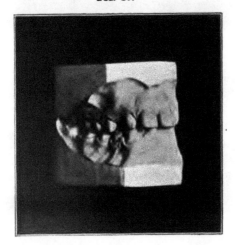

Fig. 11.

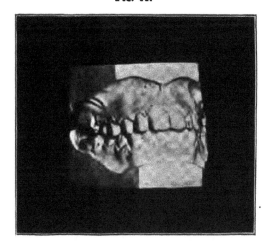

Fig. 12.

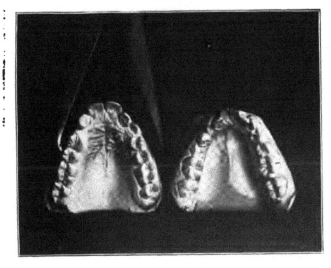

Fɪɢ. 13.

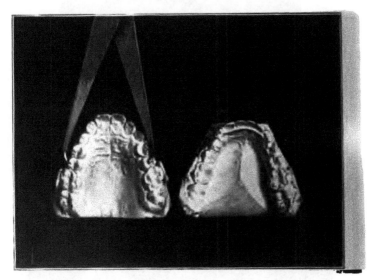

FIG. 14.

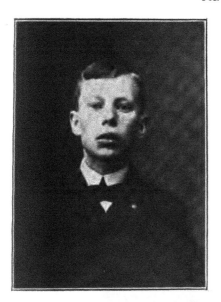
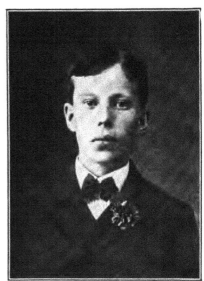
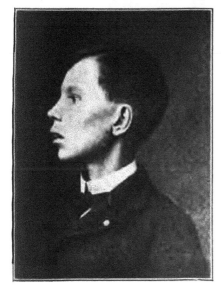
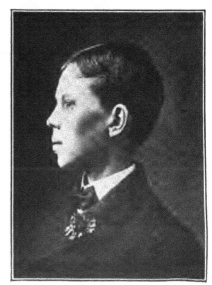

FIG. 15.

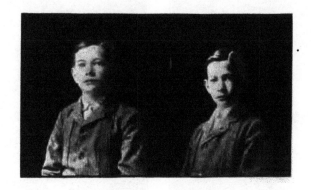

FIG. 16.

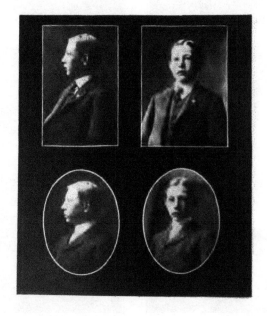

Fig. 17.

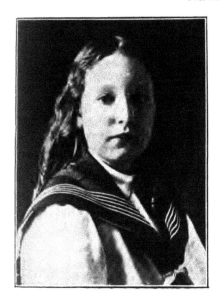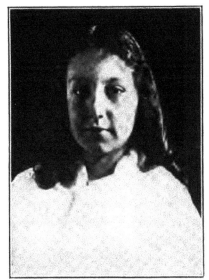

Fig. 18.

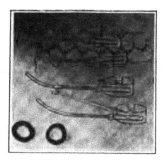

Fig. 19.

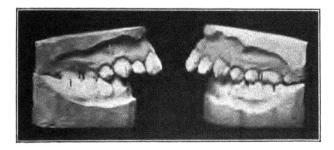

Fig. 20.

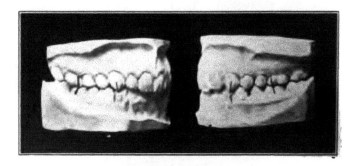

FIG 21.

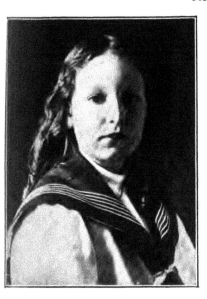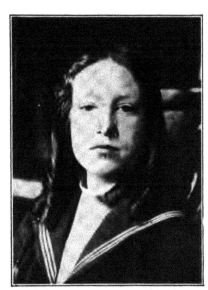

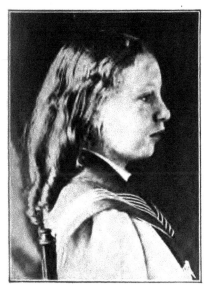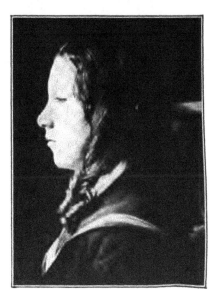

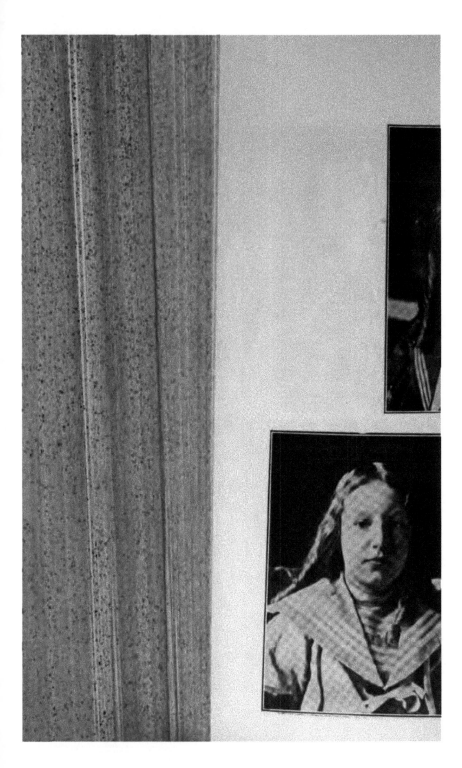

FIG. 26.

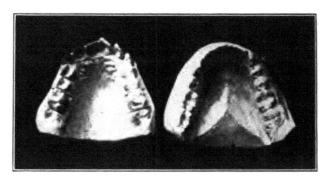

FIG. 27.

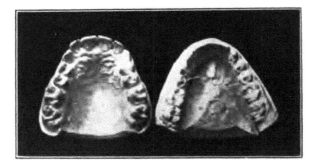

FIG. 28.

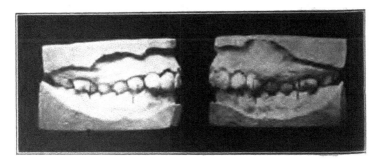

FIG. 29.

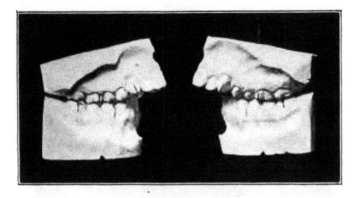

FIG. 30.

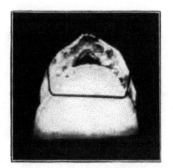

FIG. 31.

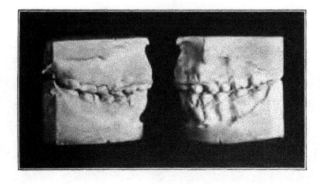

Fig. 32.

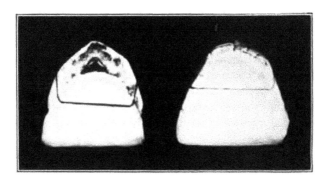

Fig. 33.

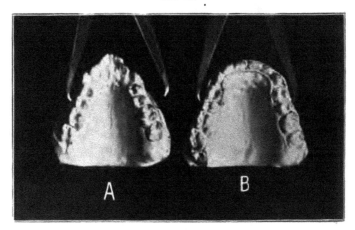

Fig. 34.

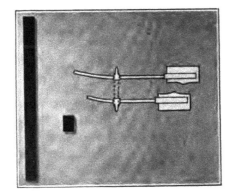

Now let us consider one or two typical examples of tooth movement accomplished with this appliance.

Fig. 2 shows a case that is a severe test for this or any appliance, a badly contracted, pinched, and distorted arch caused by adenoids and mouth breathing. Fig. 2b shows the result of the work of this appliance in its simplest form. Note the measured expansion and general enlargement of the arch, allowing room for the partially erupted cuspids to be brought into place; note also the rotation of the incisors.

Fig. 3a is another example of a condition where the tongue was noticeably cramped; Fig. 3b shows a new arch, chiselled out, we might say, by the appliance. Again note the expansion as shown by the calipers. As the arch was expanded the alveolar process followed the teeth, building in the new bony vault. So you see the law that the alveolar process is subservient to the positions and uses of the teeth is as true of applied forces as of natural forces.

The next illustration (Fig. 4) shows normal occlusion. It is the model from which I work and it is regarded as the model by all who consider orthodontia a true science. A wonderful piece of nature's work it is, wonderful from the standpoint of art and proportion, from the standpoint of hygiene and utility. However, it is not for these reasons that I spent an entire Sunday morning in obtaining this negative. The reason why I want you to see every visible line, curve, and contour is this: when the teeth are in their normal positions they are in their most retentive state, in their most retentive positions; they are in a state of equilibrium, occlusal equilibrium. There is an exact correlation of the occlusal forces which can be produced in no other conceivable arrangement of the occlusal planes. It is for this simple reason that true orthodontists consider normal occlusion their model. Without stopping to consider the law of this balance,— how and why each and every cusp is so shaped and arranged, how the muscular pressure of the lips and tongue aids in maintaining it,—I shall deduce one simple rule, a rule with few exceptions: A corrected case of orthodontia is a success in proportion to the approach or establishment of the occlusal balance.

From Fig. 4 it is also possible to see the classification which has been made by Dr. Edward H. Angle and which is perhaps the greatest step that has been taken towards placing orthodontia among the true sciences. Using normal occlusion as a working basis, with the first permanent molars as the primary landmarks, Dr. Angle has given us a most adequate classification of the various forms of malocclusion. It is the classification that I have adopted in the grouping of the cases that I am about to show you. No doubt you are all familiar with it, so I shall not consider it minutely. Roughly it is this: Class 1. Irregularities in which the first permanent molars are normal mesio-distally. Class II. Irregularities in which there is a distal displacement of one or both the lower first molars. Class III. Irregularities in which there is a mesial displacement of one or both lower landmarks. With this introduction we will now consider the cases.

Case I, Fig. 5, shows a very ordinary type of the first group. It belongs to this group because of the normal position of the molar landmarks. The antro-buccal cusp of the lower first molar one plane in advance of the upper ones as indicated by the pencil lines. The eye falls at once upon the tusk-like appearance of the upper cuspids, exaggerated perhaps by the sunken and depressed positions of the laterals. You all know that if this case were left uncorrected, the laterals, from their instanding position, would suffer sadly from dental caries, and the cutting edges would become badly worn.

Fig. 6 shows the result of the attempt at approaching our model normal occlusion. There is a marked improvement in appearance, an increase in utility, and the danger from dental caries is greatly minimized. All these result from the fact that the occlusal balance has been established.

Case II (Fig. 7) belongs in Class I because the molar landmarks are normal; otherwise it differs widely from Case I. It is a much more difficult case than the first, nearly every tooth being in malocclusion. Nature has been so interfered with that her laws of self-cleansing have been entirely overthrown. Look ahead some years and imagine the probable condition.

Fig. 8 shows the result. I am sure the occlusal balance was reached, for after I had done my best the case steadily improved and since the removal of the retainers has kept on improving. Nor was the improvement confined to the occlusion: the facial lines have improved in proportion. A sad fact regarding this case,—and the same is true of the majority of cases,—is that the deformity could have been largely prevented. Fig. 9 shows the cause, the injudicious handling of the temporary teeth. The remains of the deciduous teeth have deflected the incoming permanent teeth until these occlusal planes were forced out of the normal relation; and when once beyond the normal these same forces, instead of working for the balance, work directly against it. The result is an ever-increasing deformity.

Case III. This case is interesting because it illustrates another force of the dental arches that we have not yet considered, the mutual contact force.

Fig. 10 shows the conditions before treatment. The case belongs in the first group, since the molar landmarks on both sides are normal. Note the missing cuspid and its partly obliterated space. Above the space upon the gum is the characteristic swelling indicating the position of this impacted tooth.

The arches were enlarged to make room for the missing member, the space was retained, and the patient was dismissed for the summer. Fig. 11 reveals the condition of affairs when the boy reported for treatment this fall. The cuspid is in place and the lower retainer is doing its work admirably. My plan now is to complete the slight adjusting of the occlusal planes necessary to obtain the perfect occlusal balance.

Now comes the interesting part of the case. Fig. 12 shows the individual views of the arches before treatment. Note in the lower arch the contraction through the anterior region, a corresponding deformity which is nature's way of making up for the missing cuspid in the upper arch. It is a never-failing rule that when one arch is deformed there is invariably a corresponding deformity of the same kind in the opposing arch.

To return to the case. What I especially want to call your attention to is the width of the arch, as shown by the calipers. Compare it with the relative width of the arch after treatment in the next view.

In Fig. 13 this expansion is clearly shown. The enlargement of the arch is not remarkable in itself being about one half the width of a bicuspid; but it was maintained when once established by the natural forces and not by applied forces. The cuspid, wedging it way down into place, held the enlargement, and it was further aided by the lower arch, which, when remodeled, acted normally through occlusion. This case is presented not with the intention of giving you the idea that it is a difficult one, but as an illustration of the reward for assisting nature.

Having considered these three cases, which are fair types of the first group, we will now pass on to the second group, which to me is the most fascinating and interesting of all classes of cases that the orthodontist is called upon to treat. I doubt if within the entire province of dentistry there is a branch which is capable of such gratifying results. These cases are fascinating, interesting, and gratifying simply because of their great benefit to humanity. They benefit humanity more than any class of operations that we as dentists are called upon for treatment.

Not only do these deformities cause the greatest impairment to the functions of the teeth, jaws, and vocal organs, but they cause a most unsightly and distressing facial disfigurement.

The results of these deformities are far reaching: they go deeper than mere facial disfigurements, they penetrate even to the highest nerve centres, and I believe that there is a definite psychological effect produced by the correction of these deformities.

We are now to consider a series of faces illustrating these facts, and I want your opinion as to whether or not there is a psychological change produced in the treatment of these cases. Fig. 14 shows a subject at our clinic at the Harvard Dental School.[2]

The illustration shows a boy fifteen years of age. In the upper left-hand picture the full face is shown before treatment. It is a typical illustration of the expression of a sufferer from distal occlusion in its simplest form. Note the vacant stare. Below is the profile taken at the same time. Again see the weak expression of the mouth caused by the recession of the chin, and exaggerated by the protruding incisors. It was not possible

---

[2] It is through the courtesy of Professor E. H. Smith that I have the pleasure of presenting this particular case to you. I must digress just a moment to say one word regarding this series of photographs. The negatives were not in any way re-touched, the prints were not altered, nor were the patients posed so as to exaggerate either the deformity or the result. The patients were simply instructed to take a natural position.

for the boy to cover these teeth with his lips except by conscious effort.

On the right we see the results of treatment,—a bright, intelligent face. Below is shown a good profile caused by the restoration of the occlusal balance. The result of which is the maximum amount of masticating surface, normal respiration, normal tongue room, normal muscular pressure of lips and tongue; and above all and with all, normal facial expression. Also notice that the boy has spruced up a bit: a flower appears in his buttonhole, his collar and necktie show signs of more tidiness, his hair a little more care in arrangement; in all, a little more self respect. Is this change a coincidence or is it a result?

Figs. 15 and 16 have been lent by Dr. H. L. Howe and fine examples they are of the improvement to the facial lines.

Now, gentlemen, I want to consider with you regarding these faces. I want to get at the truth of the matter. Is there a relation between these disfigurements and the brain, or is this a mere optical illusion produced in the correction of these cases; or is the improvement due to the establishment of normal respiration, or is it due to the general effect of the full power of mastication, or is it the combined results of these factors that give the boy his manly carriage and set-up? In short I want your opinion as to whether or not a psychological change has taken place.

Figs. 16 and 17 are other examples illustrating this same point.

In each and all of these children whose faces we have just considered, not one tooth was lost through neglect, or removed for correction. The laws of occlusion were sacredly regarded, with gratifying results to the facial lines, as we have just seen.

The method used in the treatment of these cases is interesting because it is the final step that placed orthodontia among the true sciences. Like all other great advances, it is so simple that its origin is obscure. It is impossible to say who was the first to use it. However, I am pleased to state that my father, as you all know, was one of the pioneers in introducing this most valuable method. He was the first, as far as I am able to learn, to use it with marked success, the first to obtain the occlusal balance. Because of the far-reaching influence of this method in his hands, it bears the name of Baker anchorage. We must not, however, forget that Dr. Case of Chicago worked along the same lines as my father, although each was entirely independent of the other.

Fig. 18 is a diagram, original with Dr. Angle, illustrating the underlying principles of the Baker anchorage which is called by some the intermaxillary elastics. In the upper figure we see the appearance of the two arches in distal occlusion, with the appliances in position. When the lower arch is in distal occlusion, you remember it occludes one occlusal plane back of its normal place, as is clearly seen here. In the figure below, the elastic, indicated by the dotted line, is looped over the distal end of the tube of the lower anchor band, passed forward and engages in the hook on the upper arch wire. At one side are the elastics which are especially prepared for this particular use. You readily see that this is just the necessary force to correct this class of deformity, pulling forward on the lower arch and backward on the upper.

By the skilful handling of this elastic force, in combination with our three primary forces, it is possible to obtain the pleasing facial results that we have already considered, and the occlusal results that we are now to consider.

Case IV, Fig. 19, is the first case of the second group, that in which the Baker anchorage plays such an important part. This case is unmistakably different from the former cases. When we study the occlusal relations, we find that our landmarks are out of their normal position. The lower arch is one plane back of its normal place. It is in distal occlusion. The entire dental apparatus, we might say, is dislocated; the lower jaw is dislocated distally and with it naturally the lower part of the face is distorted, as you have already seen from the photographs.

This dislocation was formerly treated by mutilation. The upper arch was mutilated by extraction, two or more bicuspids being sacrificed to compensate for the malposition of the lower arch. This was before the time of the intermaxillary elastics. But now, by the aid of these elastics, the occlusal balance is made possible.

Fig. 20 shows the result of the use of the Baker anchorage,— the ever-sought occlusal balance.

Sometimes a fear is expressed that the lower jaw will fall back to its old position. It is impossible for this to occur because the upper arch has been remoulded, and widened, and the old position of the lower jaw has been destroyed. If the lower jaw falls back, the cusps will strike point to point. The patient will not tolerate this condition, but will slide the jaw forward into its normal place, where the cusps will interlock.

Figs. 21 and 22 are the photographic record of the results of the occlusal changes upon this child's facial expression.

In Fig. 21 (left) note the decided lack of balance between upper and lower portions of the face. The part above the upper lip is well-proportioned and strong, the lower part is weak and receding. The result is an inharmonious whole.

On the other side we see both views after one month's work. The lower jaw has just been brought forward, producing a great improvement in the facial contour but not so great an improvement in the expression, for there is a more or less set and constrained appearance.

Fig. 22, (lower left view,) which was taken one month later than the preceding, shows that the expression is adapting itself to the facial contour.

The next view taken just eight months after the last one. You see it is a most pleasing expression.

(Fig. 17). The comparison again. The time elapsed between these two pictures is just ten months and eighteen days. During this time the dental arches, we may say, have been remoulded, and the lower jaw rearticulated. The effect of these changes upon the facial expression you can judge for yourselves.

Case V, Fig. 23, shows a new kind of case, distal occlusion on only one side. This deformity Dr. Angle cleverly places as a subdivision of the second group.

This sub-class is considered by all difficult to treat because it is hard to make the arches normal. Each lateral half of each arch is treated differently. The distal side is treated as a simple case of distal occlusion: the normal side, as a case of the first group. In this case as in all others, it was necessary to make sure that the occlusal planes fall within the normal influence and then to allow the case to settle.

Fig. 24 shows the case when it has settled enough so that the distal side will hold in its forward position. It will hold there because the old position into which the boy used to bite has been destroyed. When he now tries to bite back, the cusps strike point to point and he unconsciously slides forward to the present position where the cusps interlock properly. Thus the occlusal balance is secured.

Case VI, Fig. 25, is an unusual case of distal occlusion and one that has aroused much interest because the distal state of the lower arch was self-correcting. It is entirely different from either of the two preceding cases, because the incisors do not protrude, by retrude. Therefore it is classified as a case of distal occlusion with retruding incisors. In Fig. 26 which shows the individual aspect of the two arches before treatment, note that the upper incisors are badly crowded, and that the lower arch is perfectly normal. In Fig. 27 which presents the same views of the corrected casts, see that the upper arch has been corrected and that the lower arch has not been altered. In fact no appliance, elastic or other mechanical force of any description was used during the progress of the case. In Fig. 28 we see that the simple rotation of the superior incisors has allowed the lower jaw to come forward to its intended place. Formerly the lower arch was forced back into its distal position by the malposition of the superior incisors. When this condition was corrected the lower jaw simply slid forward to its proper place.

This case is introduced, not so much for its unusualness but rather because it illustrates an important detail in the use of the elastics. A great many in using this method apply so much elastic force that the anchorage is disturbed. This is not necessary. It is surprising what a slight elastic force will do provided it is intelligently applied. All that is necessary is to make the arches normal, and then to guide the lower jaw forward to the occlusal balance. It is amazing how soon nature appreciates the fact that she is being assisted, and how soon the new position becomes natural.

In the last case which I have to show you this evening, the deformity was great. In order to appreciate the changes that took place, it would be well to refer to the model normal occlusion shown in Fig. 4. It is seen there that the normal position for the cuspids, the secondary landmarks, is one in which the lower cuspid occupies the space between the upper cuspid and the lateral.

Fig. 29 shows the two side views before treatment. The marked deformity is due to a decided displacement of the two arches, principally of the lower. In an ordinary case of distal occlusion the point of the lower cuspid falls one space back of the normal position; in this case this point is one plane back of ordinary distal, or between the two bicuspids. Since in this extreme case the lower jaw recedes not one but two notches, the deformity might be termed double distal.

That the deformity caused a great impairment of the function of mastication, as well as a pronounced facial disfigurement, can be judged from studying this illustration. You may be sure that I must have had great confidence in the possibilities of the intermaxillary elastics, or I should have hesitated at the responsibility of undertaking this case.

When the boy came to me the lower six-year molars were beyond saving. So, at the proper time the bits of roots were removed, allowing the then erupting twelve-year molars to come forward into the spaces of the missing six-year molars.

In Fig. 30 the effects of the extreme distal position of the lower jaw upon its function are here clearly shown. The ten or twelve anterior teeth were made entirely usless for masticating purposes. It was possible to pass the forefinger between the two arches even though they were in close apposition.

In Fig. 31 are seen the two side views after treatment. The upper arch has been made normal, and the lower jaw has been brought forward to its intended position,—one notch, to simple distal, and another notch to normal,—greatly improving the facial contour, as well as increasing the utility of the entire dental apparatus.

In this case a great many would have considered extraction in the upper arch necessary. Probably the removal of two biscuspids would have been resorted to or possibly the entire bicuspid region would have been sacrificed. That is to say, another deformity would have been created equal to the already existing one. I firmly believe that by keeping the upper arch intact and bringing the receding jaw forward not only were the jaws given full power, but the facial lines were placed in much better balance. Instead of weakening the upper part of the face by moulding it to the weak receding lower jaw, the whole face was strengthened by bringing the chin forward to harmonize with the general facial contour.

Now here is another problem for you gentlemen to solve. In producing these changes what has taken place? Study the profile of the two casts. Is this change produced by the reciprocal movement of the teeth? Is it in the body of the jaw, or has there been a change in the temporo-maxillary articulation itself? My opinion is that there is something of all of these possible movements. I am sure that in the correction of these extreme cases,—to which we might almost apply the word " dislocation,"—there is a change produced in the joint itself. This theory is strengthened by the interesting case reported before this society by my father a few years ago which some of you may remember. It was a case of an excessive protruding lower jaw in which the changes that took place were accurately recorded by an indicator. In this case there was a measured movement in the joint of at least three eighths of an inch.

My confidence in this theory was still further strengthened by a most interesting morning spent with Dr. Cryer in his museum. He was decided in his opinion that there is a migration of the condyles in this case, and to confirm his belief he showed me specimen after specimen in which there was a migration of one or both joints. In some specimens the old articulations were completely obliterated; in others the path of the condyle could be definitely traced.

Fig. 32, another comparative view of the deformity, illustrates what we have already seen many times this evening:—first, that with the occlusal balance the jaws and teeth have been brought to their maximum usefulness; second, that this great increase is the very secret of the lower jaw remaining in its new position; and third, that this occlusal balance acts as a perfect and natural retainer.

Fig. 33 shows the palatal aspects of the upper arches before and after treatment. Note the great amount of expansion. The anterior teeth are held by the retaining device indicated; but no mechanical means whatever is employed to hold the extreme amount of expansion. The occlusal balance is the lock and the occlusal balance is the key.

One difficulty connected with the case proved very instructive. It was easy to make the arches normal, it was easy to bring the lower arch forward, but it was not easy to get the proper interlocking of the cusps. They would not settle because, with the lower arch in its extreme forward place, the two arches were moulded on different curves.

Fig. 34 shows the method of overcoming this difficulty. I applied a controllable and reciprocal elastic force between the two arches. I stretched a strong elastic over these spurs on the arch wire. This force, of course, is transmitted to the ligated teeth, and the arches are brought into closer contact. In fact, this is but a natural force,—the settling force,—magnified.

Perhaps the only novel idea about this simple method is the scheme for applying this elastic force,—the spurs fastened to the arch wires. Since it was difficult to get elastics short enough and strong enough for this purpose, I made use of the ordinary rubber wedging strips with suitable holes punched in them. The hole was put over one spur, and then the elastic was stretched to the other. Of course the strength of the elastic can be varied by the thickness of the rubber and the size of the hole. This simple method is introduced because it has since proved invaluable in other cases in obtaining that final and important settlement of the cusps.

Let me close with a few statements regarding the question that is at present agitating our profession,—extracting in orthodontia.

Personally I believe that the extremists of both the old and the new schools agree better than either will admit. Each side sees the situation from such entirely different points of view that to a casual observer they seem to disagree entirely; but, as I say, in reality they agree better than they will admit. As we become familiar with this wonderful appliance, the work of which I have but feebly presented, we find that the cases requiring extraction rapidly diminish in number. When we realize what the occlusal balance is, what its powers are, and how disastrous injudicious extracting is to this great piece of nature's work, we find that the cases requiring extraction are again greatly diminished, until such cases are few and far between.

However, once in a while and only once in a while, we find a case in which all the teeth are present, where extraction seems indicated; but even these cases are decreasing in number as our knowledge of the possibilities of this appliance increases.

Then there are cases in which the arches have been badly

mutilated by the forceps, because of previous neglect. Of all cases these are the hardest and most discouraging to treat. Each of these cases is a puzzle in itself, but no law or rule can be applied to them; they are simply mutilated nature. In these cases, almost any method is admissible: extracting in some cases to balance lost planes, bridge work in others to supply lost planes; and in every case an attempt to establish a balance of some kind and remedy the facial distortion. As Dr. Smith says regarding these mutilated cases: "Obtain the best abnormal occlusion possible."

If I have been the means of causing any of you to look upon the occlusal balance with more respect I consider my efforts well rewarded; for the laws of occlusion are the very basis of the science of orthodontia: occlusion for utility, occlusion for retention, and occlusion for facial balance.

A RESUME OF THE STUDY OF SALIVA.[1]

BY SAMUEL DOSKOW, D.D.S.

MR. PRESIDENT AND GENTLEMEN: In the human economy there are, in connection with the general apparatus for the carrying on of the metabolic process, two systems that play a great part in the proper performance of that process. One, occupied in the formation of substances that do not preexist in the blood, and are employed for the purpose of serving some ulterior purpose in the economy, and which bears the name of *secretion*. To this class belong such substances as saliva, bile, pancreatic juice, etc., etc. The other tends to rid the economy of waste and injurious materials that are called excretions. The constituents of this class are urine, feces, sweat, etc.

Under normal circumstances, *i. e.*, when the food ingested is the proper amount, proper kind, and properly assimilated, both the secretions and excretions will be in proportion as regards both the quantity and composition. But when the normal is not realized, either through some fault on the part of the food or through some impairment of the digestive apparatus, the functions of both the secretory and excretory processes will be interfered with.

---

[1] Read before the Garretson Dental Society, Philadelphia, November 21, 1904.

Hence, if on examinations of the secretions or excretions, they are found to deviate from the normal, the conclusion of the existence of a defect in the metabolism of the economy is a natural corollary.

In a paper read before the Odontographic Society of Chicago, February 16th, 1903, Prof. Edward C. Kirk likens the human economy to that of a furnace; that when there is a lack of proportion between draught and fuel, the energy produced by it will not be the kind nor amount desired for the accomplishment of the work intended by it, also that the products and waste of the combustion from that furnace are good indicators in the hands of the chemist for the determination of its condition.

In the body, the alimentary tract plays the part of the furnace; the fuel is represented in the food ingested ; the draught is furnished by the secretions ; the parts absorbed by the blood represent the energy created; and the waste is found in the excretions.

This analogy falls short in this one respect, that while in the mechanical furnace the furnace itself has no influence over the place of supply of the draught, in the human economy this influence is brought about in an indirect way. For instance, should the food ingested be in some way inimical to the lining of the stomach, the effect will be that the secretions of the pyloric and cardiac glands of that organ will be greatly modified. A like effect may in turn be brought to bear on some of the larger glands. The effect then becomes double; the glands affected will produce a secretion that is not fully capable of performing the function intended, and it in turn further disables the activity of the digestive tract.

The above illustrations give proof to the statement made in the earlier part of this paper that the compositions of the secretions and excretions of the body are determining factors of the metabolic activity of the economy whether it be normal or not.

Having established the proof that the secretions and excretions are reliable means for the determination of the normal or abnormal states of the economy, I shall now devote the rest of my paper to one secretion of the body, although it has not been regarded heretofore of diagnostic value; still from the part it plays, its relation to the general metabolic activity, and especially in view of some researches that have been recently made, I think it is worthy of consideration. This secretion is saliva.

In looking over the history of the subject, we find that the study

of it dates as far back as 1838, when Dr. A. Donné published a
treatise considering saliva as a means for diagnosing certain diseases
of the stomach. He was followed by others, but it was not until
1884 that the first treatise of importance came to light. I refer
to the work of Dr. Binet, entitled "Etude sur la Sueur et la Salive."
He wanted to know what were the substances contained in sweat
and saliva under normal conditions; also the relations existing between them. In 1900, Dr. Joseph P. Michaels, of Paris, presented
before the Third International Dental Congress a large thesis—
Sialo Semeiology—of careful systematic observations made during a
period of six years. He introduced the use of the micro-polariscope
for its examination. The advantage gained by it is that the light
is changed from a ray radiating in all planes to one that radiates
only in one plane as if passing through a grating. By that means
he was able to detect crystalline substances that are not detected
by ordinary light. About this time Prof. Edward C. Kirk, of this
city, took up the study of this subject. He was at once confronted
with the difficulty that the salts were very minute owing to the
colloid substances in the saliva, and that although they presented a
beautiful view for observation from the point of view of the antiqua-
rian they did not present sufficient characteristics for the determination of their exact composition. To overcome this difficulty he
determined to remove the colloid substances from the saliva so that
they should not interfere with the proper crystallization of the salts.
This was accomplished by means of a dialyzer especially constructed
for this purpose. As a result of this, a definite work was done
on the composition of saliva in relation to erosion: "The Clinical
and Chemical Study of a Case of Erosion, March, 1902;" its
diagnostic value: "The Saliva as an Index of Faulty Metabolism,
February, 1903;" its relation to caries: "The Predisposing Factor
in Dental Caries, March, 1903."

Saliva is a mixed fluid that is secreted into the mouth from
various glands situated in the proximity of the oral cavity through
their respective ducts. It assists in articulation and deglutition, and
plays an important rôle in the first stage of digestion. It converts
the starches into sugars; first into dextrin and maltose, later
converting the dextrin into maltose. According to Michaels,
normal saliva should be transparent, clear, bluish in color, possessing neither taste nor odor, neutral in reaction, diastasic, containing sodium chlorides, but no polarizable salts.

Regarding the above as a standard guide we determine that any deviation from it means abnormal saliva. From observations made by Michaels it was found that certain characteristics of the saliva exist under certain metabolic conditions. It was also found that those characteristics are constant under similar diathetic conditions in different individuals. It was further observed by Prof. Kirk that the development of a certain abnormal metabolic condition is in a graded scale beginning with the element most abundant and easier dispensed with, and further, that in the treatment of that condition for the restoration of the economy to the normal the replacement of the elements lost is in the reverse order of the graded scale. This establishes beyond doubt the reliability of the saliva as a means for the determination of the different oscillations in the economy when external relations are not in accord with internal relations in whatever phase it may be manifested.

The disposition of the economy towards the gradual development of abnormal metabolic conditions, thereby lessening its vital resistance to the attack of specific disease, known as diathesis, is subdivided into two distinct heads: That condition in which the oxidation process is over-active, resulting in a decrease of organic acidity with a corresponding increase in saline chlorides excreted by the economy, is known as hypoacidity. This condition renders the body favorable for the development of various contagious diseases, such as scrofula, tuberculosis and syphilis. Fortunately this condition is not prevailing, or else the fate of the civilized races would be in as sorrowful a state as some of the Indian tribes on our borders, who resort to the adoption or acquisition of white children, so that the extinction of their tribes may be thereby prevented. The other diathetic condition is the reverse of the former. It is characterized by an under or suboxidation in the metabolic process; a general slowness in the biochemical changes ; the gradual deposition of acid salts in all the articular tissues, and especially in those most active ; the increase of organic acidity as a consequence. It leads to the development of gout, rheumatism, sclerosis, etc. According to Gautrelet and others, if the amount of waste products distributed through the blood-plasma and its constant increase be taken into account, the blood in this condition should be regarded as decidedly acid in reaction. It approaches senility. Many individuals are found to-day that although young in age are really old as far as their metabolic activity is concerned. This diathesis is termed hyperacidity.

The composition of the saliva under the different diathetic conditions varies with the degree or period of the diathesis. In the hypoacid diathesis, the saliva, according to Michaels, is usually abundant in quantity, opalescent, of fluid consistence, white, insipid, of nauseating odor, actively fermentative, alkaline in reaction and contains crystalline ammoniacal salts. Caries of the teeth is most abundant in this diathesis. Our experience with this kind of saliva is very limited, and I shall therefore leave it and consider more fully the saliva of the hyperacid diathesis.

As stated above, hyperacidity is characteristic by a slowness in the biochemical changes of metabolic activity, resulting in the deposition of the various crystalline salts throughout the course of the blood plasma. The casting off of the various elements from the economy is in a slow, gradual way, beginning with the element most abundant and easier dispensed with. The elements affected, and which are at the basis of the chemical construction of the body, are sodium, calcium, and magnesium. The acids connected with the precipitation of these elements that afterwards are dialyzed through the gladular structures and appear in the saliva are: phosphoric, lactic and oxalic acids. The first installment of salts that gives the indication of the existence of the diathesis in question is the phosphates of sodium, first appearing as neutral phosphates and later as the acid-sodium-phosphate. The appearance of this salt in saliva is noteworthy, inasmuch as we know that this salt in small quantity is a normal constituent of the urine. The presence of a salt that is a normal constituent of the urine has no place in normal saliva. The action of the renal epithelium upon the blood when it reaches the kidneys produces the reaction forming this salt, thereby giving the urine its acid reaction, while the blood remains alkaline in reaction.

$$Na_2HPO_4 + H_2CO_3 = NaH_2PO_4 + NaHCO_3.$$

With the advent of the diathesis, when the supply of sodium has been largely depleted the calcium is affected, and we will first get the combination of sodium and calcium and later pure crystals of the calcium acid phosphate. The condition of the teeth at this stage depends upon whether they were affected by caries prior to the development of this stage. Usually there is an absence of caries, for when the saliva reaches an acidity of this strength the development of bacteria is almost impossible. But should the teeth have been affected by caries prior to the development of this diathesis they will present certain characteristics that in themselves are determining factors. The carious matter assumes a dark brown color, of a semi-hard texture, and when the bur is applied it crumbles away like dried rotten wood. Unlike teeth that are in an acid medium, they are almost devoid of sensation. The destruction of the teeth does not seem to cease with the cessation of the development of caries; on the contrary, destruction proceeds, but from a totally different cause. They are, so to say, dissolved out.

A striking illustration of this kind presented itself at the clinic of the University of Pennsylvania, and upon careful study much valuable information was derived from it. The patient was a young man of about twenty-five years of age. Almost every tooth in his mouth was decayed. The condition of the decay was like that described. On examination of his saliva it was found to contain very large crystals and a large quantity of acid-sodium-phosphate. He showed every condition of approaching old age, and judging from the amount of phosphates in his saliva it was concluded that he was a phosphorous diabetic. He was instructed as regards habit and diet and phosphorus was administered to him in various ways and in varying doses. In a comparatively short time he showed marked signs of improvement. Unfortunately we were not able to follow this case to completion, but we learned from the student who had him in charge for the treatment of the disorders about the teeth, that he was following the instructions as outlined to him in the laboratory and is faring well.

Following up this stage in regular order come the lactates. We first have the lactates of sodium, then of calcium and magnesium. Later come the double lactates of sodium and calcium. Then we have the combination of lactates and phosphates, such as the lacto-phosphates of calcium and lacto-phosphates of magnesium. These crystals are very rich in color when viewed by porlarized light, and possess definite outlines distinct from any family of salts. The action upon the teeth is very marked. It is here that we have that class of erosion that was named by Prof. Kirk as the general erosion in contradistinction to the localized erosion that is caused by the sodium-acid-phosphate from some of the buccal glands. A systematic study of this subject had been presented by Prof. Kirk before the Second District Dental Society of the State of New York in the paper referred to above.

The third stage in the development of this diathesis is the appearance of the oxalates. So far we have only met with the oxalate of sodium. The appearance of this salt is usually a signal of nervous debility, and in many cases complete derangement of the nervous system. There are many cases to which I can refer that were analyzed at the laboratory, diagnosis determined, and for whom valuable aid was rendered towards restoring them to the normal. I shall, however, quote only one case, that I may say was nipped in the bud and which is under my observation almost every day. The case is that of a young man of about twenty-two, who complained that his appetite was not as he thought it should be and that he feels as if something is lacking. Examination was made of his saliva and urine, as is done in every case. It was found that in addition to the few diacid-phosphate crystals he had a large number of the sodium oxalates—thus proving that he was drained of his phosphates to a large extent and that his system was manufacturing oxalic acid and assisting the phosphoric acid in its destructive activity as well as acting as a toxic irritant. A diet was prescribed to him, barring all carbohydrates and such vegetables as help in the formation of oxalic acid. In addition to this he was ordered to drink hot water as many times during the day as he was able to manage and a tonic of phosphorus and arsenic in small doses, in the form of a pill, taken three times a day. He continued taking the tonic for about three months but he is still adhering to his diet. He has since gained in health, his weight has increased and he assured me many times upon questioning him in regard to it that he could not expect to feel better.

The oxalates appear sometimes as double oxalates of sodium and calcium, while the oxalate of magnesia is often found in urine. When this occurs the indications are that the individual is sliding down a steep slope, and unless efforts are made to prevent him from landing in the pit, serious complications will follow.

I acknowledge my indebtedness to Prof. Edward C. Kirk, who first advised me to follow this line of study. His personal instruction and direction in the laboratory helped to inculcate into my mind the comprehension of the vast scope of this work and to what extent mankind in general could be benefited by it; also, that there is a domain in dentistry in addition to that of filling teeth and the making of artificial appliances for the restoration of the lost organs, important as that may be. The study of prophylaxis could not in any way be undertaken or understood, unless the condition of the system is studied in a systematic and scientific manner.

BURNISHED GOLD FILLINGS IN SOFT CEMENT.[1]

BY DR. WALTER I. BRIGHAM, BOSTON, MASS.

In cement we have a valuable tooth filling. It is as compatible a substance for filling teeth as we have. Many times it meets with failure from the ease of its manipulation, so that it has been neglected, and there is trouble also from the improper preparation of a cavity. There is no filling material which we have, that requires more careful preparation of the cavity than cement. I have many times said myself, and I have heard others say, " We speak of the preserving qualities of a porcelain filling ; in reality a porcelain filling has no preserving qualities whatever, unless you consider the cement that is under the porcelain as a part of the porcelain filling. It is the cement that preserves the teeth, and it is made permanent by being covered with porcelain."

Now, in the method that I am trying to explain, we have just these same conditions. We have a lining of a compatible cement made permanent by covering it with gold. This is not original by any means with me. Many men would say that they have used cement, or cement and gold, and I do not doubt but that they have, but I have never seen it demonstrated in just the way I shall try to, unless perhaps at the hands of Dr. Taylor, of Hartford. He is a man of great resources, and I have great confidence in him. Whatever is said or done by him is surely for the best of his patients, and he was the one that encouraged me to try this method.

Now we do not depend upon the cement to hold the filling, as the filling is locked in just as if the cement was not there. In the case of an incisor where we find considerable breaking down of the tissue. We will imagine that we are looking at the mesial surface of an incisor. The preparation of this cavity is not unlike that of any other cavity, only you are not required to have any definite undercuts. In all of these cases our labial wall is the heavy enamel wall. All these cavities should be opened into from the lingual side, because the decay extends lingually more than labially, and with this method it allows us to save a great deal of the labial wall which we might otherwise have to cut off.

Now, in my method of preparation, I always carry the cervical

---

[1] Read before the Academy of Dental Science, January 4, 1905.

line across nearly straight, because it takes off the vulnerable point at the lingual angle where decay is liable to commence, because if you pack gold from the lingual surface as you should, you have no chances against that wall if curved ; if you carry it across straight, you have a chance to pack it against that wall instead of sliding it along. In the preparation of this cavity, we will remove all the decay and the cavity will be retentive. We have, perhaps, a little bit of a recess at cervical border and a little at incisal angle. The cavity, of course, is thoroughly dried out and we have left all of the labial wall that we can. Now by filling that partly full of cement, which is mixed up quite thin, we will attempt to fill it with gold.

In my burnishing method I always use a foil. The gold that I use is No. 4 foil, and it is folded until it is twenty-four thicknesses ; taking half of a sheet of gold and folding it until it is twenty-four thicknesses, it would be practically 96 foil. I generally fold it upon a piece of chamois. I fold one-half sheet so it will be three thicknesses. Fold it in the centre and you have six thicknesses. Fold it again and have twelve. Fold that again and you have your gold of twenty-four thicknesses, and that ought to be about ⅛ of an inch wide, and cut off any lengths you choose.

I feel that the gold with the crystalline surface works the best. It seems to me, to remain softer under the burnisher for a longer time than the other forms of gold. We will carry in one or two small pieces with the pliers, force it back into the cement at the cervical border and force the cement over the border. Take two or three pieces and force it under the incisal angle, forcing the cement over the enamel border. Do that while the cement is soft. We can gradually commence and in a minute anchor the two pieces together. And by this time you have forced the cement over all of the borders. Now you keep packing this gold continuously for a long time without disturbing your cement in the least. Do not break off the cement around the periphery for a long time after you think you ought to. Keep packing and burnishing the gold on little by little. After you think you have got near enough to the periphery with gold, if you will take a burnisher and carry it in from this lingual surface, you will break the surface of cement over the walls, and you will be surprised to see how closely you have forced the gold to the periphery.

I do not know how many of you burnish gold, but I imagine that this method of burnishing gold would work much better on the soft cement than a mallet would, although when the cement is hard, I do not see why you cannot mallet it if you choose. If I can claim any originality, it is the fact of keeping your burnisher blued. That is, you want to burnish with a blued surface. If they get bright, gold will stick to the burnisher, and you cannot burnish it well. Heat the gold burnisher red-hot and allow it to cool off.

The cases that you see are the distal surfaces of cuspids. You know that the labial surface of a cuspid has a very strong, heavy enamel wall, and it is liable to decay from the lingual surface and leave that wall intact. It is strong enough to stay for a long time if in any way you can support it. It is in these cases that gold in soft cement works beautifully. Now in a cuspid we would prepare the cavity just as we speak of in the central incisor of allowing the labial wall to remain in place, and filling it practically all from the lingual surface.

A few moments ago I spoke of the necessity of a thorough preparation for the reception of a cement filling, and I will come back in a minute to that. Now you have all seen many times how the enamel deteriorates from the inner surface after it has been in the presence of decayed dentine, and becomes white and chalky. Dentists remove this debris, thinking they have a surface good enough for cement. Supposing we do not remove this chalky substance from the under side of the enamel and allow it to remain and fill it with cement. The result is that pretty soon the cement wears out until it gets to the inner surface of the enamel, and then there is nothing to prevent moisture from getting between the soft deteriorated enamel and cement, working under your filling and leaving a big decayed place. How many times you have removed a cement filling like this, when it was very hard to cut on the surface, but when you got to the bottom of the cavity, it was soft and easily removed. That was because the moisture worked down from improper preparation of the cavity. But if you will take an instrument and clean this soft surface of the enamel or dentine until thoroughly clean and hard, so that when the cement gets against it, it has a tight union and will last a long while. Now we have just this same condition with a porcelain inlay, if you do not remove the deteriorated enamel and dentine wall. If you had porcelain here, after the cement worked out at the joint nothing would prevent it leaking and softening the cement in a little while. You might have the same condition with the gold in cement, if you allowed the edge of the cement to come to the enamel border.

Now we come to the bicuspids, and we use the same method. We fill in with cement, and by taking a few pieces of gold and putting them under the lingual or palatal border and pressing them back so that they will be under the walls, we can gradually anchor these two together. Sometimes we force the cement up over the cervical border, carrying it up slightly. Now we will remove the excess of cement there, and you have all the chance in the world to burnish on your gold and finish the fillings.

These are the burnishers that I use. They are very simple affairs indeed, but meet nearly all cases. There is a bicuspid that was filled, holding them in my hands and burnishing the gold into the soft cement. Then the tooth was ground off to show the anchorage which we had there. The surface of that gold where it was ground off was not burnished afterwards at all, and it was not consolidated in the least. It shows how homogeneous the filling is.

Here is an incisor that was filled the same way and ground off to show the cement underneath. At the present time I am capable of leaving more cement in a bicuspid filling than there is there. That was made a long time ago, and the cement was forced out to a great extent, and yet you can see the line of cement thoroughly around the filling.

I think it is often of advantage to use the matrix. It is a simple matter to burnish gold into a bicuspid with the matrix in place. All that you want to do is to keep that part of the gold which is next to the tooth a little bit higher than that which is next to the matrix.

I have no patience with the ruthless cutting away of a tooth substance for prevention of decay. I do believe in it to a conservative extent, but I doubt if there are many here who realize how it is done in the West. I saw there a cavity in a bicuspid that had never broken through to the occlusal surface that took six or seven sheets of gold to fill when they had it cut away. Perfectly ridiculous! They may say that it is necessary to do that to preserve the teeth, but we know it is not. Here in my method we have a cavity-filling that must hermetically seal because we have a soft, plastic substance next to the tooth surface. I believe in cutting these walls away so that they can be kept clean and contoured to hold the teeth in place, and I know of no way that you can get a contour in gold so well as burnishing it.

Dr. Wedelstædt, of St. Paul, is one of those heroic cutters with whom I have no patience whatever. He is a man who says that lots of times he has taken out fillings that other men have put in that were doing good service simply to have a gold filling there. I could put it in terms a good deal severer than I have. I ran up against him in St. Louis, and I have no respect for that method at all. He says he found that the cement had deteriorated. But what caused him to remove the filling. Cement will last under amalgam or gold indefinitely. A year ago I was called upon to fill the lower second molar mesial surface with amalgam in a tooth that I had filled seventeen years before with amalgam. There was no decay there. The filling had anchored back into the crown and broken off. I filled it again, but the cement after seventeen years was just as I left it.

The method is just the same in the crowns of molars, filling them up with cement and putting in your pieces of gold and forcing it over the walls. Of course the proximal cavities in the molars are practically the same as in the bicuspids. Now in a straight pit fissure where I wanted to put in gold, I would simply fill it with cement, and then take a few pieces of gold and pack them down into the centre of this, forcing the cement up over the walls, and we would have a great supply forced up over. As we force this down continually by forcing it into the centre, that would have the tendency to force the gold out a little bit so that it would be anchored in the cement. By cleaning off the surface we have the gold carried over the walls, and we have it anchored with just a simple layer of gold which permanently fills it. This is an ideal way for filling on the lingual surface of incisors where you have been obliged to remove the pulp.

Dr. Payne.—You generally wait until the cement is hard before you begin burnishing your original pieces?

Dr. Brigham.—Once in a while I have waited, but generally with light pressure and then with harder pressure it will harden so that you can go right along with the work.

In doing burnishing it is better to keep the instrument warm, and the heat of the instrument would have a tendency to hasten the hardening of the cement, so that you seldom wait for that.

Dr. Payne.—Isn't the cohesive property of the gold destroyed by the free liquid of the cement?

Dr. Brigham.—It seems generally to work admirably, but if the cement does act on the gold the least bit, it can be pushed off and the cohesion takes place just the same.

I burnish with both the ends and the sides of instruments, but ordinarily on the sides. In burnishing with gold, it is advisable not to cover too much of the gold with the burnisher. Where I do not go along flat with my burnisher, I do not cover so much gold, but I get a perfect adaptation. This is of great advantage in many smaller cavities in incisors where it would take heroic cutting away to get lines of margins which would be out of the zone of decay, but with this you have it as perfect as the tooth was in the first place, and you can fill this so that it will last beautifully.

Take a case of a lateral incisor that may have a great deal of lost tissue on the lingual surface, and it may be at the cervical border not a very deep cavity, but towards the incisal edge there will be a great loss of tissue, and with an overhanging enamel border. Now if this cavity were shallow, I would simply have my undercuts filled until I got down to the centre of the cavity, and put a little soft cement under this labial wall and pack gold in there, and we have strengthened that wall and used it for a retention of that filling.

Now I have described in the best way that I could other than by demonstrating it in the mouth, the way that I would insert gold fillings in soft cement. Now what are its advantages? You do not have to make any definite retention or definite undercuts. You can save walls which you otherwise could not. Burnishing gold on the cement allows you to work on walls that you would not think of working on with a mallet. You have facilitated matters. You have made it easier for your patient. In the burnishing of the gold, you can work with much less room than you can with a mallet. It is seldom that I am called on to spread teeth unless in cases where a great deal of tissue has been lost and the teeth have fallen together.

The ease to the patient is a very important factor. Another thing, you have your cavity lined with a non-conducting material and one of the most compatible materials we have.

Dr. Payne.—Some ten or twelve years ago Dr. Clapp brought

to the attention of the Academy the method of inserting gold fillings, using soft cement at the base of the cavities ; and showed us a large gold filling which he had placed in a central incisor, without undercutting, using the cement for retention. It required considerable force to remove it, more than would be exerted upon it in the mouth.

During the past few years I have used this method almost exclusively. I find it unnecessary to make undercuts in most cases, never in cavities that have four walls.

The cavity is filled about one-half full of sticky cement, being careful not to smear the edges, and DeTrey's gold is worked into the soft cement and then finished with any gold the operator chooses.

You will notice that the preparation of gold called DeTrey's has one surface very porous. That side is placed upon the soft cement, and the cement will work through or into the gold, giving a very strong adhesion. Weston's cement is used, as it is very sticky and sets quickly.

Large pluggers must be used at first, and when the cement commences to harden finer points can be used for condensing.

It has been of the greatest help to me and saves fully one-third of my time in that branch of my work.

The essayist spoke of heating his burnishers red-hot. I should consider an instrument unfit for use that had been so heated a number of times.

Dr. Brigham.—Dr. Payne illustrated his method of gold in cement. Now mine is unlike his. I think I like mine better. He depends upon the adhesiveness of his cement to hold his gold. If you will notice that bicuspid, all the powers that be cannot disturb it, yet it was lined with cement. Now by Dr. Payne's method the gold is held like porcelain fillings, which rely upon the adhesiveness of the cement. Now we do put in a good many porcelain fillings without any retention and they will last, but others will not, and I do not know why some will and some will not. But in the method that I tried to describe we force the gold in the cement and the gold is packed under the undercut.

Dr. Payne spoke of the heating of the burnishers. There is no temper in the burnishers and there was never intended to be, and it is not necessary. When I break one, I step into the laboratory and make another.

I do not know that I have anything else to say, only I feel that I have not done the subject justice. If any of you have a day off, the latchstring of my office is always out, and I should like to demonstrate it in the mouth to show how easily and beautifully it works. I have given several clinics upon this subject, and perhaps some of you may see me some time again.

ANKYLOSTOMIASIS OR UNCINARIASIS.[1]

T. M. RUSSELL LEONARD, L.R.C.P., L.R.C.S.(ED.), GRENADA, BRITISH WEST INDIES.

THIS disease, an endemic anæmia caused by the parasite, *Ankylostoma duodenale* or *Uncinaria duodenalis* and *Uncinaria americana* (Stiles), is a dangerous one both to the individual and to the community in general, leading as it does in individual cases to degeneration of important organs, resulting probably in death and to widespread infection and deterioration among the community in general.

The parasite is now too well known to need a full description; in Grenada, B. W. I., the large majority of cases show the old world parasite,—viz., *A. duodenale,* but in many cases I have come across the variety described and named by Stiles, *Ankylostoma* or *Uncinaria americana,* the new world variety. The chief differences between these two species lie in the size and the armature of the mouth, the *Ankylostoma duodenale* being larger, with a heavily armed mouth,—viz., two pairs of hook-like ventral teeth and one pair of dorsal,—the *Uncinaria americana* being smaller, with two pairs of ventral plates or lips and one dorsal pair (Stiles). Microscopically, the worms appear as short threads white or gray in color, according to the contents of the genital organs; usually I have found that the white are males and the gray colored ones females with ova; I have only occasionally seen them blood-red.

---

[1] Read in the Section on Stomatology of the American Medical Association, at the fifty-sixth annual session, July, 1905, and republished with request of the Section, through the courtesy of the Journal of the American Medical Association.

DEVELOPMENT.

The ova develop in earth under favorable conditions of humidity, temperature, and shade. I have found that a certain proportion of water is necessary. In undiluted fæces the larvæ appear but soon die; in fæces diluted with much water, in a few cases of mine the larvæ appeared, but did not live; but in the majority the ova did not develop. The ova developed at the ordinary temperature in this island,—viz., 80° to 90° F.,—but the larvæ are killed and the ova prevented from developing when placed in ice. Direct exposure to the sunlight killed the larvæ when these had developed, and also prevented the ova from developing, so that a certain amount of shade is required for the development of the larvæ from the ova. Each ovum only produces a single larva, and this never takes place within the host, but outside, so that an increase of adult worms in any particular case is impossible without reinfection from without; this point is therefore of great importance both in the treatment and in the prevention of this disease.

MODES OF INFECTION.

Two methods of infection are possible: 1. By the ingestion of the larvæ in the food or water. 2. By penetration through the skin and subsequent migration to the intestine, where the embryos mature into the adult worms.

In Grenada the class found to be chiefly affected with the disease are the laborers and agriculturists, consisting chiefly of negroes, East Indians, and poor whites. The huts occupied by them are small, raised a few feet off the ground in most cases, entirely surrounded with vegetation almost up to the walls, in this island being chiefly bananas and cocoa and other trees planted to protect the growing cocoa. Sanitation is unknown among them, and latrines are never used, the fæces being deposited on the earth among the trees, so that in time the soil around these huts and also in the fields where they work becomes heavily infected. During the rains the mobile larvæ, also ova, are washed down into the pools, shallow wells, and streams, and as most of the villages depend on such for their drinking water, it can be readily understood that infection in this manner—viz., by ingestion—can take place; helped to a very great extent by the dirty habits of the people, such as eating with soil-stained hands, improperly washed vegetables and fruit, and, as above stated, drinking water infected with the larvæ and contained a large quantity of earthy matter in suspension. I am of opinion that in this island at any rate this method of infection takes place, as the drinking-water contains to my knowledge both the living larvæ and earthy matter in suspension, so that although many observers have remarked, and I have proved to myself, that the embryos die on drying and that the earth taken in must be moist, yet in the above condition we have both earth and moisture. True geophagy is not practised to any extent in this island, chiefly among children, so that a few cases may be set down as due to this method of infection.

The second method of infection—viz., penetration of the skin by the larvæ—is without any doubt the true one, as proved by the experiments of Looss and others. In every case treated by me I have elicited the fact that the patient has suffered from a form of dermatitis known in this island as "chauffie" or "ground-itch" prior to his anæmia, the period ranging from three months to a year or two, and in advanced cases they have had attacks every year, especially during the rains. I have had ten cases of this dermatitis under treatment in the hospital, and the following were the chief characteristics: in cases of recent infection scattered vesicles were seen, many of which broke down, leaving small ulcers, usually affecting the lateral side of the feet and the urb of the toes; in older cases the ulceration was more extensive, deep cup-shaped ulcers being seen on the dorsum and lateral parts of the foot and between the toes. Some of these cases resisted treatment for some time, although in the early cases they healed quickly. These cases remained under treatment, and in about three to six months from the date of the first appearance of this dermatitis they complained of uneasiness in the epigastrium, in some cases actual pain and other dyspeptic symptoms, and on my examining the fæces later I found the characteristic ova, thus showing that this dermatitis known here as "chauffie" is caused by the penetration of the skin by these larvæ. This skin infection is widespread in the island, especially on the estates and among the villages, and nearly every adult laborer has had it, and also the children who are allowed to roll about and play in the earth around the huts.

The disease chiefly affects the country, and very few cases are seen in the larger towns, and this fact is easily explained as follows: No sanitation in the villages; fæces deposited on the earth among the bananas and cocoa trees; the ideal temperature, shade, humidity, and decaying matter being afforded by these groves for the development of the ova, and the poverty and filthy habits of the class as a whole, necessitating walking barefooted, infecting himself and then carrying it to his hut and infecting the children in turn. With regard to immunity from this disease, there is none; all classes may become infected, but the poorer classes are more liable not only from the nature of their work and poverty, but also from the inadequate diet both in quality and quantity.

SYMPTOMATOLOGY.

Within the past year, April, 1904, to April, 1905, I have had two hundred and fifteen cases under my treatment and observation at the Colony Hospital. These cases were simply admitted as they applied, and a large number also suffered from other complications. I found that uncinariasis could be divided into two distinct classes, (*a*) acute and (*b*) chronic, the acute class being further subdivided into (1) mild cases and (2) moderate. On a microscopic examination of the fæces the ova can be readily detected, but the number present in the field is no guide to the extent of the infection in many cases, although if large numbers are seen it is probable there are a large number of parasites, but the reverse is not necessarily correct. The mere presence of this parasite does not constitute the disease, and these early cases are only of importance from their being a source of danger to others and to the district or village in which they reside.

Mild Cases.—Pain or uneasiness in the epigastrium often relieved, but usually increased, by the ingestion of food. Appetite lost but in many cases ravenous. Frontal headache, dizziness and palpitation, breathlessness on exertion, and indisposition to do any work, either physical or mental. In these cases anæmia was not marked and pallor was only slight, being yellowish in whites and muddy in the colored races.

Moderate Cases.—In these cases all the above symptoms were pronounced; pallor is more marked and the anæmia prominent. The mucous membranes and conjunctivæ pale, skin dry, appetite in the majority of cases lost, nausea and vomiting present in many cases, pain in the epigastrium. Headache is very severe and continued, referred chiefly to the frontal region, often temporal, vertigo and extreme tinnitus present. Palpitation is severe, and breathlessness ensued on the slightest exertion. Great languor and lassitude is complained of, and fever of an irregular, intermittent type is present with pains in the joints.

Chronic or Very Advanced Cases.—Here the anæmia is intense and pallor very extreme, the patient having an icteric tinge of the sclera. Œdema of the feet and ankles is present, with general anasarca in the majority of cases, and in eight cases under treatment ascites was present. The digestive symptoms have changed, either becoming more pronounced, with vomiting or ingestion of food, or in many cases they disappear altogether. Precordial pain and pain in the chest is complained of, palpitation is severe, and dyspnœa comes on with the slightest exertion; the pulse is weak and compressible, and pulsation of the large veins of the neck is noticed. Vertigo and tinnitus is extreme, this latter symptom often causing sleeplessness. Dimness of sight is complained of, and in many cases the pupils are noticed to be dilated. The urine is normal in quantity, usually pale in color, and in only three cases was albumin present. On auscultation, bruits are heard over the veins, and there is a well-marked murmur on the valve areas, and the heart itself is often dilated, with the apex-beat depressed. The muscular system is weak, although the muscles appear plump and well nourished and the patient is absolutely incapacited from any kind of work. The patient is listless and apathetic and the temperature is often raised, but in the majority of cases it is subnormal.

Digestive System: Stomatitis.—In two cases only have I seen a stomatitis affecting the tongue and mucous membrane of the mouth, and both these cases were in the advanced stages. I do not attach any importance to it, as I have not seen it present in other cases. Pyorrhœa alveolaris is very common in this island among the laboring class, also caries of the teeth, and may be noticed in all the cases of the disease, but I do not see any connection between them.

Tongue.—In the acute and chronic cases the tongue is very pale, almost white in color, usually coated but often red and raw-looking and denuded of epithelium. I have remarked a peculiar pigmentation seen in every case except the poor whites. It consists of a black or blue-black pigmentation, in minute spots, either singly or in patches, usually on the tip and sides of the tongue; it is not seen, as I mention above, in cases in whites, but only in the pigmented races, negroes and East Indians. I am of opinion that there is some connection between this pigmentation and the disease, but so far I have not been able to establish it. The digestive symptoms are very similar to those due to dyspepsia, and often in the mild cases are simply treated as such, the fæces not being examined, with the result that the case steadily progresses instead of improving. Appetite is variable, being lost in many cases, but ravenous in others; pain or uneasiness in the epigastrium is a well-marked symptom, and is likened by the patient to the sensation of having a stone in the stomach; this symptom is usually increased by the food taken by the laboring class here, which is of poor quality and very coarse and bulky, quantity instead of quality being preferred. Flatulence and palpitation is very common, and the bowels are usually constipated; only in the very advanced cases have I seen diarrhœa.

Circulatory System.—On inspection, the apex-beat is found to be pronounced, especially if the patient is made to walk a little, and is usually displaced downward and to the left, but in many of the chronic cases it is feeble. On percussion, the cardiac area is found to be enlarged in the second class of cases, and in the chronic cases dilatation is present. On auscultation, bruits are heard, very marked in the third left space, and in eight cases under my treatment they were practically organic, fatty degeneration and dilatation having occurred. (Two of these cases died in hospital and enabled me to make an autopsy.) Precordial pain and pain in the chest, palpitation, and dyspnœa are present and are very distressing symptoms in chronic cases. Vertigo and tinnitus aurium are also other well-marked symptoms, especially in the later stages, and are no doubt adjuncts in causing the inability of the patient to get about and in producing the sleeplessness complained of in many cases.

Nervous System.—Symptoms pointing to this system are languor and lassitude, mental apathy, insomnia, and the severe and continued headache, usually frontal, often temporal, and sometimes the pain is referred to the whole head. Numbness of the feet and formication are complained of as well.

Integumentary System.—The skin is harsh and dry, and in the chronic cases general pruritus is often a constant and very annoying symptom; atrophy is present in chronic cases.

Fæces.—In all the above cases I have not seen any blood in the stools, but in six cases I have noticed blood-stained mucus, although it is not a constant symptom. I have mentioned that constipation is usually complained of, but diarrhœa may occur. Microscopically the ova are readily seen, in conjunction with those of *Ascaris lumbricoides* and *Tricocephalus dispar*, but I have also found them in conjunction with those of *Oxyuris vermicularis*, and in twenty cases *Rhabdonema intestinalis* was present.

Blood Examination.—On a microscopic examination the point that is noticed is an increase of the eosinophiles, but on making a count there is no marked leucocytosis; the percentage of hæmoglobin varied, but there was a slow but steady decrease as the disease advanced; it was also noticeable that after treatment and when the patient began to improve the red corpuscles increased, but the percentage of hæmoglobin often fell before it began to rise.

The following table shows the percentage obtained by me from blood-counts in twenty cases: Eosinophiles, 18; polymorphonuclear, 55; large lymphocytes, 8; small lymphocytes, 17; other cells, 2; total, 100. Hæmoglobin varied from eight to forty per cent.

Diagnosis.—The diagnosis of the disease depends not so much on the symptoms, which, although they may be well known, are very often mistaken for those of dyspeptic troubles in the mild cases and of heart disease in the advanced cases, but on the discovery of the ova in the fæces. The ova are very characteristic and cannot be mistaken for those of any other parasite, as they are unstained by bile, while those of the other parasites are usually stained yellow. The ova of the *Oxyuris vermicularis* may be mistaken by beginners for that of *Ankylostoma*, but a little practice enables them to be easily distinguished. The *Ankylostomum* ova are perfectly clear and chitinous, shelled with a granular grayish vitellum, usually segmented into four, sometimes six or eight, parts; those of *Oxyuris* are smaller and the vitellum is not segmented, but fills up the entire shell. In many cases the temperature is of an irregular intermittent or remittent type, patients complaining that the fever comes on every night or morning, and this fever often causes the disease to be mistaken for malaria. A microscopic examination of the blood soon clears this point, although malaria is very often, especially in certain districts of this island, a complication of the disease, and when the case is treated as one of malaria, without an examination of the fæces having been made, the practitioner is surprised to find that quinine has, seemingly, no effect on the temperature. (I had a case of this nature sent into hospital—*vide* report on case attached.)

MORBID ANATOMY.

The following data are taken from four autopsies made by me at the hospital on bodies of patients who died from advanced uncinariasis. One died suddenly (forty-eight hours) on the second day after admission (this case I have described separately, with a complete history).

General Condition.—The bodies appeared plump and well nourished, the skin was harsh and dry, of a dirty, muddy color, œdema of the feet and ankles with ascites was present, and there was serous effusion into the various cavities,—viz., pericardium, and ventricles of the brain; subcutaneous fat was abundant and yellow in color.

Heart.—The heart was found to be enlarged, fatty degeneration and dilatation being present with incompetence of the valves; the heart walls were thin and flabby, and patches of atheroma were present in the aorta. The cavities were found filled with soft dark clots.

Lungs.—The lungs appeared normal, although pale in color, but in one case advanced pulmonary tuberculosis was present and was no doubt the cause of death. Pleural cavities contained about a pint of clear, yellowish fluid.

Spleen.—This organ appeared normal in two cases, but in the others was enlarged and fibrous, probably due to malaria, as both cases came from a very malarious district.

Liver.—This was pale and slightly enlarged in all the cases; fatty degeneration was present and the tissue very friable.

Kidneys.—In one case the kidneys were small, pale, capsule adherent (chronic interstitial nephritis), but in the others they appeared normal although pale in hue.

Stomach.—This organ showed signs of chronic catarrh, in two cases dilatation was present, but I did not find any uncinaria in the cavity of the organ.

Intestines.—The parasite was found in large numbers, chiefly in the upper part of the jejunum, but also in the duodenum. The parasites were lying free in the lumen of the bowel, but a great many were attached to the intestinal wall. There was a large quantity of mucus present in the intestine, in which the worms were lying embedded. The mucous membrane should show minute hemorrhagic spots, as well as pigmented spots. In one case the wall itself was very thin. There was no blood in the intestines.

Brain.—The brain showed anæmia, with effusion into the ventricles of a pale yellowish fluid.

The above four cases were the only ones that died and enabled me to make an autopsy. The majority of the cases made rapid and uneventful recoveries, but a few of the very advanced cases were slow, and remained in hospital over three months before being discharged.

PIGMENTATION OF TONGUE AND ITS PROBABLE CAUSATION.

In every case of ankylostomiasis under my treatment, with the exception of the poor whites who are of European parentage, the pigmentation of the tongue is seen. It consists of minute black, blue-black, or brown spots, usually on the lip and sides of the tongue; sometimes the pigmentation is seen in larger areas. The colored races in this island—viz., the negro, East Indian, and their descendants—show this pigmentation in every case of uncinariasis, and it is especially marked in the chronic cases.

Pigmentation of the skin and mucous membranes may be derived either from the blood or bile or from external agents. In these spots the pigment is deposited chiefly in the mucosa of the papillæ in its lower layers, but also in the upper layers. There is no doubt that disturbed innervation plays a part in producing this result, as is seen in the bronzing of the skin in Addison's disease, which is probably due to inflammation of the abdominal sympathetic. The pigment melanin closely resembles hæmatin, one of the constituents of the hæmoglobin, in its composition, hence we can conclude that it is derived from that source. Its presence is usually associated with two very opposite conditions of nutrition, being sometimes an accompaniment of tissue degeneration and at others of active trophic changes. It is well known that the chlorophyl of plants and the hæmoglobin of the blood are intimately associated with respiratory changes. In the majority of cases where pigment is found some concomitant blood change is also present, as, for instance, in malaria, pigment is formed from the destruction of the red corpuscles and deposited in various organs of the body, and without doubt deposition of pigment is under the control of the sympathetic system.

In uncinariasis we have a toxin produced by the parasite and which is the true cause of the profound anæmia, blood and nervous changes. Here, therefore, we have both the necessary factors for the production of pigmentation, not only on the tongue and mucous membranes, but elsewhere,—viz., (1) blood changes in which the hæmoglobin of the red corpuscles is broken and disintegrated, as shown in the reduction of the hæmoglobin percentage as the case advances, and (2) disturbance of the nervous system by the same toxin which affects all centres, sympathetic included, as evidenced by the symptoms.

Dr. Laycock has observed that pigmentation may be regarded as having reference to the excretion of carbon after it has served its purpose in the tissues, and hence, pathologically, pigmentation may be taken to be expression of (1) imperfect oxidation of the carbon, so that it is not eliminated as carbonic acid from the body; (2) excessive production of carbon from highly carbonaceous food; (3) pigment resulting from the disintegration of the hæmoglobin of the red cells. In uncinariasis all three of these factors are present, produced by the toxin excreted by the parasites,—(1) diminished oxygenating power of the blood from destruction of the blood-cells, so that carbon waste is not got rid of; (2) presence of hæmatin from disintegration of the hæmoglobin; and in this island (3) we have the third factor,—viz., excess of carbonaceous food, as the laborers all live on coarse, bulky food, the quantity rather than the quality being the chief item of importance. The class of people in whom the disease is chiefly seen are the colored races, and, therefore, more liable to pigmentation than those races in whom pigment is not usually present in the skin. From the above facts I am of opinion that this pigmentation of the tongue and buccal mucous membranes and mucous membrane of the intestine has some connection with the disease, and may be taken as of diagnostic value, as I have never failed to find the ova and the other symptoms of the disease present in any case which showed this pigmentation.

Another view of its causation may be taken in the dermatitis or " chauffie" affecting the laboring class in this island and which without doubt is the true method of infection. Pigmentation of the skin affected takes place in this island, where the class affected are dirty in their habits and careless in regard to eating unwashed fruit and vegetables. Muddy drinking-water is one method of infection, as during the rains the water supply, which usuualy consists of shallow wells and ponds, is contaminated to a large extent. and as the larvæ do not take very long to penetrate the skin, as seen from Claude Smith's experiments, it may be possible that. when taken into the mouth, they make their way more easily and quickly into the mucous membrane, and that these pigmented areas are the points of their entrance.

CASE I.—A. J., aged nineteen, unmarried, living with his parents, laborer in cocoa estate. Admitted to Colony Hospital, February 2, 1905.

History.—Patient has been ill for the past year with general weakness, as he termed it, unable to do much work, owing to breathlessness and palpitation. Three weeks prior to admission he had a severe rigor, followed by fever and slight perspiration; fever comes on every day. Has lost flesh and is emaciated. Complexion muddy; lips and buccal mucous membranes very pale; tongue shows minute pigmented spots on lip and sides. Conjunctivæ very pale, and scleræ have an icteric tinge; appetite very poor, can only take fluid nourishment; pain and tenderness in epigastrium; nausea and vomiting after food; bowels constipated and have usually been so for the past year. Skin harsh and dry, and does not perspire very much; itching sensation over the whole body. Precorial pain and pain in the chest complained of; palpitation marked. with dyspnœa in exertion. Dimness of sight, with severe and continued frontal headache and tinnitus aurium. Vertigo and sleeplessness present. Very weak, and has not left his bed for the past three weeks. Pulsation of veins in the neck; apex-beat depressed and to the left; marked bruit in third left intercostal space. Pulse soft and compressible.

Examination of Fœces.—Ova of uncinaria present in large numbers with those of *Ascaris lumbricoides* and *Tricocephalus dispar.* No blood in the stools.

Examination of Blood.—Malaria Æstivo-autumnal parasite present. Eosinophiles, 20; polymorphonuclear, 58; large lymphocytes, 10; small lymphocytes, 12.

Temperature on admission, 102.6°, rising on the day after to 104°. No marked rigor or diaphoresis.

Diagnosis.—Ankylostomiasis or uncinariasis. Complication, malignant malarial fever.

Treatment.—Saline aperient every morning. Hypodermic injection of quinine bihydrochlor. grs. 5 every morning at ten and in the evening. Diet: Milk, beef tea, arrowroot, etc.

Course.—Temperature still continued. February 17, blood re-examined and found free of malarial parasites. Temperature, 99.8°. Fæces contained the ova in numbers. February 20, 120 grs. thymol given in cachets of 40 grs., followed by a saline aperient four hours after the last dose; stools carefully washed and found to contain large numbers of worms. Temperature reduced, but still above normal. Thymol repeated February 23 and stools examined, worms still being passed.

Repeated thymol February 26 and 28, and after the last dose only a few worms (six) were found in the last stool.

Fæces examined March 2; no ova present, but thymol repeated once more, and a week later they were again examined, but no ova present; similarly on the 17th.

The diet was now changed, as appetite had increased; after the second dose of thymol the headache disappeared and the tinnitus was very much decreased, and patient slept well at night. He was now put on the following mixture as well:

R. Tinct. ferri perchlor............................. ʒ iiss 10
Liq. arsenitis hydrochlor ....ʒ i 4
Mag. sulph... ....ʒ iv 15
Syrupi aurantii............................... ...ʒ iss 6
Aquæ, q. s. ad................................. ℥ viii 240

M. Sig.—One tablespoonful three times a day after meals.

Blood examination, March 31: Eosinophiles, 13; polymorphonuclear, 65; large lymphocytes, 10; small lymphocytes, 7. Hæmoglobin percentage, 22.

Blood examination, aMrch 31: Eosinophiles, 13; polymorphonuclear, 45.5; large lymphocytes, 14.8; small lymphocytes, 26.2.

Patient is doing well, has gained weight and flesh, all symptoms have disappeared, skin moist. Rapid and uneventful convalescence.

CASE H.—R. G., aged thirty-six, married, children, laborer.

History.—Patient has been ill for past six years, gradually getting worse each year; weakness, fever, breathlessness, and palpitation; disinclination or inability to work. Husband and children also affected similarly. Has had " chauffie" very often, particularly after or during the rains. Appearance plump and well nourished. Very anæmic; has been very ill for the past month; bedridden; brought to hospital in a chair.

Examination.—General anasarca very marked; ascites developed; face and scalp puffy and œdematous. Says she never perspires; appetite lost; pain and tenderness in epigastrium; vomiting after food. Tongue very pale and white; teeth indentations on tongue; numerous minute pigmented spots on lips and sides, with bluish streaks on side as well.

Superficial veins of abdomen distended; diarrhœa; fæces yellowish-brown, no blood; on examination ova of ankylostoma and ascarides were seen. Liver enlarged; abdomen tender on pressure; ascites present. Precordial pain and pain in the chest very severe; dyspnœa extreme, cough troublesome, bases of lungs dull on percussion.

Extreme vertigo; marked tinnitus aurium, with severe continued frontal headache; sleeplessness, and has had fainting attacks.

Vision dim, great weakness. Heart markedly dilated, with bruits, pulsation of veins in neck; apex-beat full and diffused. Pulse 110, weak and dicrotic. Urine normal; patient quite sensible, but prefers being left alone. Temperature on admission 97.8°.

Diagnosis.—Ankylostomiasis, chronic.

Treatment.—Milk and beef tea, stimulants.

Patient did not do at all well, and died suddenly on the second day after admission.

Blood Examination.—Eosinophiles, 8; polymorphonuclears, 56; large lymphocytes, 6; small lymphocytes, 30. Hæmoglobin, 10 per cent.

Morbid Anatomy.—Lungs very pale, but otherwise normal; bases œdematous, and pleural cavities contained about two pints of straw-colored fluid.

Heart: Pericardium contained four ounces of serous fluid. Heart very much enlarged and dilated; cavities filled with soft, dark clots. Fatty degeneration present in the walls; valves inefficient.

Liver enlarged, pale, and fatty degeneration present. Abdomen contained large quantity of ascitic fluid.

Spleen slightly enlarged, pale, but otherwise normal.

Intestines: Jejunum and duodenum both contained large quantities of the worms, most of which had dropped and were lying in the lumen of the bowel. Mucus present in large quantities. Large intestine contained dark yellowish-brown fluid fæces. Intestinal wall thin and atrophied in parts, presenting large numbers of minute hemorrhagic and pigmented spots.

Stomach: Signs of chronic catarrh present; no worms in the cavity itself.

Kidneys pale and otherwise normal.

Brain anæmic and ventricles filled with fluid. Pia mater stripped easily off the cortex, serous fluid beneath it filling the sulci.

Death in this case was due to mitral inefficiency, resulting from dilatation of the heart caused by chronic uncinariasis or ankylostomiasis.

TREATMENT.

Thymol is the drug employed by me, and I have had the very best results, with no single ill effect, even in children. The dose given by me always varies with the age of the patient and also his general condition; it ranges from ten grains to a child to forty grains for an adult at a single dose.

The following is the procedure adopted by me at the Colony Hospital: The patient is carefully prepared for three or four days after admission, the bowels are kept active by saline aperients administered every morning in sufficient dose to cause one evacuation, the diet is light and easily digested,—viz., milk, beef-tea, arrowroot, etc., with pepsin if required. In very advanced cases with cardiac troubles, stimulants and cardiac tonics administered. The chief object in the administration of the aperient being to get rid of the mucus with which the intestine is often loaded and in which the parasites lie buried.

At ten P.M. on the night prior to the administration of the thymol a dose of saline aperient is given, and no food except a pint of milk given to the patient next morning, and two hours afterwards the first dose of thymol is given. I give it in the form of cachets each containing five grains for a child and forty grains for an adult, and one cachet is taken every hour till fifteen grains are given to the child and one hundred and twenty grains to the adult. In old people and very advanced cases in adults I usually give thirty grains instead of forty grains. No food is allowed the patient, and four hours after the last cachet is given a saline aperient is given and the patient allowed his diet. The stools are collected and carefully washed, and invariably show a large quantity of worms. In the case (1) described by me five hundred worms were passed after the first administration of thymol. The above treatment is carried out on three alternate days, occasionally an interval of four or five days is allowed in debilitated cases; the fæces are carefully examined for ova a week afterwards and usually found free. The fæces are again examined two days before the patient is discharged, and it is my invariable practice to give another single dose of thymol and to carefully examine the stools again. The after-treatment of the case consists in the administration of tonics, chiefly iron and arsenic, often combined with strychnine; the diet is increased, but is still one which is easily digested and nourishing, and usually the patients seek their discharge in from a fortnight to three weeks after the fæces are free of ova; and are recommended to continue the tonic at their own homes for a still longer period. I usually administer the iron and arsenic in the form mentioned in the report of Case I above, as I find it gives the best results in a shorter period of time.

The saline aperient used by me, and which is preferable to any other aperient, is the following:

℞. Sodii sulphas,
  Mag. sulphas...................................āā ʒiss 6
  Aqua ....ad ℥ii 00
M. Sig.—Drink.

As I have previously stated, I have had no ill effects from administering thymol, although a few cases have complained of dizziness and a sensation of fainting, but it has gradually passed off; it is, as we know, a very insoluble drug except in spirits and oils, and therefore is not absorbed in sufficient quantity to cause toxic effects, besides which the saline purge given shortly after the last dose hurries it out of the system, although sufficient time has been given the thymol to act on the parasites, and besides this there is no doubt that sodium or magnesium appears to be an antidote.

A remarkable fact, and one which confirms me in the use of thymol, is the immediate relief given by the first administration of the drug from the severe headache and other mental symptoms, the patient next day feeling much brighter and better. Bentley recommends and prefers betanaphthol to thymol. I have not tried this drug as yet, being so far satisfied with my results from thymol, but I intend giving it a trial and comparing the results.

PROPHYLAXIS.

In this island the two chief factors in the causation of this disease are (1) muddy and infected drinking-water; (2) soil pollution and infection through the skin. With regard to the first, it has been doubted whether this factor is a true one, yet I have had two cases of this disease in which there was no history of dermatitis, the patients being fairly well to do and not exposed to the second method of infection, but they admitted that the first cause might be the real one, as the water supply was obtained from shallow wells, liable to infection, and, especially during the rains, was often muddy.

However, there are only three methods of prevention,—viz., 1, prevention of water infection; 2, prevention of soil infection; 3, treatment of all cases of the disease.

The last two are the chief ones. In this island the disease is widespread throughout all the districts, especially on the estates and in certain villages, hence the chief essential is the prevention of the fecal contamination of the soil in order to eradicate the disease; the promiscuous depositing of fæces near the huts and villages and in the fields should be prevented, but owing to habit and the low intelligence of this class it seems an impossibility.

On all estates where huts are provided for the laborers and other families easily accessible privy accommodation should be provided; pits and trenches would do, which could be filled in from time to time and fresh ones opened. Another point is to try to destroy all ova and larvæ on heavily infected fields by ploughing the earth over and burning bush fires over it and replanting, but as most of the cultivation here is cocoa this is an impossibility; these cocoa groves are the chief infected areas, as here the ova have the ideal humidity, shade, and temperature for their growth and development. The people should, therefore, be made acquainted with the danger of depositing fæces promiscuously and thus infecting the soil and the liability of their acquiring the disease owing to the nature of their work, barefooted. The next point is the proper examination and treatment of all cases of the disease. On all estates and in villages an examination of all cases of dyspeptic troubles, dermatitis, and anæmia should be made and the fæces examined, and, if the ova are found, immediate treatment of the case begun, so as to prevent their becoming a source of danger to others who are not infected. This cannot be done without an outlay on the part of the estate owner or the government itself, but there is no doubt that to thoroughly eradicate this disease such measures must be adopted; otherwise the treatment of cases individually is of little use, for as soon as they are cured and go back to their work, they are reinfected.

DISCUSSION.

Dr. V. A. Latham, Chicago, said that the southern parts of this country were now confronted with this condition. In patients with ankylostomiasis the whole system stops developing; they are anæmic, frail, and almost infantile in their actions and characteristics.

Dr. Eugene Talbot, Chicago, said that two or three similar cases have occurred in this country, but not enough to warrant the conclusions brought out by Dr. Leonard. One occurred lately in Southern Illinois.

ON THE HISTORY OF DENTISTRY FROM THE EARLIEST TIMES TO THE FOUNDING OF THE PROFESSION BY HAYDEN AND HARRIS; WITH SPECIAL REFERENCE TO THE IMMEDIATE PUBLICATION OF SUCH A WORK IN ENGLISH.[1]

DR. CHARLES M'MANUS, HARTFORD, CONN.

WHEN I promised nearly a year ago to read a paper before this Institute, I had but a very vague idea of what I could present that would be of any particular interest to the members. That it should be something of a historical character goes without saying, —for I deal in little else. That it would probably be an appeal to you to take a little interest in the early development of that art which you are all engaged in developing was very probable.

But that I should be able to come before you this evening with the surprisingly good news that the *dental history* (for which we have looked so long,—with a sort of despair,—)was an accomplished fact, was more than I could have dreamed of, when I promised to appear before you.

The work exists,—within the past week I have read it with the deepest interest and admiration. It has been written, as I have always believed it should be written, by a dentist, and what is more remarkable by a dentist with the historical instinct,—a rather rare combination.

I refer to that distinguished dental historian Dr. Vincenzo Guerini, of Naples, Italy, and his " History of Dentistry from the most ancient times to the close of the Eighteenth Century."

The period I shall allude to in my remarks is the time from the very beginnings in medicine, dentistry, civilization itself, up to the true founding of the profession in this country by Hayden and Harris. I tell of dentistry before there was a society, a journal or a college, before anæsthesia: a dentistry without cohesive gold, the rubber dam, the engine, a true cement or amalgam and with porcelain only in a sort of crude infancy.

I propose towards the close of my remarks, this evening, to tell you of this work, but before doing so I must ask your kind

---

[1] Read before the New York Institute of Stomatology, October 3, 1905.

indulgence,—perhaps endurance,—while I briefly sketch the development of the dental art during the period covered,—in a most complete, in fact, exhaustive manner, by Dr. Guerini.

The first beginnings[2] of the dental art were undoubtedly the same as those of general medicine for it is evident that in primitive times, when the healing art was still in a rudimentary stage, no divisions can have existed in it. Amongst the peoples of ancient times the Egyptian nation was without doubt the one in which civilization first took its rise and had its earliest development. The Ebers papyrus, in the library of the University of Leipsic, the oldest medical manuscript known, treats of diseases of the teeth and gums. In this very interesting book of ancient Egypt, reaching as far back as 3700 years before Christ, no less than fourteen prescriptions for the treatment of dental diseases are found. At this very remote epoch dental medicine was a part of general medicine; we say dental *medicine* because the papyrus of Ebers does not mention dental surgery.

The initiator of this lost science was undoubtedly the Greek Æsculapius who flourished thirteen centuries before the Christian era and who on account of his healing abilities was raised to the rank of a god by the gratitude of mankind. [Space will not permit[3] of the publication, in full, of the paper which was illustrated with sixty lantern slides of portraits, instruments and appliances, etc. A brief résumé will show the scope of the lecture]

After speaking of the Greeks, with a passing allusion to the lack of any dental reference in Homer, Herodotus was quoted regarding the state of medicine in Egypt in his time; when, among many other "specialists," there were those in charge of the *disorders of the teeth.* What degree of development dentistry reached among the Egyptians unfortunately, as yet, we do not know. All the assertions regarding artificial teeth, pivot teeth and particularly teeth with gold fillings that are said to have been found in Egyptian mummies are, *as yet,* entirely devoid of foundation. And yet in spite of this, it is not admissible that the Egyptians should not have known of prosthetic dentistry when their neighbors the people of Phœnicia, a country with which they had very intimate commercial relations, practiced it. Lantern

---

[2] Guerini.
[3] Note by C. M.

slides were shown of photographs of prosthetic pieces found in the Phœnician necropolis at Sidon, dating as far back as four hundred years before Christ; as well as various Etruscan pieces of even earlier date. These evidences of early dental work are authentic and to be found in the Civic Museum and the collection of Count Bruschi at Corneto, Italy. An even more interesting prosthetic piece found in an Etruscan grave at Orvieto and now in the museum of the University of Ghent, was shown, as well as a piece of Etruscan dental work from a tomb at Valsiarosa now in the museum of Pope Julius at Rome. All these ancient appliances were shown in *fac simile* at the International Dental Congress at St. Louis in the archæological collection of Dr. Guerini, who received a gold medal.

The dental art among the *Romans* was referred to with illustrations of various instruments. During the many centuries that have been called the "middle ages" dentistry was in a state of marked decline; we know very little about it and the little that was achieved must be attributed to the *Arabs*. Rhazes, the initiator of the operation of filling teeth, using for this purpose a mixture of mastic and alum, was spoken of and *Abul-casis* was quoted at some length and several illustrations of the instruments and appliances of the time were shown upon the screen. Abul-casis in the XI century was the first author who took into serious consideration dental tartar and recommended that a scrupulous cleansing of the teeth should be performed. The chapter[4] relating to this " On the Scraping of the Teeth " is worthy of attention:

" Sometimes on the surface of the teeth, both inside and outside, as well as under the gums are deposited rough scales, of ugly appearance and black, green or yellow in color. This corruption is communicated to the gums and so the teeth are in process of time denuded. It is necessary for thee to lay the patient's head upon thy lap, and scrape the teeth and molars on which are observed either true incrustations or something similar to sand and this until nothing more remains of such substances and until also the dirty color of the teeth disappears, be it black or green or yellowish or of any other color. If a first scraping is sufficient, so much the better, if not, thou *shalt repeat it on the following day or even on the third or fourth day* until the desired purpose is obtained. Thou must know however that the teeth need scrapers

---

[4] Liber I. cap 29, Guerini.

of various shapes and figures, on account of the very nature of this operation. In fact the scalpel with which the teeth must be scraped on the inside is unlike that with which thou shalt scrape the outside and that with which thou shalt scrape the interstices between the teeth shall likewise have another shape. Therefore thou must have all this series of scalpels ready if it so pleases God." Abul-casis shows in his work fourteen figures of these scalers, which were shown on the screen.

Passing on to the Fifteenth Century attention was called to *Giovanni d'Arcoli,* known under the Latinized form of Arculanus, who was the first to mention the filling of teeth with gold. In speaking of the stopping of decayed teeth, he says that it must not always be carried out with the same substance but that in making choice of the material one should have regard to the temperament of the individual and to the condition of the gums and of the tooth. He counsels filling the teeth, in certain cases, with *gold leaf.* The use of gold in dental stoppings, therefore, dates back at least to A. D. 1450. Many other writers were mentioned, particularly the great *Eustachius* and a brief account was given of *Ambroise Paré,* the " foster father of dental surgery," with several portraits and illustrations of dental instruments from his works.

A very rare and curious portrait of *Nathaniel Highmore* was shown, as well as one of the father of scientific microscopy *van Leuwenhoek,* also instruments from the work of *Pierre Dionis* (1718). After a brief glance at some of the writers of the Seventeenth Century, the "father of dental surgery," the illustrious *Pierre Fauchard* was spoken of at some length. His portrait from the original now in possession of Dr. Viau, of Paris, was shown, as well as the title page and frontispiece of his work (1728) on dental surgery with a number of the plates illustrating extracting instruments of several kinds, scalers, pluggers, and various artificial dentures.

An account of Fauchard's great work " The Surgeon-Dentist " was given with much detail and the quotation of many important passages. Two are of particular interest. In the preface to his book Fauchard says: " There does not exist any public or private course of surgery in which the theory of dental maladies is amply taught and in which one can receive fundamental instruction in this art, so necessary for the healing of these maladies and of those of the neighboring parts. This branch of the art having been but little cultivated, if not wholly abandoned, by the most celebrated surgeons their negligence has caused it to fall into the hands of persons without theory and without experience, who practice it in a haphazard fashion guided neither by principles nor methods. In Paris it is only since 1700 that people's eyes have become opened to this abuse. In this town those who intend to become dentists are now obliged to undergo an examination, but although the examiners be most learned and well versed in all the other parts of surgery, I think, if I may be allowed to express an opinion, that as they do not ordinarily themselves practice dental surgery, it would not be amiss on these occasions to admit an able and experienced dentist, who might sound the aspirants as to the difficulties which have come before him in the course of the long practice of his art and who could communicate to them the means of surmounting them. In this way one would not have to admit that the knowledge of the greater part of " dental experts " is below " mediocrity."

That this high-minded professional man was among the first to realize the necessity for a higher dental education may be seen in the following quotation:

" It is strange," writes Fauchard, " that the sovereigns of foreign countries, the heads of republics and also the administrators of our own provinces, do not provide for the expense of sending young surgeons to Paris to be instructed in a part of surgery so essential, and notwithstanding, so ignored and neglected everywhere excepting in this great city, where it has reached its highest perfection both as regards the embellishment of the mouth and the cure of diseases, often of a most serious character. These scholars would, thereafter, form others and would render great services to their nation and their fellow citizens."[*]

A mechanical device, probably the " germ " of the dental engine, described by Fauchard and illustrated by *Jourdain* in 1756, a drawing of which was shown on the screen. A brief account of *John Hunter*, with portrait, was given, as well as of other early English dentists.

The early history of dentistry in America with many por-

---

[*] 2nd Ed.   Vol. II, page 366.

traits, advertisements, etc., was considered, some of the men spoken of being Joseph Lemaire, James Gardette, Josiah Flagg, John Greenwood, Edward Hudson, John Randall, Leonard Koecker, John R. and Shearjashub Spooner, of all of whom portraits were shown as well as of a number of other prominent practitioners of the early part of the Nineteenth Century, Du Bois de Chemant,, Audibran, Serre, C. Starr Brewster, B. A. Rodrigues, Parmly, Solyman Brown, Merritt and others, ending with a brief account of the great labors of *Hayden* and *Harris.*

For the past ten years Dr. Guerini has been compiling a history of dentistry fom the earliest records down to the Nineteenth Century. As he says in the introduction to his work: " The end I proposed to myself was to write a history of dentistry that should be more complete, more circumstantial and more exact than those published hitherto and which instead of being, as are many of these works, simply a compilation, should represent in part, the fruits of personal research and scrupulous examination of a vast number of works of various kinds containing elements utilizable for a history of dental art and science."

Those who have been accustomed to regard dentistry as a modern art can have but little idea of the extent to which we are indebted to those of the middle ages and earlier for much that is woven into the fabric of our modern practice. The collecting and harmonizing of the data for this early historical record has been a labor of many years by this expert specialist. Dr. Guerini says: " I have carefully collected the greatest possible number of historical data, keeping in view the consideration that some facts, although of little value in themselves may acquire a certain referential importance for the student desirous of procuring historical notes relating to some particular point in dental science."

This work is now ready for publication in the English language. It has been the desire of its distinguished author that it shall make its first appearance in that language and under American auspices.

In a report made by the " Committee on Dental History " to the National Dental Association at the meeting held last summer at Buffalo it was stated that they were of the opinion that the National Dental Association should secure the honor of publishing this history by undertaking to guarantee the sale of a sufficient number of copies to practically cover the cost. The committee found that it would be necessary to fix the retail price of the work *fully illustrated* and bound in cloth, at $5, and that in order to guarantee the cost of an edition of 1000 copies it would require 700 subscriptions at $5 each to insure a fund of $3,500 to pay the cost of publication. It was suggested by the committee that the National Dental Association assume publication of this important work with the understanding that it shall not be published until not less than 700 subscriptions be received.

The association very willingly lent its moral support to the enterprise and the matter will soon be placed not only before the members of the dental profession in this country but of the entire world.

Reports of Society Meetings.

THE NEW YORK INSTITUTE OF STOMATOLOGY.

At a regular meeting of the Institute, held Tuesday evening, October 3, 1905, at the " Chelsea," 222 West Twenty-third Street, Manhattan, a paper was read by Dr. Charles McManus, of Hartford, on the history of Dentistry from the earliest times to the founding of the profession by Hayden and Harris, with special reference to the immediate publication of such a work in English.

(For Dr. McManus' paper see page 826.)

A meeting of the Institute was held at the Chelsea, No. 222 West 23rd Street, New York, on Friday evening, November 3rd, 1905, the president, Dr. C. O. Kimball, in the chair.

The minutes of the last meeting were read and approved.

Dr. Fossume presented for the inspection of the members some samples of removable bridgework.

Models were also presented of the jaw of a girl thirteen years of age who erupted the upper bicuspids in a completely reversed position, *i. e.*, having the lingual cusps outside.

The paper of the evening was presented, with accompanying lantern illustrations, by Dr. L. W. Baker, of Boston.

(For Dr. Baker's paper see page 784.)

Dr. S. E. Davenport.—It has been the privilege of the institute during the last three years to present some of the ablest orthodontists in this country. To-night we have had another valuable contribution to this subject, the second one from the Baker family. We feel under great obligations to young Dr. Baker for what he has done for us.

Dr. C. D. Cook.—I would like to ask Dr. Baker what influence parentage has in these cases of irregularity. We hear a great deal about the child inheriting the large teeth of one side of the family and the little mouth of the other with a resulting crowding of the teeth.

Dr. Baker.—I suppose heredity may have something to do with these malformations, but on the other hand, did you ever see one of these same children with a malformed hand or any other malformation from a cause similar to that mentioned by Dr. Cook? It hardly seems to me that nature would permit of such a discrepancy.

Dr. H. L. Wheeler.—I think there is absolutely no comparison between the development of the hands and that of the teeth. I believe that one of the reasons why the teeth are irregular and imperfectly developed is lack of use. Change in our methods of preparing and taking foods has begun to interfere with the development of the teeth. A degenerative influence has taken place because of a diminution of the work required by the jaws. This change has not taken place with regard to the work required of the hands.

Dr. F. Milton Smith.—Will Dr. Wheeler kindly explain according to this theory why it is that I have a perfectly regular arch while that of my brother, born a year and nine months before, has a very contracted arch and very irregular teeth.

Dr. Wheeler.—In a specific case I should have to know the history of the family and the environment to give any satisfactory explanation. Nature always endeavors to adapt herself to her environment but if the environment changes rapidly there may be an interval when nature will fail to succeed in her perfect adaptation.

Dr. Wilbur F. Daly.—It seems to me in all these discussions the deciduous set of teeth have been entirely overlooked. I believe that if the temporary teeth are prematurely lost we are bound to have a contracted arch. If they are retained normally we are bound always to have a normal set of permanent teeth.

Dr. Baker.—How about cases of mouth breathing where there is almost always a narrowing of the arch.

Dr. Daly.—The mouth breathing comes from enlarged tonsils and adenoids. These will not appear if the temporary teeth are normally retained.

Dr. E. A. Bogue.—I was sorry to see the discussion wandering off the subject as it did. I think perhaps what Dr. Daly meant to imply was that the deciduous teeth, just as accurately as the permanent teeth, will tell the story of impending irregularity. If he has not got as far as that, allow me to say that such is the case.

Dr. Baker asks (after showing a number of interesting specimens where there seemed to be an improvement in intelligent appearance), " Has a psychological change taken place?" As he has asked the question, it seems to me that we may try to answer it. I think such a change has taken place. I not only think so but I could point to a dozen authors who have come to the verge of this discovery,—Dr. G. V. I. Brown, Milwaukee; Dr. Swayne, New Haven; Dr. Behrens, New York, and many others.

Dr. Pfaff, of Dresden, Germany, read a paper at the International Dental Congress at St. Louis, containing the statement that partial occlusions of the nasal meatus were corrected by enlargement of the superior dental arch. In the fifteen hundred examinations or thereabouts that I have made I have found a great many cases carrying out the view that if the superior arch is regular the nasal meatuses will be regular also. In regard to lower arches the rule is that the lower teeth erupt first forming a mould into which the upper teeth erupt. There are exceptions to this rule. By just so much as the dental arch is regular, the arch of the palate regular, the palate bones sufficiently large, the sphenoid and the ethmoid bones normal, by just so much will all the cavities of the nose and pharynx be large and resonant. Now, if in a case of contracted arch this contraction is corrected, the broadening and enlarging of all these bones with a consequent enlargement of the various adjacent cavities, makes it reasonable to suppose that there is more or less of an enlargement of the cavity in which rests a portion of the brain. While I am no believer in the so-called science of "phrenology" I have no doubt but that the development in early youth of these upper maxillary bones adjacent to the brain does increase the mental capacity, and I think perhaps this explains the phenomena so nicely shown in Dr. Baker's demonstration, and presupposes a psychological change.

It is of course desirable to treat these cases of regulating as promptly as possible, so as to make use of the temporary teeth to attach the regulating fixtures. It was not ten days ago that I heard a scathing criticism of a number of cases where decay of the permanent teeth had resulted from the appliances. So I want to raise my voice against the use of regulating rings without cement. I recognize also the desirability of getting these appliances off as quickly as possible with safety to our work.

Even after we have done all that is possible in the correction of an irregularity, time must be allowed for nature to grow up to the new condition. When we say that in a few weeks we have finished a piece of regulating, we are going farther than the results will permit. Accurate retention for a certain time is absolutely necessary. I remember in one instance saying to Dr. Baker, Sr., after seeing an appliance that he had adjusted for retaining a set of teeth, that he was retaining them in an abnormal position. He acknowledged this after the retainer had been removed and nature had had time to readjust the teeth into their proper positions, the cusps occupying the sulci of the antagonizing teeth.

I want to make my acknowledgements to Dr. Angle for his classification, and also to Dr. I. B. Davenport of Paris, who in the Cosmos of July, 1887, published the first scientific article on the occlusion of the human teeth. It was this work I am told that gave Dr. Angle his first incentive in scientific orthodontia. Dr. Baker alludes to three forces, among them the expansion arch which is more than one hundred years old. He alludes to the screw. This was invented by Mr. Archimedes several centuries ago. Then he alludes to ligatures. I do not know who was the originator of these. A great deal has been accomplished by a good many men, adapting these three forms of force and that of elasticity to the regulation of teeth. I do not think that anyone has done entirely well nor anyone entirely ill. Perhaps later we shall produce an apparatus that will be far more effective than any we have yet.

Dr. Baker.—Do you suppose such an appliance can ever be discovered?

Dr. Bogue.—It is not impossible. It is not the Angle, the Coffin, the Ainsworth or the Jackson appliances, but each one of them contributing to the understanding of the *principles* underlying orthodontia, and a valuable something to the mechanical part of it that brings about advancement in the science. No apparatus in the hands of an uninformed dentist will or can be efficient.

In every one of his cases Dr. Baker alluded to the widening of the arch. There was not an exception. What does this mean? We see advertised very extensively apparatus for drawing the teeth back. How often is that needed I wonder. Every one of the cases shown us to-night was defective because there was a lack in the upper maxillary region. It shows in the nose, lip and molar region, as well as in a weak chin. I think if you will observe closely, you will find that one third of the people you meet on the streets are defective in some respect in this region and in a way that could have been corrected with proper attention early in life.

Dr. Baker mentioned that if teeth were corrected to their normal positions they would be retained by the force of occlusion after a little time had elapsed. I think the president will bear me out in the statement that was made years ago that if the lower teeth were made properly to occlude with the upper and were kept in their places, no retaining plate would be necessary for the upper teeth.

Dr. Baker also said that extraction was indicated once in a while. So is the amputation of a leg and just about as often. I have taken out one tooth for one young lady, an upper lateral incisor. It was because somebody had taken out other teeth to such an extent that they could not be brought into proper occlusion. I am very much astonished that Dr. Baker succeeded as he did in the case where the first molars were gone.

Regarding the question of the teeth not being adapted in size to the mouth they occupy, my answer is this: that the teeth are not more perfect than the rest of the body; some people are born with a club foot and some with dislocated hips. Dr. Ottolingui says that he hears a great deal about big teeth of big father and little jaw of little mother, but he has never heard of a big jaw from a big father and little teeth from a little mother. The fact is that the teeth of each individual are adapted to that individual and his size. I know of only one man who has attempted accurately to measure the teeth. This man is Dr. Hawley. I think his object was to find a method of forming the normal arch from the sizes of two erupted teeth. He has shown how we may arrange the whole arch from *three* teeth, a central, lateral and cuspid.

A vote of thanks was extended to Dr. Baker for his helpful demonstration.

Adjourned.

FRED L. BOGUE, M.D., D.D.S.,
Editor The New York Institute of Stomatology.

AMERICAN ACADEMY OF DENTAL SCIENCE,

January 4, 1905.

ADJUSTING CLASPS TO PARTIAL DENTURES.

Dr. Werner.—Mr. President and Fellows of the Academy:— I don't know that I know the best way to make these adjustments. But occasionally we make plates. At least I do. And occasionally we make difficult plates. At least I have to. About a month ago this rather difficult case, to get an accurate impression of and to adjust a partial plate nicely, came into my hands, and how did I do it? That is what I am going to tell.

First, I was careful in getting an accurate impression. Then I spent about an hour in trying that plate in, bending it and burnishing it, rebending it and reburnishing it, until I thought I had it as good as I could make it. Second, I took impressions of the three teeth to be clasped and had the clasps made.

In a lower partial case where there are two teeth on the left and

one tooth on the right to be clasped and where there is a space
between the central incisors, the first important thing is to make a
plate so low on the inside as not to come up to the teeth and show
through the spaces, and that means a narrow, thick, strong plate, a
plate of two thicknesses of No. 28 or 29 gage. Next was to adjust
the clasp to the most difficult of the teeth to be clasped, which in
this case was the left inferior third molar, which tooth was tipped
at an angle of about forty-five degrees.

We all believe in having clasps adjusted so as to do the least
harm. Now, the harm by clasps is done by molecular attraction
and retention. If your clasp fits very well all around, it has the
greatest molecular retention and attraction. A clasp need not
necessarily fit like a glove. Adjust that clasp to the most difficult
of the teeth to be clasped and hold it there with an excavator till you
have it fixed. With a little sticky wax, at once take the impression of the tooth and clasp with modelling compound. The warm
modelling compound will dissolve the wax that the clasp was stuck
by to the teeth, and it will come off in exactly the position wanted.
That clasp is then soldered to the plate. Then I proceed with
two other clasps the same way—the one on the outside and the other
on the inside.

DISCUSSION.

Dr. Horatio C. Meriam.—A good impression for partial cases,
when an impression of one side of the mouth only is needed, can
be taken by making a small cup of air-chamber metal and cutting
holes to let the remaining teeth pass through. A rough impression is modelling compound may be taken first, then removed,
cooled and trimmed. Then add a layer of soft modelling compound and replace in the mouth. A very sharp impression of the
space between molar and cuspid may be made in this way.

Dr. Bonwill some years ago described a clasp that touched
the tooth only on three points, and a few years ago Dr. Fred. Bogue
gave in New York a description of some improved wire clasps. I
am reminded to-night of the late Dr. Chandler, who insisted that
we should not say capillary attraction, for that came from the word
capillus, a hair. " It is adhesive attraction!" Professor Chandler
had been a teacher in the Latin school and often gave us a touch of
the schoolmaster.

Dr. Werner.—I know the way in which Dr. Stoddard and Dr. Dickinson do it, but it is, generally speaking, that way in which you do it well that is the best for you or for me. I was not speaking to-night so much of impressions.

Dr. Stoddard.—I have followed Dr. Werner's method of adjusting clasps to plates for a good many years, except using soft plaster instead of modelling compound to get the relation. Another method which I use in partial gold cases is, get an accurate impression with plaster of paris and when the model is being cast pour soft plaster into the teeth and put a flat pin into them, allow it to harden, and then pour the balance of the model. When it is hard the teeth may be readily removed from the model and the plate struck up and the teeth put back in position and the clasps fitted to them, so the adjustment is absolutely accurate.

Editorial.

NOTICE TO ALL INTERESTED.

AT a meeting of the Board of Directors of the International Dental Publication Company, held October 20th, it was resolved to discontinue the publication of the INTERNATIONAL DENTAL JOURNAL with the December number.

LOUIS JACK,
President.

The foregoing important notice from the President of the International Dental Publication Company is self-explanatory and requires no further comment. This journal closes its eighteen years of independent life with this number.

THE CAUSE OF THE FAILURE.

MANY of our readers connected with the National Dental Association will be mystified upon reading the announcement of the suspension of the INTERNATIONAL DENTAL JOURNAL, for they probably left the meeting at Buffalo, August last, with the full expectation that this journal would be transferred to the national organization and be continued, with some modification as to name, as its organ. They had reason to expect this, for the INTERNATIONAL had been offered free of cost by the International Dental Publication Company, provided the National Association would continue its publication in entire independence of all commercial entanglements. By a unanimous vote this proposition was accepted.

The International Dental Publishing Company had two years previously made this offer and it was held over to give the National Dental Association ample time for its full consideration. Two Presidents of that body, Dr. Noel, at Asheville, and Dr. Boardman, at Buffalo, had both advocated the transfer and the publication of a journal representing the National Association. The former appointed, at the Asheville meeting, a committee to take the matter in charge, of which the writer was chairman.

This committee made a favorable report at the Buffalo meeting and the subject was referred to the Executive Council. This body appointed a special evening for the consideration of the subject, at which prominent members of the national organization were invited to be present. At that meeting the entire subject of establishing a journal was very freely discussed. The only dissenting voices heard were not based in opposition to the proposition as presented, but the fear was expressed that its adoption would involve the Association in financial difficulties. This objection was met by the writer with the fact, that while there would be financial responsibility involved in consummating the transaction, the INTERNATIONAL DENTAL JOURNAL had for eighteen years met its own business expenses, with no year showing a deficit, and that therefore the financial risk to the Association was limited to a slight increase in expense, due to the transfer and to more extended editorial supervision. To meet this possible increase, contributions of quite large amounts were offered voluntarily by several members. After a lengthy consideration of the subject the Council felt itself unequal to deciding the question and by vote directed it be sent back to the general body with a favorable recommendation.

This was on Thursday evening, July 27th. That same evening the Secretary, Dr. Peck, states that the President of Council sent to the meeting of the general body that the "Executive Council recommends that the proceedings for the year be given to the *Dental Cosmos* for publication, which, on motion, was adopted." This fact was unknown to the writer at the time and presumably no one of the others interested, outside of the Council, was aware that such action had been taken. It will be remembered that the two bodies, the Executive Council and general meeting, were in session at the same time and the same evening. Those invited to be present were not informed that action had been taken in regard to the proceedings. This was all kept *sub rosa* and, as far as the writer was concerned, he was not aware of this action for weeks subsequently.

In ignorance of the aforesaid action, the writer, with others, went to the general meeting on Friday morning and then and there the report of the Executive Council favoring the establishing of a dental journal and the acceptance of the offer of the INTERNATIONAL DENTAL JOURNAL was received, and without discussion was unanimously adopted. The President subsequently appointed a committee of five to carry out the proposed measure, with full powers to act.

This appointment carried with it not only power to arrange the necessary procedures in starting the journal, but to secure the necessary funds to meet a possible deficit the first year. Its appointment took from the Executive Council, or the National Dental Association, the power to sell or otherwise dispose of the proceedings for the year 1905. These belonged by right of appointment to the committee. When this was named by the President, the Executive Council should have reconsidered its action in regard to the proceedings and handed these to the proper custodian, the chairman of the Committee on Journal. This was not done and the reason given why this was not even suggested was that " nothing definite would be done by that committee until the next meeting of the National Dental Association." Why the Council should have decided what the Committee on Journal could or could not do will remain an unsolved problem as far as the writer is concerned.

Whether the Committee on Journal met for organization at Buffalo is unknown. It is presumed it did not, possibly having heard of the action in regard to the proceedings. It is certainly true that nothing was heard from this committee until quite late in October. It had up to that time accomplished nothing. From what the writer has been able to learn the committee had arrived at the conclusion that the action in limiting membership in the national body to State societies would cause such a marked diminution of membership that a journal could not find proper support, and further, that the giving the proceedings to another journal made any action impossible for the present year.

That the committee has laid itself open to criticism is beyond question. It should have insisted on its rights in the premises and organized at once for active service. The managers of the INTERNATIONAL DENTAL JOURNAL were prepared to meet the members of said committee, but no official communication was received at any time as to the action proposed to be taken. The management of the INTERNATIONAL was obliged to practically force the committee to come to some decision and this, as before stated, came very late in October.

This action, or rather lack of action, made it necessary for the International Dental Publication Company to act at once, and at a meeting of the Board of Directors the offer previously made to transfer the INTERNATIONAL DENTAL JOURNAL to the National Dental Association was withdrawn.

The writer does not care to comment upon the peculiar action of all concerned in the national body. He regards the mistakes, if such they were, as very serious. It seems to involve the very life of the National Association, and unless active measures be taken to bring that organization into line with true professional progress its decline and death are assured. The dental profession cannot afford to stand still; it must advance with the spirit of the age, and if present organizations are unfaithful they must give place to others more truly representative of the professional spirit.

THE LAST WORD.

THERE is deep meaning to the last word. It may be one of affection, or one of anger. It may be the farewell of the departing guest, or the broken message of the dying, but whether these or more, it carries with it a feeling of loss, something given up, some chain of association broken and, above all, the world has in a measure changed in its relation to the individual and can never be exactly the same.

The man who has been year by year brought into close communion with his fellows through any public position of responsibility, probably feels the breaking of ties more acutely than others in the more loosely attached business relations. To this class the Editor belongs. His publication has been, to a greater or lesser extent, a centre of influence, and that influence will reflect upon him for good or ill in proportion as his power has been used intelligently. The subtile influence of editorship cannot be described in words. It holds, with ever-increasing attractiveness, its votaries and few voluntarily relinquish its arduous duties. There is probably no calling that financially pays so poorly and none that yields a greater compensation in that which money cannot buy,—that of bringing the individual in close touch with a world he may never see, or with which he is only indirectly in association. Yet it is this ever-revolving mysterious life that invigorates his being, renewing daily the old thought and infusing broader aspirations that his work may be better to-morrow than it has been to-day. To such a man the last word cannot be written without the sundering of many ties, the attenuated threads of which reach out and beyond the ordinary confines of a busy life.

The Editor-in-Chief of the INTERNATIONAL DENTAL JOURNAL has been the active supporter of its varied interests for the past now nearly sixteen years. He came into the service early in 1890, immediately succeeding Dr. Suddeth, who had charge the two previous years. It is unnecessary that the writer should recount his personal trials in the management of a periodical such as this. These have been many, but they can be left, like the flotsam of the world's wrecks, to float away and be forgotten. It may be said that the sixteen years have been hopeful years and at no period has the virus of discouragement entered the domain of the editorial sanctum. The INTERNATIONAL DENTAL JOURNAL was established on a principle and the struggle to maintain a principle always means optimism or it is valueless. The battle for progress requires faith, faith that through individual effort the world can, in degree, be made better, and this applies with full force to the development of any calling, such as ours, that has not quite outgrown the crudities of its origin.

It may be asked, and the question is a proper one, Why should the INTERNATIONAL DENTAL JOURNAL cease from its work and its influence and be lost, at this period in dentistry, where it is most needed? The answer must be that the eighteen years of experience has developed the fact that the dentists of the first decade of the twentieth century in America are not prepared to accept, much less stand, for the principles that this journal advocates. The tide of retrogression has been steadily flowing towards commercialism. The literature of dentistry to-day, in this country, is bound up in dollar journals and these constitute the intellectual pabulum of the large majority of the twenty-five thousand dentists of this country. It has been found a herculean task to meet this tendency, and while this Journal has not suffered seriously in the conflict, it was very evident that the end was not far distant when it would be forced to cease the struggle single-handed against this baleful influence that has become the dry-rot of the dental profession in America. In anticipation of this possibility, it was deemed wise, under the circumstances detailed in another article relative to the action of the National Dental Association, to close the life of this journal while still in full vigor.

The regret would be greater if it were not well understood that all reforms in the active life of the world must necessarily be slowly advanced, and the hope of the future in dentistry lies in a higher educated class. When these are in full activity a change will be manifest and the dollar will not then be the paramount motive for action.

The thanks of the Editor and his associates are due and are given freely to those who have stood faithfully by the INTER-NATIONAL DENTAL JOURNAL through all these years. The societies that have, with very few breaks, furnished their proceedings freely and at much financial sacrifice, deserve special mention, for these contain the professional germ that must eventually give life and power to the entire body. To the New York Institute of Stomatology and its succession of able editors, this journal is deeply indebted and extends most grateful thanks for its disinterested and unselfish service. The same may be said of the American Academy of Dental Science and Harvard Odontological Society, both of Boston; the Academy of Stomatology of Philadelphia; the Section of Stomatology, American Medical Association, and to other organizations and individuals who have shown their interest through repeated contributions. To all of these and a still larger contingent who have quietly expressed their satisfaction with the journal and its aims, most cordial thanks and appreciation are extended.

The Editor is, and always has been, very cognizant of his limitations. He entered upon the duty in 1890 with many misgivings, and he now retires with the feeling that at no period in the work has he reached his ideal of what a dental periodical should be. He has the consciousness, however, that his aim has been to use every effort to urge the dental profession to stand for the highest. If that work has enabled any one to cultivate loftier aspirations he will feel that he has not used mental and physical strength in vain.

It is the natural result of the editorial position that the occupant of this chair will not always be understood and his motives will often be misconstrued. This has been the experience of the present writer. This must be counted among the unpleasant things to be left upon life's troubled pathway to be forgotten.

It is doubtful whether a journal such as the INTERNATIONAL will be established for many years to come. The men behind it who have sacrificed time, energy and money, are still in the front of the battle, but they feel, with the writer, that conditions must be totally changed before success will crown a similar effort.

The writer has no harsh word to express against our contemporaries, the so-called trade journals. Many evidences of good fellowship have been experienced from these, and while it is felt that their influence has been to the demoralization of the dental profession through the insidious poison of commercialism, they have lived up to, and been consistent with, business ideals and, in their way, have contributed to the practical knowledge of dentistry and thus indirectly have made it more perfect in its mechanical and scientific progress.

The writer has nothing to add by way of regrets. The retirement to a quieter life is anticipated with some pleasure. He has not reached the period when his voice and pen are to be silenced. Other avenues for both will be found, for his interest in his profession can be extinguished only when the last glimmer of life's sunset has ceased to fall upon his pathway.

Thus may we hope that in the years to come when the higher life of dentistry has been established, that the new era will usher in a living journal that will be the organ not only of a national society, but will represent the true aspirations of the entire dental fraternity of America. For the accomplishment of this let us all unite, for in its realization lives the hope that the dental profession of this country will attain the true professional standard recognized as such in all modern civilizations.

DR. CHARLES C. CHITTENDEN.

DR. CHARLES C. CHITTENDEN, of Madison, Wis., died Friday evening, December 15, 1905.

This brief announcement, coming too late for extended notice, brought to us, as it will bring to Dr. Chittenden's friends throughout the country, a sense of unexpected loss, for it is probable few were aware of his extreme illness leading to no hope of final recovery.

His name in the dental profession was a synonym for all that stood for progress. Whenever it was deemed necessary to advance the educational standard there was always to be found Dr. Chittenden. While his work has been national, his principal effort has been in Wisconsin, his own state. There he has been able to mould professional sentiment to a standard higher than that of other sections. The impress of his energy and supreme devotion to the better professional life, has borne rich fruit, and though his voice and pen are silenced, his work and influence will remain as the standard for the dental profession of the United States to work up to and adopt.

Space will not permit at this time to enter into details of his life work. Our friend and co-worker has passed on to the road that all humanity must travel. May we all be equally able to prove, as he did, that our ambitions are based on that unselfish devotion he manifested, and in emulating his virtues, strive to finish the work he left unaccomplished.

NOTICE TO EXCHANGES.

THIS, the December number of the INTERNATIONAL DENTAL JOURNAL, will be the last issue. Exchanges will kindly take note and strike this periodical from their list.

Bibliography.

THE AMERICAN TEXT-BOOK OF OPERATIVE DENTISTRY. In contributions by eminent authorities. Edited by Edward C. Kirk, D.D.S., Professor of Clinical Dentistry in the University of Pennsylvania, Philadelphia; Editor of *The Dental Cosmos;* Officier de l'Acadèmie de France. Third edition, revised and enlarged. Illustrated with 875 engravings. Lea Brothers & Co., Philadelphia and New York, 1905.

This, the third edition of the "American Text-Book of Operative Dentistry" has necessitated some changes among the contributors. This seems a wise procedure, in view of the fact that it has become necessary to treat various subjects in dentistry in special publications. While this burdens the library with many books, it relieves, or should relieve to that extent, books supposed to be confined to one special branch. The chapter on Embryology has been omitted and new matter has been added. The very valuable chapter on the "Use of the Matrix in Filling Operations," by Dr. Crenshaw, of Atlanta, will be read with interest and profit. Some of his statements will be antagonized, such as this, quoted from his article: " It will not matter what form of cohesive gold is employed if the heat sufficent to change its molecular arrangement has been applied in annealing the gold. It is practically impossible to adapt it, unaccompanied by linings, so as to secure moisture-proof joints, and therefore permanent results." This seems to the writer an assertion directly contrary to experience. Cohesive gold foil can be laid up against walls so perfectly as to defy the inroads of moisture. To think otherwise would contradict the experience of the past forty-seven years. It all depends upon the manipulator. It is true there is more danger of fillings leaking under this material than with non-cohesive gold, the latter admitting of more careless handling, but that cohesive gold, properly annealed and properly manipulated, will preserve teeth, needs no argument at this period of practice. The author of this chapter is evidently a strong advocate for the use of non-cohesive gold, and the writer is not disposed to criticise this as he fully appreciates its value, having had long experience in both methods of practice; but he must deprecate the condemnation of a property in gold that has met all conditions in tooth structure and saved teeth impossible under older methods.

The chapter on Orthodontia has been changed by substituting Dr. E. H. Angle in the place of the late Dr. Clark L. Goddard. This was arranged previously to the death of the latter and with his " cordial consent."

Dr. Angle's work is so well known and regarded by many, including the editor of this book, as the " chief exponent of the modern trend of thought upon orthodontia as a problem of occlusion," that criticism would be out of place. It is, however, not possible to agree with all his conclusions, and the reviewer must regard some of his ideas as peculiar to his own teaching and not altogether those of some other equally prominent workers in the same direction. Readers of works on orthodontia and some other subjects are getting weary with the constant repetition of illustrations. We have become so familiar with some of Dr. Angle's patients, through the half-tones in this chapter and previous publications, that introductions would be superfluous if circumstances called for meeting them in the social circle. The introduction of the comparatively easily prepared half-tone should have caused the old method of repeating illustrations to become obsolete. It seems, however, to be growing again under a false economy to the very great detriment of interest in authors' productions.

This chapter, however, must not be judged by this criticism. It is but a small part of the 171 pages taken up by the author of the chapter—a book in itself. It is a valuable production and will appeal to the practical man, whether he agrees with all the ideas enunciated, or prefers to permit them still to remain within the domain of theory.

The book, as a whole, must appeal to every practitioner. It is the thought and practice of a number of men, and has a distinct value because of this variety. It loses, necessarily, something of the harmony of statement belonging to a work prepared by a single mind, but gains in a wider observation of the details of practice. In this respect it becomes in a measure the complete history of operative procedures from the earliest periods, and when the comparison is drawn between this book and those published a half century in the past, the progress is marked. In making this statement it must not be understood that the writer regards earlier workers deficient. for this would not be true. but in the systematic arrangement of study, the present period shows a marked advance over the period named, and this is why this volume is an epitome of all the work of the past years.

The publishers have done their part in the preparation of the book with their usual ability. It is a very satisfactory production in paper, type and illustrations where their responsibility rests with the latter.

A Text-Book of Physiology, Normal and Pathological. For Students and Practitioners of Medicine. By Winfield S. Hall, Ph.D., M.D.(Leipzig), Professor of Physiology, Northwestern University Medical School. Chicago; Member of the American Physiological Society: Member of American Association for the Advancement of Science, etc., etc. New (2d) edition, revised and enlarged. In one octavo volume of 795 pages, with 339 engravings and three full-page colored plates. Lea Brothers & Co., Publishers, Philadelphia and New York, 1905.

This, the second edition of this very valuable work of Dr. Hall, carries with it its own recommendation in its carefully prepared pages. The author writes in the preface to the first edition, that " The plan of the work adapts it to the needs of several classes of readers. Medical students will, it is hoped, find a clearly defined exposition of Physiology proper, its relevant facts from Chemistry, Physics, and Morphology and accompanying outlines enabling them to arrange their knowledge in an orderly and logical manner. Students in literary or scientific institutions who are preparing for the study of medicine or of physiology as a specialty, will find the method of the book equally adapted to their needs."

In the preface to this second edition the author has added subchapters on Pathologic Physiology. The reason for this addition is stated to be that " It is becoming apparent to medical educators that to master normal physiology alone without applying its laws to the symptomatology of disease is to miss a large part of the service which physiology should render." That this is true must be clearly evident to every student of the subject.

A careful reading of the book leaves the impression that the author has prepared it from original observations, and although he has properly made use of the investigations of others, his clear explanation of various phenomena indicates the scholarly investigator. This valuable and absolutely necessary trait in an author's character and work at times leads to the fault, by no means uncommon with some teachers, of talking beyond the comprehension of the stupid man in the class. For this reason some parts of this book seem to be better adapted to the practitioner than to the mental capacity of the average student. For the former class it must prove a storehouse of valuable knowledge upon the subject which it treats.

Individuals will take up the study of this book and find interest in those chapters more directly related to their own special studies, and it, therefore, becomes somewhat difficult to point out to our readers any part of it as superior to any other part. The reviewer, while an interested reader of all the chapters, found special satisfaction in reading the one on digestion, covering, as it does, the entire subject from Physiology of Digestion to the Pathologic Physiology of Digestion.

Chapter XI, upon "The Physiology of the Nervous System," is of peculiar value to practitioners of the healing art, as they are brought constantly in contact with the phenomena accompanying nerve lesions. This is peculiarly applicable to dental practitioners. While the latter are not supposed to be deficient in a general knowledge of the nervous system, they can learn much from this scholarly specialist.

In the former chapter on Digestion, the author antagonizes the generally accepted dictum that water should not be taken with meals and his reasons for this are worth quoting. Under the subtitle, " The Influence of Dilution," he says: "Much has been said and written against the drinking of cold water with meals and especially at the beginning of meals. There is more misconception regarding water than any other food. Without entering into a discussion of the details of the question, and without citing the numerous and reliable authorities, the author will briefly state a few of the fundamental facts regarding the relation of water to nutrition: (1) Water is a prime necessity to the animal body. Lack of sufficient water is just as certain to lead to a derangement of the nutrition of the body as is lack of sufficient solid food. Most people use too little water ; few people use too much water. (2) The free use of water does not tend directly to the accumulation of fat. The statement that it does so is a fallacy, which arises from these facts : The free use of water facilitates the processes of nutrition and economizes food by utilizing a greater proportion of it. * * * (3) Cold water stimulates the free secretion of the gastric juice. Cold water in moderate quantity at the beginning of a meal thus hastens the gastric digestion and makes more efficient the antiseptic action of the gastric juice."

Space will not permit quotations from other portions of the book, although the temptation is to give some of the author's conclusions to the reader.

This work of Dr. Hall should appeal to every critical student, for it embraces not the results of patient investigation only, but the reasoning of a philosophical thinker, and the two qualities combined have given a result valuable to the student of the subject, whether he be classed among the undergraduates or among those having had years of experience.

The work is carefully illustrated with engravings and colored plates and the general make-up is creditable alike to author and publisher.

MANUAL OF CHEMISTRY. A Guide to Lectures and Laboratory Work for Beginners in Chemistry. A text-book specially adapted for students in Medicine, Pharmacy and Dentistry. By W. Simon, Ph.D., M.D., Professor of Chemistry in the College of Physicians and Surgeons of Baltimore and in the Baltimore College of Dental Surgery; Emeritus Professor in the Maryland College of Pharmacy, Department University of Maryland. Eighth edition, thoroughly revised. Lea Brothers & Co., Philadelphia and New York, 1905.

This very valuable book is now presented in the eighth edition, a sufficient recommendation in itself without further notice.

The author says in his preface that "This Manual has been delayed for a year in order to incorporate in it the changes and additions of the new Pharmacopœia. * * * Several of the chapters on organic chemistry have been practically rewritten and the matter has been rearranged so to conform to modern views. * * * The request of teachers in dental schools to consider more fully dental metallurgy has been complied with."

This chapter, the fourth in the book, will be found of value to the dental teacher equally with the student, covering, as it does,

" metals and their combinations." It is probable that this will not take the place of special works on metallurgy, of which there are at least two in this country, but it occupies a fitting place in a text-book of chemistry written, in part, for dental students and dental teachers.

The book has been so extensively reviewed in its various editions and with a deserved reputation established, that nothing specially new relating to its value can be written. The author has not deemed it necessary, beyond changes noted, to do much more than endeavor to bring the manual, in all its parts, " up to date."

Every dentist, whether familiar with the subject or not, should have a work of this kind in his library, if not for study at least for reference, and the writer knows of no work better adapted for the latter purpose than the one under consideration.

It contains besides sixty-six illustrations, one colored spectra plate, and there are eight colored plates representing sixty-four chemical reactions.

LONG'S DENTAL MATERIA MEDICA AND THERAPEUTICS. A Text-book of Dental Materia Medica, Therapeutics and Prescription Writing. For Students and Practitioners of Dentistry. By Eli H. Long, M.D., Professor of Materia Medica and Therapeutics in the Dental and Medical Departments of the University of Buffalo, New York. New (2d) edition, enlarged and revised to accord with the new United States Pharmacopœia. In one octavo volume of 298 pages with 7 engravings and 18 colored diagrams. Cloth, $3.00 net. Lea Brothers & Co., Publishers, Philadelphia and New York, 1905.

This, the second edition of Long's Dental Materia Medica and Therapeutics, indicates its value, for a new book on this somewhat overwritten subject must present certain attractive features to make it worth while for students and teachers alike to seek its pages for instruction.

The book was reviewed very fully in the first edition and the writer has nothing more to add to the opinions then expressed, beyond the fact that, upon the whole, he considered it the best text-book on Materia Medica for students in dentistry.

. The writer did not agree with the author's method of arranging

" remedies into groups, based upon their action and uses," and he still continues to entertain this opinion. It means annoying reference to index, and that continually, in the effort to find out all the author considers important in the matter of remedies. It is very doubtful whether the " student unconsciously acquires a *comparative* knowledge of drugs and their values" by this arrangement, and it certainly adds to his labor.

While not necessarily agreeing with all the author's views in his therapeutics of the various drugs, it is with exceptional pleasure that the writer has again gone over this portion of the book. It is certainly not the least valuable portion of the 298 pages. It is anticipated that the book must be eventually adopted as a textbook in all dental colleges, for the reason it satisfies a need not heretofore met in the general text-books.

A PRACTICAL TREATISE ON ARTIFICIAL CROWN, BRIDGE AND PORCELAIN WORK. By George Evans, formerly Lecturer on Crown and Bridge Work in the Baltimore College of Dental Surgery, etc. Seventh edition. Revised and enlarged. With 734 illustrations. S. S. White Dental Mfg. Co., Philadelphia, 1905.

The author says of this, the seventh edition of " Artificial Crown, Bridge and Porcelain Work:" The endeavor has been, as in each of those which preceded it, to better meet the requirements of a practical treatise for college and post-graduate study and as well of a reference book for the practitioner. To effect this in the present state of the art has involved a revision so extensive as to make the present edition almost a new work."

That this book now covers 448 pages is sufficient to indicate the wonderful growth of this branch of dental work. When it is considered that the crown of a few years in the past was of simple construction and that bridge work was entirely unknown, it becomes difficult to realize that this branch has now reached practically the proportions of a specialty in dentistry, but such it is. The author of this work has occupied a prominent part in the upbuilding of this branch and is justly regarded as an authority.

The book has been reviewed repeatedly as each edition has appeared and the dental profession is sufficiently familiar with it to accept the fact that it has been thoroughly revised to make a demand for it as a book of reference in every office in this or other countries.

From the reader's point of view it must prove very satisfactory in type and paper, as well as in the care extended by the publisher to make it as perfect as possible in other respects.

THE PHYSICIAN'S VISITING LIST FOR 1906. Fifty-fifth year of its publication. P. Blakiston's Son & Co., Philadelphia.

This well-known visiting list needs no special notice after more than a half century of a satisfactory place in medical practice. While not quite as satisfactory for dental engagements, it has a value in other respects, and could be used for that purpose. Its tables are valuable. The "Dose Table" is worth more than the cost of the visiting list, giving the quantity in apothecaries' weight and metric system. This, if not equally important to the dentist, should be in his hands for ready reference.

Obituary.

DR. FREDERIC FRANK DURAND.

IN the sudden death of Dr. Frederic Frank Durand, at his residence in Maplewood, New Jersey, on Sunday, October 29th, 1905, the dental profession has lost another of its older practitioners, whose ranks are rapidly diminishing.

He had but recently returned from his summer home at Lake George, N. Y., apparently in the best of health, and the announcement of his sudden demise was a sad surprise to his many friends. Without warning he was stricken with heart trouble, and while conversing with his wife he succumbed immediately.

Dr. Durand was born in New York sixty-six years ago and was a son of the distinguished artist, Asher B. Durand. He was educated in private schools in that city, the preparatory school at Lee, Mass., then taking the scientific course in Civil Engineering and Architecture at Rensselaer Polytechnic Institute in Troy, N. Y.

The Civil War then coming on, and inactivity of business, decided his entering the dental profession. Dr. Edwin James

Dunning, who was a personal friend of his father, and one of the leading dentists of that day, persuaded young Durand to enter his office as a student—which at that time was known as the " Dunning School of Dentistry."

In addition to those facilities afforded under his teaching he took a course in Anatomy and Materia Medica at the College of Physicians and Surgeons, New York, completing his dental education in the Baltimore College of Dental Surgery, where he graduated in 1863.

He remained associated with Dr. Dunning until the latter retired from practice in 1874, when with Dr. George Elias Hawes, also an associate of Dr. Dunning's, under the firm name of Durand & Hawes a partnership was formed to continue the practice established by Dr. Dunning at 11 Waverly Place in 1856.

Upon Dr. Hawes's death in 1880 he was succeeded by his brother, Dr. John B. Hawes. Owing to business encroachment in the lower Fifth Avenue residential section, Durand & Hawes were compelled to leave Waverly Place, the house in which Dr. Dunning had established his practice twenty-five years before, locating at 13 West Thirty-second Street, where they remained until 1894, when conditions again required removing to their present address, 20 West Forty-seventh Street. With the death of Dr. Durand terminated a partnership of over thirty years' standing and, including the Dunning school, an established practice of half a century. Dr. Durand was in active practice over forty years and had devoted his life to the professional training of young men who were associated with him,—a worthy teacher of his predecessor's system; and a large number of dental practitioners who came in close contact with him will cherish his memory for its valued friendship and teachings. Although in his 67th year, he continued in active practice, travelling daily between his country home and New York.

Outside of his profession Dr. Durand was very much interested in art. He was one of the founders of the American Water Color Society, and devoted much of his vacations to art work, mostly landscapes.

He was also greatly interested in the welfare of his home community, where he had spent most of his life; the landed property he inherited had been in his father's family upward of one hundred and thirty years.

He was an active member of the Maplewood Improvement Association, and Chairman of the Board of Governors of its Public Building Company.

Dr. Durand was married in 1903 to Miss Helen Thompson, of Louisville, Kentucky, who survives him, also a brother, Prof. John Durand, of Paris, and one sister, Mrs. George B. Woodman, of New York.

DR. WM. N. WILSON.

DR. WM. N. WILSON, of Indianapolis, formerly of Richmond, Ind., was killed October 14th by the explosion of a milk sterilizer in that city. For many years Dr. Wilson practised dentistry at Richmond, Ind. He gave up practicing dentistry and went to Indianapolis, where he engaged in the dental supply business, later becoming an instructor in the Indiana Dental College, which position he held until 1902, when he engaged in the condensed milk business. Dr. Wilson was a highly esteemed member of the Friends' Church, being a very active participant in the affairs of the church and Sunday-school, particularly in the latter. A wife, two sons and one daughter survive him. He was 52 years old.

FRANK A. HAMILTON.

GEORGE B. HARRIMAN, D.D.S.

DIED, at Moosehead, Maine, May 22d, 1905, of pneumonia, George B. Harriman, D.D.S., of Boston, Mass.

George B. Harriman was born at Groton, New Hampshire, on March 18th, 1837. He received his preliminary education at New Hampton Institute, studied dentistry under John Clough, M.D., of Boston, in 1857, and entered practice in 1858.

After several years of practice he entered Boston Dental College as a student and graduated in 1870. The next year he was elected Dean of the College, in which capacity he served for two years; later he was chosen as Trustee and remained a member of that Board until after the school was transferred to the Tufts College Corporation.

As a student of the College he became deeply interested in microscopy under Professor Rufus King Brown and for several years was an enthusiastic student in that science, conducting certain important investigations. For a time he was Professor of Histology and Microscopy at the College.

Dr. Harriman was one of the eight graduates who met in one of the lecture rooms of the old College at No. 5 Hamilton Place on March 4th, 1872, and founded this association. He was chairman of the Executive Committee during the first two years of its existence, was President in 1897, again chairman of the Executive Committee in 1898, and an active member until his death.

For a long time he had suffered from asthma and had gradually withdrawn in part from active practice. Last March he closed his office on Park Street and went to California, returning early in May. It had been his custom for several years to visit the Moosehead region on the opening of the fishing season in the Spring; and though urged by friends not to do so this year, he went to Moosehead Lake on May 13th, accompanied by Mrs. Harriman. There pneumonia supervened, and he died on the 22d. As has been beautifully said, "The Call of the Wild led him back close to Nature's heart, and with his head on her bosom, he slept."

Dr. Harriman was a prominent Freemason, a life member of Boston Commandery, an earnest supporter of the First Free Baptist Church, of Roxbury, and though he never aspired to salaried political office he was at one time active in Republican politics, serving as a member of the State Central Committee. He was a man of moderate wealth, of sterling character and Christian brotherhood. He leaves a widow, his second wife, and three sons.

In respect to his memory, the Boston and Tufts Dental Alumni Association adopted the following resolutions on October 11th:

WHEREAS, the hand of Providence has removed from us our honored member and colleague, Dr. George B. Harriman; and

WHEREAS, in his decease we have lost one of the founders of our association, who in committee, as President, and as an active member until his death, evinced a warm interest in its welfare; who as Dean, as Professor, and as Trustee of our Alma Mater gave to her freely of his wisdom; and who in many years of practice set before us a worthy example of fidelity to his patients, of fairness toward his colleagues, and of kindly interest in his younger professional brethren; therefore, be it

Resolved, that we desire to express to the bereaved family our sympathy and sorrow in their affliction, and our admiration for the professional and personal qualities of our colleague; and

Resolved, that these resolutions be spread upon the records of our association, a copy sent to the family of our departed brother, and others to the dental journals for publication.

FRED'K S. FOGG,

E. W. BRANIGAN,

JAMES R. PIPER,

Committee.

MARION L. WOODWARD,

Recording Secretary,

Boston and Tufts Dental Alumni Association.

Current News.

SOUTH DAKOTA STATE BOARD OF DENTAL EXAMINERS.

NOTICE.

THE next meeting of the South Dakota State Board of Dental Examiners will be held at Sioux Falls, S. D., January 16th, 1906, beginning at 1.30 P.M. sharp. All applicants for examination must bring diplomas from reputable dental colleges or affidavit of having been engaged in the practice of dentistry for at least three years immediately preceding said examination. Instruments and materials necessary to do all kinds of operative and prosthetic work will be needed at this examination. Vulcanizer and lathe will be furnished by the Board. All applications must positively be in the hands of the Secretary by January 9th.

G. W. COLLINS, *Secretary,*

Vermillion, S. D.

AMERICAN SOCIETY OF ORTHODONTISTS.

AT the fifth annual meeting of the American Society of Orthodontists in Chicago, September 28th to 30th, inclusive, the election of officers was announced, as follows: President, Dr. R. Ottolengui, New York, N. Y.; Vice-President, Dr. Herbert A. Pullen, Buffalo. N. Y.; Secretary-Treasurer, Dr. F. S. McKay, St. Louis, Mo.; Member of the Board of Censors, Dr. Milton T. Watson, Detroit, Mich.

F. S. McKAY,

Secretary.

INDEX TO VOLUME XXVI.

A

B

Lightning Source UK Ltd.
Milton Keynes UK
UKHW020604261118
332889UK00009B/957/P